Computerized Medical Office Procedures

A Worktext

FOURTH EDITION

Computerized Medical Office Procedures

A Worktext

Using Medisoft v18

William D. Larsen, MBA, CMA

Timothy Hartman, MSHSA, MBA
Technical Editor
Accounting & Business Instructor
Metro Business College

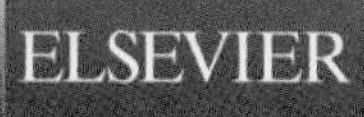

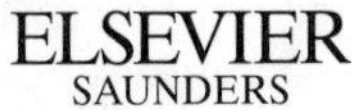

3251 Riverport Lane
St. Louis, Missouri 63043

COMPUTERIZED MEDICAL OFFICE PROCEDURES: A WORKTEXT, FOURTH EDITION ISBN: 978-1-4557-2620-2

Notices

Knowledge and best practice in this field are constantly changing. As new research and experience broaden our understanding, changes in research methods, professional practices, or medical treatment may become necessary.

Practitioners and researchers must always rely on their own experience and knowledge in evaluating and using any information, methods, compounds, or experiments described herein. In using such information or methods they should be mindful of their own safety and the safety of others, including parties for whom they have a professional responsibility.

With respect to any drug or pharmaceutical products identified, readers are advised to check the most current information provided (i) on procedures featured or (ii) by the manufacturer of each product to be administered, to verify the recommended dose or formula, the method and duration of administration, and contraindications. It is the responsibility of practitioners, relying on their own experience and knowledge of their patients, to make diagnoses, to determine dosages and the best treatment for each individual patient, and to take all appropriate safety precautions.

To the fullest extent of the law, neither the Publisher nor the authors, contributors, or editors, assume any liability for any injury and/or damage to persons or property as a matter of products liability, negligence or otherwise, or from any use or operation of any methods, products, instructions, or ideas contained in the material herein.

ISBN: 978-1-4557-2620-2

Executive Content Strategist: Jennifer Janson
Associate Content Development Specialist: Elizabeth Bawden
Content Coordinator: Laurel Berkel
Publishing Services Manager: Julie Eddy
Design Direction: Margaret Reid

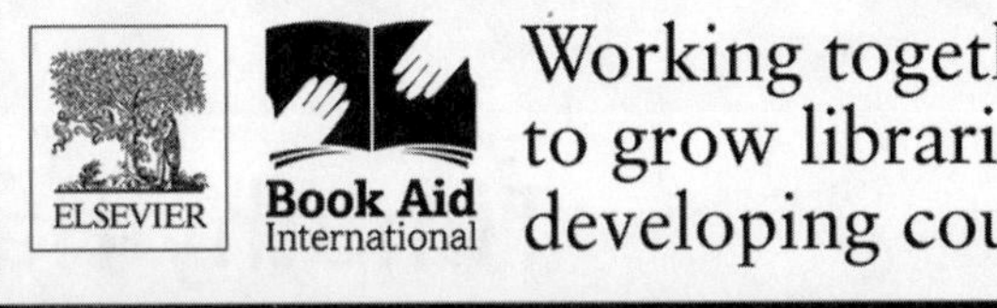

Printed in the United States of America

Last digit is the print number: 9 8 7 6 5 4 3 2 1

To my family, ***Traci***, ***Zachary***, *and* ***Anna-Marie***, *without whose support, love, and encouragement, this textbook would have never been written.*

Editorial Review Board

Preface

You are about to start using a tool that will enable you to maintain your medical office billing practices effectively and efficiently. Administrative duties in health care offices have changed because of technological advances in the use of computers. Computer knowledge is often the prerequisite to obtaining a job in health care. Students who successfully complete this textbook will have learned basic computerized administrative skills that will be transferable to other applications.

Computerized Medical Office Procedures: A Worktext introduces the student to common administrative procedures performed in both small and large medical practices. Students will learn to input patient information, bill insurance companies, and schedule appointments. Finally, the student will be able to run common reports associated with the medical practice. Day sheets, patient ledgers, and other financial reports that are important to the day-to-day financial operations of the medical practice are discussed.

Many assumptions were made in writing this worktext. One assumption is that the student will have already taken or will be taking a basic computer course. Such a course may teach the student basic computer operations (e.g., how to turn the computer on and off and the booting process), how the Windows operating system functions and the resources available for the operating system, and how to run basic word processing and spreadsheet programs.

Certain regions of the United States and other countries have different perceptions and definitions of the size of a medical practice; this text portrays a medium-sized medical practice with seven providers.

In addition, this worktext does not attempt to cover in detail all aspects of *International Classification of Diseases, Ninth Revision*, (ICD-9) and Current Procedural Terminology (CPT) coding and insurance. It is assumed that the student has taken a prior course in coding or is taking a concurrent course that will provide the student with more detailed information about coding and insurance.

Although this worktext features Medisoft, its concepts are general enough to cover most medical practice software available to medical practices. Students who complete *Computerized Medical Office Procedures: A Worktext* should be able to transfer their knowledge to other medical practice software, thus decreasing training time in the workplace.

The chapters begin with the objectives that will be acquired by studying the material contained in the chapter. The terminology list contains the most important vocabulary terms found in the chapter. Numerous figures and tables are provided for reference. Important ideas and tips are presented in a *Notes* box. Each chapter provides step-by-step procedures for the student to gain understanding of the specific concepts. Directions for the steps to be performed in the procedure are presented in *Procedures* boxes. Occasionally, alternate methods of performing procedural steps will be highlighted in *Another Way* boxes.

Each chapter also includes terminology review and checking your understanding. Each chapter ends with *Putting It into Practice*, which is an exercise that allows the student to perform the skills taught in the chapter without rote exercises. In other words, the student needs to perform the exercises based on the knowledge gained. If needed, the student should go back through the chapter to review the concepts. Finally, each chapter lists many references to further a student's studies in computerized medical office procedures.

Medisoft has made some changes on where to enter and find information between version 16 and 18. Most of the changes occurred in version 17, this text uses the *Student Demo Version of Medisoft v18*.

Note: The installation instructions in this worktext apply only to the *Student Demo Version of Medisoft v18* software. Many different versions of Medisoft v18 are available. Please confirm that you have the *Student Demo Version of Medisoft v18* if using these instructions.

I need to thank several people in preparation of this worktext. The first person is Tim Hartman who tested the exercises in Medisoft and provided guidance in writing the worktext. In addition, I would like to thank Jennifer Janson who helped us on so many details of the book, along with providing support. Finally, thanks to Elizabeth Bawden who kept us on track for the deadlines that were always looming.

William D. Larsen

INSTALLATION AND SET UP

If any previous version of Medisoft is loaded on the computer, completely REMOVE the Medisoft and MediData files BEFORE installing Medisoft, version 18. If it is unknown whether previous versions exist on a computer, then look at the contents of the C: drive and both "Program File" folders on the C: drive. Remove any Medisoft and MediData files.

Note: The following installation instructions apply only to the *Student Demo Version of Medisoft v18* software. Many different versions of Medisoft v18 are available. Please confirm you have the *Student Demo Version of Medisoft v18* if using the following instructions.

To install, perform the following:

1. Insert the Medisoft Student disk into the CD or DVD drive on your system.
2. The following screen will open on your system. Click "Install Medisoft."

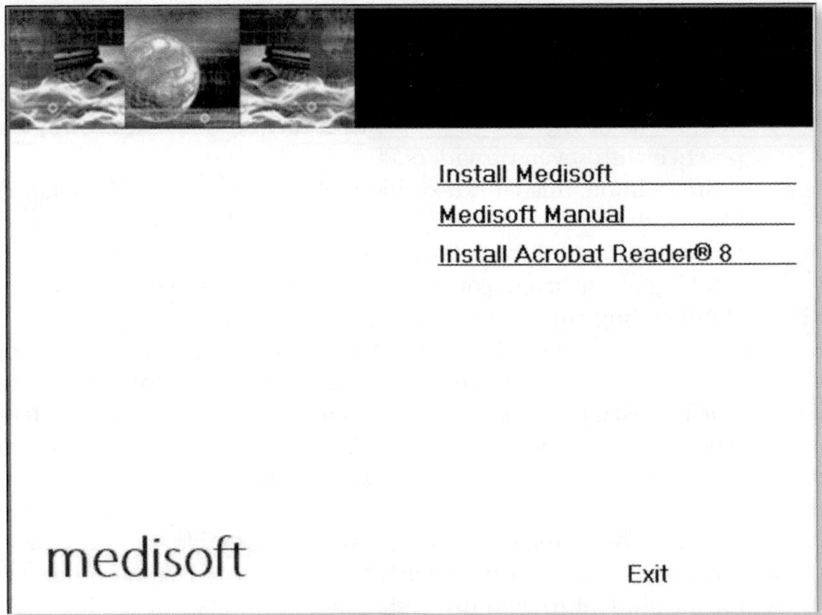

3. Depending on your system configuration, you may be asked to grant permission for the program **PAForschooldemoinstall.exe** to make changes to your hard disk drive. Answer "Yes." It is possible that anti-virus software may need to be temporarily turned off (disabled) or a firewall may need to be bypassed to install the software.
4. The next screen will ensure that all Windows programs are closed before continuing. If they are, then click "Next."

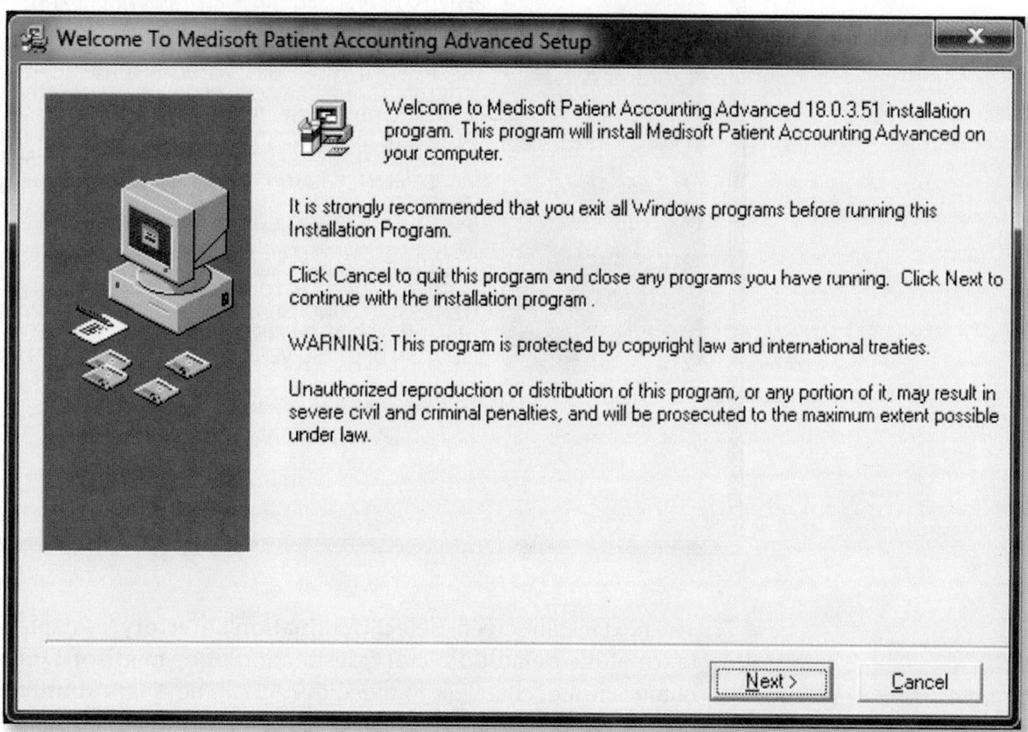

5. For the next screen, the **End User License Agreement,** select "I accept the agreement." After clicking the "I accept the agreement" button, click the "Next" button.

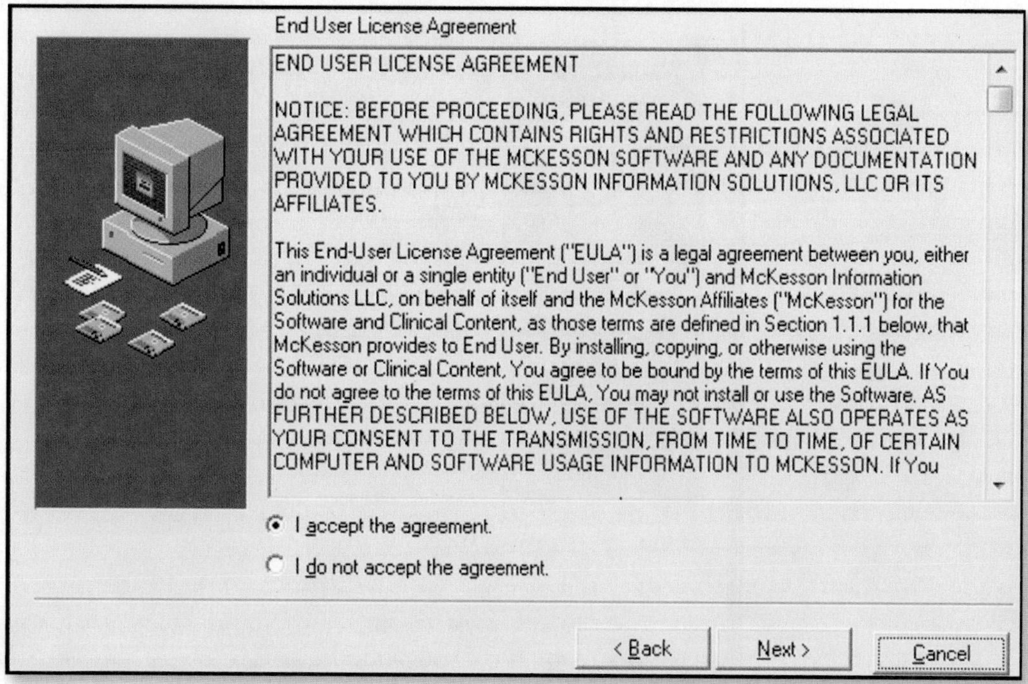

6. The next screen is the **Subscription Agreement**. Select "I accept the agreement." Then click the "Next" button.

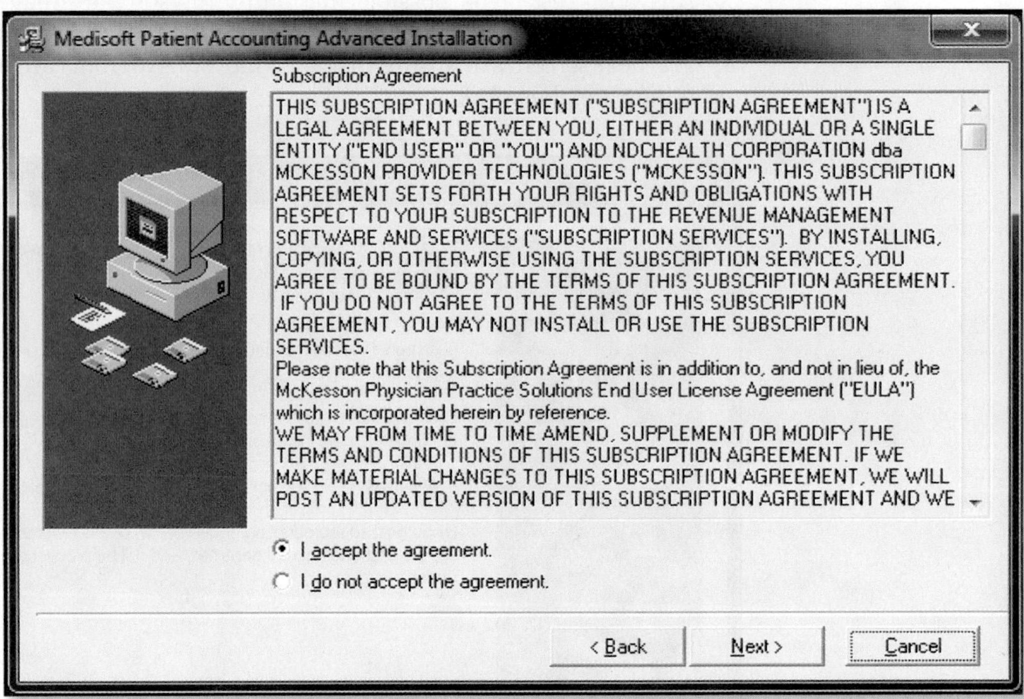

7. The next install screen, **Select Destination Directory**, is displayed to confirm your acceptance of the default directory destination of **c:\medisoftDEMO**. If any other directory name is listed, change it to the above. Click the" Next" button at the bottom right.
8. Click the "Next" button on the screen below to begin the installation process. Do not interrupt the installation process. If a problem appears, alert your instructor before doing anything.

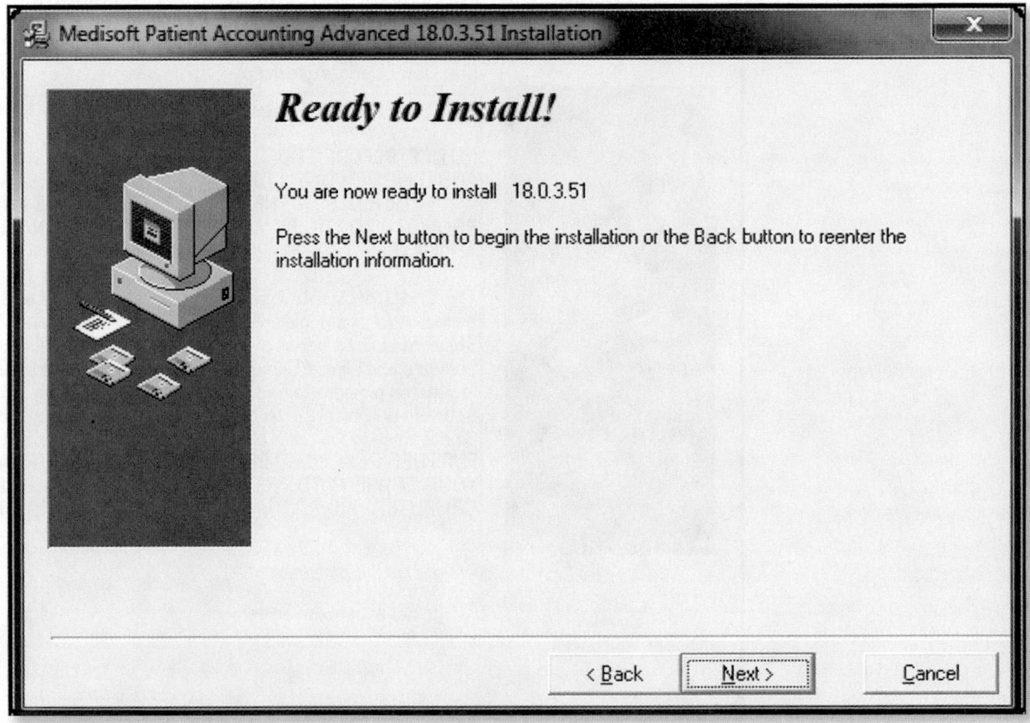

9. On the **Installation Completed** screen, select "Launch Medisoft Patient Accounting Advanced Demo" and click "Finish." Medisoft will automatically start.
10. Finally, please refer to the Evolve site for the 4th edition of *Computerized Medical Office Procedures*. Find the student link for downloading the **Larsen Data Executable: *Elsevier Clinic***. Please refer to the download instructions provided on the same page as the link. It is very important that Medisoft v18 not be open when downloading the executable. Please close Medisoft.

KEYBOARD SHORTCUTS IN MEDISOFT

The following keyboard shortcuts can save you time when using Medisoft:

F1: Access the Medisoft Help files.

F3: Save the data entered in a dialog box.

F7: Open the Quick Ledger dialog box where you can get up-to-date information about a patient or guarantor and print statements.

F8: Access a dialog box to create a new record without closing the current dialog box. For example, suppose you are entering a transaction and need to enter a new patient. Pressing F8 in the Chart field will open the Patient/Guarantor dialog box without closing the Transaction Entry dialog box.

F10: Open the Eligibility Results dialog box. If you are set up to access insurance carrier eligibility information for patients, this information will display on the screen.

F11: Open the Quick Balance dialog box to access up-to-date account balance information on a patient.

Alt + F4: Exit the Medisoft program.

There is also a Shortcut Key bar at the bottom of the screen where you can see what other shortcut keys are available for the particular area of Medisoft Advanced and Office Hours that you are currently operating.

Note: The procedures in this worktext apply to the *Student Demo Version of Medisoft v18* software.

Contents

Chapter 1 Introduction to Computerized Medical Office Procedures

chapter 1

Introduction to Computerized Medical Office Procedures

Objectives

1. Describe the medical information cycle in a medical office.
2. List the main functions used in Medisoft that are performed in a medical office.
3. Start Medisoft.
4. Describe the primary features used to operate Medisoft.
5. Enter practice information.
6. Add provider information, and print the Provider List report.
7. Add facility and address information.
8. Create records for new patients.
9. Locate and edit an existing patient's record.
10. Print the Patient List report.
11. Backup data files, and exit Medisoft.

Terminology

backup: Process of copying computer files and storing them on a disk or another electronic device for safekeeping

BillFlash: Able to bill and send statements to patients through this online service

case: Group of transactions related to a specific medical condition for which a patient seeks treatment

chart number: Set of digits or letters assigned to a patient's medical record for identification purposes

clearinghouse: Company that provides services to medical practices, which include verifying and transmitting claims to insurance carriers

encounter form: Document used by a provider during a medical examination to indicate the patient's type of illness or injury and the medical procedures performed; also called a *superbill*

front desk: Area of the medical office where patients check in for their appointments

guarantor: Person who is responsible for paying the patient's bill

Health Insurance Portability and Accountability Act (HIPAA): Federal legislation that provides guidelines for transmitting electronic data and protecting patients' privacy

medical information cycle: Series of steps performed before, during, and after a patient has been seen by a provider

medical practice management software: Computer programs used to schedule patient appointments, submit electronic claims to insurance companies, and perform basic accounting procedures

Medisoft: Type of medical practice management software widely used in medical offices

menu bar: Long, rectangular bar at the top of the main Medisoft window that displays menu names

patient registration form: Document containing personal, financial, and insurance information needed to complete insurance claims for a patient

provider: General term referring to someone who charges for health care services

side bar: Optional, navigational feature that allows quick access to the most frequently used Medisoft menu items

toolbar: Row of buttons with icons that allow quick access to many Medisoft features

Employment advertisements reveal that most health care facilities require job seekers to know how to use computer programs called **medical practice management software**. This software is essential to the business operations of medical offices because it enables staff to perform routine tasks more accurately and efficiently. For example, medical practice management software is used to schedule appointments, track patient data, perform basic accounting procedures, and submit electronic claims to insurance companies.

This textbook provides hands-on experience with **Medisoft**, one type of medical practice management software. Learning how to use Medisoft will help you build essential scheduling, accounting, and other data processing skills needed to work in a medical office. Whether your medical office uses Medisoft, these skills will make it easier for you to learn other computerized systems.

MEDICAL INFORMATION CYCLE OVERVIEW

Before you start learning to use Medisoft, you need to understand how information in a medical office is collected, processed, and retrieved. This process, sometimes called the **medical information cycle**, is a series of steps performed before, during, and after a patient has been seen by a **provider**. The term *provider* typically refers to someone who charges for health care services, such as a physician, chiropractor, nurse practitioner, or physical therapist. The medical information cycle can vary according to the size and type of medical office. However, this cycle can be divided into two major parts (1) gathering patient information and (2) processing and tracking the data.

Gathering Patient Information

The medical information cycle is initiated when a patient makes an appointment with the medical office assistant. The medical office assistant may be a medical assistant, a medical receptionist, or any member of the health care team who performs **front desk** duties. The front desk is the area adjacent to the patient reception area where patients check in, telephone calls are received, and appointments are scheduled. Depending on the size and type of practice, some activities, such as answering the telephone and scheduling patients, may be done in another area. For instance, many fertility clinics often place their appointment scheduling in another part of the building, away from the reception area. Therefore patient confidentiality is reasonably maintained.

A patient who has not been previously seen by a provider in a specific practice is considered a new patient. An established patient has previously received services at the practice. New patients need to fill out a **patient registration form** (Figure 1.1), which contains personal, financial, and insurance information needed to complete insurance claims. Patient registration forms may vary in appearance in different medical offices.

Often, new patients are preregistered over the telephone, and basic information is provided when the appointment is made. Later, when the patient arrives at the medical office, this information can be verified or added to as needed. Even established patients are routinely asked to confirm whether their address, telephone, employer, and other information have changed since their last visit. Patients sometimes change insurance companies without informing the medical office, which causes medical billing claims to be rejected (unpaid).

During new patient check-in, the medical office assistant usually photocopies the patient's insurance card and asks the patient (or patient's guardian) to sign the patient registration form. This signature often serves a dual purpose (see Figure 1.1). It allows payments to be sent from the insurance carrier to the provider instead of to the patient.

Patient Registration Information

Account # : ______
Insurance # : ______
Co-Payment: $ ______

Please PRINT AND complete ALL sections below!

PATIENT'S PERSONAL INFORMATION Marital Status ❑ Single ❑ Married ❑ Divorced ❑ Widowed Sex:❑ Male ❑ Female

Name: ______ (last name) ______ (first name) ______ (initial)

Street address: ______ (Apt # ____) City: ______ State: ______ Zip: ______

Home phone: (____) ______ Work phone: (____) ______ Social Security # ____-____-____

Date of Birth: ____ / ____ / ____ (month / day / year)

Employer / Name of School ______ ❑ Full Time ❑ Part Time

PATIENT'S / RESPONSIBLE PARTY INFORMATION

Responsible party: ______ Date of Birth: ______

Relationship to Patient: ❑ Self ❑ Spouse ❑ Other ______ Social Security # ____-____-____

Responsible party's home phone: (____) ______

Address: ______ (Apt # ____) City: ______ State: ______ Zip: ______

Employer's name: ______ Phone number:(____) ______

Address: ______ City: ______ State: ______ Zip: ______

Name of Parent/Guardian: ______

PATIENT'S INSURANCE INFORMATION Please present insurance cards to receptionist.

PRIMARY insurance company's name: ______

Insurance address: ______ City: ______ State: ______ Zip: ______

Name of insured: ______ Date of Birth: ______ Relationship to insured: ☐ Self ☐ Spouse ☐ Other ☐ Child

Insurance ID number: ______ Group number: ______

Does your insurance cover medication? ______

EMERGENCY CONTACT

Name of person not living with you: ______ Relationship: ______

Address: ______ City: ______ State: ______ Zip: ______

Phone number: (____) ______

Assignment of Benefits • Financial Agreement

I hereby give lifetime authorization for payment of insurance benefits to be made directly to ______, and any assisting physicians, for services rendered. I understand that I am financially responsible for all charges whether or not they are covered by insurance. In the event of default, I agree to pay all costs of collection, and reasonable attorney's fees. I hereby authorize this healthcare provider to release all information necessary to secure the payment of benefits.
I further agree that a photocopy of his agreement shall be as valid as the original.

Date: ______ Your Signature: ______

FORM # 58-8423 • BIBBERO SYSTEMS, INC.• PETALUMA, CA.• TO ORDER CALL TOLL FREE :800-BIBBERO (800-242-2376) • FAX (800) 242-9330 (REV.7/94)

Figure 1.1 Patient registration form. (Courtesy Bibbero Systems, Inc., Petaluma, Calif, 800-242-2376; www.bibbero.com.)

The signature also signifies that the patient will accept responsibility for charges that the patient's insurance does not pay.

Before a patient sees a provider, the medical office assistant prepares an **encounter form** (Figure 1.2). This document contains common codes used by the medical office. An encounter form is used by the provider during the medical examination to record the patient's type of illness, injury, and any medical services performed. The encounter form is also called a *superbill* because it indicates the fees charged for the services provided. These two terms are frequently used interchangeably.

When the medical examination is over, the patient may be asked to return to the front desk or another appropriate area where follow-up appointments can be scheduled or payments made. Depending on the practice, the patient may be asked to pay on his or her account when checking in for the appointment or after the examination.

Elsevier Clinic
1234 College Avenue
Saint Paul, Minnesota 55316

Phone: (555) 555-1234
Fax: (555) 555-5678

PATIENT NAME	CHART #	DATE	☐ MEDI-MEDI ☐ SELF PAY ☐ MEDICARE	☐ MEDICAL ☐ PRIVATE ☐ HMO_____

CPT/Md	DESCRIPTION	FEE
OFFICE VISIT - NEW PATIENT		
99202	Focused Ex.	
99203	Detailed Ex.	
99204	Comprehensive Ex.	
99205	Complex Ex.	
OFFICE VISIT - ESTABLISHED PATIENT		
99212	Focused Ex.	
99213	Expanded Ex.	
99214	Detailed Ex.	
99215	Complex Ex.	
PREVENTATIVE MEDICINE - NEW PATIENT		
99381	< 1 year old	
99382	1-4 year old	
99383	5-11 year old	
99384	12-17 year old	
99385	18-39 year old	
99386	40-64 year old	
99387	65 + year old	
PREVENTATIVE MEDICINE - ESTABLISHED PATIENT		
99391	< 1 year old	
99392	1-4 year old	
99393	5-11 year old	
99394	12-17 year old	
99395	18-39 year old	
99396	40-64 year old	
99397	65 + year old	

CPT/Md	DESCRIPTION	FEE
LAB STUDIES		
36415	Venipucture	
81000	Urinalysis	
81003	- w/o Micro	
84703	HCG (Urine, Pregnancy)	
82948	Glucose	
82270	Hemoccult	
85025	CBC -diff.	
85018	Hemoglobin	
88174	Pap Smear	
87210	KOH/ Saline Wet Mount	
87430	Strep Antigen	
87070	Throat Culture	
80053	Chem profile	
80061	Lipid profile	
82465	Cholesterol	
99000	Handling fee	
X-RAY		
70210	Sinuses	
70360	Neck Soft Tissue	
71010	CXR (PA only)	
71020	Chest 2V	
72040	C-Spine 2V	
72100	Lumbrosacral	
73030	Shoulder 2V	
73070	Elbow 2V	
73120	Hand 2V	
73560	Knee 2V	
73620	Foot 2V	
74000	KUB	

CPT/Md	DESCRIPTION	FEE
PROCEDURES		
92551	Audiometry	
29705	Cast Removal Full Arm/Leg	
2900__	Casting (by location)	
92567	Ear Check	
69210	Ear Wax Rem. 1 2	
93000	EKG	
93005	EKG tracing only	
93010	EKG Int. and Rep	
11750	Excision Nail	
94375	Respiratory Flow Volume	
93224	Holter up to 48 hours	
10060	I & D Abscess Simple	
10061	I & D Abscess Comp.	
94761	Oximetry w/Exercise	
94726	Plethysmography	
94760	Pulse Oximetry	
11100	Skin Bx	
94010	Spirometry	
99173	Visual Acuity	
17110	Wart destruction up to 14	
17111	Wart destruction 15 lesions +	
11042	Wound Debrid.	

CPT/Md	DESCRIPTION	FEE
INJECTIONS		
90655	Influenza 6-35 months	
90656	Influenza 3 years +	
90732	Pneumoccal	
J0295	Ampicillin, 1.5 gr	
J2001	Liocaine for IV infusion 10mg	
J1885	Toradol 15mg	
90720	DTP - HIB	
90746	HEP B - HIB	
90707	MMR	
86580	PPD	
90732	Pneumovax	
90716	Varicella	
82607	Vitamin B12 Inj.	
90712	Polio oral use (OPV)	
90713	Polio injection (IPV)	
90714	Td preservative free 7 yrs +	
90718	Td 7 years +	
95115	Allergy inj., single	
95117	Allergy inj., multiple	
OTHER		

DIAGNOSTIC CODES (ICD-9-CM)

789.0__	Abdominal Pain	564.0	Constipation	784.0	Headache	782.1	Rash or ezanthem
682.__	Abscess/Cellulitis	692.6	Contact dermatitis due to plants	414.9	Heart Dis., Coronary	714.0	Rheumatoid Arthritis
995.3	Allergic Reaction	692.9	Contact dermatitis, NOS	599.70	Hematuria	V70.0	Routine general exam
331	Alzheimer's	V25.09	Contraceptive management	455.6	Hemorrhoids	V76.10	Screen, breast
285.__	Anemia, other & unspec	923.10	Contusion, forearm	573.3	Hepatitus, NOS	V76.2	Screen, cervix
280.9	Anemia-iron deficiency	434.91	CVA	V03.81	HIB	V76.44	Screen, prosate
281.0	Anemia-pernicious	266.2	Deficiency, folic acid B12	V65.44	HIV counseling	V76.47	Screen, vagina
285.9	Anemia-unspecified	311	Depression	401.1	Hypertension, benign	216.5	Sebaceous cyst
413.9	Angina, pectoris, oyher/unspecified	250.01	Diabetes, type I, juvenile type	401.9	Hypertension, unspecified	706.2	Sebaceous cyst
300.00	Anxiety state, NOS	787.91	Diarrhea	401.0	Hypertension, malignant	786.05	Shortness of Breath
300.4	Anxiety reaction	780.4	Dizziness	V04.81	Influenza	701.9	Skin tag
716.90	Arthritis, NOS	V06.1	DTP	271.3	Lactose intolerance	845.00	Strain, ankle
493.20	Asthma; chronic obstruction	V06.3	DTP + polio	573.9	Liver Disease	307.81	Tension headache
493.00	Asthma; extrinic	536.8	Dyspepsia	724.5	Low Back Pain	V06.5	Tetanus - distheria (Td)
493.10	Asthma; intrinsic	788.1	Dysuria	346.9	Migraine	305.1	Tobacco dependence
493.90	Asthmas; unspecified	782.3	Edema	V06.4	MMR	788.41	Urinary frequency
427.31	Atrial fibulation	530.81	Esophageal reflux	278.01	Obesity/Morbid	599.0	Unrinary tract infection, NOS
724.5	Backache, unspecified	530.11	Esophagitis reflux	715.90	Osteoarthritis	V05.3	Viral hepatitis
790.6	Blood chemistry	530.10	Esophagitis, unspecified	719.43	Pain in joint, forearm	368.40	Visual field defect, unspecified
E906.3	Cat bite	780.6	Fever	625.4	PMS	V20.2	Well Child Exam
786.50	Chest Pain	789.07	Generalized abdominal pain	486	Pneumonia		
428.0	CHF	V72.3	Gynecological examiniation	V25.01	Prescription of oral contraceptivess		

DIAGNOSIS: (IF NOT CHECKED ABOVE)		RECEIVED BY:	TODAY'S FEE	
		☐ CASH	AMOUNT RECEIVED	
PROCEDURES: (IF NOT CHECKED ABOVE)	RETURN APPOINTMENT INFORMATION: (DAYS) (WKS.) (MOS.) (PRN)	☐ CREDIT CARD ☐ CHECK #_______	BALANCE	

Figure 1.2 Encounter form (superbill).

Processing and Tracking Data

After information has been collected about the patient and his or her office visit or encounter, the medical office assistant uses the practice's computer system to enter and process the data. In addition to entering patient and office visit data, this process also includes recording payments made by the patient, producing statements of the patient's accounts, submitting claims to his or her insurance company for payment, and printing various reports needed by the medical office staff. Information from both the patient registration form and the encounter form or superbill is used to accomplish these tasks.

It may also be the responsibility of the medical office assistant to follow up on patient accounts with unpaid, overdue amounts. In addition, insurance claims that are not paid in a reasonable amount of time need to be investigated. Depending on the reason for non-payment, insurance claims may need to be resubmitted.

Remember, medical offices come in many different sizes and types. Your responsibilities may include performing some or all of the steps previously described (except for, of course, the actual medical examination) to complete the medical information cycle. As you will see, the focus of this textbook is showing you how to process and track data using Medisoft.

GENERAL MEDISOFT FUNCTIONS AND FEATURES

Computers have simplified the accounting and scheduling procedures for a medical office. Software programs such as Medisoft make it easy to enter information from the patient registration form, encounter form, and other forms used in the medical office. After the information is in the computer system, it can be accessed for scheduling, billing, insurance, and practice analysis with a few keystrokes. Medisoft can be used to perform the following tasks:

- Enter patient information.
- Schedule appointments for patients, and reserve rooms designed used to perform special procedures.
- Enter charges and payments to patient accounts.
- Submit claims to insurance companies.
- Print an assortment of reports.
- Follow-up unpaid patient accounts and insurance claims.

Before a medical office can fully utilize Medisoft's features, some basic information must be entered about the practice and its patients. The author of this textbook has created a small amount of data to get you started. Before you begin to do any of the textbook procedures, check first with your instructor to make sure this sample data has been previously loaded on your computer. If not, you will need to visit the Evolve Learning Resources site for this textbook and follow the directions to load the data.

How to Start the Medisoft Program

The first step in using a software program is learning how to start it. The following procedure shows one way to start Medisoft. Medisoft version 18 is supported by the following operating systems.

- Windows XP SP3
- Windows Vista 32 bit
- Windows Vista 64 bit
- Windows 7 32 bit
- Windows 7 64 bit

This text is written to reference the Student Demo Version of Medisoft version 18 on the Windows 7 operating system. At the end of this chapter, you will also learn how to exit the program.

PROCEDURE 1.1 STARTING MEDISOFT

1. Click the *Start* button on the taskbar, located in the bottom-left corner of your computer's desktop. The Start menu displays.
2. Point to or click *All Programs* on the Start menu. A list of available programs displays.
3. Click *Medisoft* on the All Programs menu. A list of Medisoft-related programs displays.
4. Click *Medisoft Advanced Demo.* (In some situations, the program name may be *Medisoft Network Professional*; ask your instructor.) The program opens on your computer and displays the main Medisoft window (see Figure 1.3) on the computer screen.
5. Look at the horizontal title bar that runs along the top of the window. The name of the software program and the name of the current medical practice displays.

Another Way
You can also launch Medisoft by double-clicking the Medisoft icon located on the computer desktop.

Another Way
An underlined letter in a menu name indicates that you can use the keyboard to display menu options. Press and hold down the ALT key while pressing the letter that corresponds to the menu. For example, ALT+F displays the File menu.

The main Medisoft window (see Figure 1.3) provides a variety of ways to select various Medisoft program commands. The **menu bar** (Figure 1.4) is the long, rectangular bar at the top of the main Medisoft window. It displays the names of the Medisoft menus. When you click any one of these menu names, a list of options displays. Just below the menu bar is the **toolbar**, a row of buttons with icons (Figure 1.5). These toolbar buttons are frequently used as shortcuts for accessing menu options.

Another navigational tool that you may choose to include on the main Medisoft window is called the **side bar**. To display the optional side bar on the left side of the window, first click Window on the menu bar and then click Show Side Bar on the list of menu options. The side bar is simply another way to access quickly the most frequently used Medisoft menu options.

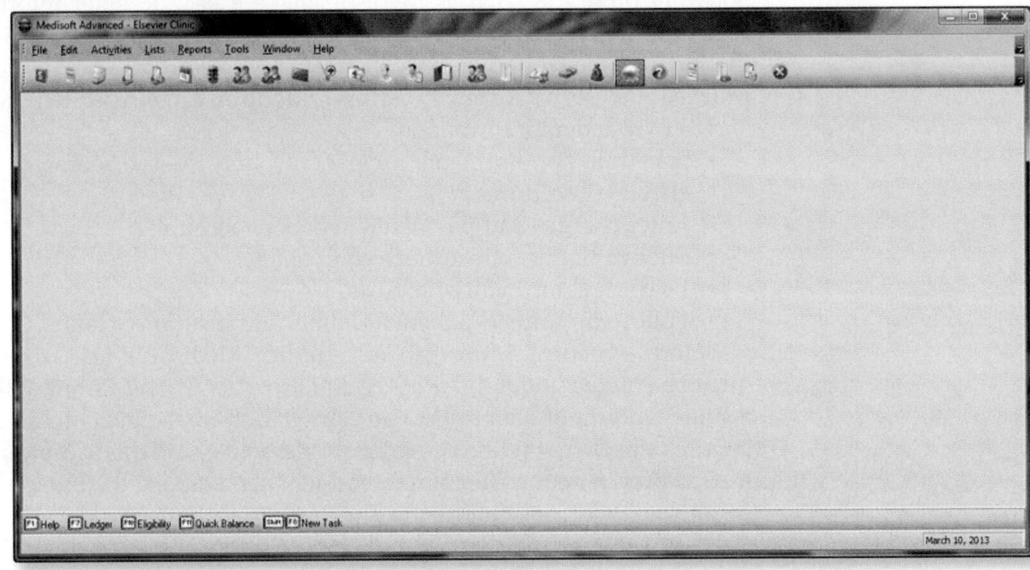

Figure 1.3
Main Medisoft window.

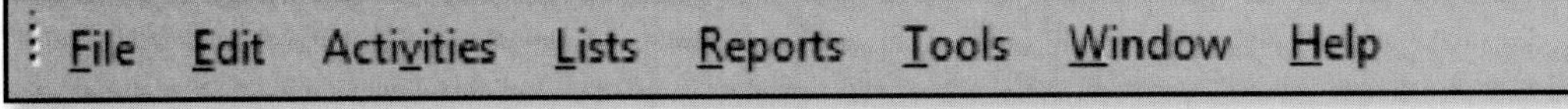

Figure 1.4
Menu bar.

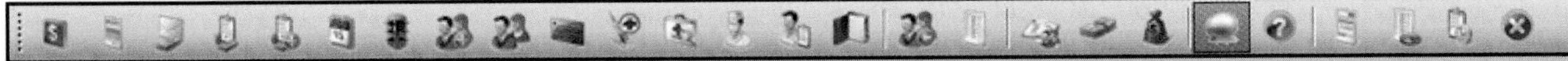

Figure 1.5 Toolbar.

Menu Bar and Side Bar

Eight Medisoft menus are located on the menu bar: File, Edit, Activities, Lists, Reports, Tools, Window, and Help. The File menu (Figure 1.6) contains the basic operations of opening practices, creating new practices, backing up and restoring data, setting the program date, entering practice information, setting up security and login options, and exiting the program.

The Edit menu (Figure 1.7) contains the editorial options Cut, Copy, Paste, and Delete. This menu is used to change, move, or alter information.

The Activities menu (Figure 1.8) is used to enter various transactions, manage insurance claims and collections, create patient statements, enter deposits or payments, schedule appointments, and verify insurance eligibility. From this menu, you can also access the Revenue Management system. This feature enables you to send electronic insurance claims to a clearinghouse or directly to insurance carriers. A **clearinghouse** is a company that provides services that include verifying patients' insurance eligibility, checking insurance

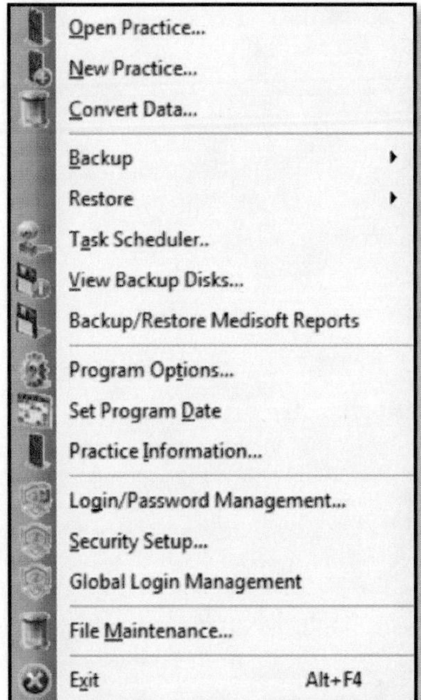

Figure 1.6
File menu.

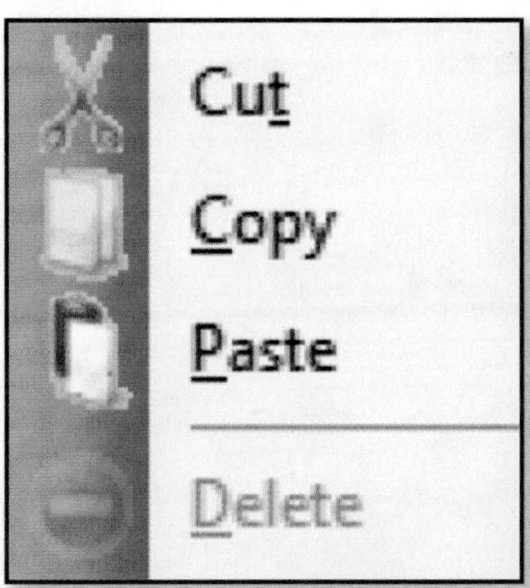

Figure 1.7
Edit menu.

claims for accuracy, and transmitting claims to insurance carriers. Medisoft uses **BillFlash** for patient statements, which was first used in Medisoft version 17. BillFlash enables users to process statements through Medisoft's online billing application. Several submenus are located under BillFlash. They include Approved Statements, View Statements, Reports, My Account, and Enroll. Before the first use of BillFlash, the practice will need to enroll. Once enrolled, the practice can print and send statements to their patients.

The Lists menu (Figure 1.9) is used to access information on patients, patient recall (follow-up appointments), patient treatment plans, diagnosis codes, insurance carriers, addresses, providers, and billing codes. The Lists menu is also used to enter case information. In Medisoft, a case is used to group transactions related to a specific medical condition for which a patient seeks treatment. You will learn more about setting up cases in Chapter 2.

The Reports menu (Figure 1.10) generates different reports that are used by administrators, physicians, and other medical office staff. For example, you can print reports that show which patients were seen on a given day, various analysis reports used to evaluate the practice's financial status, superbills, and many more reports. You can also create custom reports, based on the particular reporting requirements of the practice. Notice that some Medisoft menus, such as the Lists and Reports menus, display a small arrow beside certain options. Pointing to, or clicking, one of these options will cause a submenu to display with additional choices.

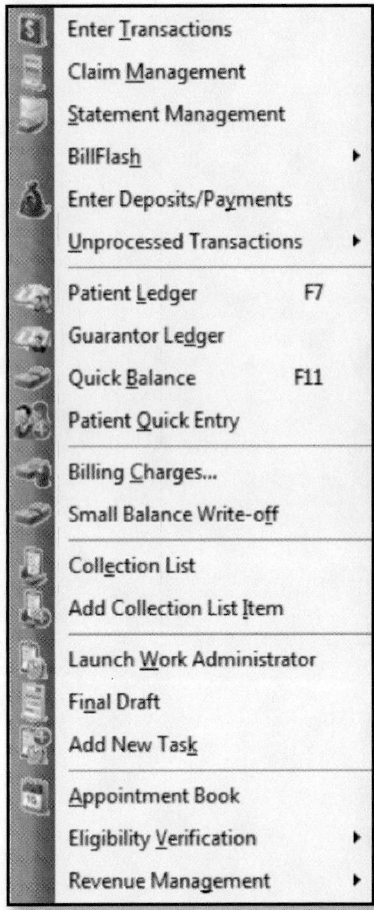

Figure 1.8
Activities menu.

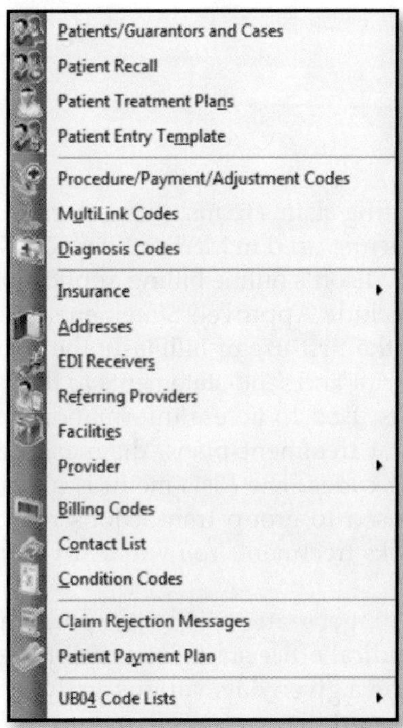

Figure 1.9
Lists menu.

The Tools menu (Figure 1.11) enables you to access information about your computer system such as the current operating system, memory, central processing unit (CPU), printers, and drives. Providers' notes and narratives for patient records can also be entered

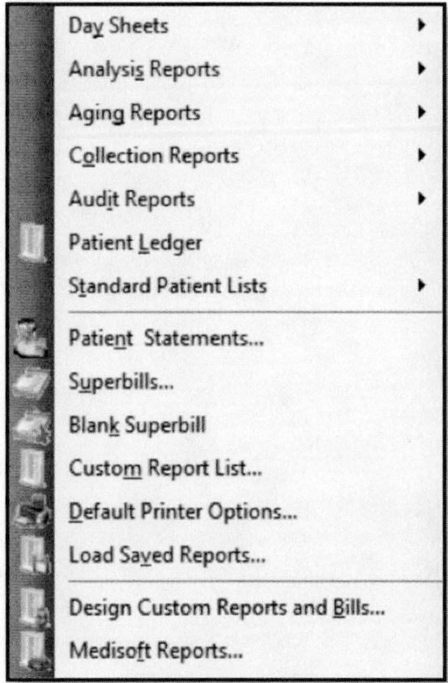

Figure 1.10
Reports menu.

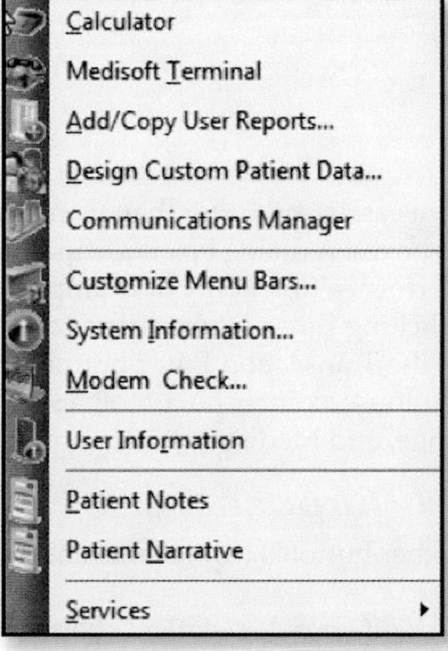

Figure 1.11
Tools menu.

using the Tools menu. Services options on the Tools menu are used to submit electronic prescriptions and to check for software updates.

The Window menu (Figure 1.12) allows you to tile (arrange) open windows, minimize windows, or close windows. If you have several windows open at one time, then you can switch back and forth between them by using this menu. One of the items on the Window menu is Show Side Bar, previously introduced. This option acts like a toggle switch. Clicking it once displays the side bar in the main Medisoft window. Likewise, clicking it again removes the side bar from the main window. The side bar lists four menu names Accounting, Patient Management, Office Management, and Daily Reports. When clicked, each one displays a list of related menu options that are typically used the most in Medisoft.

The Help menu (Figure 1.13) gives you access to information on how to use Medisoft. A built-in, searchable library provides everything from general overviews of processes to step-by-step procedures. The Help menu also provides links to Medisoft's Web site where you can obtain training and product information, as well as technical updates and customer support.

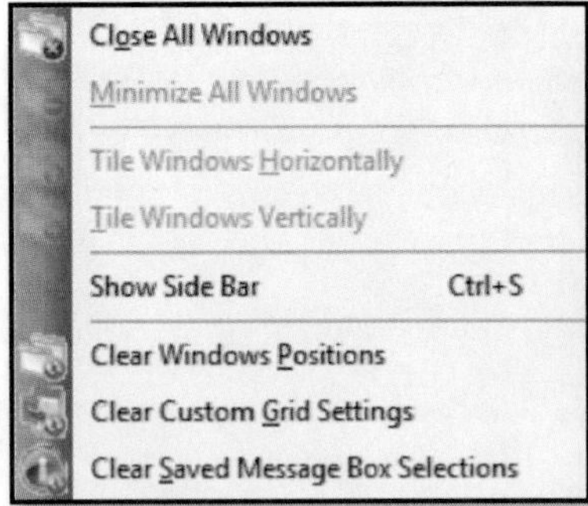

Figure 1.12
Window menu.

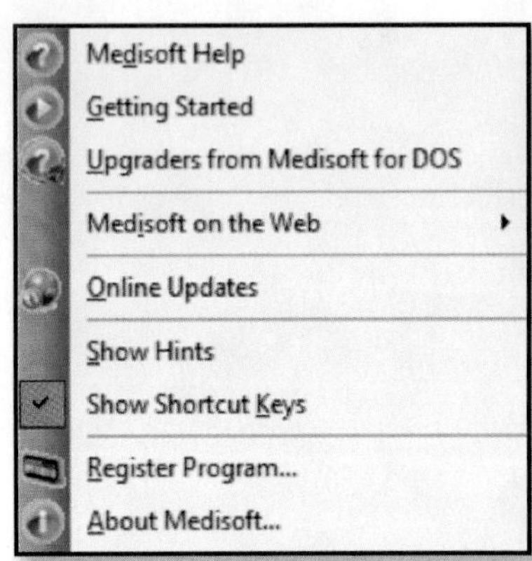

Figure 1.13
Help menu.

Toolbar

Using the Medisoft toolbar is often easier and faster than using the menu bar to access certain program features and dialog boxes. A dialog box is a window in which you can add or change data or tell Medisoft to perform a function. For example, instead of clicking Activities on the menu bar and then clicking Enter Transactions to open the Transaction Entry dialog box, you can simply click the Transaction Entry button on the toolbar (first one on the left). When you position the mouse pointer on a toolbar button, the color behind the button changes from blue to orange, and Medisoft displays the button's name.

Toolbar Icon Name & Purpose

The following is a list of each toolbar button's icon, name, and purpose

Transaction Entry. Enter, edit, or delete patient charges and payments.

Claim Management. Process insurance claims for the practice.

Statement Management. Create and review statements of patient accounts.

Collection List. Follow up on financial transactions that need to be collected.

Add Collection List Item. Add reminder notes to the Collection List.

Appointment Book. Open the Office Hours system to schedule patients' appointments and set up providers' schedules.

View Eligibility Verification Results. Results of an eligibility inquiry. Checks the status of a patient's insurance.

Patient Quick Entry. Create a customized template for adding new patient records more efficiently.

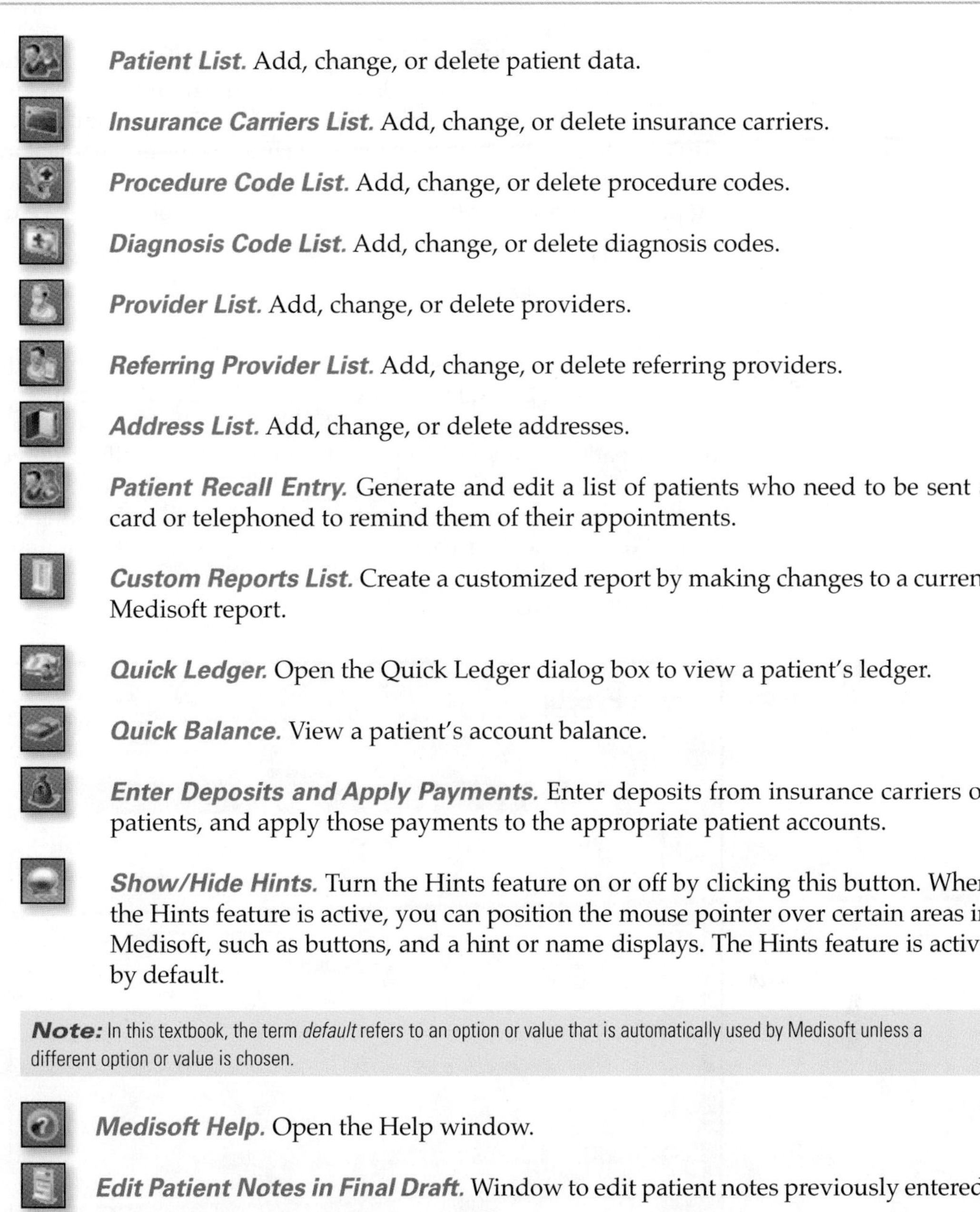

Patient List. Add, change, or delete patient data.

Insurance Carriers List. Add, change, or delete insurance carriers.

Procedure Code List. Add, change, or delete procedure codes.

Diagnosis Code List. Add, change, or delete diagnosis codes.

Provider List. Add, change, or delete providers.

Referring Provider List. Add, change, or delete referring providers.

Address List. Add, change, or delete addresses.

Patient Recall Entry. Generate and edit a list of patients who need to be sent a card or telephoned to remind them of their appointments.

Custom Reports List. Create a customized report by making changes to a current Medisoft report.

Quick Ledger. Open the Quick Ledger dialog box to view a patient's ledger.

Quick Balance. View a patient's account balance.

Enter Deposits and Apply Payments. Enter deposits from insurance carriers or patients, and apply those payments to the appropriate patient accounts.

Show/Hide Hints. Turn the Hints feature on or off by clicking this button. When the Hints feature is active, you can position the mouse pointer over certain areas in Medisoft, such as buttons, and a hint or name displays. The Hints feature is active by default.

Note: In this textbook, the term *default* refers to an option or value that is automatically used by Medisoft unless a different option or value is chosen.

Medisoft Help. Open the Help window.

Edit Patient Notes in Final Draft. Window to edit patient notes previously entered.

Launch Medisoft Reports. Launch the Medisoft Reports Engine, a feature that allows additional reporting options and views of data that are not available on the regular Medisoft Reports menu.

Launch Work Administrator. Assign a to-do list for yourself or other Medisoft users.

Exit Program. Close the Medisoft program.

You now have a general overview of the Medisoft program and can start using it to enter practice and provider information.

PRACTICE INFORMATION ENTRY

Medisoft allows you to set up one or more medical practices, each with its own set of separate data. In situations in which multiple practices have been set up, you can easily tell which practice is currently open by looking at the horizontal title bar at the top of the main

Medisoft window. This bar displays the name of the active practice. You can switch to a different practice by clicking File on the menu bar and then clicking Open Practice. These actions cause the Open Practice dialog box to display (Figure 1.14). If multiple practices display in this dialog box, then you can click the desired name and click the OK button to open it. Notice, you can also create new practices via the Open Practice dialog box by clicking the *New* button. For the purposes of this textbook, a practice has been created for you to use when completing practice exercises.

Practice Information Dialog Box

Part of the process of setting up a new practice involves entering information in the Practice Information dialog box. For Figure 1.15 they have added email as one of the dialog boxes. When a new practice is first created, this dialog box automatically opens after entering the data path (place where the practice information will be stored in the computer). For practices already established, this dialog box is also used to edit addresses, phone numbers, or other types of practice information, when necessary. Looking at Figure 1.15, notice that dialog boxes show their name in the upper-left corner. Some dialog boxes also have tabs that display just below the box's name. The Practice Information dialog box has four tabs Practice, Practice IDs, Practice Pay-To, and Statement Pay-To.

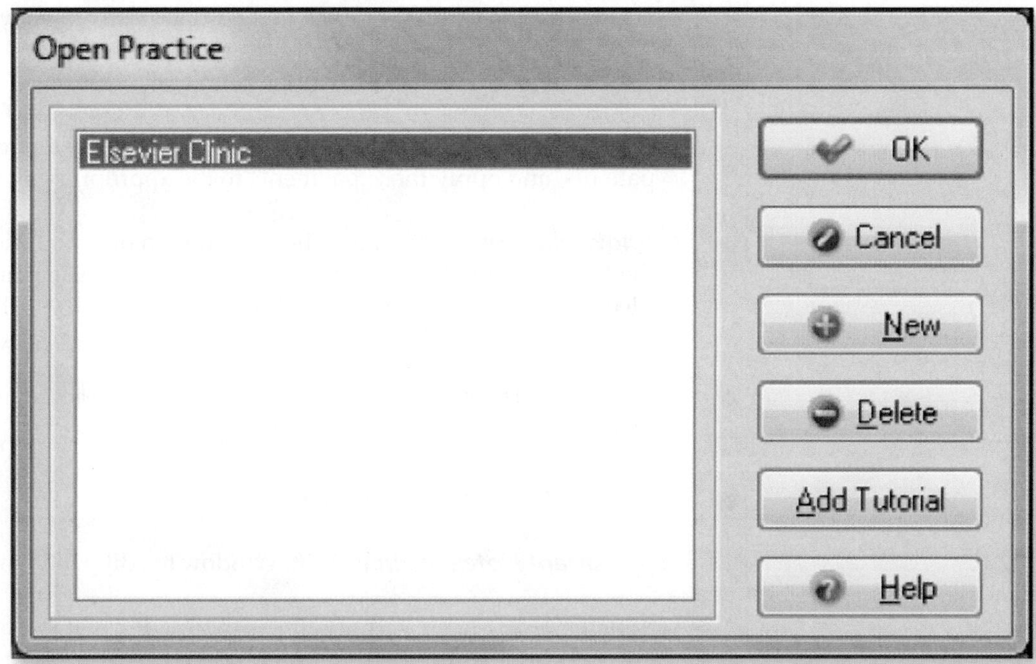

Figure 1.14
Open Practice dialog box.

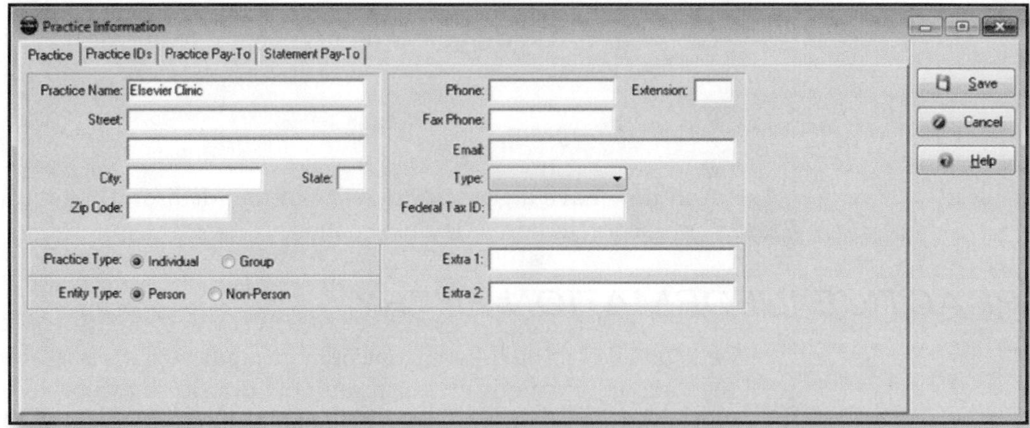

Figure 1.15
Practice Information dialog box with Practice tab displayed.

Practice Tab

Clicking a tab's name causes Medisoft to display a group of related fields where data can be entered (see Figure 1.15). For example, City and Zip Code are two fields in the Practice tab. Fields usually have text boxes in which you can key data. Some of these boxes have an arrow beside them. When this arrow is clicked, a drop-down box with options will display.

You can enter or change a field's information by clicking in the box beside the field's name. You can delete text in a field by pressing the Delete key or the Backspace key; or you can double-click a word to highlight it and then key new text.

In most dialog boxes, you can press the Tab key or Enter key on your keyboard to move the cursor from one field to the next. In some situations, pressing these keys will activate Medisoft's auto-populate feature. Auto-populated fields are ones that Medisoft automatically fills in, based on information previously entered. Consider, for example, dialog boxes with address-related fields. After keying the street address and pressing the Enter key, the cursor will move to the Zip Code field, skipping the City and State fields. If you enter a Zip Code that has been previously entered somewhere in Medisoft, the program will automatically complete the City and State fields. If the Zip Code has not been previously entered, the cursor will move to the City field so that you can enter the information.

Instead of boxes in which text is keyed, some fields have round shapes called *radio buttons*. For example, look at the Practice Type field in Figure 1.15. Instead of keying information, you click the desired radio button to select it. If the practice consists of a single provider, then the Individual radio button should be selected. If the practice is made up of multiple providers, then the Group radio button should be selected. The same principle applies to the Entity Type field. You should click the Person radio button if the practice name is a person's name (such as Dr. Jane Smith). However, if the practice name is, for example, Elsevier Clinic or Midwestern Medical Offices, the Non-Person radio button should be clicked.

Next, notice the Type field in Figure 1.15. When you click the arrow beside this field, a drop-down box displays with a list of options: Anesthesia, Chiropractic, or Medical. Depending on the option you click, Medisoft may alter fields in the Practice Information dialog box, as well as other dialog boxes within the program. For the purpose of this textbook, the Medical option is used.

Many dialog boxes also contain Save, Cancel, and Help buttons. You must click the Save button to keep and store the data entered. Clicking the Cancel button closes the dialog box *without* saving any new or edited data. Clicking the Help button displays information about the dialog box and how to use it.

Practice IDs Tab

The Practice IDs tab in the Practice Information dialog box shows a feature, called a *grid*, that you will see in many other Medisoft dialog boxes (Figure 1.16). Medisoft grids look somewhat like charts or tables because they have columns and rows. This layout allows

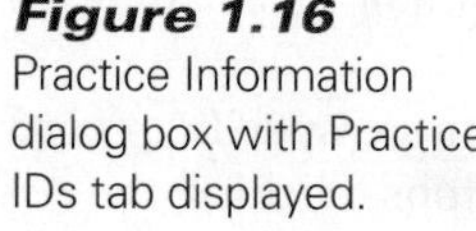

Figure 1.16 Practice Information dialog box with Practice IDs tab displayed.

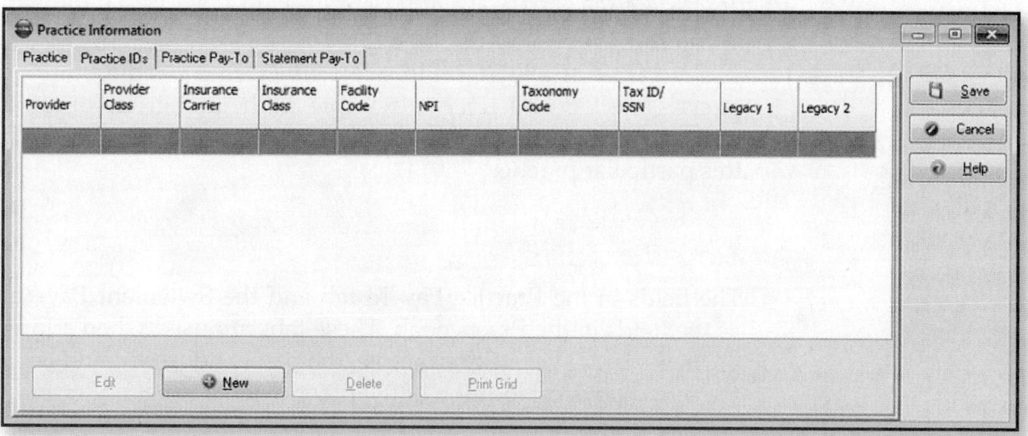

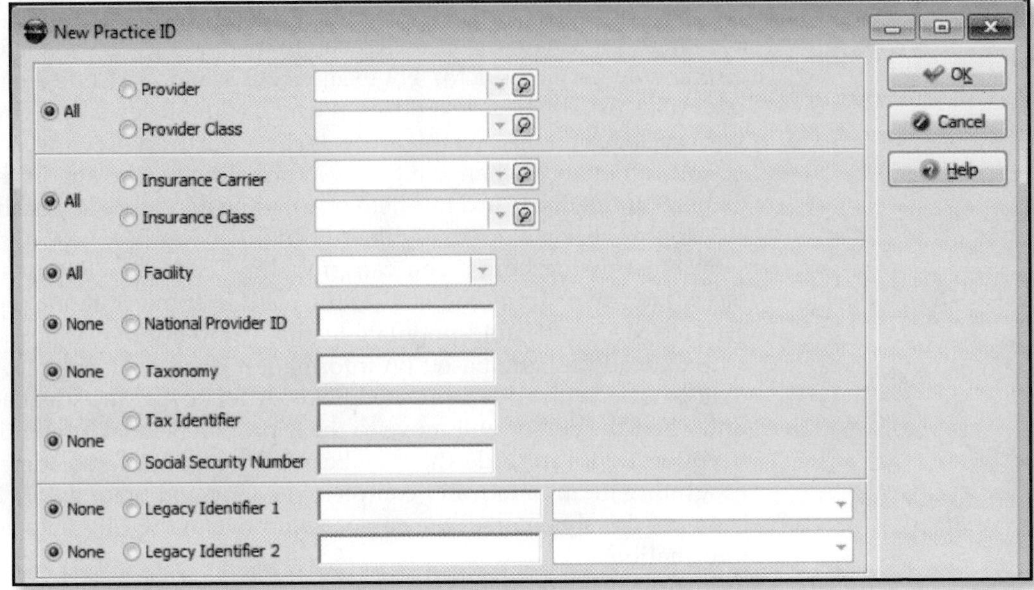

Figure 1.17 New Practice ID dialog box.

you a great deal of flexibility for setting up rules and records so that reports and claims generated by Medisoft reflect the practice's particular billing needs. To edit an existing entry in a grid, you click the desired row to highlight it, and then click the Edit button. To make a new entry, click the New button.

Clicking the New button in the Practice IDs tab opens the New Practice ID dialog box (Figure 1.17). The possible scenarios for setting up a practice are too varied to describe fully in this textbook. To keep things simple, assume that your practice is a group practice with multiple providers but that those providers submit all their insurance claims as a group, rather than as individuals. That means that only one entry, with the group's identification numbers, has to be added to the Practice IDs grid. If, for example, a provider were required by an insurance company to submit claims using individual identification numbers, then more grid entries would be needed. The following is a description of several main types of identification numbers

- National Provider Identifier (NPI). Every health care provider in the United States is assigned an NPI, which is a unique 10-digit number.
- Taxonomy codes. Providers use taxonomy codes to identify their specialty area, such as pediatrics, gynecology, dermatology, oral surgery, or general practice, among others.
- Federal tax identification (ID) number. The U.S. federal government requires a federal tax ID number for businesses. If an individual is a one-person business and does not have a federal tax ID number, then the Social Security number (SSN) may be used.

Several fields allow you to select either an All radio button or a more specific record or class (see Figure 1.17). For example, in the first group of radio buttons, clicking the All radio button will apply this claim-generation rule to all of the providers associated with this particular practice.

Pay-To Tabs

The fields in the Practice Pay-To tab and the Statement Pay-To tab are almost the same as the fields in the Practice tab. These tabs are used when address information for billing purposes is different. For example, the pay-to address could be a post office box instead of the actual physical location of the practice (e.g., street address).

PROCEDURE 1.2 ENTERING PRACTICE INFORMATION

In the following exercise, you will add information for a practice that is only partially set up.

1. Click *File* on the menu bar. The File menu displays.
2. Click *Practice Information* on the File menu. The Practice Information dialog box opens with the Practice tab displayed.
3. In the Practice Name field, replace Elsevier Clinic with *[your last name] Associates Clinic*; for example, Smith Associates Clinic.
4. In the Street field, key *1234 College Avenue*. Then press the Enter key twice. The cursor skips down to the Zip Code field.
5. In the Zip Code field, key *55316*. Then press the *Enter* key. Once a zip code has been entered into Medisoft, the program automatically populates (completes) the State field and the City field. Since this is the first time zip code 55316 has been used, you must hit the *enter* key to go back to the city and state and fill in St. Paul, MN. From now on each time you key *55316* in the zip code field, Medisoft will populate the city and state with St. Paul, MN. The city and state may populate after the zip code is entered. If it does not, please enter the city and state as instructed in step 5.
6. In the Phone field, key *5555552133*. Then in the Fax Phone field, key *5555552134*. Medisoft automatically inserts parentheses and hyphens to separate the digits in these numbers.
7. Click the arrow beside the Type field. A list box with options displays.
8. Click *Medical* in the list box if it is not already showing. Medisoft inserts the selected option in the Type field.
9. In the Federal Tax ID field, key *32-4514552*.
10. In the Practice Type field, click the *Group* radio button to select it.
11. In the Entity Type field, click the *Non-Person* radio button.
12. Click the *Practice IDs* tab. The Practice IDs grid displays.
13. Click the *New* button. The New Practice ID dialog box displays.
14. Click the *National Provider ID* radio button to select it. Then key *6789012345* in the box outlined in red.
15. Click the *Taxonomy* radio button. Then key *208D00000X*.
16. Click the *Tax Identifier* radio button. Then, key *324514552*.
17. Leave the rest of the fields alone, accepting the default selections of All and None.
18. Click the *OK* button. The New Practice ID dialog box closes, and the new entry appears in the Practice IDs grid.
19. Click the *Save* button. Medisoft saves your changes and closes the Practice Information dialog box.

Note: Including your last name in the practice name will help you more easily find your printouts when using a network printer shared with other students.

PROVIDER INFORMATION ENTRY

In Medisoft, the term *provider* is not exclusive to medical physicians. For example, a provider could also be a nurse practitioner or a physical therapist. Although a provider is typically an individual who charges for health care services, the term can also refer to a

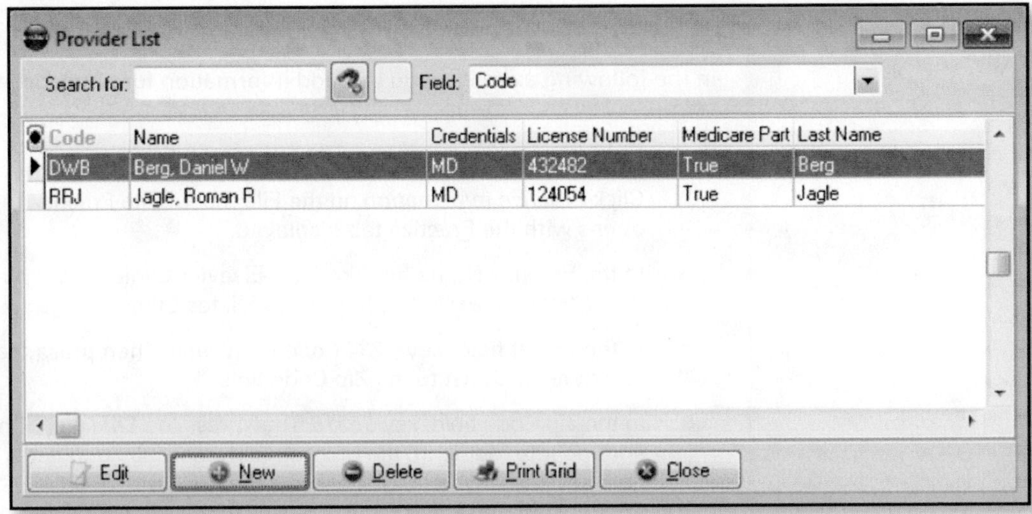

Code	Name	Credentials	License Number	Medicare Part	Last Name
DWB	Berg, Daniel W	MD	432482	True	Berg
RRJ	Jagle, Roman R	MD	124054	True	Jagle

Figure 1.18
Provider List dialog box.

non-person entity, such as a laboratory or medical supplier. A practice typically assigns a code to each provider for billing purposes. Even if a provider is part of a group practice that submits insurance claims as a group, a record is still set up for each provider.

The sample data that comes with this textbook has two providers already set up. In the next few pages, you will add three more providers. Figure 1.18 shows the Provider List dialog box where you can view the list of providers previously entered, as well as add or edit, delete, and print provider records. Notice that the Provider List dialog box has a grid layout similar to the grid you saw in the Practice Information dialog box. Some of the buttons associated with the Provider List grid are also similar, but others are different.

The following text provides a brief description of the primary features in the Provider List dialog box:

Search for. This field works along with the field beside it, named Field. The ability to search for a provider record is especially helpful in practices with many providers. Depending on the option you choose in the Field box, you can type in a provider's last name or a provider code to display the corresponding provider record in the grid below.

Field. You can display the list of providers in two ways: (1) alphabetical order by last name or first name or (2) the provider code.

Edit. To edit an existing provider's record, click the desired provider in the list, and then click this button to open the record.

New. Click this button to add a new provider.

Delete. Click this button to delete a provider. If the provider has appointments scheduled in Medisoft, then a message will appear warning you that all information and appointments associated with this provider will be lost if the provider is deleted. You may then choose to go ahead with the deletion or cancel the operation.

Print Grid. Click this button to open the Print Grid Columns dialog box where you can choose what information to print. For example, if you do not want the provider code to print on the report, then you can remove that field from the Print Grid Columns dialog box. Similarly, you can add fields to the report.

Close button. Click this button to close the Provider List dialog box.

Provider Dialog Box

If you click the Edit button or the New button in the Provider List dialog box, then the Provider dialog box will open with three tabs Address, Reference, and Provider IDs. The tab displayed by default is the Address tab (Figure 1.19).

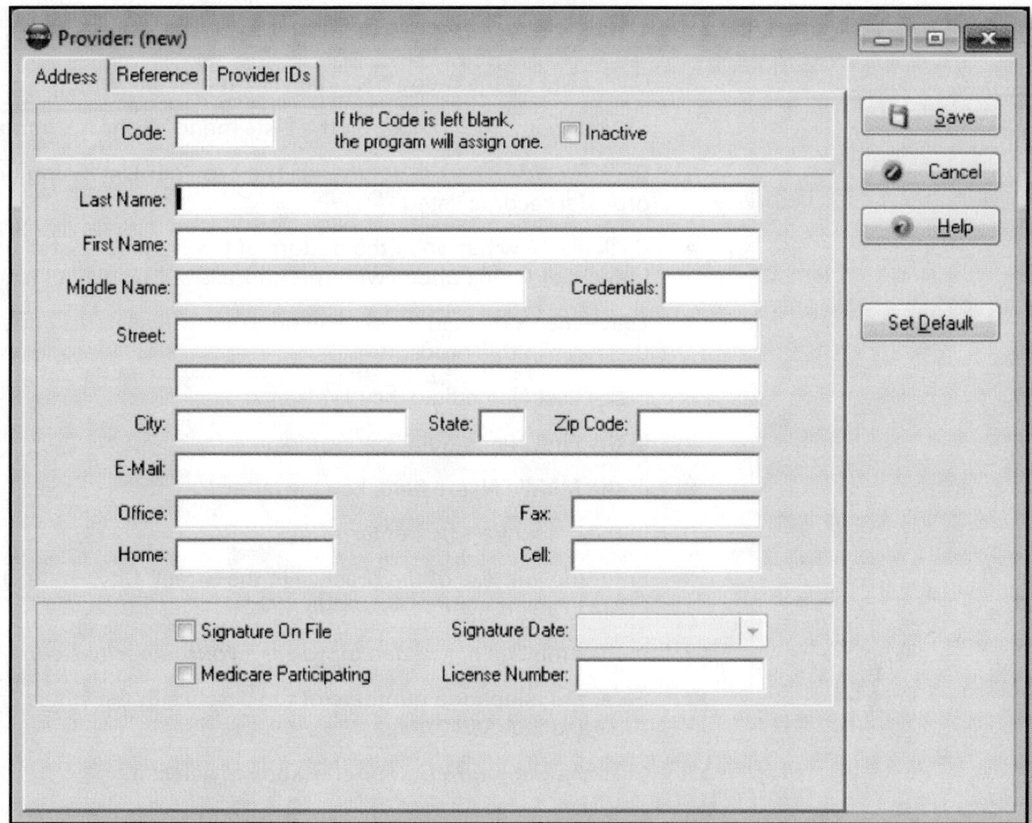

Figure 1.19
Provider dialog box with Address tab displayed.

Address Tab

The following list describes the fields contained in the Provider dialog box's Address tab

Code. This alphanumeric code is used to identify or locate a provider in Medisoft. If a code is not entered, then Medisoft automatically assigns one using the provider's initials.

Inactive. Click this checkbox to deactivate a provider; the provider's record will not be deleted.

Last Name, Middle Initial, First Name. Enter the parts of the provider's name.

Credentials. Enter the provider's credentials, for example, MD, NP, and PNP, among others.

Street, City, State, Zip Code. Enter the address where the provider's practice is located.

E-Mail. Enter the provider's e-mail address, if known. For the purpose of this textbook, the following convention will be used first.last@elsevierclinic.com (e.g., daniel.berg@elsevier.com).

Office, Fax, Home, Cell. Enter the provider's office, fax, home, and cellular telephone numbers.

Signature on File. If the provider has signed an agreement with Medicare to accept its charge amounts, then click this checkbox. Doing this will later print the words "Signature on File" on the CMS-1500 insurance claim forms (discussed further in Chapter 2).

Signature Date. This field becomes available when the Signature on File checkbox is selected. Enter the date when the provider's signature was placed on file.

Medicare Participating. If the provider is a participating Medicare provider, then click this checkbox.

License Number. Enter the provider's state license number.

PROCEDURE 1.3 ADDING A NEW PROVIDER

1. Click *Lists* on the menu bar. The Lists menu displays.
2. Click or point to *Provider* on the Lists menu. A short, submenu displays.
3. Click *Providers* on the submenu. The Provider List dialog box displays with two provider records listed.
4. Click the *New* button at the bottom of the Provider List dialog box. The Provider (new) dialog box opens with the Address tab displayed (see Figure 1.19).
5. Leave the Code field blank. The program will assign a code after you complete the steps in this procedure.
6. In the Last Name field, key *Walker.*
7. In the First Name field, key *Daniel.*
8. In the Middle Name field, key the letter *I.*
9. In the credentials box enter *MD.*
10. Enter the address of the practice in the Street, City, State, and Zip Code fields (*1234 College Avenue, St. Paul, MN 55316*).
11. In the email field, key *daniel.walker@yournameclinic.com.*
12. Enter the telephone numbers of the practice in the Office and Fax fields (*555-555-2133* and *555-555-2134*).
13. Click the *Signature On File* checkbox to select it.
14. In the *Signature Date* field, key *1/15/2009.*
15. Click the *Medicare Participating* checkbox to select it.
16. In the License Number field, key *114653.*
17. Click the *Save* button to save the data you have entered, and then the Provider dialog box will close. The Provider List dialog box now shows three provider records.
18. Click the *Close* button at the bottom of the Provider List dialog box to close it.

Reference Tab

The Reference tab is primarily used for reference purposes. This tab contains fields that were previously used in the Provider dialog box in Medisoft, version 15. When medical offices upgrade to the current version, the values in the previous version are converted and placed on the Reference tab. With the exception of the Provider Class field, none of the data in the Reference tab's fields is used when insurance claims are generated by Medisoft. Setting up provider classes is optional, allowing a practice to categorize or group providers, if desired.

Although the Reference tab is not critical for billing purposes, data can still be entered in its fields for reference purposes. Some of these fields relate to PINs. *PIN* is an acronym that means *provider identification number*. In the past, it was common for each type of major insurance carrier to issue a unique PIN for every provider. However, now each provider is assigned a National Provider Identifier (NPI) number, which is used in place of all previous PINs.

Provider IDs Tab

The Provider IDs tab (Figure 1.20) contains another grid that Medisoft uses when claims are created. Similar to most grids, it has Edit, New, Delete, and Print Grid buttons. When the New button is clicked, the New Provider ID dialog box displays (Figure 1.21).

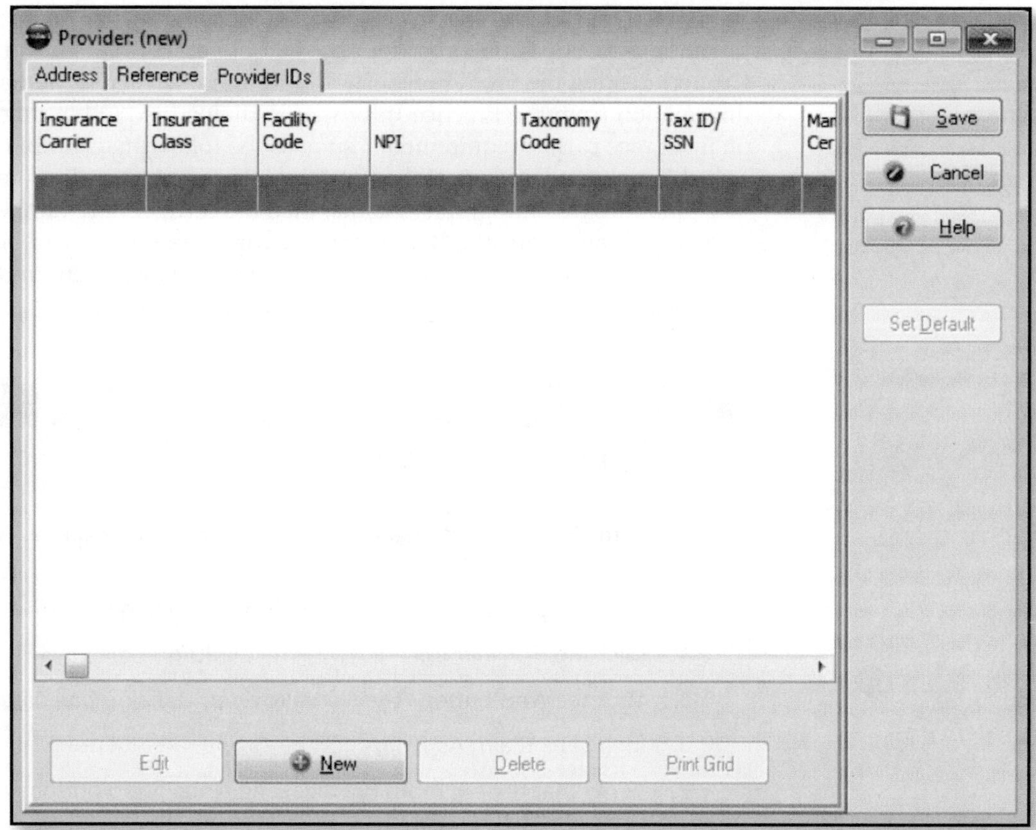

Figure 1.20 Provider dialog box with Provider IDs tab displayed.

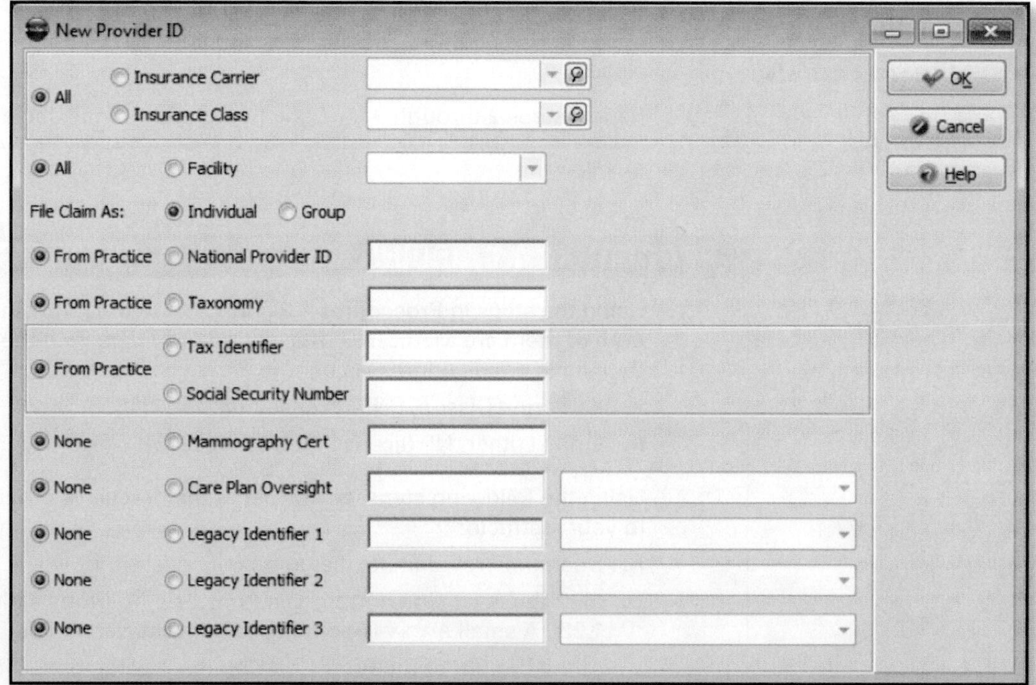

Figure 1.21 New Provider ID dialog box.

Some of the fields in the New Provider ID dialog box (see Figure 1.21) are similar to the fields in the New Practice dialog box that you previously set up. For instance, you can choose to apply this provider rule to all insurance carriers associated with the provider or to a specific one.

Because you are setting up a group practice, which files all of its claims as a group rather than as individual providers, the File Claim As radio button that should be clicked is Group. Clicking the From Practice radio buttons will cause Medisoft to pull identification information from the Practice Information dialog box. Other field choices are dependent on insurance carrier requirements, such as the following examples

- Mammography Cert. If the provider is certified to perform mammogram procedures and files mammography claims, then the certification number is entered in this field.
- Care Plan Oversight. If an insurance carrier requires a care plan oversight (CPO) number for a provider involved in supervising a patient under the care of a home health agency, then that number is entered in this field.

PROCEDURE 1.4 EDITING AN EXISTING PROVIDER

1. Click *Provider* on the Lists menu. Then click *Providers* on the submenu that displays.
2. In the Provider List dialog box, click the record for Daniel Walker (if not already highlighted).
3. Click the *Edit* button to open the Provider dialog box.
4. Click the *Provider IDs* tab. The Provider ID grid displays.
5. Click the *New* button. The New Provider ID dialog box displays.
6. In the File Claim As field, click the *Group* radio button.
7. Verify that the All, From Practice, and None radio buttons are selected for the remaining fields.
8. Click the *OK* button. The New Provider ID dialog box closes, and the new entry displays in the Provider IDs grid.
9. Click the *Save* button. The data entered are saved, and the Provider dialog box closes.
10. Repeat steps 2 through 9 for Daniel Berg and Roman Jagla.

Another Way
To open an existing record, double-click the line related to the provider in the Provider List dialog box.

PROCEDURE 1.5 ADDING AND PRINTING PROVIDERS

1. Using the steps in Procedures 1.3 and 1.4, add the following two new providers. Both of them are Medicare Participating providers with their signatures on file. Both have e-mail addresses per the e-mail convention.
   a. Katherine Olsson, PNP (license number 434839)
   b. Emily Luther, NP (license number 129835)
2. Using the following steps, print a list of the practice's providers, to be handed in to your instructor
   a. Open the Provider List dialog box, if necessary.
   b. Click the *Print Grid* button. The Print Grid Columns dialog box opens (Figure 1.22). A small arrow is pointing to the Last Name field.
   c. At the bottom of the Print Grid Columns dialog box, click the up arrow two times. Notice how the program moves the Last Name field to a new location.

Note: You can click on any field in the print grid to select it, and then use the up and down arrows to reposition the field where you want it to print on the report.

d. With the Last Name field still selected (small arrow pointing at the field name), click the *Remove Field* button at the bottom of the dialog box. The Last Name field is removed from the print grid.
e. Click the *OK* button. The Print Report Where? dialog box displays (Figure 1.23). The report is viewed on the computer screen and then sent to a printer or exported to a file.
f. Click the *Print the report on the printer* radio button.
g. Click the *Start* button. The Print dialog box opens.
h. Select the printer where you want the report to print. (Your report should list five providers.)

Note: To restore the print grid to its original settings, the Restore button can be clicked.

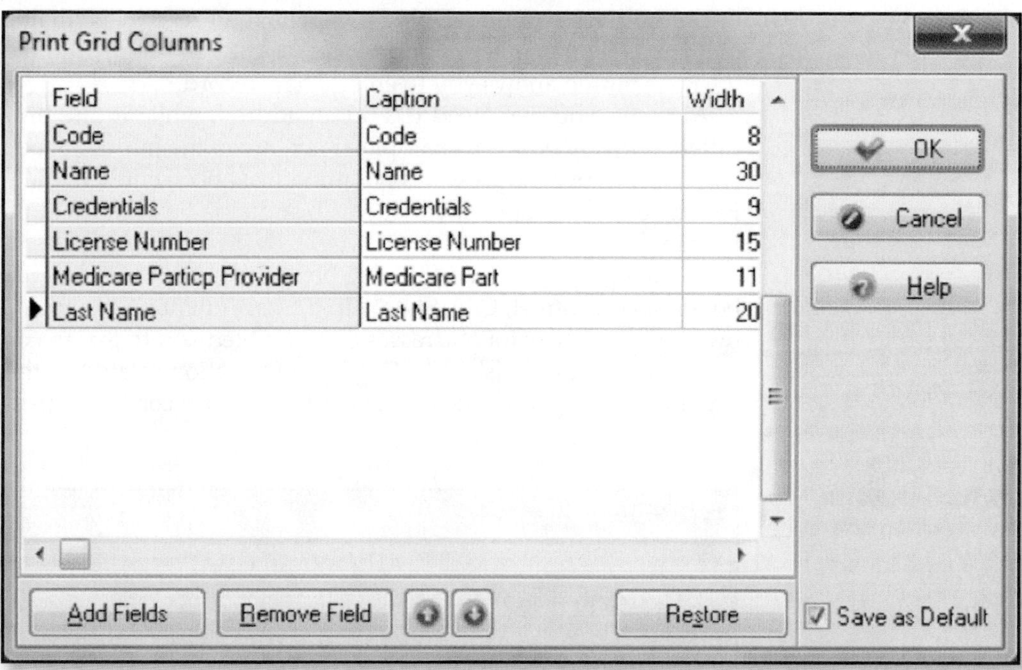

Figure 1.22 Print Grid Columns dialog box.

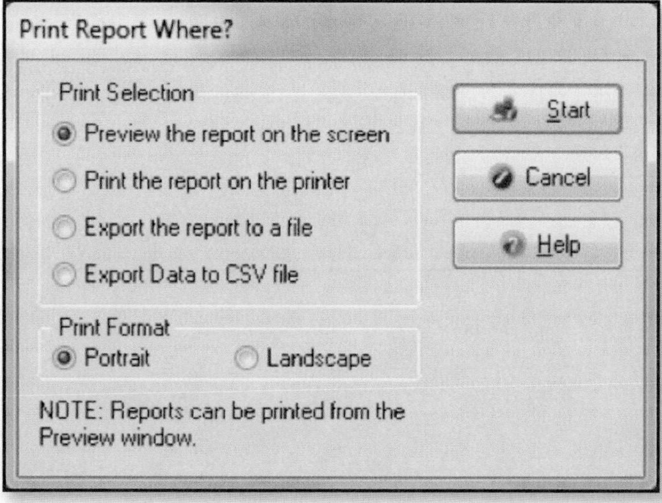

Figure 1.23 Print Report Where dialog box.

Referring Providers

If a patient is referred to your clinic by a provider in another medical practice, information on the referring provider can be entered by clicking Referring Providers on the Lists menu. This action will open the Referring Provider List dialog box, which is similar to the Provider List dialog box. When you click the New button to add a referring provider, the Referring Provider dialog box displays with two tabs (1) Address and (2) Referring Provider IDs. These tabs are similar to the tabs found in the Provider dialog box, which you have already learned to use.

FACILITY AND ADDRESS INFORMATION ENTRY

The Facility dialog box (Figure 1.24) is used to enter information for each facility, such as a hospital or laboratory, which is affiliated with or attached to the medical practice. The Address dialog box (Figure 1.25) is used to add addresses for the practice's attorney, patients' employers, and referral sources, as well as miscellaneous addresses.

You can access either dialog box using the Lists menu, by clicking the Facilities option, or the Addresses option. Doing so opens the Facility List dialog box or the Address List dialog box, both similar in appearance to the Provider List dialog box. Likewise, clicking the New button allows you to enter a new record.

At times, you may need to add an address while in the process of entering data in a different dialog box. For example, if you are in the middle of adding a new patient record and the employer address has not previously been entered, then you can simply press the F8 key to directly open the Address List dialog box. You will practice using this shortcut later in the chapter.

The fields in the Address dialog box are similar to fields you have seen in other dialog boxes, such as Street, City, State, Zip Code, and Phone, among others. You can create your own code numbers for addresses or allow Medisoft to assign codes for you.

You have now finished setting up information related to the medical practice and its providers. Next, you will enter and edit patient records and print a list of patients.

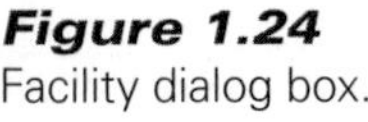
Figure 1.24
Facility dialog box.

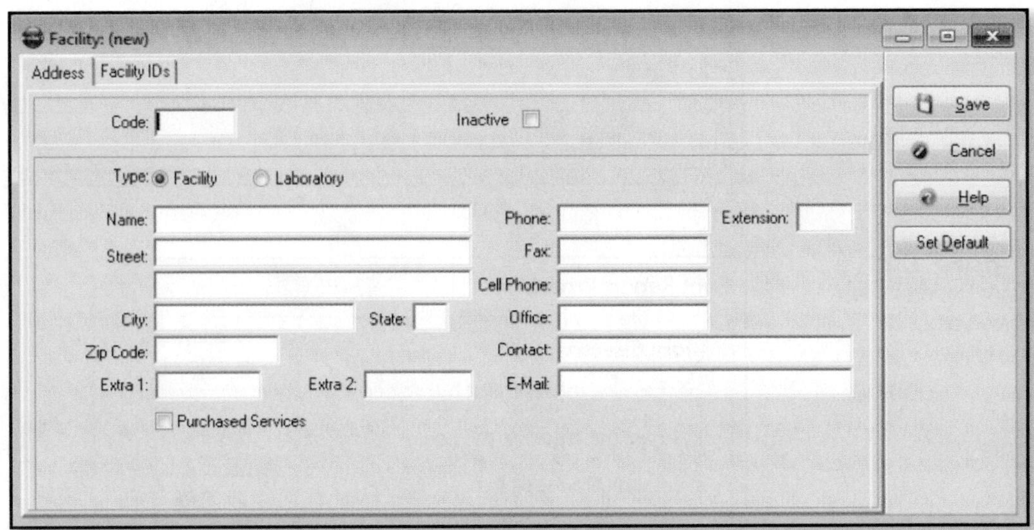

PATIENT INFORMATION ENTRY

In Medisoft, patient information is entered through the Patient List dialog box (Figure 1.26). This dialog box is divided into two main parts. On the left side, there is a window for displaying a list of patient records. The right side of the dialog box is for case records. As

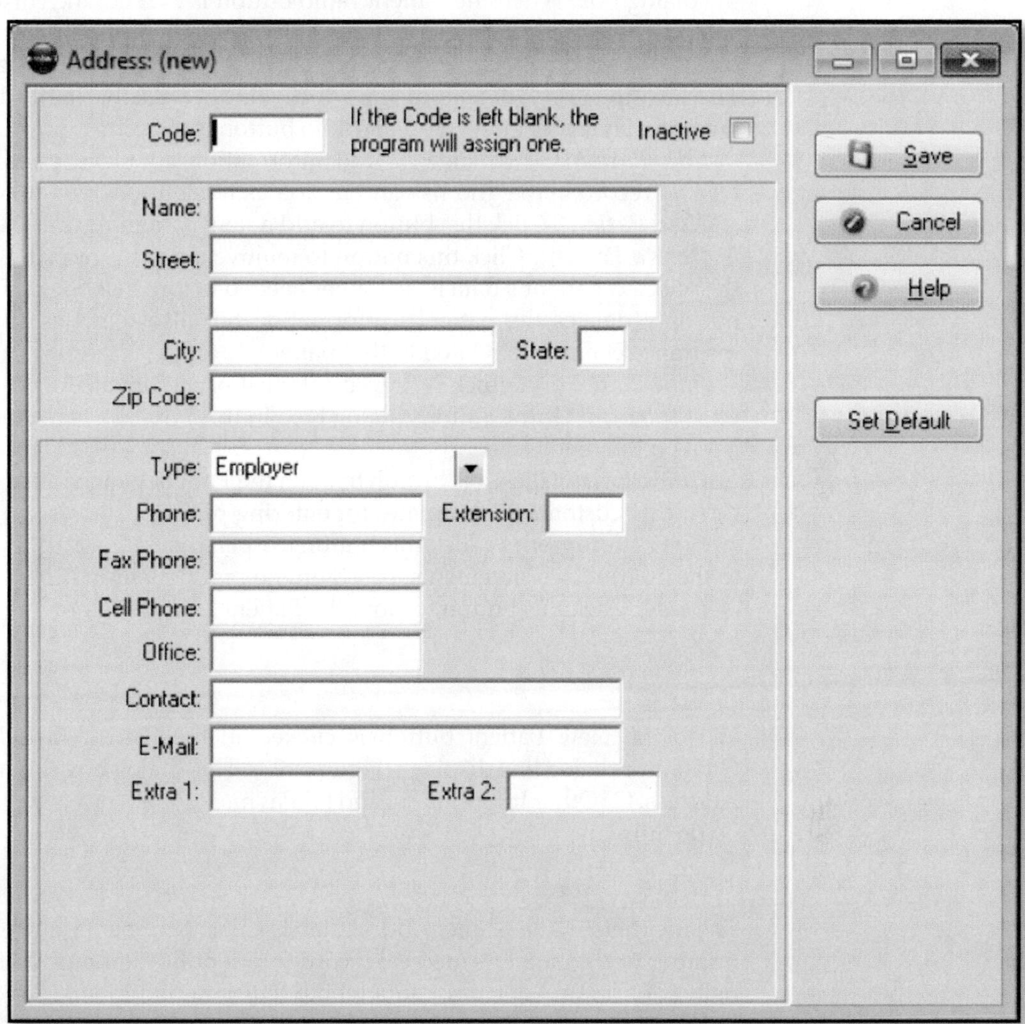

Figure 1.25
Address dialog box.

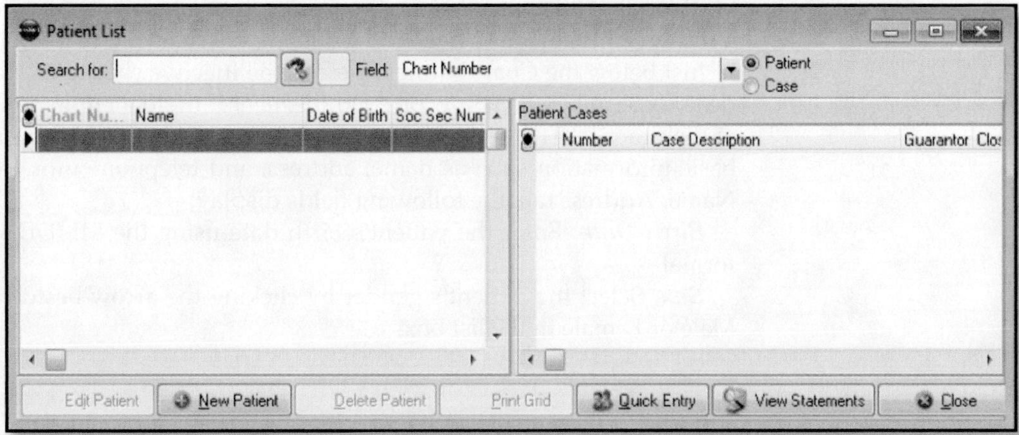

Figure 1.26
Patient List dialog box.

explained previously, a case is used in Medisoft to group transactions related to a specific medical condition for which a patient seeks treatment. For example, if Jane Doe is treated for a sinus infection and then visits the practice next week with a broken ankle, each condition is a separate case. If the patient changes insurances, then that is another case as well. (A more detailed explanation of cases is provided in Chapter 2.)

In Figure 1.26, notice the two radio buttons, Patient and Case, are located near the top of the dialog box. When the Patient radio button is clicked, the corresponding window (left side) becomes active. Likewise, when the Case radio button is clicked, the right side of the dialog box becomes active. At the bottom of the Patient List dialog box is a row of buttons. These buttons vary, depending on which window is active in the dialog box. The following buttons display when the Patient radio button is clicked:

Edit Patient. To change or add information about an established patient, click the desired record in the grid list, and then click this button to open the record.

New Patient. Click this button to add a new patient record.

Delete Patient. Click this button to remove a patient record. Be absolutely certain that the selected patient's data is no longer needed before deleting it. The Delete Patient option not only deletes the patient's information but also removes any case, transaction, and insurance claim data related to that patient.

Print Grid. For a quick way to print a list of the practice's patients, click this button to open the Print Grid Columns dialog box. In this box, you can choose the data you wish to print on the report.

Quick Entry. Click this button to open the Patient Quick Entry dialog box in which you can create customized templates for entering patient data.

View Statements. Click this button to open the BillFlash eView page. A page will open to the guarantor's statements, based on the case default in Program Options, Data Entry.

Close. Click this button to close the Patient List dialog box.

Patient/Guarantor Dialog Box

When the New Patient button is clicked in the Patient List dialog box, the Patient/Guarantor dialog box displays (Figure 1.27). This dialog box contains three tabs: (1) Name, Address; (2) Other Information; and (3) Payment Plan. The Name, Address tab is displayed by default.

Name, Address Tab

The first field in the Name, Address tab is Chart Number. Medisoft assigns a unique **chart number** to the patient's medical record for identification purposes, unless you do so manually. Chart numbers may contain both letters and numbers, although some practices use only letters or numbers. When Medisoft assigns a chart number, it uses the first three letters of the patient's last name and the first two letters of the patient's first name, and then adds three zeros. For example, the chart number for Michael Smith will appear as SMIMI000, if this patient is the first person by that name to be entered into the program. If a second Michael Smith becomes a patient, his chart number will be SMIMI001.

Just below the Chart Number field is the Inactive checkbox. Clicking the checkbox will deactivate this patient's record. Do this *only* if the patient is no longer receiving services at the practice! The next group of the fields in the Name, Address tab allows you to enter basic information such as name, address, and telephone numbers. At the bottom of the Name, Address tab, the following fields display:

Birth Date. Enter the patient's birth date using the MMDDYYYY (month/day/year) format.

Sex. Select the patient's gender by clicking the arrow beside this field, and then click Male or Female in the list box.

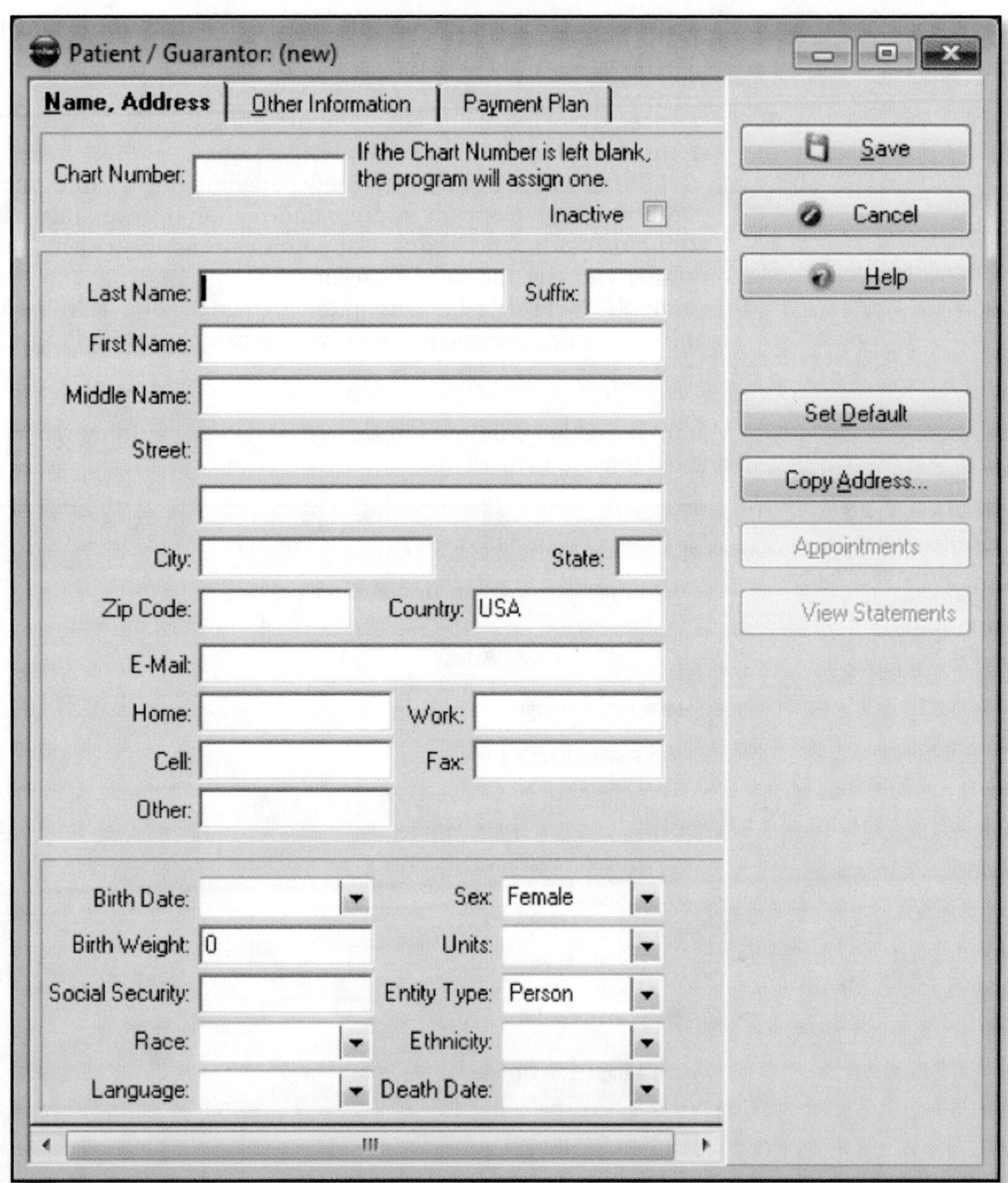

Figure 1.27 Patient/Guarantor dialog box with Name, Address tab displayed.

Birth Weight. If the patient is a newborn, enter the birth weight in this field.

Units. Indicate the unit of measurement used in the Birth Weight field by clicking Pounds or Grams in the list box.

Social Security. Enter the patient's Social Security number.

Entity Type. In this field's list box, click Person if the patient is a human being, or click Non-Person if the "patient" is a company.

Race. Enter the patient's race from the drop-down menu.

Ethnicity. Enter the patient's ethnicity from the drop-down menu.

Language. Enter the patient's primary language from the drop-down menu. The language field can assist in determining whether an interpreter is needed.

Death Date. If the patient is deceased, enter the date of death (if known) in this field.

The buttons on the right side of the Patient/Guarantor dialog box continue to display, no matter which one of the three tabs is selected:

Save. Save the data entered in the patient's record.

Cancel. Close the dialog box without saving the data entered.

Help. Access Medisoft's built-in Help database.

Set Default. Set a default for all new patients using the information currently displayed.

Copy Address. Copy the address information from another patient's record.

Appointments. Check current appointments for the patient. This button becomes active only after you save the patient's record.

View Statements. Click this button to open the BillFlash eView page. A page will open to the guarantor's statements, based on the case default in Program Options, Data Entry.

Other Information Tab

Within the Other Information tab, employment and emergency contact information is entered (Figure 1.28).

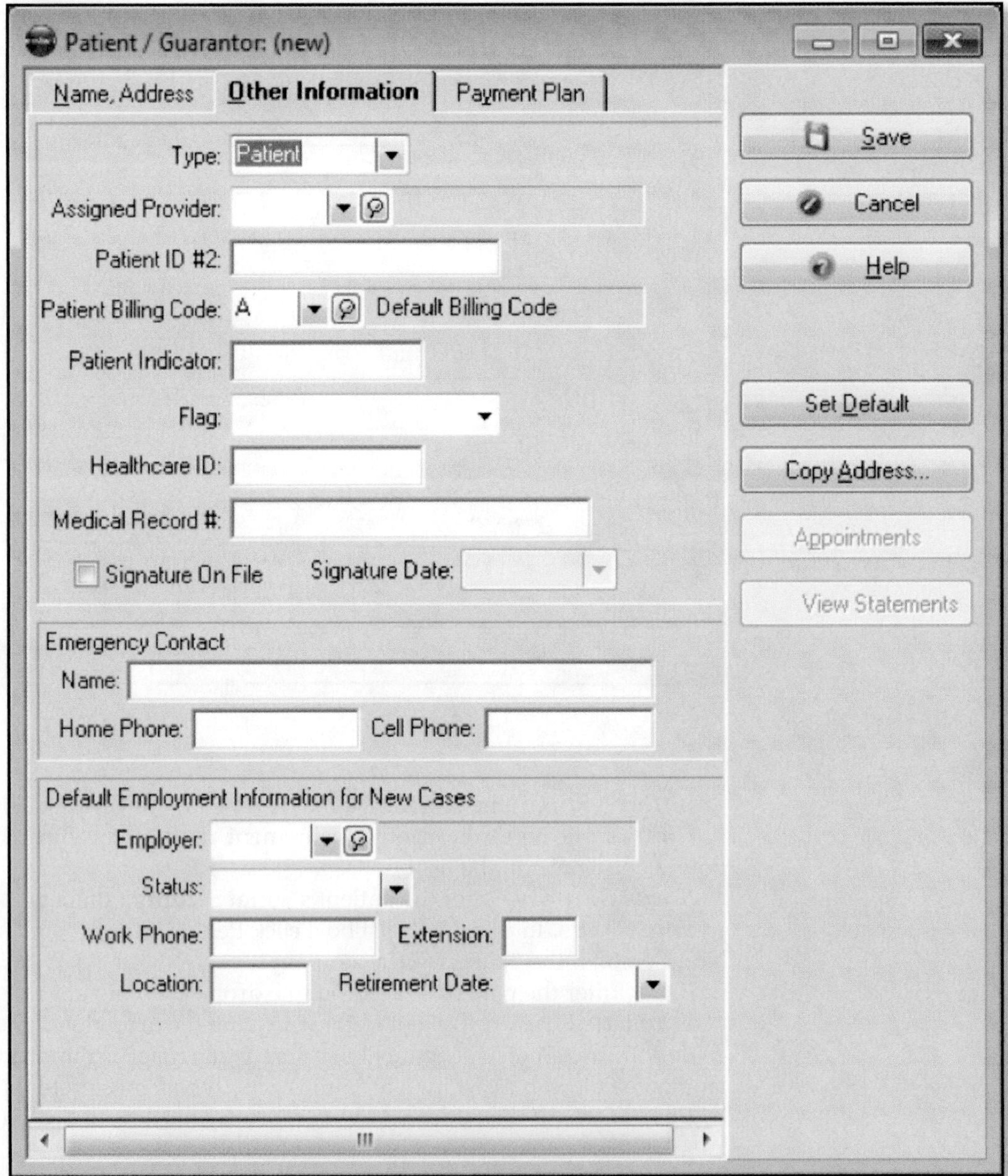

Figure 1.28
Patient/Guarantor dialog box with Other Information tab displayed.

Type. There are two choices for this field: Patient or Guarantor. A **guarantor** is the person who is responsible for paying a patient's medical bill. This person is normally the one who purchased the insurance policy. So, if a patient is a child, spouse, or other dependent who is covered under another person's insurance policy, you must set up two records: one for the guarantor and one for the patient. If a patient is responsible for his or her own medical bills, then Patient should be selected for the Type field.

Assigned Provider. The list box for this field shows all the providers associated with the practice. Choose the provider who is normally the patient's main provider. This does not mean, however, that other providers in the practice cannot see the patient.

Patient ID #2. Some medical clinics use this field for a second identification number.

Patient Billing Code. Billing codes can be used to sort patient records in specific ways. For instance, your practice may wish to differentiate between patients who have insurance coverage and patients who pay in cash. Clicking Billing Codes on the Lists menu sets up these codes.

Patient Indicator. This field is used as another way to classify and sort patients; for example, classifying and sorting patients who are diabetic.

Flag. Color-coded flags are used to alert medical office staff about certain situations or conditions. Clicking Program Options on the File menu and then clicking the Color-Coding tab in the Program Options dialog box set up these flags. After a flag has been assigned to a patient's record, that person's name is shaded in the assigned color in various Medisoft dialog boxes.

Healthcare ID. This file is not currently used but is reserved space for a future unique number that will be assigned to the patient for HIPAA purposes. **HIPAA** is an acronym for **Health Insurance Portability and Accountability Act** of 1996. This federal legislation provides guidelines for transmitting electronic data and protecting patients' privacy.

Medical Record #. This field is used by providers who wish to assign a patient identification number in addition to the patient's chart number.

Signature On File. Clicking this checkbox indicates that the patient's signature is on file. This field refers to a form that the patient has signed authorizing the release of medical information needed to file an insurance claim on behalf of the patient. If no signature appears on file, then the patient will need to sign an authorization form before a claim can be submitted to the insurance carrier for payment.

Signature Date. When the Signature On File field is checked, the Signature Date field becomes available. Enter the date when the patient signed the insurance release form (often a part of the patient registration form).

Emergency Contact Fields. Enter the name and phone number(s) of the person to be contacted in case of an emergency involving the patient.

Default Employment Information for New Cases. The data entered in these fields will be used as default information when new case records are created for the patient. If the patient's employer does not appear in the Employer field's list box, then it will need to be added first. You can do this by clicking Addresses on the Lists menu, or you can simply press the F8 key to open the Addresses dialog box. In the Status list box, click the appropriate option not employed, full time, part time, retired, and unknown. Be sure to enter the work phone number and location since some employers have multiple sites. If you clicked *retired* in the Status field, then you can enter the official retirement date in the Retirement Date field. Do not enter an anticipated future retirement date.

Payment Plan Tab

The Payment Plan tab in the Patient/Guarantor dialog box is used for patients whose accounts are overdue. You can create a payment plan to satisfy the outstanding amount—for example, a payment due on the first day of every month in the amount of $30.00. (This subject is further discussed in Chapter 5.)

PROCEDURE 1.6 ENTERING A NEW PATIENT

1. Click *Patients/Guarantors and Cases* on the Lists menu. The Patient List dialog box displays.
2. Click the *New Patient* button. The Patient/Guarantor dialog box opens with the Name, Address tab displayed.
3. Leave the Chart Number field blank, and make sure the Inactive checkbox is not checked.
4. Using the patient registration form for Charles Weber in **Figure C.1 in Appendix C**, enter the patient's name, address, and telephone numbers. You can click in a field to key the information or press the *Enter* key or the *Tab* key to move from one field to the next.
5. In the Birth Date field, enter the patient's birth date from the patient registration form using the MMDDYYYY format.
6. Click *Male* in the Sex field's list box.
7. In the Social Security field, enter the patient's Social Security number listed on the patient registration form.
8. Click *Person* in the Entity Type list box, if necessary.
9. Click the *Other Information* tab. A different set of fields displays.
10. Click *Patient* in the Type list box if it is not already displayed.
11. In the Assigned Provider field's list box, click the line displayed for Dr. Walker.
12. Leave the following fields blank or as they default: Patient ID #2, Patient Billing Code, Patient Indicator, Flag, Healthcare ID, and Medical Record #.
13. Click the *Signature on File* checkbox to select it.
14. Key *3/1/2010* in the Signature Date field.
15. Key the name and telephone number for the Emergency Contact as indicated on the patient registration form.
16. Mr. Weber's employer is not listed in the Employer list box. Therefore click in the box beside the Employer field, and then press *F8* to open the Address dialog box. Use the information on the patient registration form to enter the employer:
    a. Leave the Code field blank, and allow Medisoft to create one for you.
    b. Enter the name, address, and telephone number of the employer.
    c. In the Type field's list box, click *Employer* if not already displayed. Leave the remaining fields blank.
    d. Click the *Save* button. The Address dialog box closes. The Work Phone field is automatically completed.
17. In the Status field's list box, click *Full time*.
18. Compare the data you entered on the Name, Address tab, and Other Information tab with the data shown in Figures 1.29 and 1.30. If necessary, make corrections.
19. Click the *Save* button. The Patient/Guarantor dialog box closes, and the new record displays in the Patient List dialog box.
20. Click the *Close* button to close the Patient List dialog box.

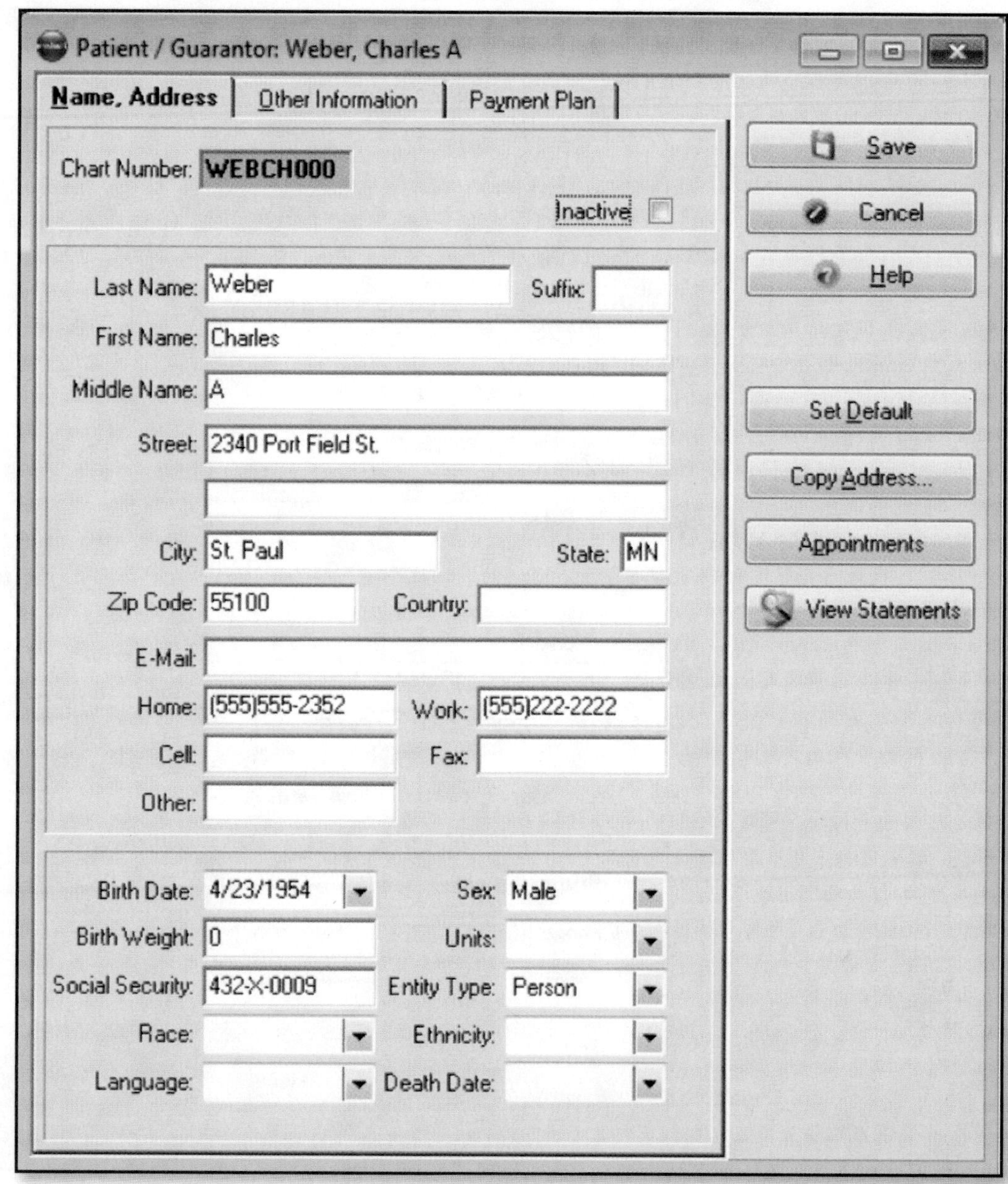

Figure 1.29
Completed Name, Address tab.

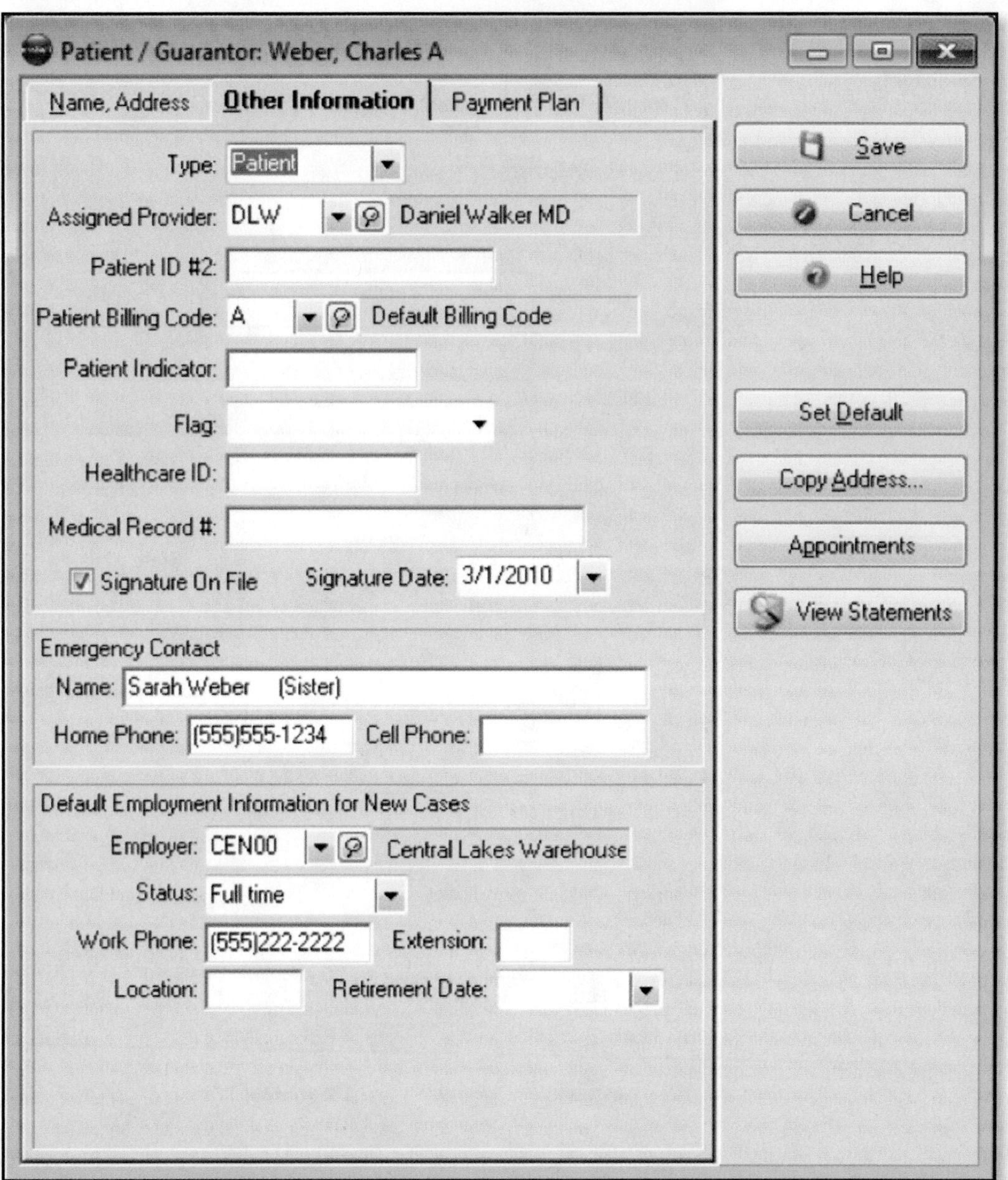

Figure 1.30
Completed Other Information tab.

PROCEDURE 1.7 ADDING A NEW PATIENT WHO HAS A GUARANTOR

This exercise involves the scenario in which the patient, a child named Carlos Hernandez, has a guarantor (his father). Guarantors should be entered in Medisoft before the patient(s) with whom they are associated.

1. Open the Patient List dialog box.
2. Click the *New Patient* button. The Patient/Guarantor dialog box opens with the Name, Address tab displayed.
3. Leave the Chart Number field blank, and make sure the Inactive checkbox is not checked.
4. Using the patient registration form for Carlos Hernandez in **Figure C.2 in Appendix C**, enter the guarantor's name, address, telephone numbers, date of

birth, and Social Security number. (This data is provided under the Patient's/Responsible Party Information section on the registration form.)

5. In the Sex field's list box, click *Male*.
6. In the Entity Type field's list box, click *Person*, if necessary.
7. Click the *Other Information* tab to display its fields.
8. In the Type field's list box, click *Guarantor*.
9. Enter the guarantor's Healthcare ID number and employer information. Often, Healthcare ID and Insurance ID are referring to the same information.
10. Click the *Signature on File* checkbox, and enter the date, 01/01/2010, when the registration form was signed.
11. Enter the guarantor's full-time employment information, adding a new Address record as needed.
12. Click the *Save* button. The guarantor's record is saved and appears in the Patient List dialog box.
13. Continuing to use the same patient registration form in **Figure C.2 in Appendix C**, add a new patient record for Carlos Hernandez. His assigned provider is Dr. Walker. Enter the appropriate information in both the Name, Address tab, and Other Information tab.
14. Click the *Save* button.

Another Way

Instead of keying an identical address twice, you can click the Copy Address button in the Patient/Guarantor dialog box. This button opens the Copy Demographics Information From dialog box where you can click the record from which to copy the address.

You have now finished entering a new patient into the system. In the next chapter, you will learn how to enter the patient's insurance and case information.

Locating and Editing Patient Records

Searching for an existing patient is an easy task in Medisoft. You access the information in the same manner as if you were entering a new patient into the system—by first opening the Patient List dialog box. Before entering a new patient, it is recommended that you search for that patient's name first. This is to avoid accidentally creating unnecessary, multiple records that can cause billing confusion. You will also need to locate patient records in order to edit them.

Searching for patient information in the Patient List dialog box can be done one of two ways: (1) use the fields called Search for and Field (Figure 1.31), or (2) use the Locate buttons. The fields, Search for and Field, work together as a filter. First, you click the arrow beside Field to display a group of search options in the list box. Depending on the option you choose, you next key the desired data in the box next to Search for. For example, if you selected the Last Name–First Name option, you would then key the name of the patient you wish to locate.

Clicking the Locate button directly to the right of the Search for field displays the Locate Patient dialog box (Figure 1.32). The Locate button is identified by a capital letter "A" and a magnifying glass. This dialog box allows you to define search restrictions. For example, you can key the last name of the patient in the Field Value field, click one of the three radio buttons (e.g., Exact Match, Partial Match at Beginning, or Partial Match Anywhere), and then choose what field (e.g., Last Name) in the patient records to search.

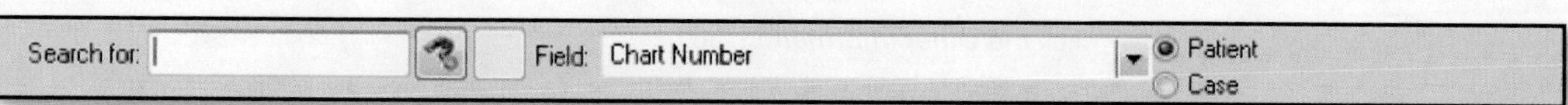

Figure 1.31 Search tools in Patient List dialog box.

Figure 1.32
Locate Patient dialog box.

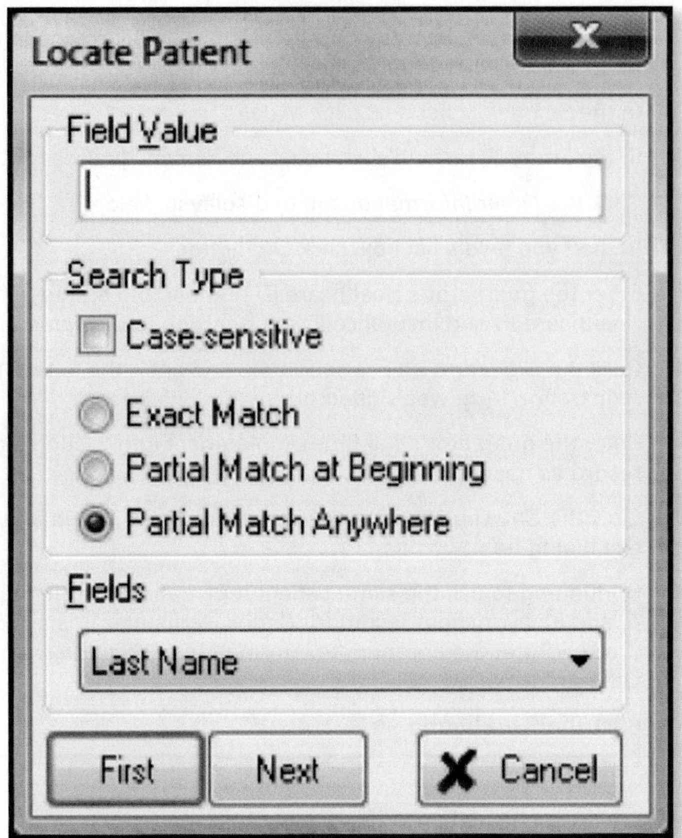

PROCEDURE 1.8 LOCATING AND EDITING A PATIENT RECORD

Use the following steps to search for Charles Weber's record

1. Open the Patient List dialog box, if necessary.
2. Click *Last Name, First Name* in the Field list box if not already selected.
3. Key *Weber* in the Search for field. Any other records will disappear, leaving only Mr. Weber's record displayed.
4. Delete the name in the Search for field. The full patient list is restored.
5. Click the *Locate* button. The Locate Patient dialog box displays.
6. Key *Weber* in the Field Value field.
7. Leave the Case-sensitive checkbox unchecked.
8. Click the *Exact Match* radio button.
9. Click *Last Name* in the Fields list box, if not already displayed.
10. Click the *First* button. The Locate Patient dialog box closes, and Mr. Weber's name is highlighted in the Patient List dialog box.
11. Click the *Edit Patient* button. The Patient/Guarantor dialog box for Mr. Weber opens.
12. Click the *Other Information* tab.
13. Change the emergency contact information to *Bob Weber, (555) 555-5678.*
14. Click the *Save* button to save your changes.

PROCEDURE 1.9 PRINTING THE PATIENT LIST REPORT

Print a list of the patients, and hand it in to your instructor.

1. Open the Patient List dialog box, if necessary.
2. Click the *Print Grid* button. The Print Grid Columns dialog box opens.
3. Click *OK*. The Print Report Where dialog box opens.
4. Click the radio button for *Print the report on the printer.*
5. Click the *Start* button.
6. Select the printer where you want the report to print.
7. Click *Close* to close the Patient List dialog box.

HOW TO SAVE DATA AND EXIT MEDISOFT

Because it is tedious and time consuming to reenter important data if the computer crashes or if a power outage occurs, it is a good idea to save your work on a regular basis. In other words, click the Save button to close the dialog box you are working in before getting up and leaving your desk. Many medical practices save their data to a hard drive. For this textbook, your instructor will tell you how and where to save your data. You may save to a hard drive, a network drive, or some other type of storage media (e.g., flash drive, portable hard drive, or other device). Always make sure you save your data!

Before exiting the Medisoft program, it is always wise to **backup** your data—the process of copying your computer files and storing them on a disk or other electronic device for safekeeping. Medical offices backup their data files on a regular schedule. This schedule may be daily, once a week, such as every Friday afternoon, or once a month. The reason for backing up data is simple computer storage devices (e.g., hard drives, external disks) can fail or a natural disaster, such as an earthquake, tornado, or flood, can strike.

If you have a problem with your current data files or experience a hard disk failure, then you can restore those backup files by using the Restore Data option on the File menu. The current working date will be overwritten with the backup data. Therefore any data you have entered since the last backup will be lost, and you will have to reenter the data in Medisoft. For this reason, it is recommended that you perform frequent backups. Backing up data is generally performed using disks, tape drives, or recordable CDs that can be stored in different locations other than the medical office.

When you exit Medisoft, the program will remind you to backup your data (Figure 1.33). Three options are provided: Back Up Data Now, Exit Program, and Cancel. If you

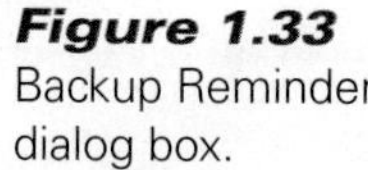

Figure 1.33 Backup Reminder dialog box.

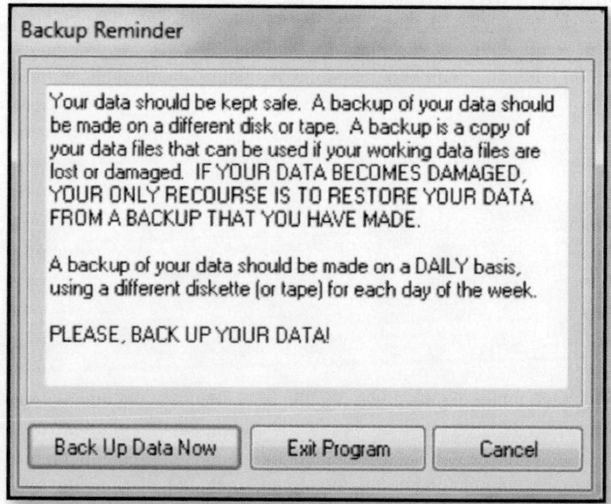

click the Back Up Data Now button, a warning will display that asks all users in the practice to log off the system in order to backup the data. Clicking the OK button will then open the Backup dialog box (Figure 1.34). In the Backup dialog box, you can select a destination drive and name the backup file. You can also create a password to protect the data.

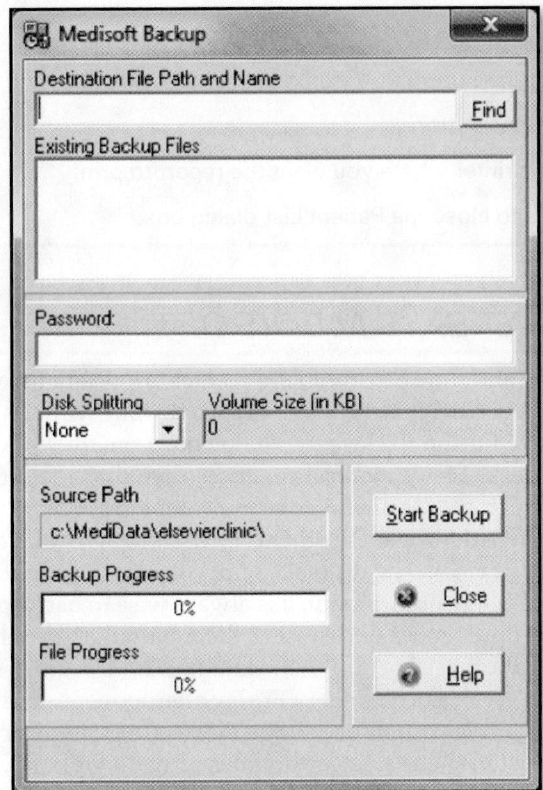

Figure 1.34 Medisoft Backup dialog box.

PROCEDURE 1.10 EXITING MEDISOFT

1. Close all open dialog boxes.
2. Click *File* on the menu bar to display the File menu.
3. Click *Exit*. The Backup Reminder dialog displays.
4. Click the *Exit Program* button (unless your instructor tells you to do otherwise). The main Medisoft window closes.

Another Way
Instead of using the menu bar, you can also exit the Medisoft program by pressing and holding down the Alt key, and then pressing the F4 key.

Using Terminology

Match the terms on the left with the definitions on the right.

____ **1.** chart number
____ **2.** patient registration form
____ **3.** menu bar
____ **4.** encounter form
____ **5.** front desk
____ **6.** guarantor
____ **7.** medical information cycle
____ **8.** Medisoft
____ **9.** medical practice management software
____ **10.** side bar
____ **11.** provider
____ **12.** clearinghouse
____ **13.** backup
____ **14.** BillFlash
____ **15.** case
____ **16.** toolbar
____ **17.** HIPAA

a. Area in a medical office where patients check in for appointments

b. Set of digits and/or letters assigned to a patient's medical record

c. Computer programs used to schedule patient appointments, submit electronic claims, and perform basic accounting procedures

d. Series of steps performed before, during, and after a patient has been seen by a provider

e. Row of buttons with icons that allow quick access to many Medisoft features

f. Group of transactions related to a specific medical condition for which a patient seeks treatment

g. Type of medical practice management software widely used in medical offices

h. Optional, navigational feature that allows quick access to the most frequently used Medisoft menu items

i. Company that provides services, including verifying and transmitting insurance claims, to medical practices

j. Process of copying and storing computer files for safekeeping

k. Document used by a provider during a medical examination to indicate the patient's illness or injury and the medical procedures performed

l. General term referring to someone who charges for health care services

m. Long, rectangular bar at the top of the main Medisoft window that displays menu names

n. Person who is responsible for paying a patient's bill

o. Federal legislation that provides guidelines for transmitting electronic data and protecting patients' privacy

p. Document containing personal, financial, and insurance information needed to complete insurance claims

q. Able to bill and send statements to patients through this online service

Checking Your Understanding

1. Describe the medical information cycle.
2. List the main functions that Medisoft performs in a medical office.
3. Explain how to start and exit Medisoft.
4. List the primary features used to operate Medisoft.
5. Describe how you would set up a medical practice.
6. List the steps involved in adding a new provider.
7. Explain how to create, edit, and search for a patient's record.
8. Describe the steps used to print the Patient List report.
9. Name two reasons why you should perform regular data backups.

Putting It into Practice

1. Enter the following new patients' data into Medisoft, using the completed patient registration forms in Figures C.3, C.4, and C.5 in Appendix C.
   a. William O'Connor; Dr. Berg, assigned provider
   b. Cindy Wixen; Henry Wixen, guarantor; Dr. Jagla, assigned provider
   c. Ronald Baxter; Emily Luther, assigned provider
2. Print the Patient List report, and hand it in to your instructor.
3. Before you exit Medisoft, create a backup of your data. For easy identification, you can use your name and the chapter number to name the backup file (e.g., SmithTom-Ch1.mbk). However, be sure to check first with your instructor for specific directions.

References

Adams DM: *Diagnosis documentation and coding,* New York, 1997, McGraw Hill.
Flight M: *Law, liability, and ethics for medical office procedures,* ed 3, Albany, NY, 1998, Delmar.
Fordney MT: *Insurance handbook for the medical office,* ed 11, Philadelphia, 2010, Saunders–Elsevier.
HealthCare Consultants of America: *Healthcare fraud and abuse,* Augusta, Ga, 1997, The Consultants.
Holmes DLL: *Practical guide to medical billing,* Springfield, Ill, 1997, US Department of Commerce.
Kuehn L: *Health information management medical records process in group practice,* Englewood, Colo, 1997, Center for Research in Ambulatory HealthCare Administration.
Moini J: *Glencoe medical assisting review passing the CMA and RMA exams,* New York, 2001, Glencoe.
Redman B, editor: *Life and health insurance,* ed 4, Chicago, 1998, Dearborn Financial Institute.
Reid J: *A telemedicine primer understanding the issues,* Billings, Mont, 1996, Artcraft Printers.
Rizzo C: *Uniform billing a guide to claims processing,* Albany, NY, 2000, Delmar.
Ross A, Pavlock E, Williams S: *Ambulatory care management,* ed 3, Albany, NY, 1998, Delmar.
Rowell J: *Understanding health insurance a guide to professional billing,* ed 5, Albany, NY, 2000, Delmar.

chapter 2

Basic Concepts of Coding and Insurance

Objectives

1. Describe the main differences between fee-for-service plans and managed care plans.
2. List the primary government health care programs and the basic eligibility requirements for each.
3. Enter and change insurance carrier information in Medisoft.
4. Describe the difference between Current Procedural Terminology (CPT) coding and International Classification of Diseases, Ninth Revision (ICD-9) coding.
5. Explain the process used to identify Evaluation and Management (E/M) codes.
6. Set up diagnosis and procedure codes in Medisoft.
7. Create Medisoft cases.

Terminology

capitation fee: Fixed prepayment made to a provider by an insurance carrier for supplying services to a patient during a specified time period, regardless of how many times the patient is seen by the provider

copayment: Small, fixed fee paid by the patient or guarantor each time the patient visits the provider

Current Procedural Terminology (CPT): Numerical codes used to designate procedures or services performed in a health care setting

deductible: Amount that must first be paid by the insurance policyholder before the insurance carrier will begin to issue payments for medical services

electronic data interchange (EDI): Process of exchanging information, such as business transactions, in a standardized format from one computer to another

Evaluation and Management (E/M) codes: Procedure codes used to identify the level of service performed by a provider

fee-for-service plan: Type of insurance in which the carrier pays specific amounts for specific medical services covered in the policy

health insurance: Protection for patients against the financial consequences of illness, injuries, and disabilities

health maintenance organization (HMO): Type of managed care system that hires providers who agree to be paid on a regular, fixed payment per patient instead of on a fee-for-service basis

International Classification of Diseases–Ninth Revision–Clinical Modifications (ICD-9-CM): System used to code patient diagnoses and to facilitate the payment of health care services

managed care: System of prepaid health plans that provides health care services at a negotiated cost

Medicaid: Joint federal and state government program that pays health care benefits for people with low incomes or limited resources

Medicare: Federal health insurance program, primarily for people aged 65 and older and those who are disabled

modifier: Two-digit code used to clarify or modify a CPT code's description, usually to indicate some alteration to the procedure performed

policyholder: Person who purchased a health insurance plan

preferred provider organization (PPO): Type of managed care organization that uses the fee-for-service concept by predetermining a list of charges for all services

premium: Periodic payment made to an insurance carrier to maintain health care insurance coverage

primary care provider (PCP): Physician or other provider who is selected by a patient enrolled in a managed care plan and who is responsible for coordinating the patient's health care treatment

third-party payer: Public or private organization that pays health care expenses for patients who have received services from providers

TRICARE: Health care plan that provides benefits for members of the U.S. military and their dependents; administered by the U.S. Department of Defense

workers' compensation: Insurance that protects employees against lost wages and medical costs resulting from work-related illnesses and injuries

This chapter provides a basic overview of the main types of health insurance plans and a brief description of diagnostic and procedural coding. This chapter also explains how insurance and coding information is linked to patient records. However, it makes no attempt to give you detailed coverage of the insurance industry or the medical coding process. Because these concepts are so important in a medical office setting, if you are not currently enrolled in a medical assistant program, then you may want to pursue additional coursework at a local technical or community college.

OVERVIEW OF HEALTH INSURANCE

Health insurance provides protection for patients against the financial consequences of illness, injuries, and disabilities. Health insurance plans are agreements in which a person, or policyholder, buys insurance coverage or benefits. A payment for health insurance is typically referred to as a **premium**. The degree of coverage varies, depending on the type of insurance plan. An insurance carrier is referred to as a **third-party payer** because it is a private company or public (government) program that pays health care expenses for patients (the first party) who have received services from providers (the second party).

Major Types of Insurance Plans

There are many different health insurance plans available. Two of the most common types are fee-for-service plans and managed care plans.

Fee-for-Service Plans

In a **fee-for-service plan**, the insurance carrier pays specific amounts for specific medical services covered in the insurance policy. Each individual policy identifies the various types of covered medical services and how much of the charges are paid by the insurance carrier. Although some services are covered 100%, only a portion of others may be paid. For example, a policy with an 80/20 rule for a particular type of service will pay 80% of the charges, and the policyholder will pay 20%. In most fee-for-service plans, a **deductible** amount must first be paid by the **policyholder** before the insurance carrier will begin to issue payments.

Managed Care Plans

Managed care is a system of prepaid health plans that provides health care services at a negotiated cost. In broad terms, managed care can refer to organizing providers into groups to help improve the quality and cost-effectiveness of medical services. Managed care organizations typically employ providers and health care workers and also assume some of the responsibilities of an insurance carrier. For example, a managed care organization processes claims; provides member services to its patients; and assists providers in referral and authorization information, utilization review, and eligibility. Most individuals with insurance coverage under a managed care plan are required to choose a **primary care provider (PCP)**. Typically a physician, the PCP helps coordinate the patient's health care treatment.

One type of managed care is the **health maintenance organization (HMO)**. An HMO hires providers who agree to be paid on a per-patient basis instead of the traditional fee-for-service basis. The HMO then contracts with employers to provide health care services, and each employee selects a PCP from a medical group (owned by the HMO). In return, the provider receives a capitation fee. A **capitation fee** is a fixed prepayment per month or year based on several factors, including the number of plan members. This fee is paid, regardless of whether the patient receives care during the time period covered by the payment. The provider does not receive any additional fees if the patient is seen more often. Some HMOs also require the patient to pay a **copayment**, or *copay* for short, which is a small, fixed amount such as $20 or $25. The copayment is paid each time the patient visits the provider.

Another type of managed care is the **preferred provider organization (PPO)**. This type of managed care plan keeps the fee-for-service concept intact. The providers involved with this type of plan agree on a predetermined list of charges for all services. A PPO is not prepaid, such as the case with an HMO. When a patient with a PPO plan comes to a member provider, the provider treats the patient and then bills the PPO. Sometimes, the patient may be responsible for a deductible.

Government Programs

Major health insurance programs administered by the U.S. federal government or state governments include Medicare, Medicaid, Medi/Medi, TRICARE, CHAMPVA, and workers' compensation.

Medicare

Medicare is a federal government health insurance program, primarily for people aged 65 years or older. Others who may qualify for this type of insurance are those with certain disabilities or conditions, such as end-stage renal disease.

Medicare is a fee-for-service plan with two main parts. Medicare Part A is hospital insurance. Medicare Part B is a medical insurance option that pays for outpatient services, as well as other provider services and medical supplies obtained outside the hospital setting. The patient can choose any provider who accepts Medicare.

Although Medicare is a government plan, it does not cover all medical expenses. Individuals with Medicare Parts A and B may also purchase a supplemental Medigap policy, so named because it is intended to help fill in the "gaps" of insurance coverage. In other words, a Medigap policy will help pay some of the health care costs not covered by the original Medicare plan.

Medicare Advantage plans are optional plans approved by Medicare but administered by private companies such as HMOs and PPOs. Joining a Medicare Advantage plan generally means that a patient gets all of the Part A and Part B Medicare coverage through that particular plan. Some Medicare Advantage plans offer extra benefits, and costs may also be lower than in the original Medicare plan. However, patients may be required to go to certain hospitals and physicians that belong to the specific Medicare Advantage plan rather than choose their own provider.

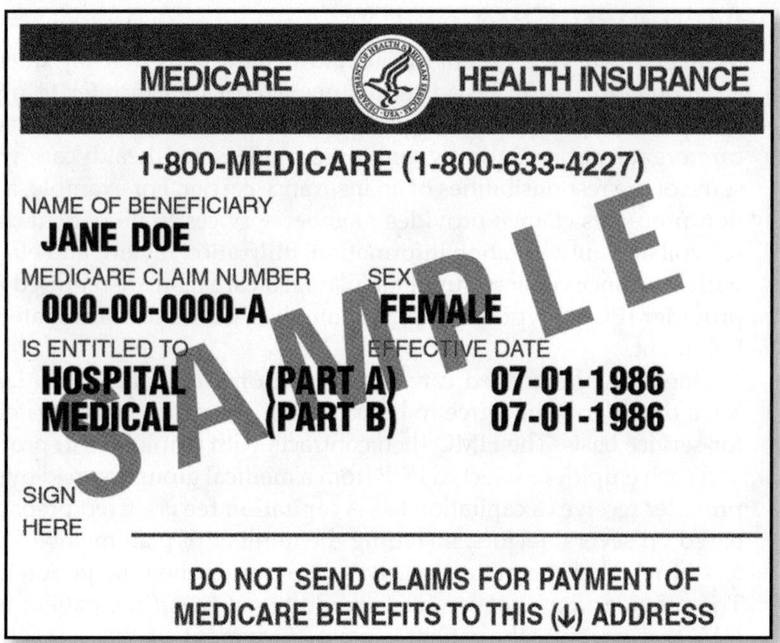

Figure 2.1
Medicare insurance card. (Courtesy of www.medicare.com.)

Figure 2.1 is an example of the Medicare insurance card. This card includes the name of the insured person, their Medicare number, the type of Medicare coverage, and the date(s) when the coverage started. For more details on eligibility and the various Medicare plans, visit the Web site, www.medicare.gov.

Medicaid

The purpose of the **Medicaid** program is to help pay health care benefits for low-income families and people with limited resources who meet specified criteria. Medicaid is a joint government program, which means that basic guidelines are provided by the federal government. However, each state government sets its own rules that specify eligibility and determine the type and extent of medical care coverage. For more information on Medicaid, visit the Web site, www.cms.hhs.gov/home/medicaid.asp.

Medi/Medi

In some cases, patients cannot afford to pay the portion of their bill unpaid by Medicare. They may qualify for both Medicare and Medicaid benefits. In that case, Medicare is the primary insurance, and Medicaid covers any leftover payment due.

TRICARE

TRICARE, formerly called Civilian Health and Medical Program of the Veterans Administration (CHAMPUS), was originally created by Congress in 1966. TRICARE is a health care program administered by the U.S. Department of Defense, which combines military health care resources with civilian medical services. Benefits are provided for members of the U.S. military in Active Duty and Activated Guard and Reserves. TRICARE also includes benefits for the families of active duty service members, as well as military retirees and their dependents.

The three main plans under the TRICARE program are Prime, Extra, and Standard. Active service members are automatically eligible for the Prime plan. Military dependents and retirees may select from the various plans. Unlike the other two plans, the Prime plan has no annual deductible. Military Treatment Facilities (MTFs) are the main source of health care used in the Prime plan. However, this plan does have a point-of-service option that allows patients to receive care from authorized civilian providers.

TRICARE Extra is similar to a PPO plan. TRICARE Standard, the original CHAMPUS program, is a fee-for-service plan. The Extra plan allows the patient to get services from any provider in the TRICARE Extra network. It is often less expensive than the Standard plan. However, TRICARE Standard is the most widely available plan with the largest number of providers from which to choose. For more details about the three primary TRICARE plans and other TRICARE options, visit the Web site, www.military.com/benefits/tricare.

CHAMPVA

The CHAMPVA program is available for the spouses and dependent children of veterans who have died from service-related disabilities. The dependents of veterans with permanent service disabilities are also eligible. However, if an individual is eligible for TRICARE, that person cannot also be eligible for CHAMPVA. For more information about CHAMPVA, visit the Web site, www.military.com/benefits/veterans-health-care/champva-overview.

Workers' Compensation

State-mandated **workers' compensation** programs require employers to buy insurance coverage for employee work-related injuries and illnesses. These laws help protect workers against medical costs and wages lost while unable to work. Workers' compensation coverage varies from state to state. The Web site, www.workerscompensationinsurance.com, provides an overview of each state's workers' compensation laws, as well as various articles about this type of insurance. The federal government also has a number of workers' compensation programs available. Visit the website, www.dol.gov/owcp.

Patients with workers' compensation programs must make periodic visits to their provider to check on their ability to return to work after an injury on the job. When dealing with a workers' compensation claim, keep the following items in mind:

- When a patient schedules an appointment, ask if the illness or injury is related to their work. If so, make sure the patient provides the workers' compensation claim number. The workers' compensation insurance should be billed instead of the patient's primary health insurance for job-related injuries.
- Obtain the workers' compensation fee schedule(s) for your state.
- Use the correct fee schedule to bill accurately for services.
- Any charges in excess of the fee schedule need to be supported in writing by the provider, and a copy needs to be kept in the patient's medical record.
- If you have any questions, contact the patient's workers' compensation insurance carrier. Make sure to use the proper forms required by the insurance carrier for all workers' compensation claims.

CMS-1500 Claim Form

Most providers typically use the Centers for Medicare and Medicaid Services–1500 (CMS-1500) claim form when filing insurance claims. Although this form is always used for Medicare and Medicaid claims, most commercial and other third-party payers also accept the CMS-1500. Appendix B provides detailed instructions for completing this claim form. Medisoft automatically generates claims based on the CMS-1500 format.

INSURANCE CARRIER INFORMATION ENTRY

Medisoft allows you to add as many insurance carriers as needed. The sample data that comes with this textbook includes three insurance companies. In the next few pages, you will add four more insurance carriers. Figure 2.2 shows the Insurance Carrier List dialog box, which is accessed from the Lists menu. In the window of this dialog box, you can view a list of the current insurance carriers in the Medisoft system. Five buttons display along the bottom of the dialog box: Edit, New, Delete, Print Grid, and Close. These buttons work similarly to the ones in the Provider List dialog box.

Figure 2.2 Insurance Carrier List dialog box.

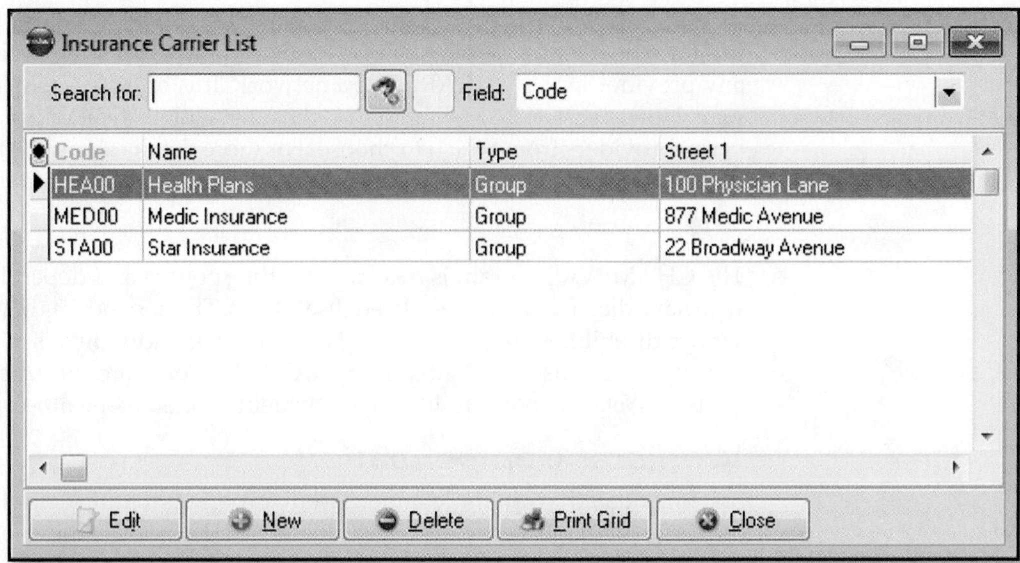

Insurance Carrier Dialog Box

If you click the New button in the Insurance Carrier List dialog box, the Insurance Carrier dialog box opens with four tabs: Address, Options and Codes, EDI/Eligibility, and Allowed. By default, the Address tab displays when this dialog box is opened (Figure 2.3).

Address Tab

The Address tab in the Insurance Carrier dialog box allows you to enter basic address and plan information such as the carrier's name, street, city, state, zip code, telephone numbers, and the plan name administered by the carrier. In the Code field, you can enter a unique alphanumeric code for the insurance carrier, or you can allow Medisoft to assign one automatically. The Inactive checkbox should only be clicked (to insert a checkmark) when an insurance carrier is no longer actively needed in Medisoft.

The Class field is an optional field used by some practices or clinics to group insurance carriers for particular searching or reporting needs. After adding a list of Class codes to represent practice-defined categories, these codes can be entered in the insurance carrier records.

PROCEDURE 2.1 ADDING INSURANCE CARRIER NAME AND ADDRESS INFORMATION

1. Start Medisoft, and click *Lists* on the menu bar.
2. When the Lists menu displays, click *Insurance*. A submenu displays two options: Carriers and Classes. (The Classes option is used to enter optional Class codes.)
3. Click *Carriers*. The Insurance Carrier List dialog box opens with three insurance carriers displayed (see Figure 2.2).
4. Click the *New* button. The Insurance Carrier dialog box opens with the Address tab displayed (see Figure 2.3).
5. Leave the Code field and Inactive field blank.
6. In the Name field, key *Metro Healthcare*.
7. In the Street field, key *245 Franklin Avenue*.
8. In the Zip Code field, key *55418*.

9. In the City field, key *Rice Lake.*
10. In the State field, key *MN.*
11. In the Phone field, key *555-638-7643.*
12. Leave the Extension, Fax, and Contact fields blank.
13. In the Plan Name field, key *MH-123.* CAUTION: Do not key in the code field as the program will automatically assign the code.
14. Click the *Save* button. The data is saved, the Insurance Carrier dialog box closes, and the new record appears in the window of the Insurance Carrier List dialog box. Notice that Medisoft assigned the code MET00 to the new carrier based on its name.
15. Leave the Insurance Carrier List dialog box open for the next exercise.

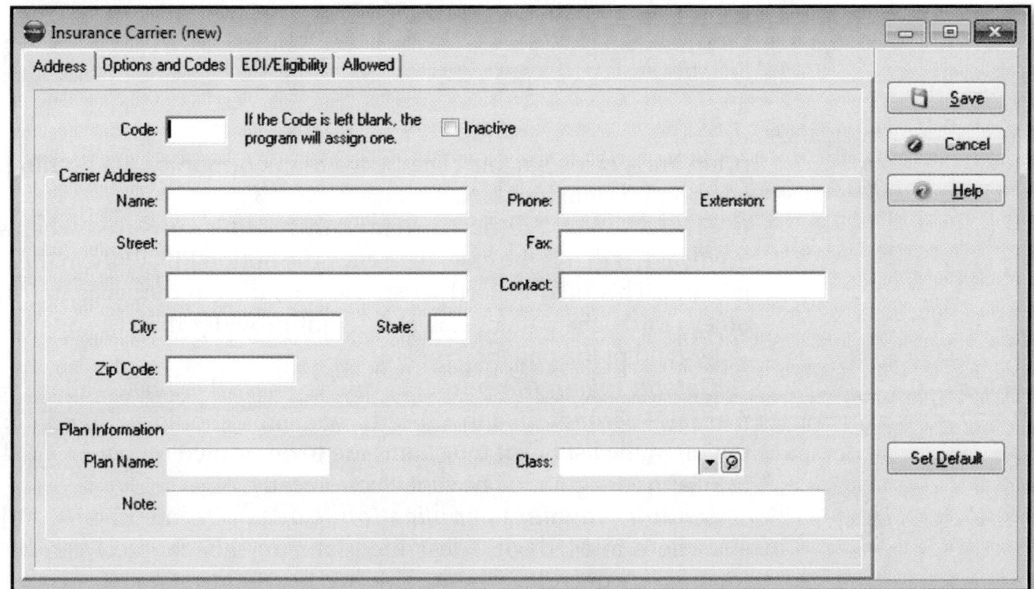

Figure 2.3
Insurance Carrier dialog box with Address tab displayed.

Options and Codes Tab

Some of the fields in the Options and Codes tab (Figure 2.4) are referenced by Medisoft when you do billing tasks, such as entering charges for services performed and generating insurance claims. Other fields in this tab are referenced by Medisoft when you apply payments or adjustments received from the insurance carrier. Following are descriptions of the fields in this tab:

Procedure Code Set and Diagnosis Code Set. In both of these fields, Medisoft allows you to select "1," "2," or "3" from the list box. These numbers correspond to procedure and diagnosis codes stored in the Medisoft system, which you will learn more about later in this chapter. Various insurance carriers may use a different code to identify the same service procedure. Likewise, some carriers may use different codes to identify the same medical diagnosis. Therefore Medisoft provides the ability to set up a procedure or diagnosis with up to three different codes.

Patient, Insured, and Physician Signature on File. These fields control what is printed in the signature boxes (e.g., 12, 13, and 31) of the CMS-1500 claim form. Each of these three fields has the same options from which to choose in their list boxes. The Signature on File option prints "Signature on File" on the claim form, but only if the Signature on File checkboxes have been selected in the patient and provider records. The Print Name option

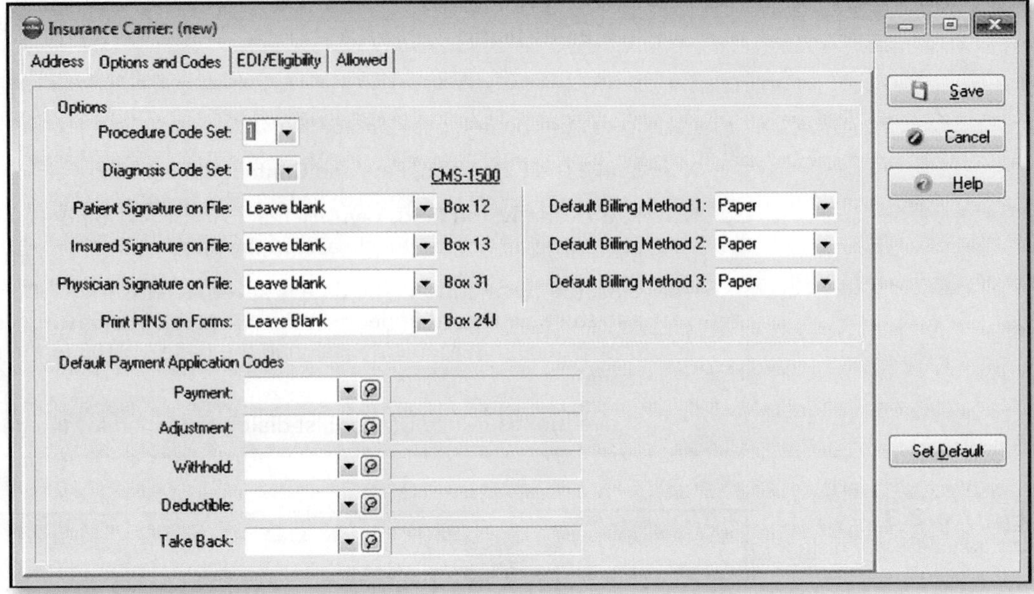

Figure 2.4 Insurance Carrier dialog box with Options and Codes tab displayed.

prints the person's name. The Leave Blank option prints nothing in the claim form's corresponding signature box.

Print PINS on Forms. Currently, this field is only used when setting up Medicare and Medicaid. If that is the case, then click the option PIN Only in the list box. Otherwise, leave it blank. This field is used when the attending provider is not the assigned provider. In other words, the patient saw a different provider than the one listed in the Assigned Provider field of the patient's record.

Default Billing Method 1, 2, and 3. These three fields allow you to define how (1) primary, (2) secondary, and (3) tertiary claims should be handled; that is, click the Paper option in the list box if the claims are to be printed on paper. Click the Electronic option if the claims are going to be sent electronically.

Default Payment Application Codes. Payment and Adjustment codes set up elsewhere in Medisoft (described later in this chapter) can be entered in these fields to serve as defaults when applying payment-related transactions from the insurance carrier.

PROCEDURE 2.2 DEFINING INSURANCE CARRIER OPTIONS

1. If necessary, open the Insurance Carrier List dialog box.
2. Click the line for *Metro Healthcare* to select it. The line appears highlighted.
3. Click the *Edit* button. The Insurance Carrier dialog box opens, and the record for Metro Healthcare displays.
4. Click the *Options and Codes* tab.
5. Leave the Procedure Code Set and Diagnosis Code Set fields at the default value (*1*).
6. In the list boxes for Patient Signature on File, Insured Signature on File, and Physician Signature on File, click *Signature on File.*
7. Leave the Print PINs on Forms field at the default value (*Leave blank*).
8. Leave all three of the Default Billing Method fields at the default value (*Paper*).
9. Click the *Save* button, or press the *F3* key, to save your work.
10. Click the *Close* button to close the Insurance Carrier List dialog box.

EDI/Eligibility Tab

Electronic data interchange (EDI) is the process of exchanging information, such as business transactions, in a standardized format from one computer to another. The EDI/ Eligibility tab (Figure 2.5) is used to enter information for submitting claims electronically to a clearinghouse or directly to the insurance carrier. This tab is also used for verifying insurance eligibility online. The Type field on the EDI/Eligibility tab has a list box with the various kinds of insurance, such as HMO, PPO, Medicare, Medicaid, and TRICARE. The insurance carrier will provide guidelines and ID numbers for completing most of this tab's fields.

Allowed Tab

Each procedure code previously set up in Medisoft (explained later in this chapter) appears in this tab (Figure 2.6). There are two ways to populate the fields in the Allowed tab. You can use the information from the carrier's remittance report to enter the allowed amounts manually for each procedure. However, normally you would let Medisoft do it automatically when you enter payments received.

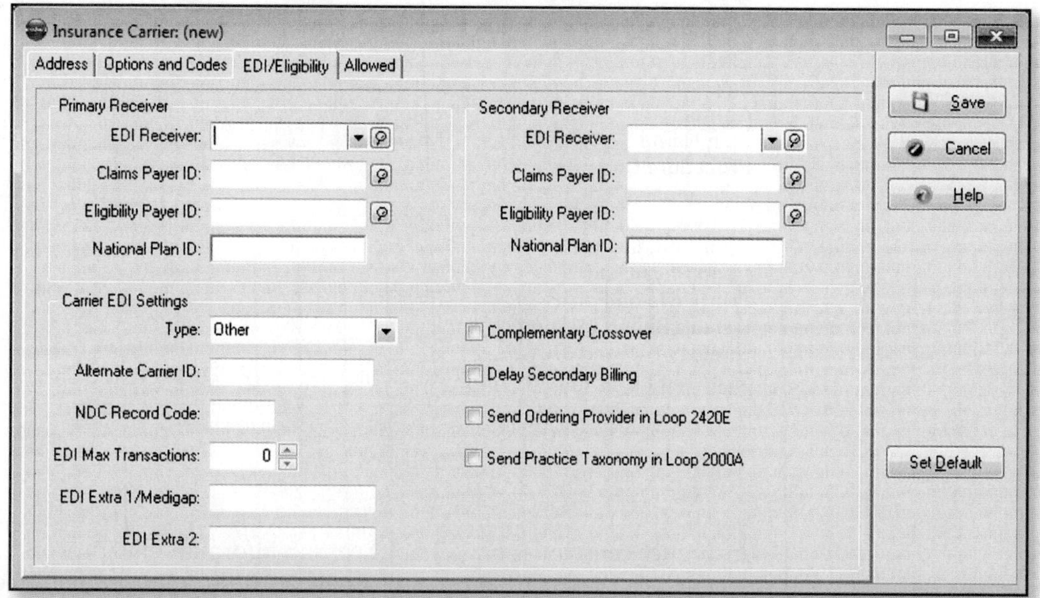

Figure 2.5
Insurance Carrier dialog box with EDI/Eligibility tab displayed.

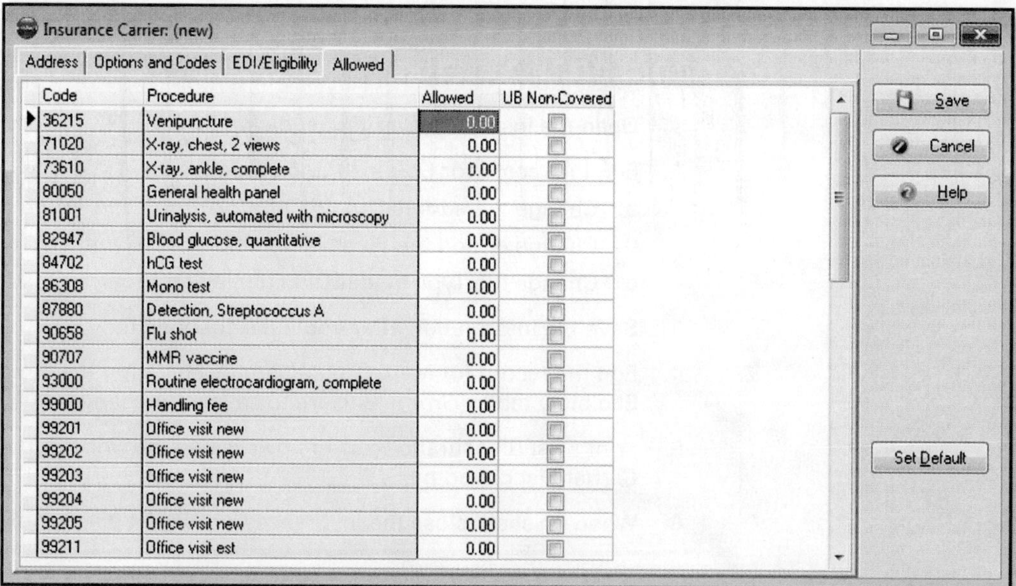

Code	Procedure	Allowed	UB Non-Covered
36215	Venipuncture	0.00	
71020	X-ray, chest, 2 views	0.00	
73610	X-ray, ankle, complete	0.00	
80050	General health panel	0.00	
81001	Urinalysis, automated with microscopy	0.00	
82947	Blood glucose, quantitative	0.00	
84702	hCG test	0.00	
86308	Mono test	0.00	
87880	Detection, Streptococcus A	0.00	
90658	Flu shot	0.00	
90707	MMR vaccine	0.00	
93000	Routine electrocardiogram, complete	0.00	
99000	Handling fee	0.00	
99201	Office visit new	0.00	
99202	Office visit new	0.00	
99203	Office visit new	0.00	
99204	Office visit new	0.00	
99205	Office visit new	0.00	
99211	Office visit est	0.00	

Figure 2.6
Insurance Carrier dialog box with Allowed tab displayed.

PROCEDURE 2.3 SETTING UP THREE INSURANCE CARRIERS

1. Open the Insurance Carrier List dialog box.
2. Use the information in Table 2.1 to enter three additional insurance companies that your medical practice now accepts. If a field is not listed in the table, leave it blank or use the default setting that displays. Notice that you will enter values in the Code field on the Address tab, instead of letting Medisoft assign the codes for you.
3. When finished, save your work and close the Insurance Carrier List dialog box.

TABLE 2.1 Three Insurance Companies to Enter

	Medicare	Blue Cross and Blue Shield	First Med
Code	MCARE	BCBS	FM
Name	Medicare	Blue Cross and Blue Shield	First Med
Street	233 N. Michigan Av	Blue Cross Road	7 Medical Blvd
City	Chicago	St. Paul	Detroit
State	IL	MN	MI
Zip Code	60601	55122	48266
Phone	555-555-1000	555-555-1110	555-555-2220
Extension	123	345	678
Fax	555-555-1001	555-555-1112	555-555-2223
Contact	Carol Smith	Elena Romero	Tom Higgins
Plan Name	Medicare	BCBS	FM
Procedure Code Set and Diagnosis Code Set	1	1	1
Signature on File fields (Patient, Insured, and Physician)	Signature on file	Signature on file	Signature on file
Print PINs on Forms	PIN Only	Leave Blank	Leave Blank
Default Billing Method fields (1, 2, and 3)	Paper	Paper	Paper
Type (on EDI/Eligibility tab)	Medicare	Blue Cross/Shield	Group

EDI, Electronic data interchange; *PINs*, personal identification numbers.

Editing Insurance Carrier Data

Insurance companies may change certain information to process claims in a more effective manner, or they may start using a new address, telephone number, or other information. The same dialog boxes used to enter a new insurance carrier are used to change carrier information.

PROCEDURE 2.4 CHANGING INSURANCE CARRIER INFORMATION

1. Open the Insurance Carrier List dialog box.
2. Edit the record for Star Insurance as follows:
   a. Change the address to: *45 Country Farm Lane, Woodsfield, MN 55432.*
   b. Change or add the Plan Name field to: *SI Contract.*
   c. Change the Type field (EDI/Eligibility tab) to: *HMO.*
3. Save the information after you have changed it.
4. Edit the record for Metro Healthcare by changing the Type field on the EDI/ Eligibility tab to *Group.* Be sure to save your change.
5. Print a list of insurance carriers by clicking the *Print Grid* button in the Insurance Carrier List dialog box.
6. When finished, close the Insurance Carrier List dialog box.

OVERVIEW OF DIAGNOSIS CODING

The **International Classification of Diseases–Ninth Revision–Clinical Modifications (ICD-9-CM)** is the system currently used to code diagnoses. The World Health Organization (WHO) developed this system of coding for statistical purposes. The ICD-9-CM (frequently shortened to ICD-9) is used to facilitate the payment of health care services. In addition, the ICD-9 may be used to study health care costs and to conduct research.

To code diagnoses accurately, you must have a working knowledge of medical terminology and understand the guidelines, language, and conventions of the ICD-9. This chapter is not designed to provide a detailed description of coding. Instead, it provides a general background needed to complete the exercises and simulations in this textbook. For more information on coding, refer to the references at the end of this chapter.

Many versions of the ICD-9 codes exist, but all are based on the official government version. It is important to use the most current version of the ICD-9 available. The ICD-9 manual is divided into three sections, or volumes. Volumes 1 and 2 are the sections primarily used in medical offices:

- Volume 1–Diseases: Tabular List and Numerical Index. This volume includes the disease and condition codes with descriptions. It also includes factors influencing health status and contact with health services (V codes) and external causes of injury and poisoning (E codes).
- Volume 2–Diseases: Alphabetical Index. Volume 2 is an alphabetical index for Volume 1.
- Volume 3–Procedures: Tabular List and Alphabetical Index. This volume contains coding procedures for surgical, therapeutic, and diagnostic procedures used and provided by a facility, such as a hospital.

Each disease has been assigned a three-digit number. For example, ICD-9 code 749 is cleft palate and cleft lip. A fourth digit is used to provide more detail regarding the site or symptom. For example, the code 749.0 is used for a patient with a cleft palate. A fifth digit may be required to classify the disease or condition further. Using the previous example, if the patient has a bilateral cleft palate, the proper ICD-9 code is 749.03. It is important to use the most extended version of the code number (fourth or fifth digit) that is appropriate for the diagnosis.

Steps in Diagnosis Coding

The following steps are general guidelines used for identifying the appropriate ICD-9 code. Keep in mind that completing these steps will not make you proficient in coding; it merely provides an introduction to the coding process. Further education and experience are required to become an expert coder.

1. Identify the main medical terms related to the diagnosis in the patient's medical record. Even if you have been given a superbill, double-check it with the progress notes in the patient's medical record to confirm the main diagnosis.
2. Locate the main term in the alphabetical index, Volume 2, of the ICD-9 book. Remember to refer to any notes under the main term and read any terms enclosed in parentheses. Do not skip any subterms indented under the main term, and follow any cross-referenced instructions.
3. Verify the code number by reading the code's description in the numerical index, Volume 1.

Entering ICD-9-CM Codes

Medisoft allows you to add as many diagnosis codes as needed. The sample data that comes with this textbook includes a number of diagnosis codes. In the next few pages, you will add a few. Figure 2.7 shows the Diagnosis List dialog box, accessed by clicking

Diagnosis Codes on the Lists menu. From this dialog box you can add, edit, delete, and print diagnosis codes.

When the New button or Edit button is clicked in the Diagnosis List dialog box, the Diagnosis dialog box opens (Figure 2.8). The following is a description of the fields:

Code 1. Enter the diagnosis code in this field as it appears in the ICD-9.

Description. Enter the ICD-9 description of the code. For example, the description for code 780.7 is Fatigue. Even though it appears that there is room for only one line of text, this field is 100 characters in length. When an extensive description is required, the text in the field will scroll as the data is entered.

Alternate Code Sets (Code 2 and Code 3). Sometimes insurance carriers use a code for the same description that is different from the ICD-9 code entered in the Code 1 field. In that case, the Code 2 and Code 3 can be used as alternate code numbers. You may recall, when you previously entered information in the Options and Codes tab of the Insurance Carrier dialog box, there was a Diagnosis Code Set field (see Figure 2.4). That field has a list box with three options: 1, 2, or 3. Those options correspond to the Code 1, Code 2, and Code 3 fields in the Diagnosis dialog box. Let us say, for example, that a specific insurance carrier uses a code number for Fatigue that is different from the ICD-9's code, 780.7. You would first enter the alternate code in the Code 2 field of the Diagnosis dialog box and save the change. Next, you would open the insurance carrier's record, and click the 2 in the Diagnosis Code Set field's list box.

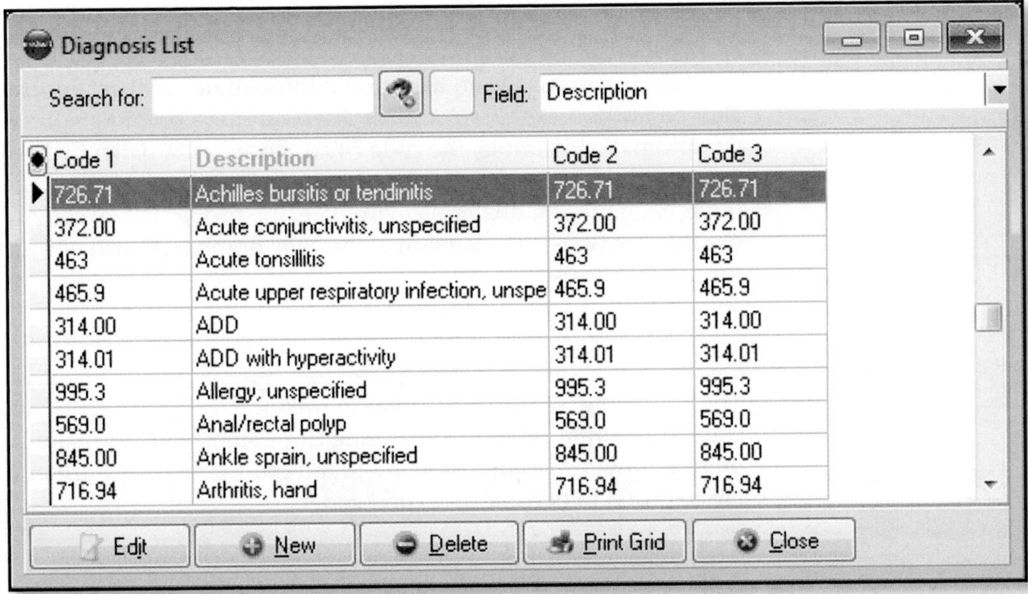

Figure 2.7
Diagnosis List dialog box.

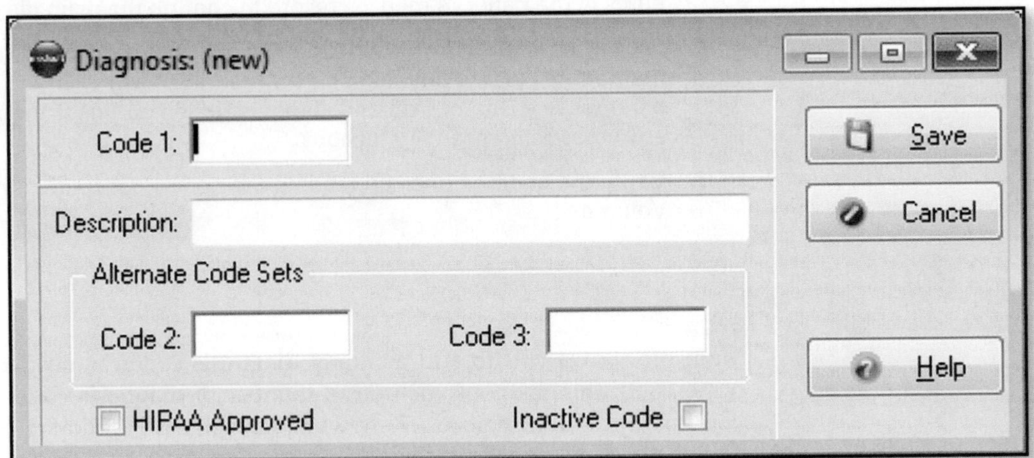

Figure 2.8
Diagnosis dialog box.

HIPAA Approved. Click this checkbox to select it, if the code is HIPAA approved.

Inactive Code. Click this checkbox to select it, if the code is no longer active or valid. If you try to select an inactive code elsewhere in Medisoft, a message will display.

PROCEDURE 2.5 ADDING DIAGNOSIS CODES

ICD-9 codes are used to give a numerical value to a diagnosis.

1. Click *Lists* on the menu bar.
2. Click *Diagnosis Codes* on the Lists menu. The Diagnosis List dialog box displays.
3. Click the *New* button. The Diagnosis dialog box opens.
4. In the Code 1 field, key *250.00.*
5. Press the *Enter* key. Notice that Medisoft automatically populates the Code 2 and Code 3 fields with the same number.
6. In the Description field, key *Diabetes mellitus, without complication, type II or unspecified, not stated as uncontrolled.* (Note: Although the field appears too small for this description, you can key up to 100 characters.)
7. Click the *HIPAA Approved* checkbox to select it.
8. Click the *Save* button. The Diagnosis dialog box closes, and the code just entered displays in the window of the Diagnosis List dialog box. The code just entered displays in the list of those diagnosis codes into the program. Scroll to find.
9. Add or edit the diagnosis codes listed below, and save your work. For all of these entries, the values in the Code 1, Code 2, and Code 3 fields should match. Also, make sure that the HIPAA Approved checkbox is selected.
   a. Add a new code *041.5* with the description *H. influenza infection, NOS.*
   b. Change the description of code 314.00 to *Attention deficit disorder without mention of hyperactivity.*
   c. Change the description of code 314.01 to *Attention deficit disorder with hyperactivity.*
   d. Make code 574.2 Gallstones inactive by clicking the *Inactive Code* field.
   e. Add a new code *574.20* with the description *Calculus of gallbladder, without cholecystitis, without obstruction.*
10. When finished, use the *Print Grid* button to print a list of diagnosis codes.
11. Click the *Close* button to close the Diagnosis List dialog box.

ICD-10-CM Update

ICD-10-CM is currently scheduled for implementation in the United States on October 1, 2014. Several countries have already adopted ICD-10. You may have the opportunity to work with a practice starting the process or near the end of the process. Medisoft version 18 currently works with ICD-9; until ICD-10 is adopted, you will not have to enter those codes in this version of Medisoft.

MEDICAL PROCEDURE AND SERVICE CODING

The **Current Procedural Terminology (CPT)** was established in 1966 by the American Medical Association (AMA) as a means to describe services and procedures performed by providers. The CPT is updated and published annually to meet the changing demands of the medical industry. Again, a general overview is presented here only for informational purposes, not to educate you as a CPT coder. The following six categories are in the CPT manual:

- **Evaluation and Management (E/M) codes** are listed first in the manual for convenience. These codes (99200–99499) are used to identify the level of service performed by a provider.

- Anesthesia (00100–01999) includes codes for the delivery of general, regional, and supportive anesthesia services to patients. These codes include the administration of fluids and blood and necessary monitoring as related to anesthesia.
- Surgery (10000–69999) is listed by anatomical site; it is the largest section in the CPT manual.
- Radiology (70000–79999) includes codes for diagnostic and therapeutic radiology, nuclear medicine, magnetic resonance imaging (MRI), and ultrasound.
- Pathology and Laboratory (80000–89999) are used to report services provided by technologists or pathologists. These codes include diagnostic studies, consultations, toxicology, hematology, immunology, and anatomical or surgical pathology.
- Medical services (90700–99999) includes codes for injections, psychiatry, ophthalmology, pulmonary, allergy, neurology, and special services.

Process Used to Identify E/M Codes

E/M codes are used to classify patients with their level of service. The three main steps used to determine the proper E/M code are as follows:

1. Identify the extent of the history obtained from the patient.
2. Identify the extent of the physical examination of the patient.
3. Determine the degree of medical decision making necessary to manage the patient's care.

History

History is subjective information provided by the patient. The patient's history has four elements: chief complaint; history of the present illness; review of the systems; and past, family, or social history. History taking is important to the provider in correctly diagnosing the disease or illness and determining the correct E/M code. After the history is obtained, there are four different history levels:

- Problem focused
- Expanded problem focused
- Detailed
- Comprehensive

Each of the different history levels contains a portion or all of the four elements. For example, at the problem-focused level, the provider notes the chief complaint, a brief history of the present illness, and a review of systems compared with the affected body system. On the other hand, a comprehensive history contains the chief complaint; a comprehensive history of the present illness; a review of systems; and past, present, family, or social history. Complete descriptions of every history level are included in the Evaluation and Management section of the CPT manual.

Examination

The physical examination of the patient is objective information. The examination levels are named exactly the same as the history titles:

Problem Focused. The provider performs a limited examination of the affected body area or organ system.

Expanded Problem Focused. The provider performs a limited examination of the affected body area or organ system and other symptomatic or related organ systems.

Detailed. The provider performs an extended examination of the affected body organs and other symptomatic or related organ systems.

Comprehensive. The provider performs a general multisystem examination or a complete examination of a single organ system.

Decision Making

The final step in obtaining a correct E/M code is the level of decision making involved in making a diagnosis. Decision making is based on the following three elements:

1. Number of diagnoses or management options made during the visit, the type of problems, and the complexity of making those diagnoses
2. Amount or complexity of data to be reviewed by the provider, based on the types of tests ordered, and the provider obtaining pertinent medical information from past medical records
3. Risk of complications, morbidity, or mortality of the patient, including the risks of the present illness, the diagnostic procedures being performed on the patient, and the type of treatment that will be given to the patient

After each of these three elements is determined, the different levels of decision making can be determined. The four levels of decision making are as follows:

1. Straightforward decision making
2. Low-complexity decision making
3. Moderate-complexity decision making
4. High-complexity decision making

Straightforward decision making includes a minimal number of diagnoses or management options, a minimal review of past data, and minimal risk of complications to the patient. High-complexity decision making includes an extensive number of diagnoses or management options, an extensive amount of data to be reviewed, and a high risk of complications or death to the patient.

The examination of all three categories—history, examination, and decision making—determines the following selection of E/M codes. These codes are used in the simulation presented in this textbook and list the level, code, history level, examination level, and decision-making level.

New patient codes are:

- Level 1: 99201 (problem focused; problem focused; straightforward)
- Level 2: 99202 (expanded problem focused; expanded problem focused; straightforward)
- Level 3: 99203 (detailed; detailed; low complexity)
- Level 4: 99204 (comprehensive; comprehensive; moderate complexity)
- Level 5: 99205 (comprehensive, comprehensive; high complexity)

Established patient codes are:

- Level 1: 99211 (minimal with all three levels; many medical offices will consider this a nurse visit or a laboratory visit)
- Level 2: 99212 (problem focused; problem focused; straightforward)
- Level 3: 99213 (expanded problem focused; expanded problem focused; low complexity)
- Level 4: 99214 (detailed; detailed; moderate complexity)
- Level 5: 99215 (comprehensive; comprehensive; high complexity)

Modifiers

A **modifier** is a two-digit code used to clarify or modify a procedure's description, when necessary. When a modifier is added to a regular five-digit CPT code, it generally indicates that some special circumstance applies, usually an alteration to the procedure performed by the provider. For example, –50 indicates bilateral procedures, –79 indicates an unrelated procedure, –56 indicates a preoperative management only, and –53 indicates a discontinued procedure.

Procedure/Payment/Adjustment Dialog Box

Using correct CPT codes is important for obtaining proper reimbursement. Moreover, it is required by law to use correct CPT codes. In Medisoft, transaction codes not only include the CPT codes but also any financial codes needed by the medical office. For example,

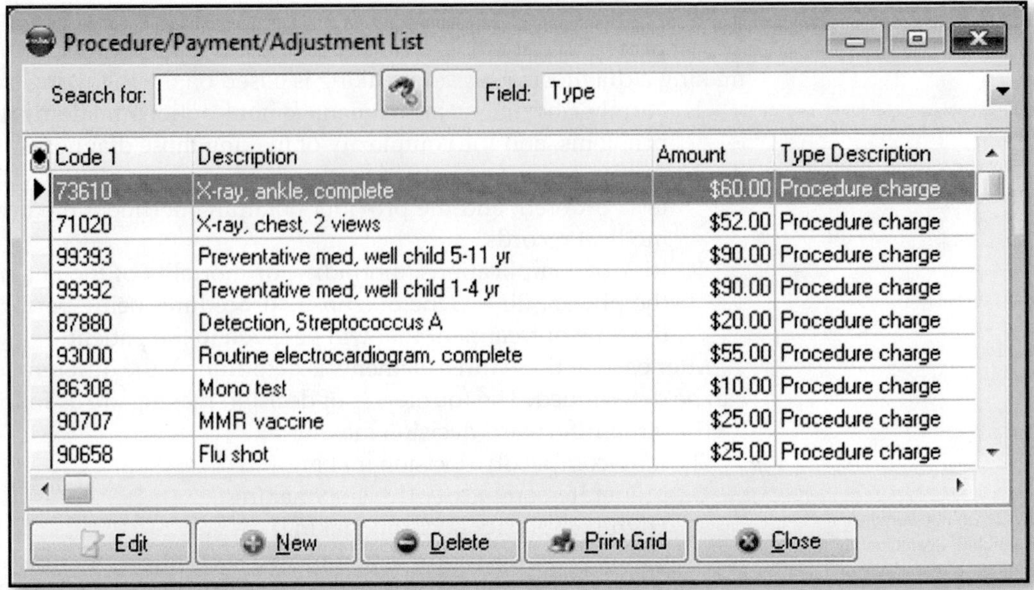

Figure 2.9
Procedure/Payment/Adjustment List dialog box.

write-off codes (forgiving debt) or patient payment codes (how patients pay for their bills) are all considered transaction codes in Medisoft. You can also set up managed care codes and finance charge codes. All CPT codes and other transaction-related codes are entered by clicking Procedure/Payment/Adjustment Codes on the Lists menu. This action opens the Procedure/Payment/Adjustment List dialog box (Figure 2.9).

The buttons along the bottom of this dialog box operate similar to the buttons in the Insurance Carrier List dialog box and the Diagnosis List dialog box. Clicking the New button opens the Procedure/Payment/Adjustment dialog box, which has three tabs: General, Amounts, and Allowed Amounts.

General Tab

The General Tab (Figure 2.10) is the default tab that displays when the Procedure/Payment/Adjustment dialog box is opened. Following is a descriptive list of this tab's fields:

Code 1. This code can be a CPT code for medical procedures/services; or it can also be any other code that your medical clinic uses to identify payments and adjustments that are associated with procedures. For example, "CASH" could be used to identify cash payments, and "WROFF" could be used to identify a patient account write-off.

Alternate Codes. When a value is entered in the Code 1 field, the same code automatically displays in the fields for Alternate Codes 2 and 3. The values for these alternate codes can be changed if an insurance carrier uses a code (with the same description) that is different from the value entered in the Code 1 field. You may recall, when you previously entered information in the Options tab of the Insurance Carrier dialog box, there was a Procedure Code Set field (see Figure 2.4). That field has a list box with three options: 1, 2, or 3. These options correspond to the Code 1 field and Alternate Codes 2 and 3 in the Procedure/Payment/Adjustment dialog box. For example, if necessary, you would first enter an alternate code in the Alternate Code 2 field in the Procedure/Payment/Adjustment dialog box and save the change. Then, you would open the insurance carrier's record and click the 2 in the list box of the Procedure Code Set field.

Inactive. To deactivate a code, click this box to select it. You may need to make a code inactive when a CPT code is deleted, but there are still outstanding (unpaid) claims that are related to the code.

Description. Enter the CPT description or a payment/adjustment description, depending on the value entered in the Code 1 field. For example, Flu shot is the description for CPT code 90658. Check payment is a payment-related description.

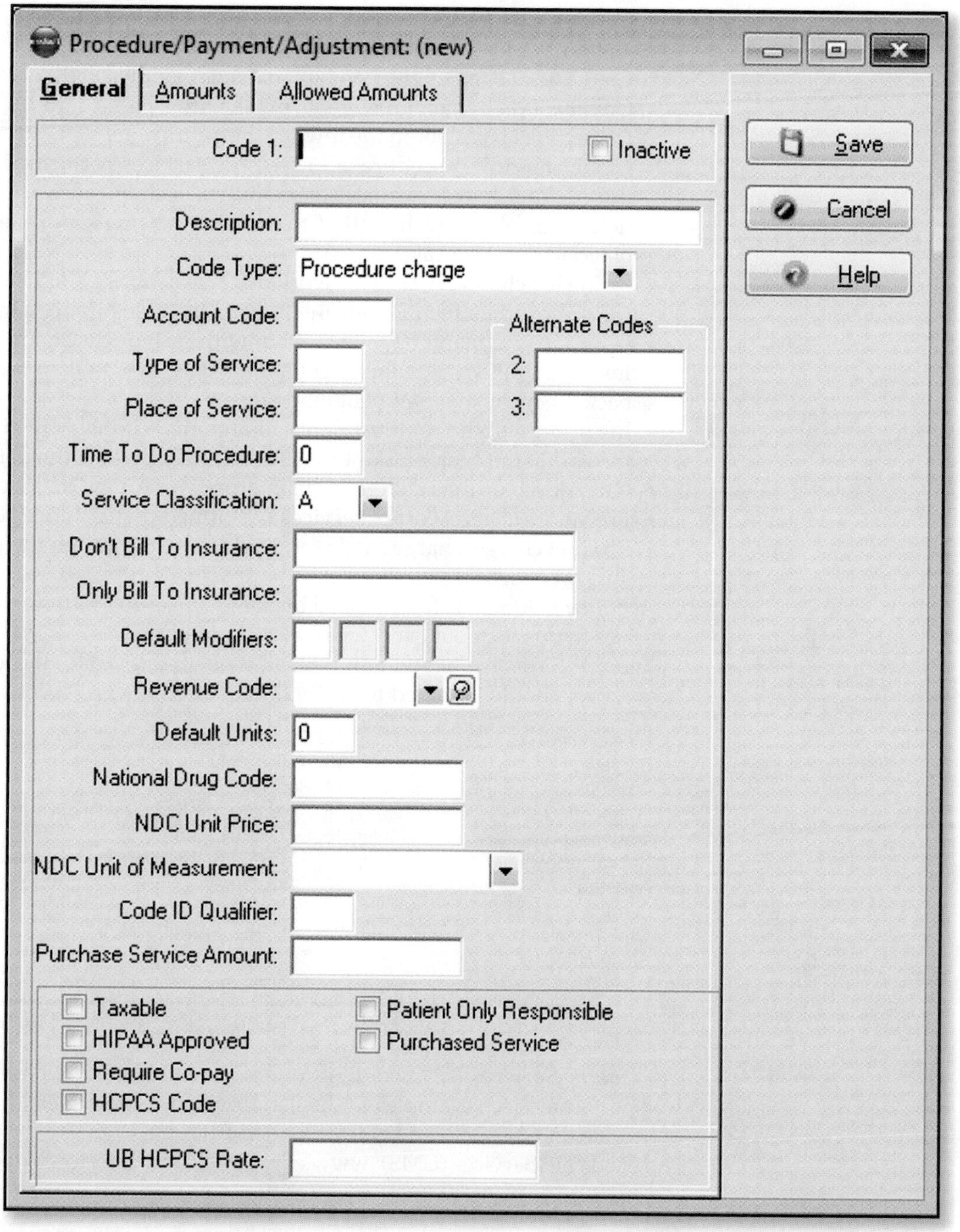

Figure 2.10 Procedure/Payment/Adjustment dialog box with General tab displayed.

Code Type. Click the arrow beside this field to select an option that correlates to the type of code. The most common code type will be Procedure charge. This charge code is used for all CPT codes, as well as other services such as a charge for a blood draw. Depending on which of the following types are clicked in the Code Type list box, some of the other fields originally displayed in the dialog box may be hidden by Medisoft because they do not apply:

- Adjustment: changes (debits or credits) in a patient's account
- Billing charge: charge applied to an account
- Cash copayment: copayment made with cash
- Cash payment: payment made with cash
- Check copayment: copayment made with a check
- Check payment: payment made with a check

- Comment: notes regarding a transaction; selection causes the Amounts and Allowed Amounts tabs to be hidden
- Credit Card copayment: copayments made with a credit card
- Credit Card payment: payments made with a credit card
- Deductible: payment made toward the deductible
- Global surgical procedure: all necessary services performed by the provider before, during, and after a surgical procedure; selection causes the Global Period X Days field to display, which is used to indicate the length of time that charges should be billed to this surgical procedure
- Inside lab charge: charge for work done by a lab within the medical office
- Insurance adjustment: adjustment made by an insurance carrier
- Insurance payment: payment, either with cash or check, toward an insurance charge
- Insurance take back adjustment: adjustment made when the insurance carrier takes back a portion of a payment made for services
- Insurance withhold adjustment: an amount withheld by an insurance carrier until the end of the year; amount must be adjusted against the patient's account
- Outside lab charge: charge for laboratory work done outside the medical office
- Procedure charge: cost of services performed that is added to the patient's account
- Product charge: charge made for products sold through the practice
- Tax: tax charge

Account Code. This field is used by some offices to group procedures together. For the exercises in this textbook, you will leave this field blank.

Type of Service. Following is a list of type of service (TOS) codes. However, the insurance carrier should be asked to verify the required or correct code to use.

1: Medical care	12: DME purchase
2: Surgery	13: ASC facility
3: Consultation	14: Renal supplies in the home
4: Diagnostic x-ray	15: Alternate method dialysis payment
5: Diagnostic lab	16: CRD equipment
6: Radiation therapy	17: Preadmission testing
7: Anesthesia	18: DME rental
8: Surgical assistance	19: Pneumonia vaccine
9: Other medical	20: Second surgical opinion
10: Blood charges	21: Third surgical opinion
11: Used DME	99: Other (e.g., prescription drugs)

ASC, Ambulatory surgical center; *CRD,* chronic renal disease; *DME,* durable medical equipment.

Place of Service. This two-digit code is used to identify where the procedure or service was performed (see examples in the list provided). A complete, more detailed list of Place of Service (POS) codes can be downloaded from the Web site for the Centers for Medicare and Medicaid Services (CMS): www.cms.gov/PlaceofServiceCodes/03_POSDatabase.asp.

11: Office	41: Ambulance—land
12: Home	42: Ambulance—air or water
13: Assisted living facility	50: Federally qualified health center
14: Group home	51: Inpatient psychiatric facility
15: Mobile unit	52: Psychiatric facility—partial hospitalization
20: Urgent care facility	53: Community mental health center
21: Inpatient hospital	54: Intermediate care facility/mentally retarded
22: Outpatient hospital	55: Residential substance abuse treatment facility
23: Emergency room—hospital	56: Psychiatric residential treatment center
24: Ambulatory surgical center	60: Mass immunization center
25: Birthing center	61: Comprehensive inpatient rehabilitation facility
26: Military treatment facility	62: Comprehensive outpatient rehabilitation facility
31: Skilled nursing facility	65: End-stage renal disease treatment facility
32: Nursing facility	71: State or local public health clinic
33: Custodial care facility	72: Rural health clinic
34: Hospice	81: Independent laboratory

Time to Do Procedure. Enter the average time (in minutes) that it usually takes to perform the procedure.

Service Classification. Enter the service classification in which this code belongs, a letter from A to H. These classifications are further defined in the Policy tabs of the Case dialog box, described later in this chapter.

Don't Bill to Insurance. Enter the insurance carrier code to prevent this code from being included on a claim to that insurance carrier.

Only Bill to Insurance. Enter the insurance carrier code to include a transaction code for specific insurance carriers.

Default Modifiers. Enter modifiers for codes that have them.

Revenue Code. This field is typically used by institutional providers, such as hospitals and skilled nursing facilities, to bill claims using the UB-04 form. A list of revenue codes can be entered by clicking UB-04 Code Lists on the Lists menu, and then clicking the Revenue Codes option. For more information, visit the Web site for the National Uniform Billing Committee at www.nubc.org.

Default Units. Enter the common number of units associated with this code.

National Drug Code. This code is used for reporting prescribed drugs when sending electronic claims.

NDC Unit Price. The price of the drug is applicable for sending electronic claims.

NDC Unit of Measurement. This code is used for reporting the unit of measurement for the drug.

Code ID Qualifier. This code is used when sending electronic claims. It tells the insurance carrier what type of claim is being sent.

Purchased Service Amount. An amount you pay a lab or other vendor for technical and professional services they performed for you for procedures such as x-rays or labs. This amount will appear on the Transaction Entry window and on the Claim window.

Taxable. If this code needs a tax charge, click the checkbox to select it.

HIPAA Approved. This checkbox should be selected if the code is HIPAA compliant.

Require Copay. Click this checkbox if a copayment should be applied to this code.

HCPCS Code. When a code is entered in the Code 1 field, this checkbox is automatically selected and the Healthcare Common Procedure Coding System (HCPCS) Rate field is automatically filled in with the same code.

Patient Only Responsible. If this checkbox is selected, the code will not print on insurance claims; only the patient is responsible for the charge.

Purchased Service. Clicking this checkbox indicates that the service is bought from a third party, such as an independent laboratory.

Amounts Tab

The Amounts tab is shown in Figure 2.11. Charge Amounts field A is where the standard charge for the procedure is entered.

Allowed Amounts Tab

The Allowed Amounts tab is used to set up procedure charges for insurance carriers (Figure 2.12). In Medisoft, all of the insurance carriers that have been set up will be listed in the Allowed Amounts tab. You should see seven insurance carriers listed. Because Medisoft will calculate each time a carrier makes a payment for a particular procedure code, it is not necessary for you to enter anything in this tab.

The Allowed Amounts tab in the Procedure/Payment/Adjustment dialog box corresponds to the Allowed tab in the Insurance Carrier dialog box (see Figure 2.6). The Insurance Carrier dialog box lists all of the procedures, whereas the Allowed Amounts tab in the Procedure/Payment/Adjustment dialog box lists all of the insurance carriers.

PROCEDURE 2.6 ADDING A NEW PROCEDURE CODE AND AN ADJUSTMENT CODE

1. Click *Lists* on the menu bar.
2. Click *Procedure/Payment/Adjustment Codes* on the Lists menu. The Procedure/Payment/Adjustment List dialog box displays.
3. Click the *New* button. The Procedure/Payment/Adjustment dialog box opens, displaying the General tab.
4. In the Code 1 field, key *29130.*
5. In the Description field, key *App. of finger splint, static.*
6. In the Code Type field, verify the *Procedure charge* is showing in the list box.
7. In the Type of Service field, key *1* (representing "Medical care").
8. In the Place of Service field, key *11* (representing "Office").
9. Click the *Amounts* tab to display its fields.
10. In field A, key *30.00.* Leave the rest of the fields blank.
11. Click the *Save* button.
12. Click the *New* button in the Procedure/Payment/Adjustment List dialog box.
13. In the General tab, enter the following values in the specified fields. Leave the other fields blank.
    - Code 1: *MISSAPPT*
    - Description: *Missed appointment*
    - Code Type: *Adjustment* (After you click this option in the list box, Medisoft hides fields that do not apply to this type of code.)
14. Click the *Save* button.
15. Leave the Procedure/Payment/Adjustment List dialog box open for the next exercise.

PROCEDURE 2.7 ENTERING AND EDITING PROCEDURE/PAYMENT/ ADJUSTMENT CODES

1. If necessary, open the Procedure/Payment/Adjustment List dialog box.
2. Use Table 2.2 to enter additional codes. Leave blank any fields not listed in the table, or use the system default values. Also, fields in the Allowed Amounts tab will not be entered.
3. Use Table 2.3 to make corrections to existing codes' descriptions, and key a value in the Type of Service field and the Place of Service field.
4. When finished, use the *Print Grid* button in the Procedure/Payment/Adjustment List dialog box to print a current list of codes to hand in to your instructor.

Several computer software programs, such as Encoder Pro, are designed to assist you in choosing the correct CPT and ICD-9 codes. Generally, medical offices use programs such as these, along with Medisoft, to choose and enter the correct codes for procedures and diagnoses.

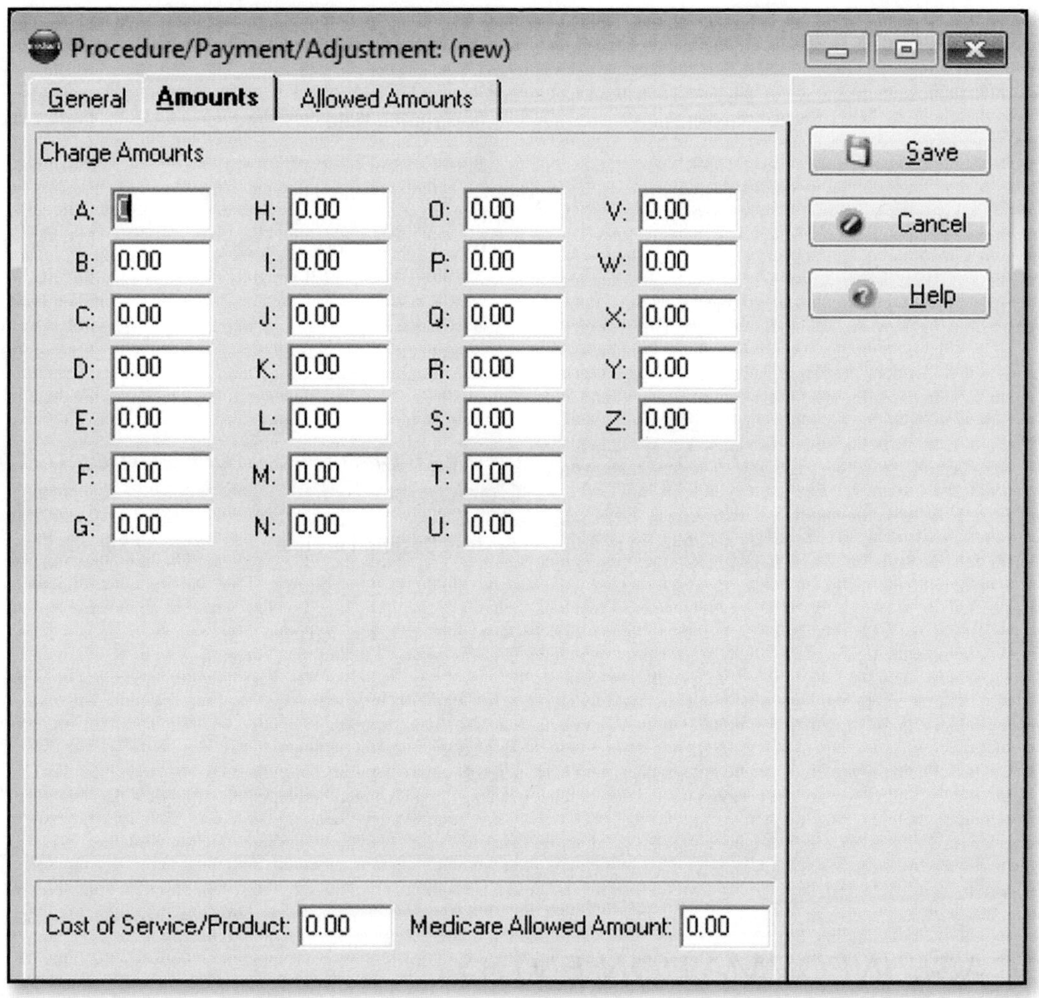

Figure 2.11 Procedure/Payment/Adjustment dialog box with Amounts tab displayed.

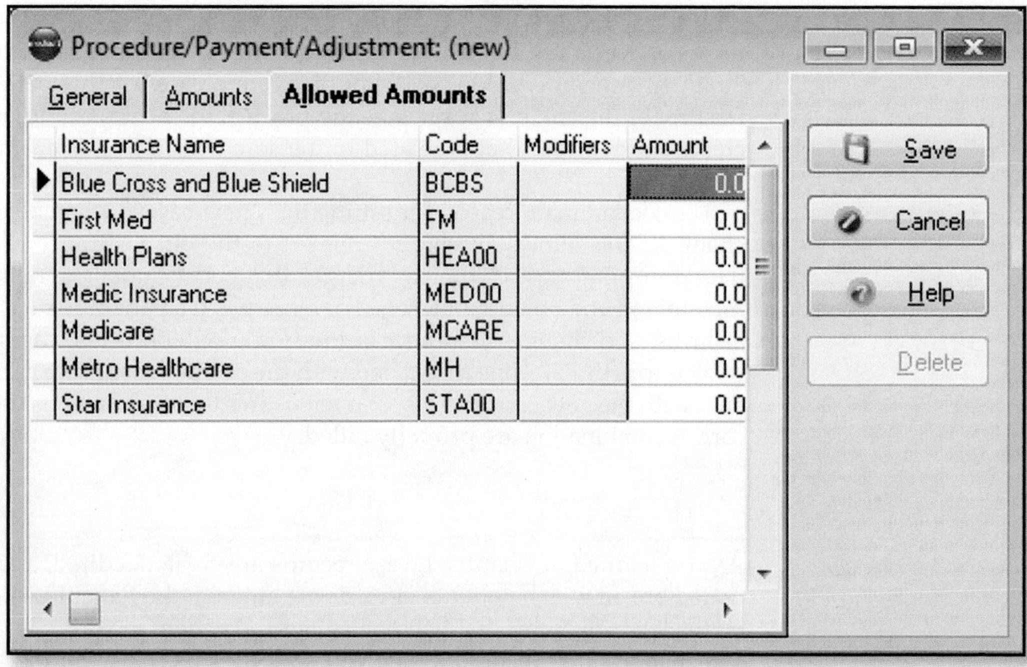

Figure 2.12 Procedure/Payment/Adjustment dialog box with Allowed Amounts tab displayed.

TABLE 2.2 *New Procedure/Payment/Adjustment Codes to Add*

Code 1 Field	Description Field	Code Type
BCBSPAY	Blue Cross/Shield payment	Insurance payment
BCBSADJ	Blue Cross/Shield adjustment	Insurance adjustment
BCBSWH	Blue Cross/Shield withhold	Insurance withhold adjustment
BCBSTB	Blue Cross/Shield take back	Insurance take back adjustment
MCAREPAY	Medicare payment	Insurance payment
MCAREADJ	Medicare adjustment	Insurance adjustment
MCAREWH	Medicare withhold	Insurance withhold adjustment
MCARETB	Medicare take back	Insurance take back adjustment

TABLE 2.3 *Existing Procedure/Payment/Adjustment Codes to Edit*

Code Record to Edit	Revised Description Field	Type of Service Field	Place of Service Field
99211	Office visit, est pt, level 1	1	11
99212	Office visit, est pt, level 2	1	11
99213	Office visit, est pt, level 3	1	11
99214	Office visit, est pt, level 4	1	11
99215	Office visit, est pt, level 5	1	11
99201	Office visit, new pt, level 1	1	11
99202	Office visit, new pt, level 2	1	11
99203	Office visit, new pt, level 3	1	11
99204	Office visit, new pt, level 4	1	11
99205	Office visit, new pt, level 5	1	11

pt, Patient; *est,* established.

CASE INFORMATION ENTRY

Cases are situations or conditions for which a patient seeks treatment or services. In Medisoft, cases are used to group together transactions that apply to specific encounters with a provider. There are two main reasons for setting up a new case. First, a case is set up whenever a patient is treated for a new and different condition. For example, if Tom Smith fractures his ankle, you would create a case for this patient that is related to the fracture of the ankle. If Tom visits the practice the next week for a sore throat, you would create another case that is related to the sore throat. In this example, the patient has two open cases.

The second main reason for setting up a new case is when a patient's insurance carrier changes. This allows all charges related to the old insurance to remain associated with the appropriate cases, whereas charges that occur under the new insurance coverage are maintained and billed separately. For example, if a patient has a chronic condition, such as arthritis, and changes insurance carriers, you will need two cases for that patient that are related to arthritis—one associated with the original insurance carrier and the other associated with the new carrier. This system ensures that transactions for each patient-condition-carrier combination are properly billed.

Patient List Dialog Box

As you learned in Chapter 1, case records are created, edited, and printed using the same dialog box in which patients' records are entered: the Patient List dialog box. The window on the left side of this dialog box displays the patient records, and the window on the right side displays case records. When you click the Case radio button in the upper-right corner of the box, the case window becomes active, and the buttons along the bottom of the box change (Figure 2.13).

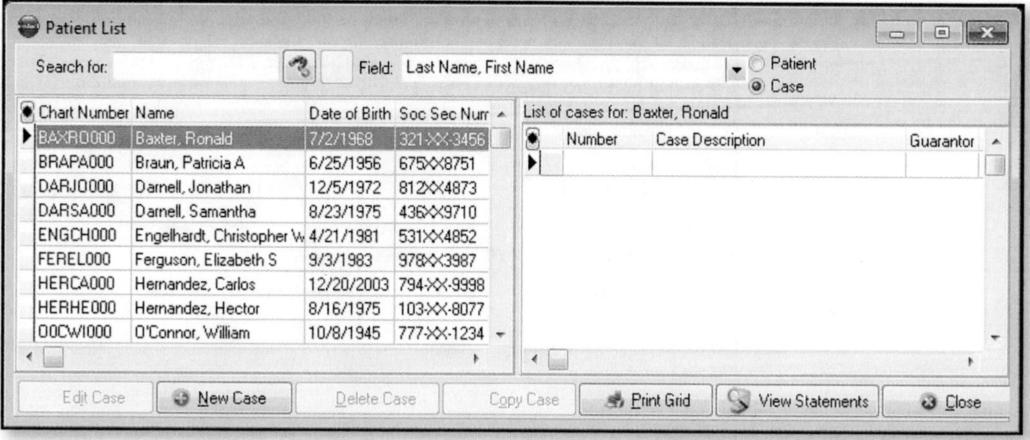

Figure 2.13
Patient List dialog box with Case radio button selected.

The buttons are similar to the ones used for patient records. The case-related buttons include Edit Case, New Case, Delete Case, Copy Case, Print Grid, View Statements, and Close. Two of them warrant further explanation:

Delete Case. You can only delete cases that have no open transactions (unpaid charges). Use extreme caution whenever deleting cases. All information on them will be removed from the system and cannot be restored unless you have a data backup containing those records. You should follow the medical office's guidelines when deleting patient information, as well as state and federal laws.

Copy Case. The Copy Case feature allows you to copy the information in an existing patient case and use it to create a new case. This saves time because you will not need to reenter case information that is identical. Instead, you edit only the data that needs changing, while checking each tab in the Case dialog box (which will be described later in this chapter) to ensure all information is indeed correct.

Case Dialog Box

To create a new case for a particular patient, you first click the patient's record in the left window of the Patient List dialog box. Next, you click the Case radio button, and then click the New Case button. This opens the Case dialog box with the following tabs: Personal, Account, Diagnosis, Policy 1, Policy 2, Policy 3, Condition, Miscellaneous, Medicaid and TRICARE, Comment, and EDI. The Personal tab (Figure 2.14) displays by default when the Case dialog box is opened. For the purposes of this textbook, if the information for any of the fields in these tabs is not available to you when completing exercises, leave the fields blank. However, in a medical office setting, you should check with your supervisor.

At the bottom of the Case dialog box, previously entered patient information is displayed, no matter which tab is selected. In a vertical column along the right side of the Case dialog box is a group of buttons that display no matter which tab is clicked. A number of these buttons you have seen in other dialog boxes, such as Save, Cancel, Help, and Set Default. Others are different. Clicking the UB-04 button allows you to enter information used to process UB-04 claims. The Eligibility button is used to verify insurance eligibility for this patient and case, and the Face Sheet button is used to print case information. In the bottom-right corner of the Case dialog box, there is also a Case field. Clicking the arrow beside this field allows you to select another one of this patient's cases without going back to the Patient List dialog box.

Personal Tab

The following is a descriptive list of the fields in the Personal tab:

Case Number. Medisoft assigns a unique, sequential number to each case; no case numbers are repeated.

Description. A brief description of the case is required, for example, "Broken ankle."

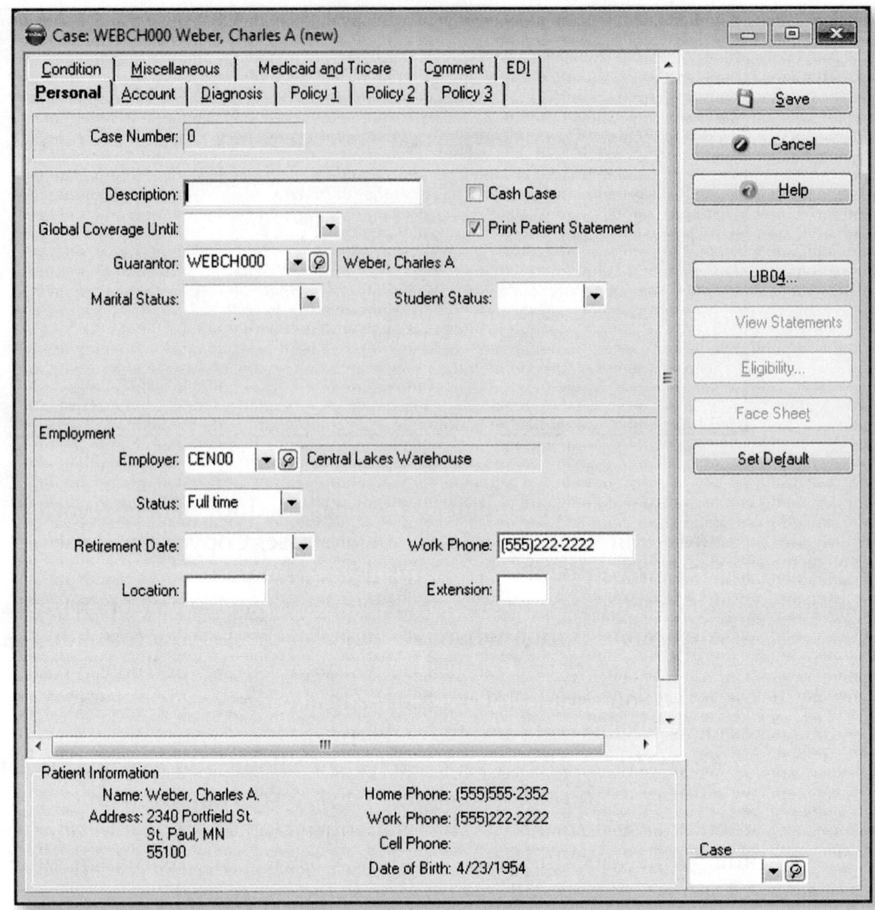

Figure 2.14
Case dialog box with Personal tab displayed.

Cash Case. If the patient operates on a cash basis and has no insurance coverage, then the Cash Case checkbox should be clicked to select it.

Global Coverage Until. If global coverage (a package of services) applies to this case, enter the date when global coverage will end.

Print Patient Statement. If this checkbox is selected, you will be able to print a patient statement when appropriate.

Guarantor. Select a guarantor, if needed, from the list box. If the patient is also the policyholder, select the patient. By default, Medisoft enters the patient's name. If the patient is not responsible for the bill, then click the proper person in the list box. This person should have been already entered into the system. If not, you can press the F8 key to open the Patient/Guarantor dialog box and add the guarantor.

Marital Status. Click the marital status of the patient in the list box. The choices are Divorced, Legally Separated, Married, Single, Unknown, or Widowed.

Student Status. Click the appropriate status in the list box: Non-student, Full time, or Part time.

Employer. If any employment information was previously entered in the Patient/Guarantor dialog box, Medisoft automatically displays it in the Case dialog box. If a new employer needs to be added, it can be done from this screen by pressing the F8 key to open the Address dialog box.

Status. If not displayed, click the work status of the patient in the list box: Not employed, Full time, Part time, Retired, or Unknown.

Retirement Date. Enter the retirement date only if the patient is retired, otherwise leave this field blank.

Work Phone. The telephone number where the patient works is entered here.

Location. The work location for the patient is listed here.

Extension. The patient's telephone number extension is listed here, if applicable.

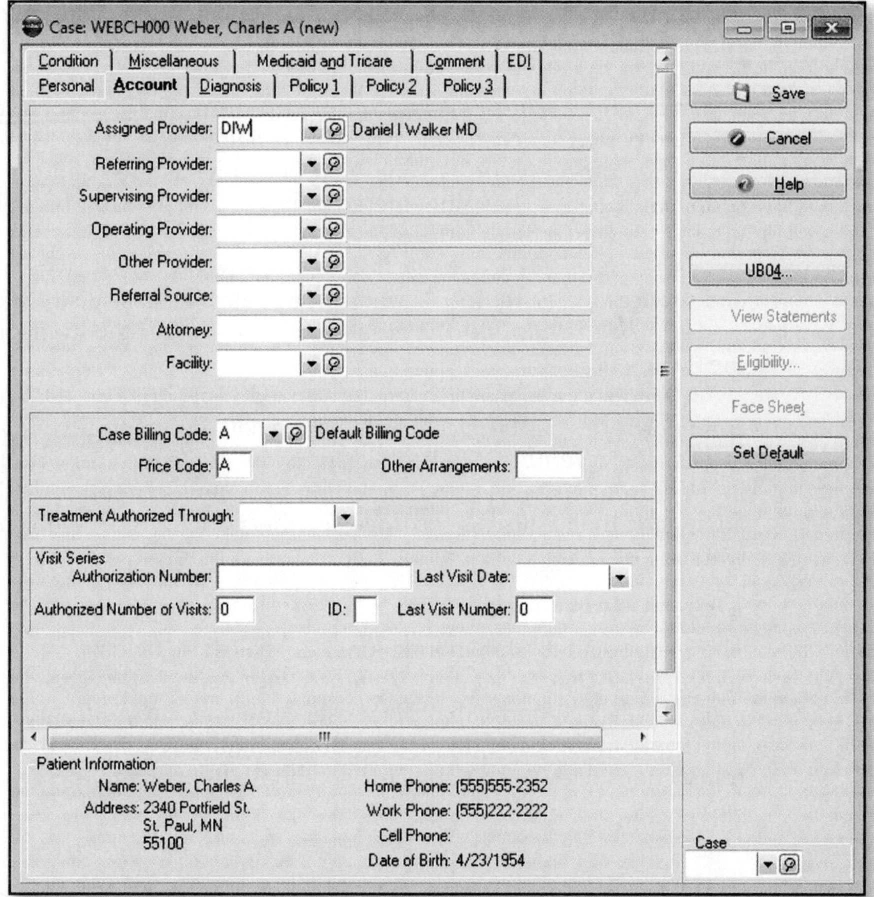

Figure 2.15
Case dialog box with Account tab displayed.

Account Tab

The Account Tab, shown in Figure 2.15, has the following fields:

Assigned Provider. Medisoft automatically displays the assigned provider's code if it was previously entered in the Patient/Guarantor dialog box. If the patient was seen by a different provider for this case, click that provider in this field's list box.

Referring Provider. The name of the provider who referred the patient to the assigned provider is selected. If the provider does not appear in the list box, you will need to add the provider. Click in the field, and press the F8 key to open the Referring Provider dialog box.

Supervising Provider. When the assigned provider is being supervised, click the supervising provider in this field's list box.

Operating Provider. This field is used for UB-04 claims. Click the operating provider in this field's list box.

Other Provider. This field is also used for UB-04 claims. In the field's list box, click another provider who provided services to the patient for this case.

Referral Source. If applicable, click the patient's referral source in the list box.

Attorney. Use this field for accident-related cases or if an attorney has been assigned to the case.

Facility. If applicable, click the facility's name where the patient received treatment. If treatment was provided at the practice's office(s), leave this field blank.

Case Billing Code. This optional field can be used by the practice to sort patients by insurance, billing cycle, or some other means. Press the F8 key to open the Billing Code dialog box, and add a new code.

Price Code. A code from A to Z can be entered in this field based on the pricing structure set up in the Procedure/Payment/Adjustment dialog box's Amounts tab (see Figure 2.11). The Price Code field allows the practice to group patients according to the price level for which they qualify.

Other Arrangements. Any special arrangement for billing can be entered in this field, such as student discount. The four-character code used is an internal, practice-defined value.

Treatment Authorized Through. If the insurance carrier has authorized treatment for a certain period, enter the end date in this field.

Authorization Number. The Visit Series fields are used for preauthorized visits for certain treatments. The value entered in the Authorized Number field is the preauthorization number provided by the insurance carrier.

Last Visit Date. Each time a transaction is recorded (i.e., when the patient visit occurred and services were provided), Medisoft updates the Last Visit Date field.

Authorized Number of Visits. If it applies, enter the number of visits authorized for the treatment.

ID. Medisoft assigns each preauthorized visit series an ID. The default is the letter A. After one series has been completed, Medisoft automatically moves to the next letter.

Last Visit Number. Medisoft keeps count of the number of authorized visits that occur in the current visit series. When setting up a new series, this field defaults to zero. Thereafter, each time a visit is recorded for this patient/case, Medisoft increases the number by one.

Diagnosis Tab

The Diagnosis Tab, shown in Figure 2.16, has these fields:

Principal Diagnosis and Default Diagnosis fields. These fields with list boxes are used to select the principal diagnosis code and any additional default diagnosis codes that apply to this case. Medisoft will automatically display these values when you enter transactions. However, you can also choose to override these values during transaction entry.

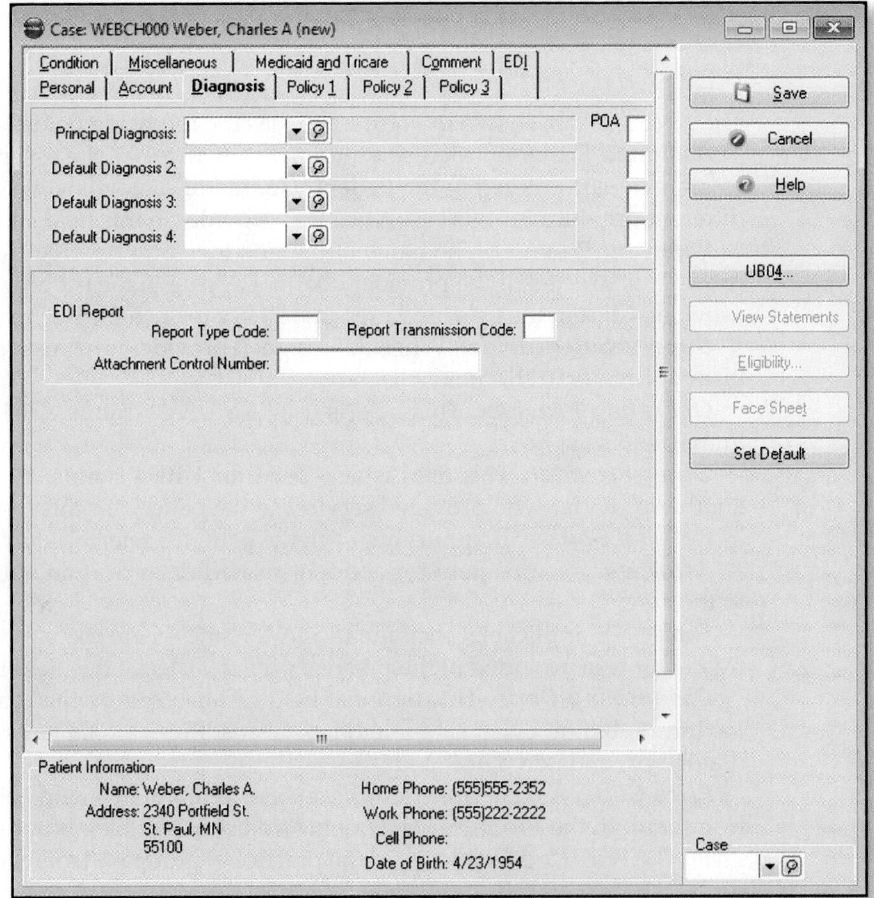

Figure 2.16 Case dialog box with Diagnosis tab displayed.

POA. These fields are used for UB-04 claims to indicate whether the diagnosis was present when the patient was admitted to the facility (e.g., hospital, skilled nursing facility).

EDI Notes. Enter any additional information that might be required by the insurance carriers to submit the claim electronically.

Note: In Medisoft version 17 and 18, Allergies and Notes and EDI Notes have been moved to the Comment tab. See the Comment tab section for further information.

EDI Report fields. The Report Type Code is a two-character code that indicates the contents of a document, report, or supporting file sent with electronic claims. The Report Transmission Code describes the format, timing, and transmission method of reports sent with electronic claims. The Attachment Control Number is the practice's own unique number.

Policy Tabs

There are three tabs used to enter insurance policies that cover the selected patient: Policy 1, Policy 2, and Policy 3. In Figure 2.17, the Policy 1 tab is shown.

The Policy 1 tab is used to enter information about the patient's primary insurance carrier. The Policy 2 tab is used for the secondary carrier, and the Policy 3 tab is used for the tertiary carrier. The fields for all three Policy tabs are similar. Following is a description of the fields in the Policy 1 tab:

Insurance 1. Click the primary insurance carrier for the patient in this field's list box. If you do not see the insurance carrier, press F8 and enter the new carrier. Save the new carrier, and then select it in the list box.

Policy Holder 1. Click the policyholder's name in the list box. Again, if the name is not there, press F8 to enter the policyholder.

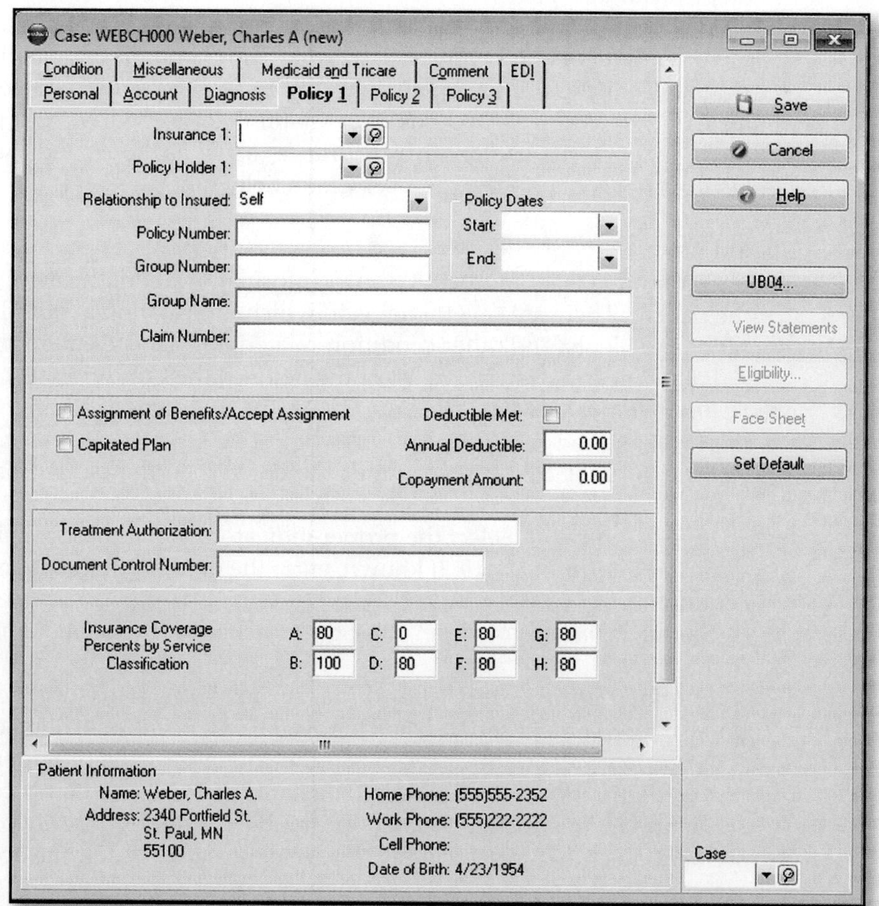

Figure 2.17
Case dialog box with Policy 1 tab displayed.

Relationship to Insured. Click the appropriate option in the list box to identify the relationship of the patient to the insured person (guarantor). If the patient is the policyholder, then the Self option should be selected.

Policy Number. Enter the policy number listed on the insurance card.

Group Number. Enter the group number listed on the insurance card.

Claim Number. This number is typically used on workers' compensation, automobile, and liability claims. Enter the number for the claim in this field.

Policy Dates. Enter the effective dates of the policy. If you do not know the effective dates, enter the date when the patient first came to the practice.

Assignment of Benefits/Accept Assignment. Click this checkbox if the patient/guarantor has authorized payments to go directly to the practice from the carrier and the provider is willing to accept those benefits.

Deductible Met. Click this checkbox if the deductible has been met for the year.

Capitated Plan. Click this checkbox if the patient is on a capitated plan. Capitation occurs when payments are made to the clinic from a managed care plan for each patient who selects the provider as the PCP. The capitation fee is paid, regardless of whether the patient receives care during the designated time period. The provider does not receive any additional fees if the patient is seen more often.

Annual Deductible. If applicable, enter the annual deductible amount in this field.

Copayment Amount. If applicable, enter the copayment amount from the insurance card.

Treatment Authorization. If applicable, enter the Treatment Authorization number in this field. For example, insurance plans often require prior authorization for surgical procedures.

Document Control Number. This field is used to enter the original control number of a claim when processing a replacement or voided claim.

Insurance Coverage Percents by Service Classification. The percentage of fees that the insurance carrier covers is entered in this field. These percentages will change, based on the insurance plans.

The Policy 2 and Policy 3 tabs are similar to the Policy 1 tab. There are, however, some minor differences. The Policy 2 tab does not contain Capitated Plan, Deductible Met, Annual Deductible, and Copayment Amount fields. It does, however, include a checkbox for Crossover Claim. The Crossover Claim field is used when a patient has Medicare as the primary carrier and another insurance carrier as the secondary insurance. The Policy 3 tab does not contain the Crossover Claim field; otherwise, it is the same as the Policy 2 tab.

Condition Tab

The Condition tab (Figure 2.18) shows information about the medical condition or status of the patient. There are several fields in which information about illness, workers' compensation, accidents, and other condition-related data can be entered.

Following is a descriptive list of the fields in the Condition tab:

Injury/Illness/LMP Date. Enter the date (if known) of a patient's injury, illness, or last menstrual period (LMP).

Date Similar Symptoms. Enter the date when the patient had similar symptoms, if applicable.

Illness Indicator. Select the proper indicator from the list box: illness, LMP, or injury.

Initial Treatment Date. If known, enter the date when the patient was first seen for this condition.

Same/Similar Symptom. Click this checkbox if the patient has had similar symptoms in the past.

Employment Related. Click this checkbox if the injury or illness is work related. If so, the workers' compensation fields in this tab will need to be filled out.

Emergency. Click this checkbox if the patient saw the provider on an emergency visit.

Accident fields. The Accident fields are used if the patient's condition is related to an accident. Options for the Related To field are No, Yes, or Auto. If the condition was an accident other than a vehicle-related accident, select Yes. If the accident was auto-related,

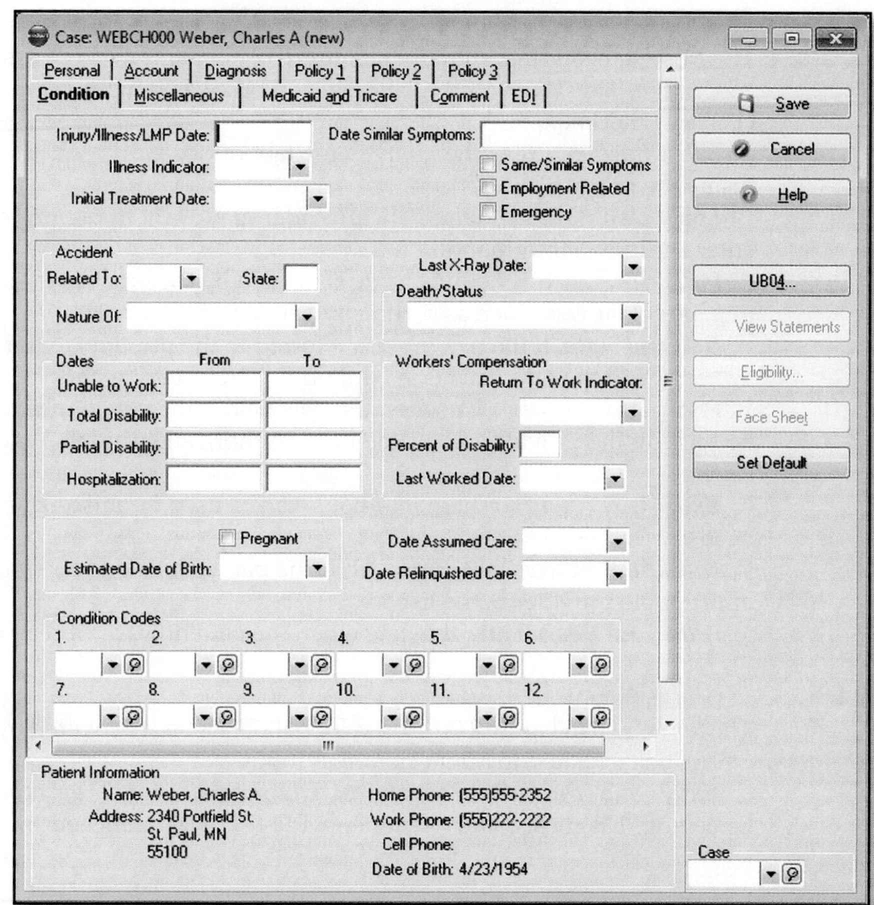

Figure 2.18 Case dialog box with Condition tab displayed.

select Auto. In the State field, enter the postal abbreviation for the state where the accident occurred. In the Nature Of list box, choose from the following options: Injured at home, Injured at school, Injured during recreation, Work injury/self-employed, Work injury/non-collision, Work injury/collision, or Motorcycle injury.

Last X-Ray Date. Select the date when the last x-ray(s) for the current condition were taken.

Death/Status. Based on the Karnofsky Performance Status scale, there are eleven options: Moribund, Very Sick, Severely Disabled, Disabled, Requires Considerable Assistance, Requires Occasional Assistance, Cares for Self, Normal Activity with Effort, Able to Carry On Normal Activity, Dead, and Normal.

Dates fields. Enter the From and To dates that apply to this case, such as when the patient was unable to work, totally disabled, partially disabled, or hospitalized.

Workers' Compensation fields. Enter the workers' compensation information in these fields, if you previously selected the Employment Related field. In the Return To Work Indicator list box, select Limited, Normal, or Conditional. In the Percent of Disability field, enter the percentage of the patient's disability upon returning to work. In the Last Worked Date field, select the last date the patient worked.

Pregnant. If the patient is pregnant, select this checkbox, and then enter the Estimated Date of Birth.

Date Assumed Care. Enter the date when the provider assumed care for this patient. This field is used when two providers share the care for the patient.

Date Relinquished Care. Enter the date when the provider turned the patient's care over to another.

Condition Codes. These codes were previously were under the UB-04 screen. They have since been moved to the Condition window, which allows the codes to be used in professional claims.

Miscellaneous Tab

The Miscellaneous tab, shown in Figure 2.19, contains a mixed assortment of fields.

Outside Lab Work. If the laboratory work was done outside of the provider's office, click this checkbox.

Lab Charges. Enter the charges for laboratory work, whether performed outside or inside the practice.

Local Use A and B fields. The provider may want to use one or both of these fields to enter additional information.

Indicator. Use this field if a code is needed by the practice to sort or categorize patients in a particular way, such as sorting by primary diagnoses.

Referral Date. If the patient was referred to the provider, enter the date of the referral.

Prescription Date. This is a required field for hearing and vision claims.

Prior Authorization Number. Use this field if the patient needed prior authorization to be seen by the provider. Enter the prior authorization number supplied by the insurance carrier.

Extra 1, 2, 3, and 4. These four fields can be used for miscellaneous provider or practice needs.

Outside Primary Care Provider. If the patient's PCP is outside your practice, click the appropriate provider in the list box.

Date Last Seen. Enter the date when the patient was last seen by the outside provider.

Medicaid and TRICARE Tab

The tab shown in Figure 2.20 is used for patients who are covered by Medicaid or TRICARE.

The fields related to Medicaid are as follows:

Early and Periodic Screening, Diagnosis, and Treatment. Early and Periodic Screening, Diagnosis, and Treatment (EPSDT) was launched in 1967. States that receive

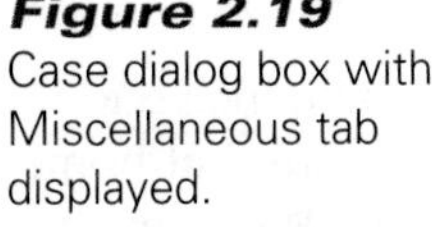

Figure 2.19
Case dialog box with Miscellaneous tab displayed.

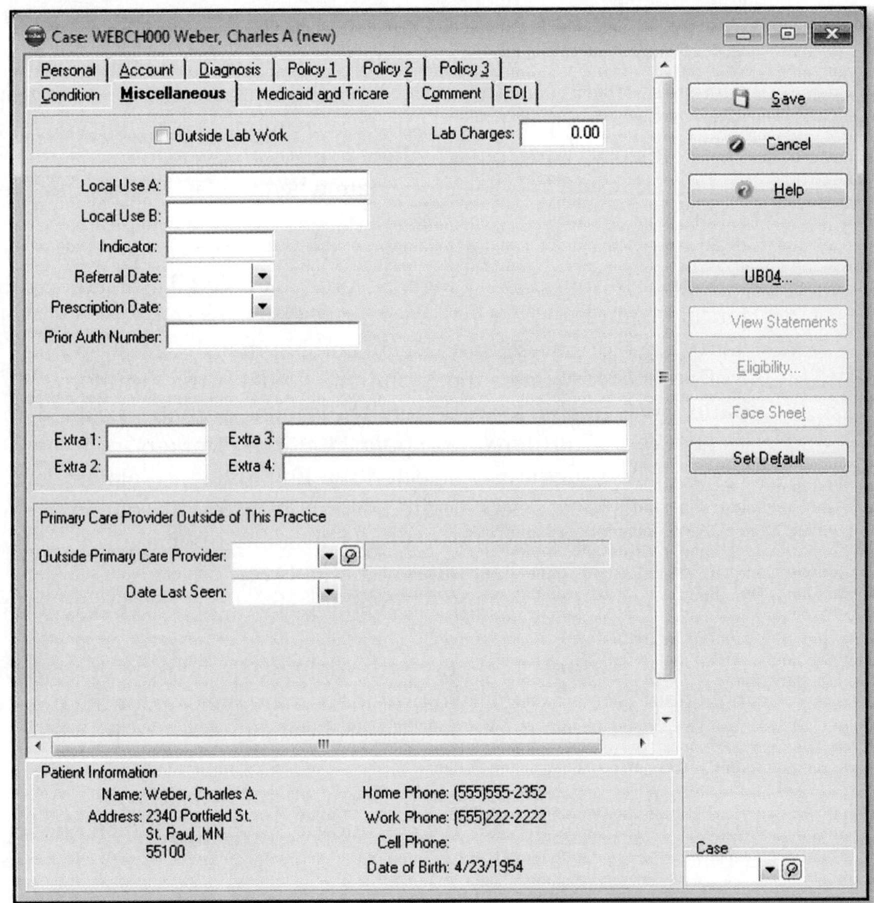

federal funds are required to provide routine pediatric (well-child) check-ups to all children enrolled in Medicaid. Select this checkbox if the patient is part of the EPSDT program.

Family Planning. Click this checkbox if the patient's condition is related to family planning.

Resubmission Number. Enter the resubmission number if the claim is being resubmitted.

Original Reference. Enter the original reference number if the claim is being resubmitted.

Service Authorization Exception Code. This code is required for some Medicaid claims. If the code was not obtained before the patient's visit, use one of the following codes:

1: Immediate/Urgent Care
2: Services Rendered in a Retroactive Period
3: Emergency Care
4: Client as Temporary Medicaid
5: Request from County for Second Opinion so Recipient Can Work
6: Request for Override Pending
7: Special Handling

Special Program Code. Code used for Medicaid claims.

EPSDT Referral Code. Values used for the Early and Periodic Screening Diagnosis and Treatment.

Below the group of Medicaid-related fields on this tab is another set of fields used for TRICARE, previously called CHAMPUS (see Figure 2.20). Following is a descriptive list of the TRICARE-related fields:

Non-Availability Indicator. The options available in this field's list box are as follows:

- NA statement not needed.
- NA statement obtained.
- Other carrier paid at least 75%.

NA is the required preauthorization issued at the treatment facility when a particular health care service cannot be performed at a military treatment facility. The patient has

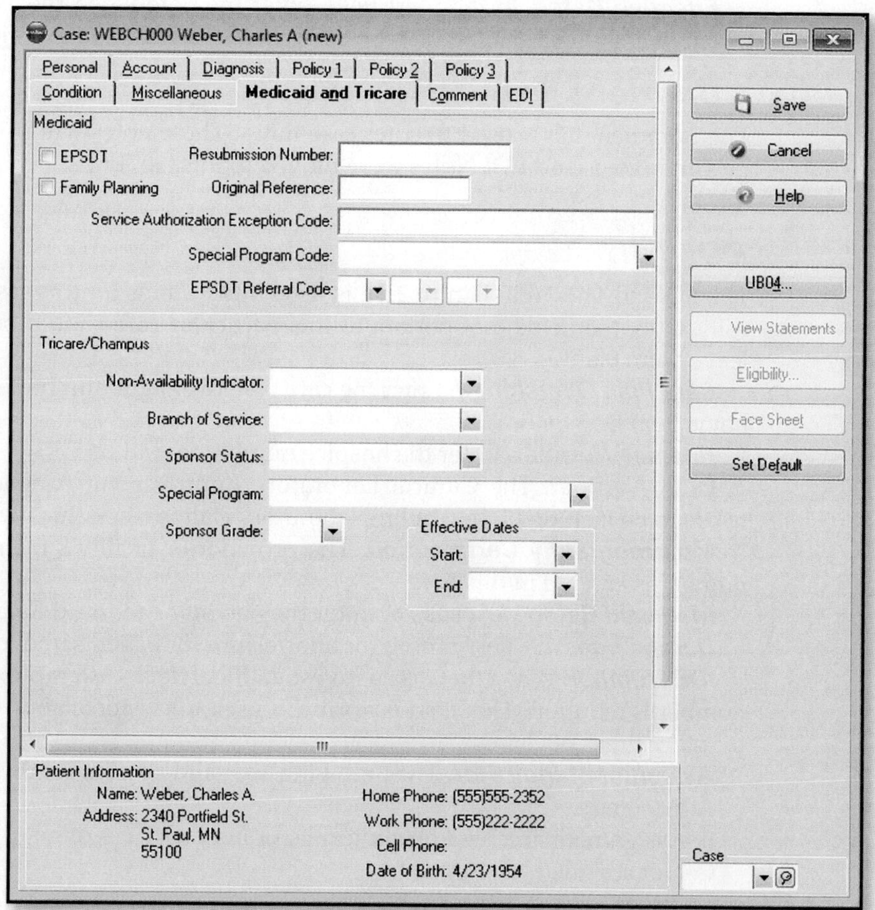

Figure 2.20 Case dialog box with Medicaid and TRICARE tab displayed.

30 days to see a civilian health care provider after the military treatment facility entered the NA. No NA is needed for emergency care if the patient resides outside the catchment area (an area defined by postal zip code boundaries within a 40-mile radius of a government medical treatment facility) or if the patient is covered by a civilian commercial insurance plan that covers 75% or more of the TRICARE Standard covered benefits.

Branch of Service. Select the branch of service: Army, Air Force, Marines, Navy, Coast Guard, Public Health Service, National Oceanic and Atmospheric Administration (NOAA), and CHAMPVA.

Sponsor Status. The sponsor is the active duty member. Select from the following:

Active	100% disabled
Recalled to active duty	National Guard
Civilian	Temporarily disabled
Deceased	Retired
Former member	Foreign military
Medal of honor	Reserves
Permanently disabled	Other
Academy student/Navy OCS	Unknown

OCS, Officer Candidate School.

Special Program. Click a code in the list box if the patient is on a special program.

Sponsor Grade. Select the patient's military grade from these options in the list box:

W1–W4: Warrant Officer	41–58: GS1 to GS18
E1–E9: Enlisted	G1: G1
01–11: Officer	S1: S1
VA: CHAMPVA	90: Unknown
19: Academy student/Navy OCS	99: Other

OCS, Officer Candidate School; *VA*, Veterans' Administration.

Effective Dates. In the Start field, enter the date when the TRICARE policy became effective. If there is an end date for the policy, enter it in the End field.

Comment Tab

The Comment tab is used to enter case notes. These notes will print on statements. Allergies and Notes and EDI Notes were moved to this tab. Enter any special conditions under this tab.

EDI Tab

The EDI tab, shown in Figure 2.21, is used if the claims for this case will be filed electronically. Only the fields that pertain to this particular case should be completed; otherwise, leave them blank.

Care Plan Oversight #. Enter the care plan oversight number in this field for billing for home health.

Hospice Number. Enter the hospice number for billing.

CLIA Number. The Clinical Laboratory Improvement Amendments (CLIA) number needs to be included when billing laboratory claims electronically.

Mammography Certification. The provider or facility's mammography certification number is entered in this field.

Medicaid Referral Access #. Enter the patient's Medicaid Referral Access number.

Demo Code. This field is used for filing claims for patients under a demonstration project.

IDE Number. When there is an investigational device exemption (IDE) on the claim, the number is required. This field is normally used for vision claims but can also be assigned for other types of claims.

Assignment Indicator. The following are valid choices for this field:

A: Assigned.

B: Assignment accepted on clinical laboratory services only.

C: Not assigned.

P: Patient refuses to assign benefits.

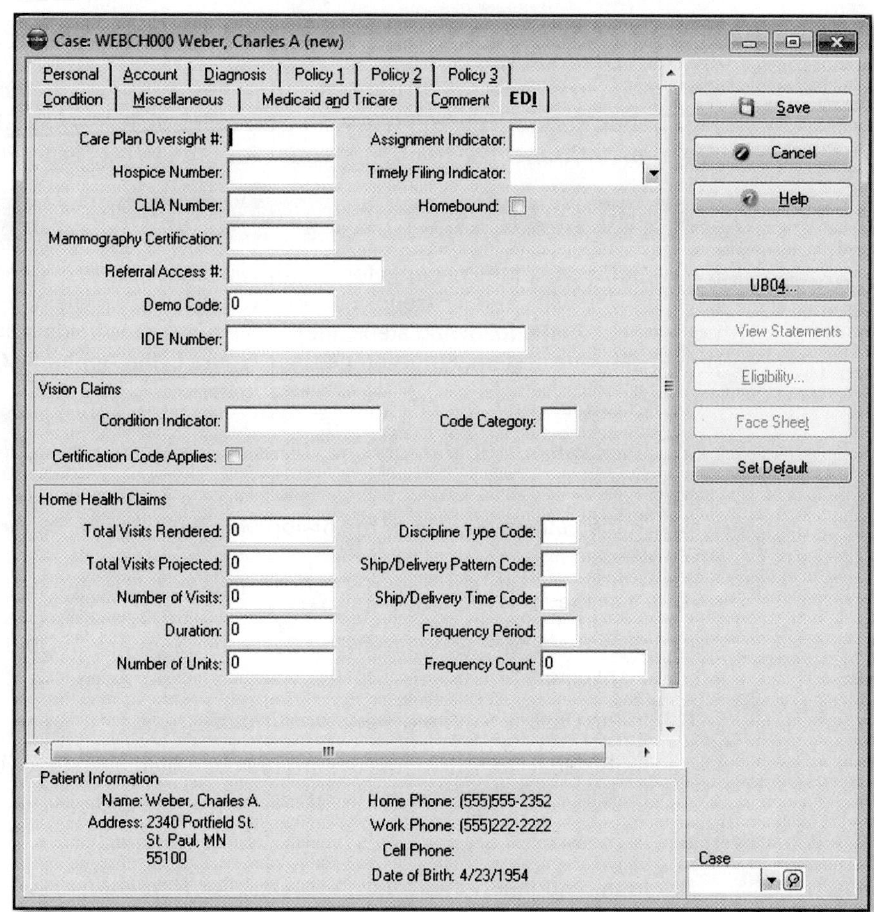

Figure 2.21
Case dialog box with EDI tab displayed.

Timely Filing Indicator. When filing a claim late, enter the reason for the delay using one of the following codes:

1: Proof of eligibility unknown or unavailable
2: Litigation
3: Authorization delays
4: Delay in certifying provider
5: Delay in supplying billing forms
6: Delay in delivery of custom-made appliances
7: Third-party processing delay
8: Delay in eligibility determination
9: Original claim rejected or denial due to a reason unrelated to the billing limitation rules
10: Administration delay in the prior approval process
11: Other

Homebound. Click the Homebound checkbox if the patient is under homebound care.

In the EDI tab, there are three fields related to vision claims:

Condition Indicator. Enter the condition indicator code in this field, which the insurance carrier should provide—for example, L5: replacement because of medical reason.

Certification Code Applies. If there is a certification code, enter it in this field.

Code Category. Enter the code for the vision device—for example, E2: contact lenses.

The EDI tab also has a number of fields related to home health claims. These fields are used as follows:

Total Visits Rendered. Enter the total number of visits rendered.

Total Visits Projected. Enter the total number of visits projected.

Number of Visits. Enter the total number of visits.

Duration. Enter the duration of the visits in this field.

Number of Units. Enter the number of units.

Discipline Type Code. Enter the discipline type code—for example, AI: Home Health Aide.

Ship/Delivery Pattern Code. Enter the pattern codes—for example, 1: first week of the month and D: Monday.

Ship/Delivery Time Code. Enter the time code in this field—for example, E: PM.

Frequency Period. The frequency code for home visits is entered in this field. WK: week.

Frequency Count. The frequency count for home visits is entered in this field.

PROCEDURE 2.8 ENTERING A CASE RECORD FOR MR. WEBER

Mr. Weber is one of the patients for whom you entered data in Chapter 1. In the following exercise, you will enter a case for Charles Weber. If a tab or field in the Case dialog box is not included in the following steps, then leave those tabs/fields blank, or keep the defaults provided by the system. For reference, see **Figure C.1 in Appendix C**.

1. Click *Lists* on the menu bar.
2. Click *Patients/Guarantors and Cases* on the Lists menu. The Patient List dialog box opens.
3. In the Patient window of the dialog box, locate and click the record for *Charles Weber.*
4. Click the *Case* radio button.
5. Click the *New Case* button. The Case dialog box opens with the Personal tab displayed.
6. In the Description field, key *Sore throat.*
7. In the Guarantor field, make sure the code displayed is for Charles Weber since he is both the patient and the guarantor.
8. In the Marital Status field's list box, click *Married.*
9. In the Student Status field's list box, click *Non-student.*
10. Information on Mr. Weber's employment is already filled in (Figure 2.22), based on the entries you made in Chapter 1.
11. Click the *Account* tab.
12. In the Assigned Provider field, Mr. Weber's assigned provider is already listed as Dr. Daniel Walker (Figure 2.23).
13. Click the *Policy 1* tab.
14. In the Insurance 1 field, click *STA00* in the list box to designate Star Insurance as the primary insurance carrier.
15. The Policy Holder 1 field should already be completed. Keep Mr. Weber as the correct entry.
16. Make sure the Relationship to Insured field displays *Self.* If not, click that value in the list box.
17. In the Policy Number field, key *SI-938102.*
18. In the Policy Dates Start field, key *1/1/2010.* Leave the Policy Dates End field blank.
19. Click the *Assignment of Benefits/Accept Assignment* checkbox to select it.
20. In the Copayment Amount field, key *20.00.*
21. Key *100* in each of the fields related to Insurance Coverage Percents by Service Classification.
22. Check your work (Figure 2.24).
23. Click the *Save* button. The Case dialog box closes, and the case record appears in the Patient List dialog box as case number 6.
24. Leave the Patient List dialog box open for the next exercise.

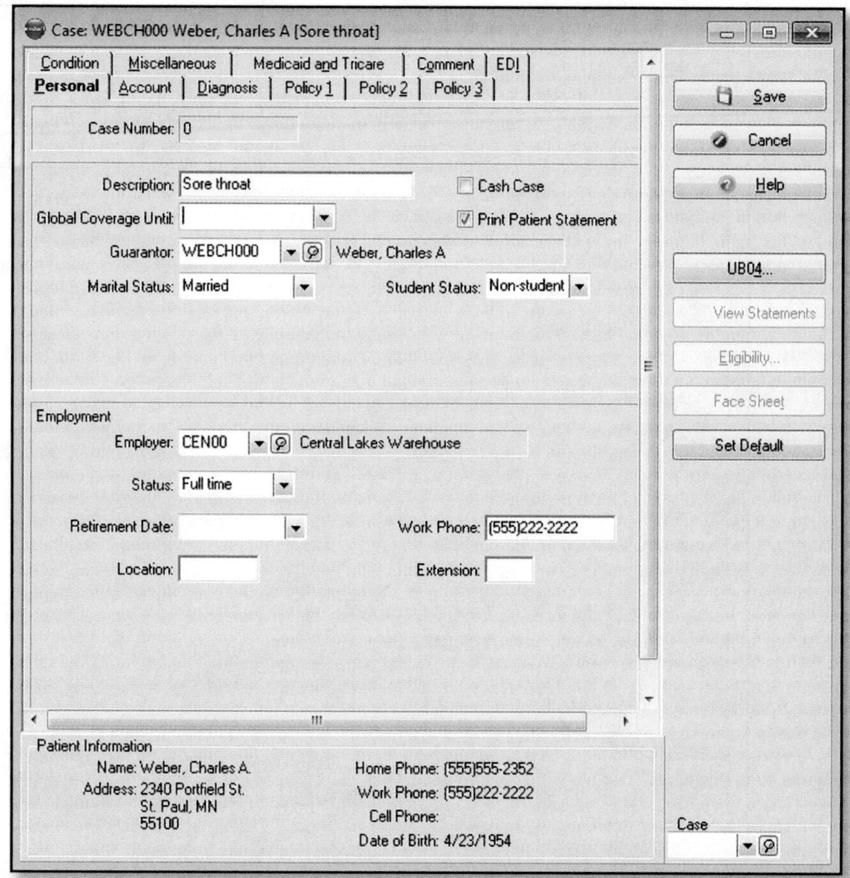

Figure 2.22
Personal tab for Mr. Weber's case record.

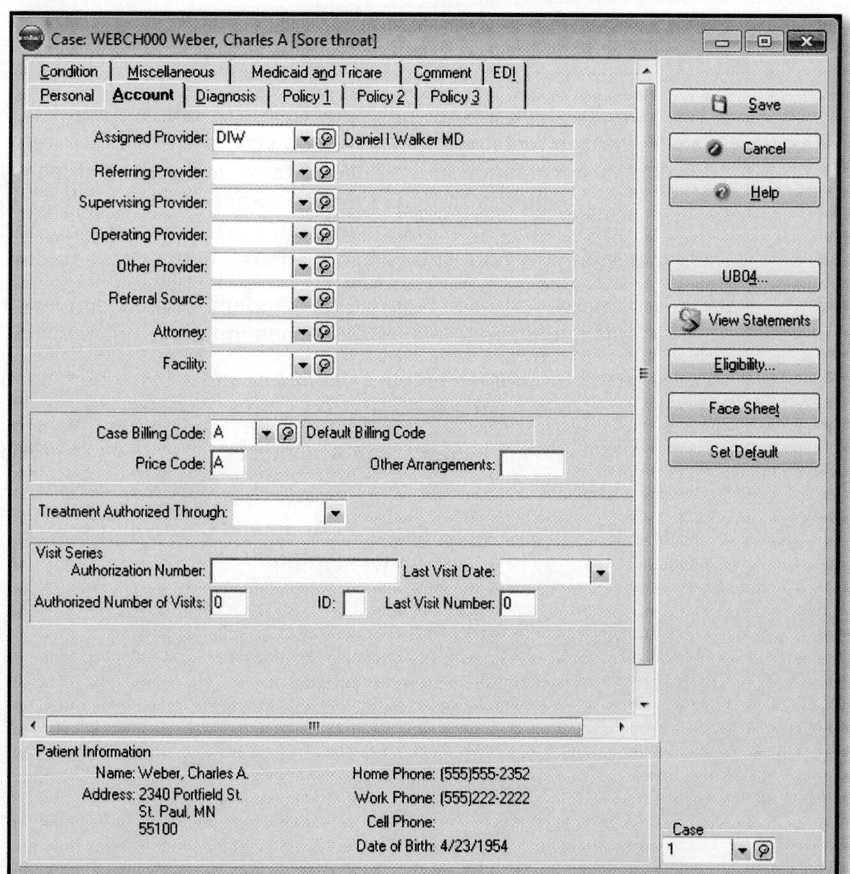

Figure 2.23
Account tab for Mr. Weber's case record.

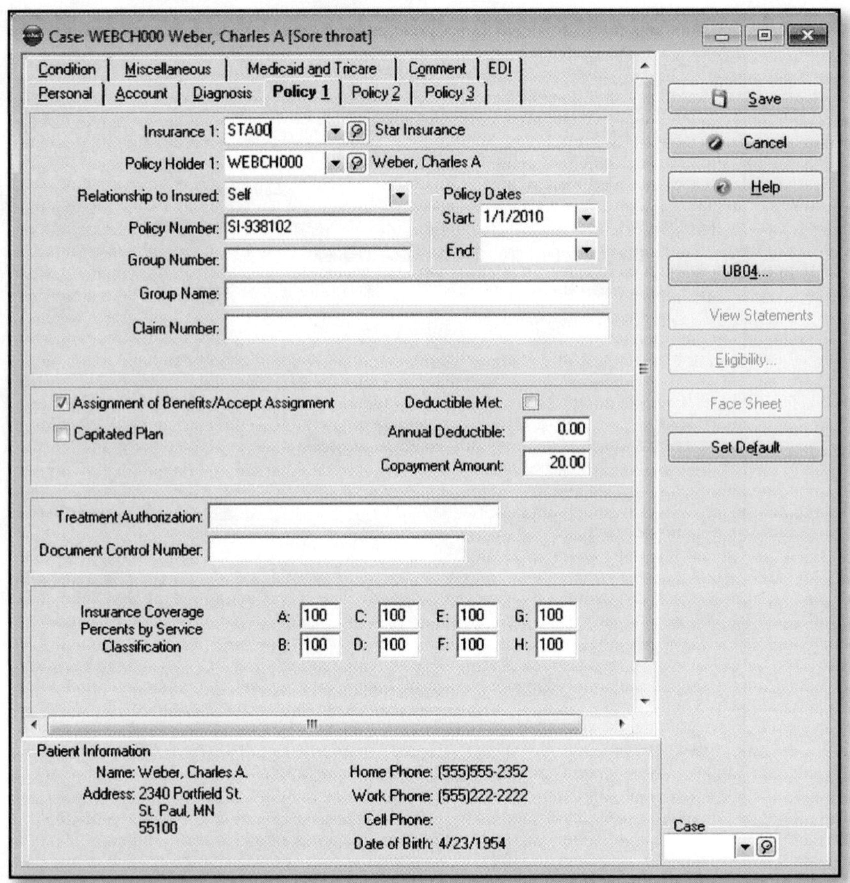

Figure 2.24
Policy 1 tab for Mr. Weber's case record.

PROCEDURE 2.9 CREATING CASE RECORDS FOR OTHER PATIENTS

Using similar steps already practiced in Procedure 2.8, create new cases for four more patients whose registration information you entered in Chapter 1. Complete the insurance policy information in the Policy 1 tab (see figure references in the list provided). Use 1/1/2010 as the start date of their insurance policies. Also, check for the marital status and any indication of student status on the registration forms for these patients and make sure the correct values are entered in their case record.

- Carlos Hernandez (see **Figure C.2 in Appendix C**) is being seen for a sore throat. The insurance policy requires a $20.00 copayment for office visits.
- William O'Connor (see **Figure C.3 in Appendix C**) is being seen for a blood pressure recheck. No copayment is required.
- Cindy Wixen (see **Figure C.4 in Appendix C**) is being seen for an ankle sprain. No copayment is required.
- Ronald Baxter (see **Figure C.5 in Appendix C**) is being seen for a routine physical examination. No copayment is required.

You now have five registered patients with case records on file. In the next chapter, you will make appointments for these patients.

Using Terminology

Match the terms on the left with the definitions on the right.

____ **1.** premium
____ **2.** CPT
____ **3.** E/M codes
____ **4.** health insurance
____ **5.** ICD-9-CM
____ **6.** managed care
____ **7.** Medicare
____ **8.** modifier
____ **9.** preferred provider organization
____ **10.** third-party payer
____ **11.** TRICARE
____ **12.** workers' compensation
____ **13.** capitation fee
____ **14.** deductible
____ **15.** electronic data interchange
____ **16.** copayment
____ **17.** health maintenance organization
____ **18.** primary care provider
____ **19.** policyholder
____ **20.** fee-for-service plan
____ **21.** Medicaid

a. Person who purchased a health insurance plan
b. Insurance that protects employees against lost wages and medical costs resulting from work-related illnesses and injuries
c. Numerical codes used to designate procedures or services performed in a health care setting
d. Health care plan that provides benefits for members of the U.S. military and their dependents; administered by the U.S. Department of Defense
e. System used to code patient diagnoses and facilitate the payment of health care services
f. Two-digit code used to clarify or to alter a CPT code's description, usually to indicate some alteration to the procedure performed
g. Type of managed care organization that uses the fee-for-service concept by predetermining a list of charges for all services
h. System of prepaid health plans that provide health care services at a negotiated cost
i. Procedure codes used to identify the level of service performed by a provider
j. Protection for patients against the financial consequences of illness, injuries, and disabilities
k. Federal health insurance program primarily for people aged 65 and older
l. Small, fixed fee paid by the patient or guarantor each time the patient visits the provider
m. Amount paid by the insurance policy holder before the insurance carrier will begin to issue payments
n. Fixed prepayment made to a provider by an insurance carrier for supplying medical services during a specified period
o. Joint government program that pays health care benefits for people with low incomes or limited resources
p. Type of managed care system that pays providers a regular, fixed payment per patient
q. Process of exchanging information from one computer to another in a standard format
r. Periodic payment made to an insurance carrier to maintain health care insurance coverage
s. Public or private organization that pays health care expenses for patients who have received services from providers
t. Type of insurance in which the carrier pays specific amounts for specific medical services covered in the policy
u. Physician responsible for coordinating a patient's health care treatment in a managed program

Checking Your Understanding

1. In general, explain how fee-for-service plans operate versus managed care plans.
2. How do PPOs and HMOs differ from each other?
3. Name three government health care programs and who, in general, qualifies for them.
4. Tell how to set up insurance companies in Medisoft.
5. Describe the difference between CPT coding and ICD-9 coding.
6. Explain the general process used to identify E/M codes.
7. List the steps involved in setting up diagnosis codes and procedural codes in Medisoft.
8. When should a new case be set up?
9. List the steps involved in setting up new cases.

Putting It into Practice

You have now learned how to set up and edit insurance companies, diagnosis and procedure codes, and cases in Medisoft. The following tasks need to be completed before moving on to Chapter 3.

1. Enter and save the following new patients' data using the patient registration forms in Appendix C, (see Figures C.6 and C.7). Also, enter a case for each patient:
   a. Jerry Silversmith; Dr. Walker, assigned provider; diabetic recheck; no copayment required
   b. Peter Portman; Dr. Walker, assigned provider; ear ache; no copayment required
2. Print the Patient List report, and hand it in to your instructor.
3. Before exiting Medisoft, backup your data as designated by your instructor.

References

Adams DM: *Diagnosis: documentation and coding,* New York, 1997, McGraw Hill.
Flight M: *Law, liability, and ethics for medical office procedures,* ed 3, Albany, NY, 1998, Delmar.
Fordney MT: *Insurance handbook for the medical office,* ed 11, Philadelphia, 2010, Saunders–Elsevier.
HealthCare Consultants of America: *Healthcare fraud and abuse,* Augusta, Ga, 1997, The Consultants.
Holmes DL: *Practical guide to medical billing,* Springfield, Ill, 1997, US Department of Commerce.
Kuehn L: *Health information management: medical records process in group practice,* Englewood, Colo, 1997, Center for Research in Ambulatory Health Care Administration.
Moini J: *Glencoe medical assisting review: passing the CMA and RMA exams,* New York, 2001, Glencoe.
Redman B: *Life and health insurance,* ed 4, Chicago, 1999, Dearborn Financial Institute.
Reid J: *A telemedicine primer: understanding the issues,* Billings, Mont, 1996, Artcraft Printers.
Rizzo C: *Uniform billing: a guide to claims processing,* Albany, NY, 2000, Delmar.
Ross A, Pavlock E, Williams S: *Ambulatory care management,* ed 3, Albany, NY, 1998, Delmar.
Rowell J: *Understanding health insurance: a guide to professional billing,* ed 5, Albany, NY, 2000, Delmar.

chapter 3

Appointment Scheduling

Objectives

1. Describe common types of medical office appointments.
2. List tasks used to prepare for and follow up a patient's office visit.
3. Explain the purpose for setting up a scheduling matrix.
4. Describe different types of scheduling methods used in a medical office.
5. Explain the primary features of Office Hours, and perform set-up tasks in Office Hours.
6. Locate available time slots, and enter new appointments in Office Hours.
7. Find and edit existing appointments.
8. Create repeating appointments.
9. Reschedule appointments.
10. Print schedules and superbills.

Terminology

cluster scheduling: Method that schedules similar procedures together at the same time or same day of the week

consultation appointment: Office visit in which a patient or provider seeks the advice or opinion of another provider

double-booking: Scheduling two patients in the same time slot for the same provider

emergency appointment: Office visit requested by a patient that requires a quick response from the medical office staff; takes priority over other appointments

modified wave scheduling: Variation of the wave scheduling method in which patients are scheduled at regular intervals within a given hour

new patient appointment: Office visit scheduled for someone being seen at the practice for the first time

no-show: Patient who does not show up for a scheduled appointment

open office hours: Scheduling system in which patients are seen in the order they arrive at the medical office, with the exception that patients with a serious or life-threatening condition will be given priority

physical: Routine examination to determine a patient's overall health

preoperative appointment: Office visit scheduled for a patient prior to surgery

resource: Item in Office Hours, such as a room or piece of equipment, which can be associated with a particular patient's appointment or provider's activity

routine appointment: Office visit scheduled for an established patient to follow-up a previous diagnosis or treat new acute symptoms

scheduling matrix: Pattern of working and nonworking hours for the medical office

stream scheduling: Method in which each patient is scheduled in a predetermined time slot, based on status and need; is sometimes referred to as *individual scheduling*

time study: Data collected during a certain time period to determine whether changes should be made to a system in current use

triage: Process of prioritizing patients according to the severity of their conditions

walk-in: Patient who arrives at the medical office without an appointment

wave scheduling: Method in which a group of patients is scheduled at the top of the hour and seen in the order of arrival

There is much more to scheduling patient appointments than simply plugging a patient's name into a time slot. Different kinds of appointments require different amounts of time. Also, each provider's schedule and the manner in which the medical office operates must be considered. This chapter will help you understand the most common types of appointments and scheduling methods. You will also learn how to use Medisoft's Office Hours program to perform various scheduling tasks.

COMMON TYPES OF APPOINTMENTS

Handling a practice's schedule is usually the responsibility of a medical office assistant who works at the front desk. Part of this job involves determining the kind of appointment required. The following sections describe the most common types of appointments.

Routine Appointments

A **routine appointment** is scheduled for patients who have been seen before at the medical practice. This type of appointment includes:

- Follow-up visits for previous diagnoses, including continual or persistent (chronic) conditions
- Visits scheduled because of a sudden (acute) onset of symptoms such as sore throats, ear infections, and so on

New Patient Appointments

A **new patient appointment** is scheduled for someone who is being seen at the practice for the first time. Also, in some medical practices, a patient who has not been seen in over 3 years may be considered new. More time must usually be allowed for new patient appointments than for routine appointments so that registration forms, personal and family history information, and billing and insurance information can be gathered from the patient.

Sometimes medical offices ask new patients to preregister. Required paperwork is mailed to the patient to complete and return prior to the appointment. This policy can help reduce the amount of time needed for new patient appointments.

When scheduling a new patient, make sure you obtain his or her correct name, address, and telephone number. Ask for preliminary information, such as the nature of the illness or injury, type of insurance coverage, and the best times for the patient to be seen by the provider. At this time, you may also want to give out information about the medical office, such as billing policies, hours of operation, and the different types of providers that your medical office employs.

Emergency Appointments

Sometimes, a patient will telephone or arrive at the practice hoping to be seen right away because of an injury or severe illness. The request for an **emergency appointment** requires a quick response from the medical office staff. A true emergency takes priority over other appointments, even if it means delaying or rescheduling other patients' visits.

Most medical offices have established protocols for handling emergencies. **Triage** is the process of prioritizing patients according to the severity of their conditions. Depending on the situation, some of the questions that may need to be asked include: What is the chief complaint? Are any other problems associated with the chief complaint? What medications is the patient taking? What was the onset of the complaint (when and how)? How has the illness progressed? Does the patient have a fever? All this information needs to be given to the provider who then assesses the case and advises what to do. The provider's most immediate goal is to determine whether the patient can be treated at the medical office or should be taken to a hospital emergency department.

If an emergency occurs, other patients whose appointments will be affected by the unexpected delay should be contacted. Most patients will understand the need to reschedule their appointments. You may also wish to suggest the option of seeing a different provider in the practice, if available.

Preoperative Appointments

A **preoperative appointment**, often called *pre-op* for short, is scheduled for a patient who is going to have surgery within the next week. The preoperative appointment determines whether the patient is in good enough condition to undergo a particular procedure. This type of appointment usually includes a complete physical, electrocardiogram (ECG), and blood work. Depending on the type of surgical procedure, the surgeon may require additional information or tests.

Walk-In Appointments

A patient who arrives at the medical office without a scheduled appointment is called a **walk-in**. Depending on the practice's policies, a walk-in may or may not be given an appointment. Walk-in appointments are common in urgent care centers where patients with a wide variety of illnesses are usually seen on a first-come, first-served basis. However, walk-ins are not common in most medical offices.

Triage methods are commonly used to evaluate a walk-in's status. For example, a patient arriving with chest pain will most likely be seen right away and, if necessary, transported (by paramedics) to a hospital. However, if the patient does not need immediate care, then an appointment can be made for a later date. In general, the medical office's protocols should be followed.

Appointments for Physicals

A **physical** is a routine examination to determine a patient's overall health. Many different types of physicals are performed in the medical office. For example, infant and child physicals, sometimes called *well-child examinations*, check for growth and mental progression. Adult physical examinations, which should be performed annually, check for any abnormalities. A physical for an adult woman is sometimes called a *well-woman examination*. Sports physicals check athletes to determine whether the body can withstand the rigor of a particular sport. Many sports physical examinations are performed in late summer and early fall when schools are back in session.

Consultation Appointments

A provider treating an illness or disease who seeks the advice or opinion of another provider requests a **consultation appointment**. Consultations are useful for obtaining another opinion or more information on a particular illness or disease. The consultation provider is often a specialist or has extensive experience in treating a particular illness or disease. A consultation appointment may also be scheduled for a patient seeking a second or third opinion about a particular problem or to discuss various treatment options with a provider.

APPOINTMENT PREPARATION AND FOLLOW-UP TASKS

The medical office assistant typically performs a series of tasks before a scheduled appointment and at the beginning and end of the appointment itself. These appointment preparation and follow-up duties are similar in most medical offices, although they may vary somewhat between practices.

Before the Patient Arrives

It is common practice for medical offices to send a card or telephone patients to remind them of their appointments a few days in advance. Confirming appointments helps avoid no-shows. A **no-show** is a patient who does not show up for a scheduled office visit. Other tasks that should be performed before a patient arrives for a scheduled appointment include the following:

- Pull the patient's chart (medical record), or request the chart from the medical records department.
- If tests or lab procedures were previously ordered, find out if the results are available. If the results have not yet been reviewed by the provider, attach them to the patient's chart.
- Put the patient's chart or test results in the correct provider's slot or tray or in an area predetermined by the medical office.

When the Patient Arrives

The following tasks should be performed after a patient arrives at the medical office:

- Verify the patient's insurance information on record with the patient's current insurance card.
- Verify the patient's current address and telephone number.
- Collect the copayment fee if applicable to the patient's insurance policy. Some practices ask the patient to pay the copayment upon arrival for the appointment. Other practices may collect the copay at the end of the appointment. Under special circumstances, a few offices may bill the copayment. However, billing a copayment is highly discouraged.
- Print an encounter form (superbill), and attach it to the patient's chart. A superbill is not usually printed until the patient checks in for his or her appointment. This is because the patient may not show up for the appointment, or the patient's insurance policy may have changed. Because insurance information often appears on the superbill, corrections may need to be made before this form is printed.
- Give the patient's chart directly to the medical assistant, or put it in the proper area to notify the medical assistant that the patient has arrived. Some clinics notify the appropriate medical assistant of a patient's arrival by checking in the patient using the office's computer system. The medical assistant can keep track of who has arrived by looking at a digital screen.

Before the Patient Leaves

When an appointment with a provider is concluded, the patient normally checks out before leaving the medical office. The following tasks should be performed during check-out:

- Schedule a follow-up appointment for the patient, if required, per the provider's orders. Give the patient an appointment card with the provider's name, the medical office telephone number and address, and the date and time of the follow-up appointment.
- Collect any required copayment for the visit, if not already done at the beginning of the appointment.

TYPES OF SCHEDULING METHODS

A common complaint of patients is the length of time spent waiting to see the provider. Established scheduling policies and procedures can help a clinic plan for many uncertainties. For example, most scheduling systems allow extra time for walk-in patients, emergency patients, late arrivals, new patients, and other situations that might arise.

Typically, most clinical offices have a high volume of patients in the morning, less at lunchtime, a slightly higher volume after 1:00 PM, and then another drop around 4:00 PM. Many practices also have evening and weekend appointments, which may be used for urgent care visits. Evening and weekend appointments may also be scheduled for regular care visits to accommodate patients who work during the day and need to be seen outside of normal business hours.

The medical office assistant is often the first person to talk with the patient, so it is important to project a professional image. Patients should be welcomed and kept informed of delays. If a delay occurs, the patient should be offered the opportunity to reschedule the appointment, make alternative arrangements for child care, or leave the medical office and return later. Providing these options helps patients avoid long waits for their visits.

Scheduling systems should be evaluated periodically. A **time study** can help determine whether changes need to be made to the system. For example, during a certain time period, the following items might be tracked:

- Patients' arrival times compared with actual appointment times
- Overall length of office visits based on patients' arrival and departure times
- Amount of time that passes before patients are called back to an examination room
- Amount of time a provider spends with patients for different types of appointments
- Days of the week and times during a day with the most and least number of appointments

Based on the results of a time study, changes can be made to improve the efficiency of the practice. Once a scheduling method is determined by the medical office, a scheduling matrix should be established. A **scheduling matrix** identifies a pattern of working and nonworking hours for the medical office. This matrix can be used with both manual and computerized appointment systems. Using a scheduling matrix, the medical office assistant can set appointments based on providers' preferences and needs by avoiding times used for hospital rounds, dictation time, or other blocked-off periods.

A scheduling system should create an organized patient flow through the medical office. If a manual system is used instead of a computerized one, an appointment book should be chosen to suit the particular office. For example, if several providers are practicing in the medical office, then the appointment book should provide room for multiple schedules and allow the medical office assistant to see all of those schedules at once. Following are some common scheduling methods used to meet the needs of various types of medical offices:

- Stream scheduling
- Wave scheduling
- Modified wave scheduling
- Cluster scheduling
- Double-booking
- Open office hours

Stream Scheduling

In **stream scheduling**, sometimes called *individual scheduling*, each patient is given a predetermined appointment time based on status and need. The stream scheduling method blocks off an appropriate length of time according to the type of patient (new or established) and the patient's reason for visiting the office. This type of individual scheduling allows for a steady *stream* of patients. Following is an example of stream scheduling:

1:00 PM: Fluery, Alice (established patient; blood pressure follow-up)
1:15 PM: Carter, Bob (new patient; complete physical)

2:00 PM: Patterson, Susan (established patient; birth control questions)
2:30 PM: Lawson, Nicole (established patient; sore throat)
2:45 PM: Rose, Diane (established patient; dermatitis follow-up)

As you can see, a new patient arriving for a complete physical requires more time than the established patients also being seen at the medical office. The time required for a complete physical may vary from practice to practice, but the general time frame for a complete physical is approximately 30 to 60 minutes. A complete physical usually includes a complete family history, personal history, habits, inspection from head to toe, eye examination, urinalysis, ECG, and blood work.

Wave Scheduling

Wave scheduling assigns a group of patient appointments to the top of each hour. Patients are scheduled for the same time slot but seen in the order in which they arrive. This, of course, means that some patients will have a longer wait time than other patients.

Wave scheduling assumes that some patients will arrive late and some will require more time than scheduled. To use this type of method, the medical office needs to determine how many patients can generally be seen within 1 hour's time. Every new hour starts a new group of patients. So, the goal is to see all the patients in a particular group by the time the hour ends. Following is an example of wave scheduling:

9:00 AM:
Simpson, David (established patient; follow-up emergency department visit)
Jones, Melissa (established patient; ear check-up, age 5 months)
Schaffer, Luke (established patient; vasectomy follow-up)
Carlson, Matthew (established patient; sore throat)

10:00 AM:
Hughes, Patrice (established patient; sore throat)
Davis, Carmen (established patient; obstetric-gynecologic [OB-GYN] examination)

Based on the preceding example, each patient has 15 minutes for the 9:00 AM hour time slot. The theory is that the time will average out and someone will be early. If Mr. Simpson arrives 5 minutes early, Ms. Jones comes on time, Mr. Schaffer comes several minutes later, and Mr. Carlson arrives 15 minutes late, all can be seen within the 1-hour time frame.

A disadvantage to using wave scheduling is, if more than one patient within a particular hour's group arrives late, the rest of the day's appointments could potentially be put behind schedule. For example, suppose Mr. Simpson arrives at 9:05, Ms. Jones arrives at 9:10, Mr. Schaffer comes around 9:20, and Mr. Carlson arrives at 9:40. If all the patients require 15 minutes with the provider, the next hour's group of appointments scheduled for 10:00 AM will also be delayed. Even if one of the 9:00 AM patients needs only 10 minutes with the provider but another in that group requires 20 minutes, the problem remains the same. The only way to get back on track is if several patients in a row need less time than expected.

Modified Wave Scheduling

A variation of wave scheduling that tries to eliminate some of the waiting time for patients is called **modified wave scheduling**. This method schedules patients at regular intervals within a given hour. Like wave scheduling, the success of this modified system depends on an accurate estimate of how many patients can be seen in 1 hour. Following are examples of how modified wave scheduling could be used:

- Patients are scheduled every 15 minutes.
- A small group of patients is scheduled at the beginning of the hour, followed by individual appointments every 15 minutes for the remainder of the hour.

Cluster Scheduling

Cluster scheduling (also called *grouping procedures*) groups similar procedures together at the same time or day of the week. For example, a provider may see patients with OB/GYN issues only on Tuesday and Wednesday mornings and see pediatric patients only on Thursday afternoons. The rest of the provider's schedule could be acute visits. Acute visits are typically short in nature and usually address minor problems, although not necessarily. Cluster scheduling can be more appropriate for medical offices with specialized equipment, such as a flexible sigmoidoscope that is used to examine the lower third of the colon.

Double-Booking

Double-booking is the method of scheduling two patients in the same time slot for the same provider. Double-booking needs approval from the provider. This type of scheduling could be used for the first appointment time slot in the morning and the first time slot after lunch. Basically, it ensures that the provider will have a patient to see. Unfortunately, double-booking can also cause a provider to get behind schedule and without enough time to see all patients adequately.

Open Office Hours

Open office hours are different from the other scheduling methods in that all patients are walk-ins and are seen in the order in which they arrive. Of course, patients with serious or life-threatening conditions are given priority. This is the type of scheduling system commonly used in an urgent care clinic. A log is kept of each patient seen, which usually requires patients to indicate the time they arrived when they sign in. Patients may have to wait for a long time, depending on the workload of the clinical staff.

PRIMARY FEATURES OF OFFICE HOURS

Medisoft's appointment scheduler program is called Office Hours. There is more than one version of Office Hours available. The content and exercises in this textbook are based on Office Hours, which has fewer features than are available in other versions.

Opening the Program

You can access Office Hours from within the Medisoft window or without starting the primary Medisoft program, as described here:

Click the Appointment Book button on the Medisoft toolbar, or

Click the Appointment Book option on Medisoft's Activities menu, or

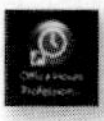

Double-click the Office Hours icon on the Windows desktop, or

Click the Start button in the bottom-left corner of the Windows desktop, click All Programs on the Start menu, click the Medisoft folder, and then click the Office Hours option.

Using the Main Window

Office Hours has its own window (Figure 3.1) with a menu bar and toolbar (Figure 3.2). These features work in a similar manner to the menu bar and toolbar in the Medisoft window. You can click a menu name to display a list of options, or you can click a toolbar button to open its corresponding dialog box.

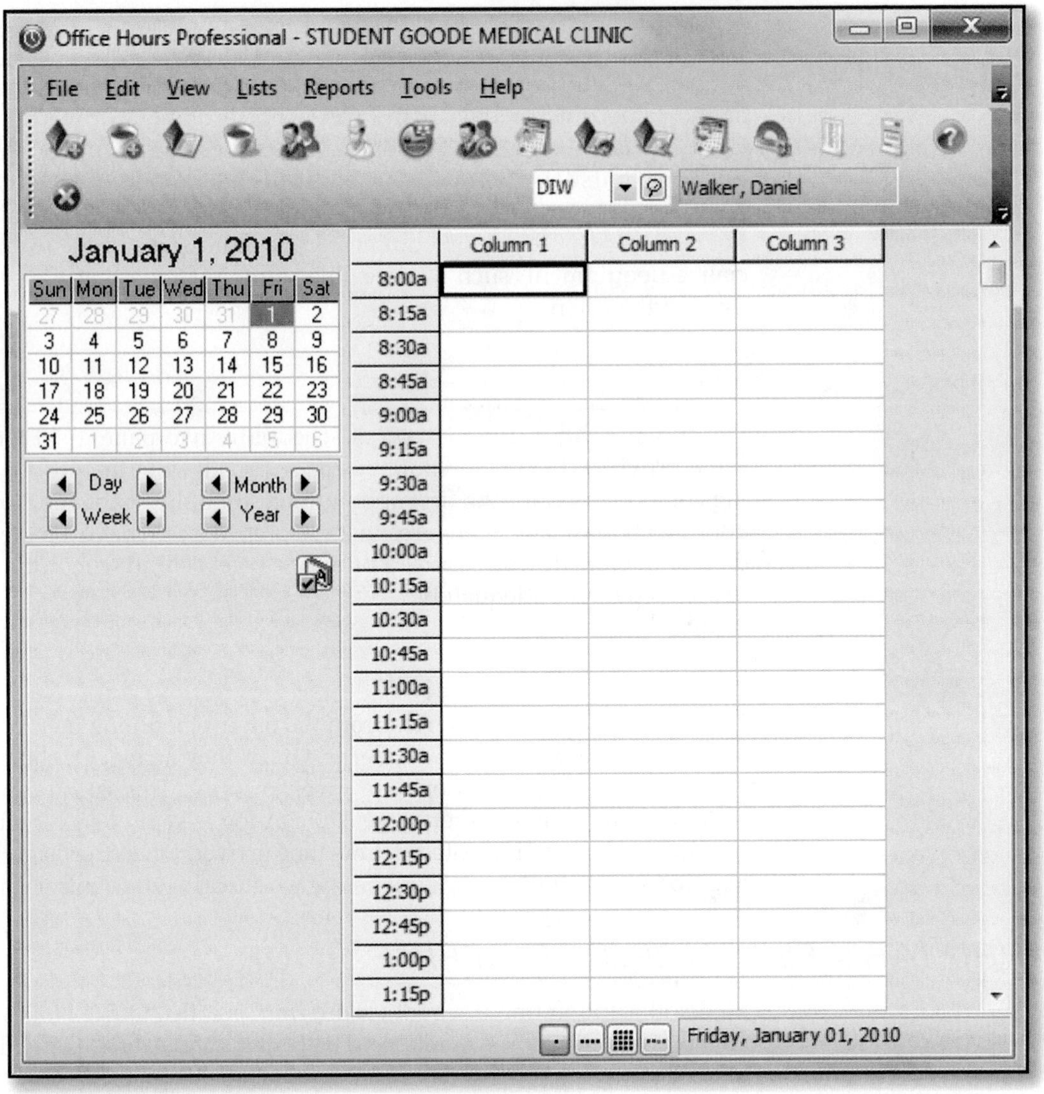

Figure 3.1 Main Office Hours window.

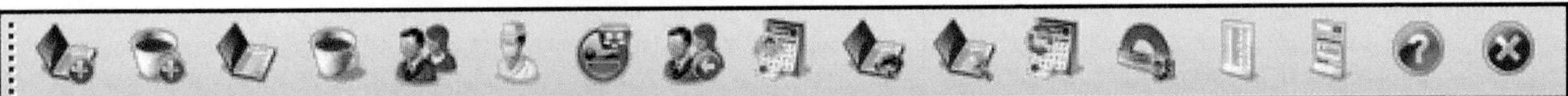

Figure 3.2 Menu bar and toolbar for Office Hours.

Below the menu bar and toolbar, the window is divided into two main parts. The left side of the window displays a calendar. (It also displays patient information associated with a particular appointment after the appointment has been entered and selected). When Office Hours is first opened, the calendar defaults to the current date. You can click on a different day in the calendar to change the date, or you can use the left and right arrows just beneath the calendar to move forward and backward by a day, month, week, or year. Whenever you change the date in the calendar, the date that displays in the bottom-right corner of the Office Hours window also changes.

The right side of the window displays the appointment grid of the provider selected for the date shown in the calendar. You can choose a different provider in the list box located at the right end of the toolbar. The default appointment interval in the appointment grid is 15 minutes. However, you can change this interval, as well as other default settings.

Also by default, the appointment grid displays three columns. This means that up to three patients can be scheduled in the same time slot for the selected provider. To add or delete a column, right-click a column heading. This action causes a pop-up menu to appear with two options: Add Column or Remove Column.

The buttons on the Office Hours toolbar provide shortcuts to various functions in the program. Each button's icon illustrates a particular activity. However, as with the Medisoft toolbar, you can also display the name of a button by using the mouse to point to the icon. Following is a brief description of each toolbar button (in order from left to right):

Another Way
Double-clicking a time slot in the appointment grid will also open the New Appointment Entry dialog box.

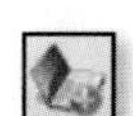

Appointment Entry. Enter an appointment. Clicking this button opens the New Appointment Entry dialog box.

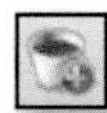

Break Entry. Create a new break. Breaks may be meetings, dictation time, or anything that makes a provider unavailable during the workday.

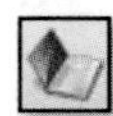

Appointment List. Open the Appointment List dialog box to display a list of appointments previously entered, as well as add new ones.

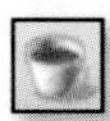

Break List. Open the Break List dialog box to display a list of breaks previously entered, as well as add new ones.

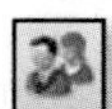

Patient List. Open the Patient List dialog box. You can add or edit patient records without going back into the main Medisoft window.

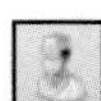

Provider List. Open the Provider List dialog box to see a list of provider records previously entered. You can edit these records or add a new one without going back to the main Medisoft window.

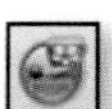

Resource List. Open the Resource List dialog box in which you can add, edit, or delete resources. A **resource** is an item that can be associated with a particular patient appointment or with a provider activity. For example, if a specific clinic room or a certain piece of equipment will be needed for the appointment, that resource can be identified when the appointment is set up. Or, if a provider spends certain blocks of time in the office lunchroom, in a conference room for meetings, or in other locations, a resource code can be set up for each of those purposes.

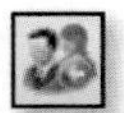

Patient Recall List. This button only appears if using Office Hours Professional. Open the Patient Recall list.

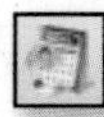

Go to a Date. Go to a specific date in Office Hours, and display that day's schedule in the appointment grid beside the calendar. This feature is another way to change the calendar to a different date, as opposed to using the left and right arrow buttons displayed beneath the calendar itself.

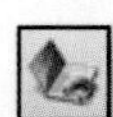

Search for Open Time Slot. Locate the first open time slot for a particular day of the week and time.

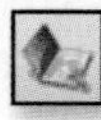

Search Again. Find the next available time slot that matches the most recent values used with the Search for Open Time Slot function.

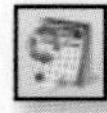

Go to Today. Change the Office Hour's calendar to the current date, and display its appointments.

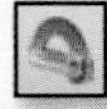

Edit Template. New Template window opens and is part of Office Hours Professional.

Quick Appointment List. Print the appointments list for a certain date or time.

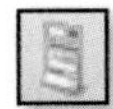 ***Edit Patient Notes in Final Draft.*** Opens Final Draft so you can edit patient notes or add patient notes.

Another Way
You can also close Office Hours by clicking the Exit option on the File menu.

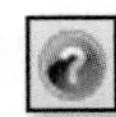 ***Help.*** Access more information about the various Office Hours dialog boxes, features, and functions.

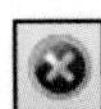 ***Exit.*** Close the Office Hours window and program.

SET-UP TASKS FOR OFFICE HOURS

If you go to work for a medical office that uses Office Hours, the program's options and codes will probably have already been customized to suit the practice. However, it is still a good idea to become familiar with set-up tasks in case options ever need to be changed or new codes need to be added.

Changing Program Options

Clicking Program Options on the File menu opens the Program Options dialog box. Changing fields in this dialog box will affect how Office Hours operates and how it displays information. There are three tabs to change Program Options. Those tabs are Options, Multi View, and Appointment Display (Figure 3.3).

Multi View. This setting displays a column for each provider and each resource set up in the practice. The view can be modified by selecting Edit, Delete, or New. Each view can be specific to the end user of the program.

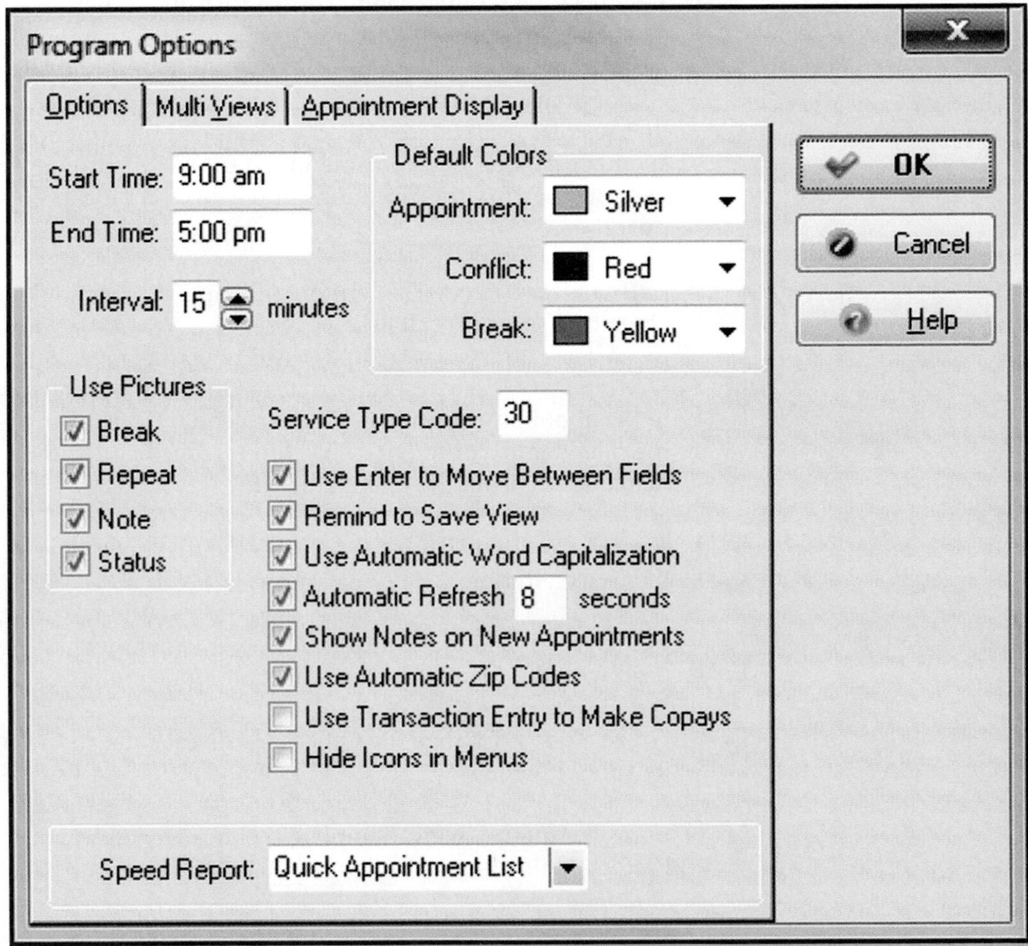

Figure 3.3 Program Options dialog box with Options tab displayed.

Appointment Display. Designate up to five rows of information to display in the appointment grid. Rows 1 through 5 can be used to select what you require to be displayed in the appointment grid.

Options. Initially, the fields in the Options tab default to the values shown in Figure 3.3. Following is a brief description of these fields:

Start Time and ***End Time.*** These two fields allow you to set the standard opening and closing times of the medical office. The initial defaults are 8:00 AM and 5:00 PM. The values in these fields affect what time slots display on the right side of the Office Hours window (appointment grid).

Interval. This field is used to define the standard or most common length of time for an appointment. The value defined affects the time-slot intervals that display in the appointment grid. The initial default is 15 minutes, but you can change it to any value from 1 minute up to a maximum of 240 minutes.

Default Colors. Use the list boxes for these fields to select the colors that display in the appointment grid for appointments, conflicts (overlap) in appointments, and breaks.

Use Pictures. Display pictures in the appointment grid.

Service Type Code. Enter the code for the type of eligibility inquiry being performed. Eligibility transaction code 30 will be used most of the time. Code 30 represents *Health Benefit Coverage*.

Use Enter to Move Between Fields. A checkmark in this field allows you to use the Enter key to move from one field in a dialog box to the next field.

Remind to Save View. Save changes to the view.

Use Automatic Word Capitalization. If this checkbox is selected, the program will automatically capitalize the first letter of each word that you key.

Automatic Refresh. Select this checkbox if you want the schedule to refresh or update itself automatically. You may also enter or change the number of seconds between each update.

Show Notes on New Appointments. If this option is checked, any data previously entered in the Allergies and Notes field of the most current case for a selected patient will automatically display when a new appointment is created for that patient.

Use Automatic Zip Codes. Selecting this checkbox allows for the automatic population of the City and State fields.

Use Transaction Entry to Make Copays. Select this option to enter deposits in Transaction Entry when you click Enter Copays in the Appointment window.

Hide Icons in Menus. If this field is unchecked, icons will display beside the options on program menus. If checked, those icons will be hidden.

Speed Report. This is a drop-down box with the following options: Quick Appointment List, Appointment List, Appointment Grid, or No-Show Report. Select which report to print when you select the Print button.

PROCEDURE 3.1 CHANGING DEFAULT OPTIONS

1. Use one of the following methods to open the Office Hours window:
   - If the Medisoft program is already open, click *Activities* on the menu bar, and then click *Appointment Book* or click the *Appointment Book* button on the Medisoft toolbar.
   - If the Medisoft program is not open, double-click the *Office Hours* icon on the Windows desktop. Or do the following: click the Windows *Start* button, click *All Programs*, click *Medisoft*, and then click *Office Hours*.
2. Notice the current defaults at work in the Office Hours window. The first horizontal time slot is 8:00 AM, and the last slot is 4:45 PM. These rows reflect the default values of a 15-minute standard interval used with an 8:00 AM start time and a 5:00 PM end time.

3. Click *File* on the Office Hours menu bar, and then click *Program Options.* The Program Options dialog box opens.
4. Change the value in the Start Time field to *9:00 AM.*
5. Change the Break color to *Yellow.*
6. Leave the rest of the defaults unchanged.
7. Click the *OK* button. The Program Options dialog box closes, and the rows in the appointment grid reflect the 9:00 AM start time.
8. Leave the program open for the next exercise.

Creating Resource Codes

If a specific medical office resource, such as a room or a piece of equipment, is needed for a particular patient visit, that resource can be associated with the appointment when it is made. You can add, edit, delete, or print resource codes by clicking the Resource List button on the Office Hours toolbar or by clicking the Resource List option on the Lists menu. Either of these actions opens the Resource List dialog box (Figure 3.4).

When you click the New button in the Resource List dialog box, the Resource dialog box opens (Figure 3.5). Here you can enter a code for the resource, or allow Medisoft to assign one, and then key a description of the resource. After the Save button is clicked, the resource record will display in the Resource List dialog box.

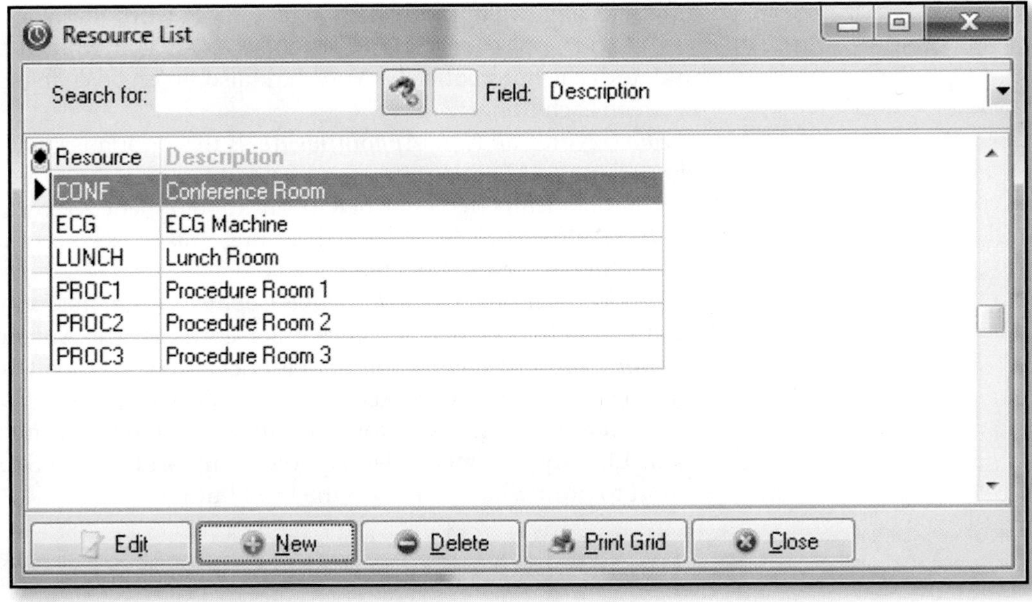

Figure 3.4 Resource List dialog box.

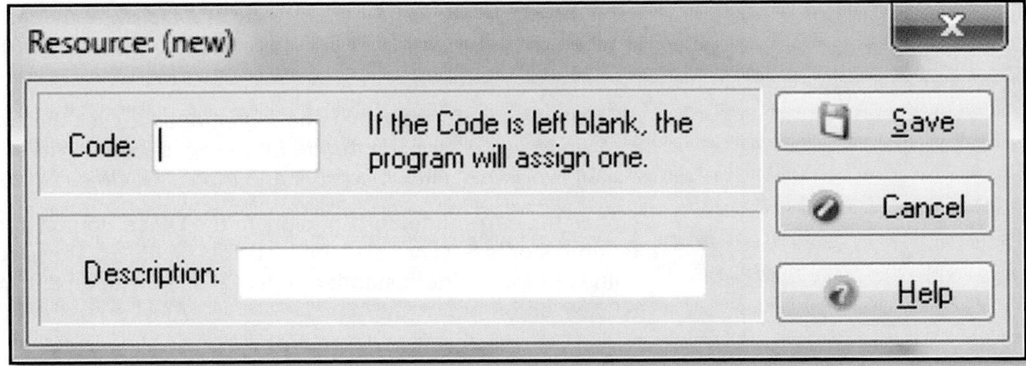

Figure 3.5 Resource dialog box.

PROCEDURE 3.2 CREATING NEW RESOURCE CODES

1. Click *Lists* on the menu bar, and then click the *Resource List* option. The Resource List dialog box opens.
2. Click the *New* button. The Resource dialog box opens.
3. In the Code field, key *LAB*, and then press the *Enter* key to move to the next field.
4. In the Description field, key *Lab Room*.
5. Click the *Save* button. The data is saved, the Resource dialog box closes, and the new resource code displays in the Resource List dialog box.
6. Using steps 2 through 5, create the following resources:
   - Code: *PROC1* (Description: *Procedure Room 1*)
   - Code: *PROC2* (Description: *Procedure Room 2*)
   - Code: *PROC3* (Description: *Procedure Room 3*)
   - Code: *CONF* (Description: *Conference Room*)
   - Code: *LUNCH* (Description: *Lunch Room*)
   - Code: *ECG* (Description: *ECG Machine*)
7. Click the *Close* button to close the Resource List dialog box.
8. Leave Office Hours open for the next exercise.

Creating Reason Codes

Reason codes are optional codes than can be associated with each appointment. These codes provide another way for a medical office to group and evaluate appointment data. Reason codes can also serve as *rules* that providers want to apply to their schedules. For example, Dr. Smith only wants to perform physicals between 9:00 AM and 10:30 AM.

To create a reason code, the Reason List option is clicked on the Lists menu to open the Reason List dialog box. This dialog box looks similar to the Resource List dialog box, with buttons for adding, editing, deleting, and printing codes. When the New button is clicked, the Appointment Reason Entry dialog box displays (Figure 3.6). You may enter

Figure 3.6 Appointment Reason Entry dialog box.

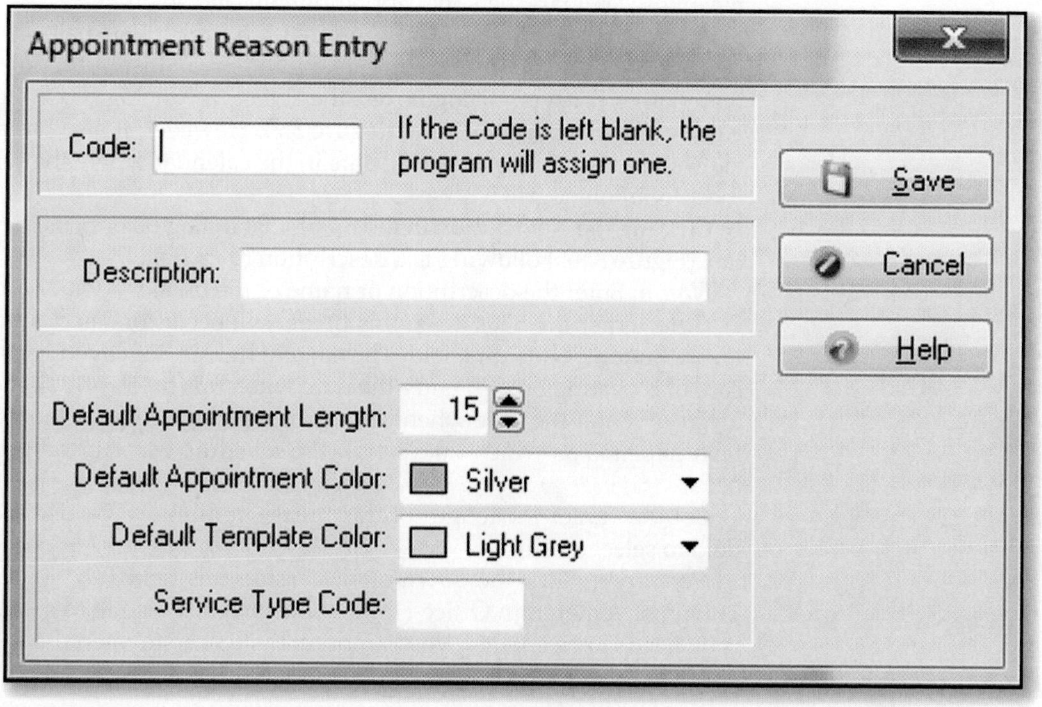

a specific code, or allow the program to create one for you. Other fields are used to enter a description and set various default values for appointment length, color, and select service type code.

PROCEDURE 3.3 CREATING NEW REASON CODES

1. On the Lists menu, click *Reason List*. The Reason List dialog box opens.
2. Click the *New* button. The Appointment Reason Entry dialog box opens.
3. In the Code field, key *RECHECK*.
4. In the Description field, key *Routine Glucose or BP Recheck*.
5. Enter *11* in the service type code field.
6. Leave the default fields unchanged and click *Save*. The Appointment Reason Entry dialog box closes, and the new reason code displays in the Reason List dialog box.
7. Use the preceding steps to create the following reason codes and use service type code 11. Adjust the value in the Default Appointment Length field, as indicated:
   - Code: *SHOT* (Description: *Flu or Allergy Shot*); 15 minutes
   - Code: *FOLLOW* (Description: *Follow-up Visit*); 15 minutes
   - Code: *ACUTE* (Description: *Acute Symptoms*); 15 minutes
   - Code: *URGENT* (Description: *Urgent Visit*); 30 minutes
   - Code: *CONSUL* (Description: *Consultation Visit*); 30 minutes
   - Code: *PHYS* (Description: *Routine Physical*); 45 minutes
8. Click the *Close* button to close the Reason List dialog box.
9. Leave Office Hours open for the next exercise.

Setting Up Breaks

Breaks are used in schedules to block off time when a provider is unavailable to see patients. Examples of breaks include holidays, vacations, lunchtime, hospital rounds, surgeries, meetings, seminars, personal appointments, and so on.

To create a new break, you can open the Break List dialog box by clicking the Break List button on the toolbar or by clicking the Break List option on the Lists menu. As with many other list-type dialog boxes, the Break List dialog box contains buttons for adding, editing, deleting, and printing (Figure 3.7). However, it also has a Jump To button, which allows you to move to a specific date in the calendar where the selected break is located in the appointment grid.

Clicking the New button in the Break List dialog box opens the New Break Entry dialog box (Figure 3.8). Following is a description of its fields:

Name. Enter the description or name of the break.

Date. Enter the date when this break will occur, or select a date by clicking the down arrow button beside this field. The current date is displayed in this field by default. In the case of repeating breaks, enter the date when this break will first occur.

Time. Enter the time when this break will begin. The default time that displays in this field depends on which time slot in the schedule was clicked prior to opening the dialog box.

Length. Enter the length of this break, in minutes. Or use the arrow keys beside this field to select a value.

Resource. Click the down arrow beside this field to display a list of resource codes previously entered in Office Hours. You can click a code to select it. Or if a new resource code needs to be entered, you can press the F8 key to open the Resource dialog box.

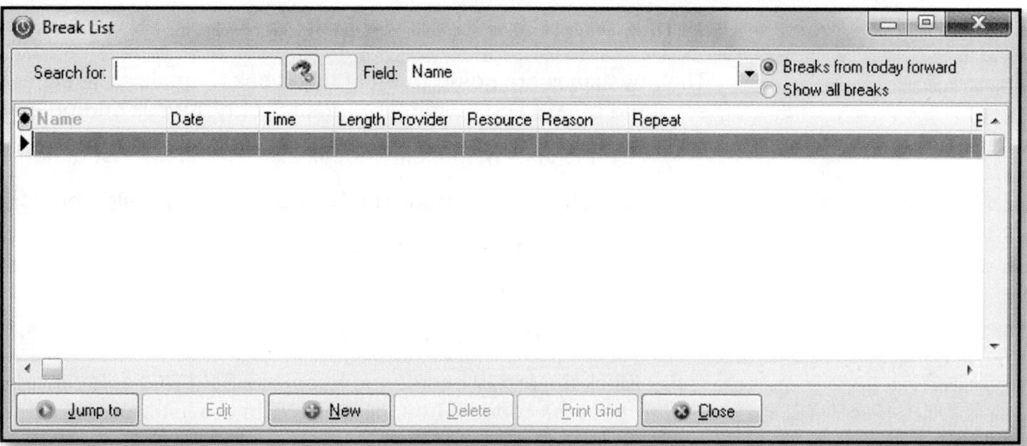

Figure 3.7
Break List dialog box.

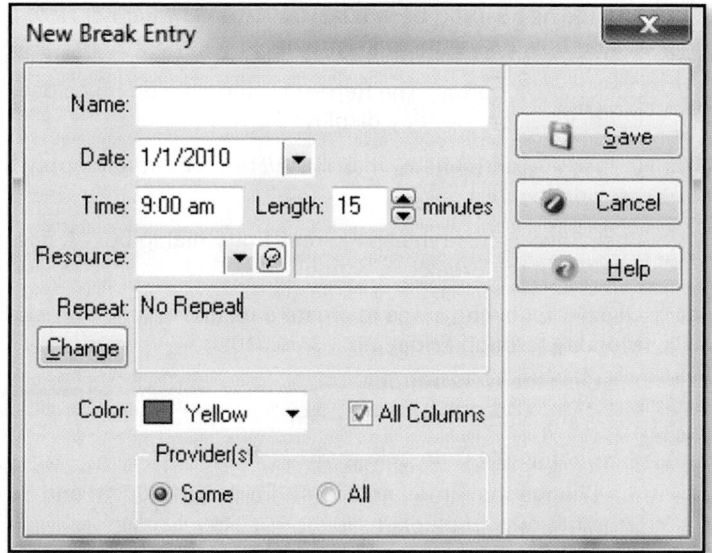

Figure 3.8
New Break Entry dialog box.

Repeat/Change. The Repeat field indicates whether the break is scheduled to repeat. The default is No Repeat. Recurring breaks can be created by clicking the Change button, which opens the Repeat Change dialog box. There are five radio buttons in the Repeat Change dialog box: None, Daily, Weekly, Monthly, and Yearly. None is the default value. If any of the other radio buttons are clicked, additional fields display so you can further define the time interval.

Color. Different colors can be selected to represent this break on the appointment grid. The default color displayed in this field is the one currently selected in the Program Options dialog box for breaks.

Provider(s). The three radio buttons associated with this field are used to indicate whether this break applies to the Current provider (the provider selected in the main Office Hours window), Some providers, or All providers. If the Some radio button is selected, a Provider Selection dialog box will appear after the Save button is clicked. In that case, you should click only the appropriate providers, and then click the OK button. Keep in mind that the Provider(s) field displays differently, depending on the method used to open the New Break Entry dialog box. If the Break Entry button is clicked on the toolbar, this field displays all three radio buttons. However, if the Break List dialog box is opened first, and then the New button is clicked, only the Some and All radio buttons will display. This is because breaks for all providers are included in the Break List window.

PROCEDURE 3.4 CREATING BREAKS

The physicians are going to meet in 1 week to finalize the schedule. For now we will schedule breaks and hospital rounds for only 1 week ending on 3/8/2010.

1. On the Lists menu, click *Break List*. The Break List dialog box opens.
2. Click the *New* button. The New Break Entry dialog box opens.
3. In the Name field, key *Provider Meeting*.
4. Change the value in the Date field to *3/1/2010*.
5. Confirm that the Time field is *9:00 AM*, and change the Length field to *30*.
6. Click the arrow beside the Resource field to display a list of previously entered resource codes. Then, click *CONF* in the list box.
7. Click the *Change* button. The Repeat Change dialog box opens.
8. Click the *Weekly* radio button. (The checkbox labeled *M* for *Monday* should already be checked because 3/1/2010 is a Monday.) Now click in the End on dialog box, delete the date shown, and key 3/8/2010.
9. Click the *OK* button. The Repeat Change dialog box closes. In the Repeat field, Every week on Monday displays.
10. In the Provider(s) field, click the *All* radio button to apply this break to all providers.
11. Click *Save* to close the New Break Entry dialog box. A new break for each provider is listed in the Break List window.
12. Use the following steps to create a recurring lunch break for Katherine Olsson, Monday through Friday until 3/8/2010:
    a. Click the *New* button.
    b. In the Name field, key *Lunch*.
    c. Change the Date field to *3/1/2010*.
    d. Change the Time and Length fields to *12:00 PM* and *30* minutes.
    e. In the Resource field's list box, click *LUNCH*.
    f. Make sure the *Some* radio button is selected for the Provider(s) field.
    g. Click the *Change* button to open the Repeat Change dialog box.
    h. Click the *Weekly* radio button. Then, click the check boxes for Tuesday through Friday. (Monday should already display a checkmark.) Now click in the End on dialog box, delete the date shown, and key 3/8/2010.
    i. Click *OK*. Then, click *Save*. The Provider Selection dialog box displays.
    j. Click the grid row with *Olsson* to highlight it. Then, click *OK*.
13. Starting on 3/1/2010, create a recurring break called *Hospital Rounds* for Dr. Walker and Dr. Berg every day but Sunday at 1:00 PM for 90 minutes. Click End on, and key a date of 3/8/2010. Leave the Resource field blank.
14. Click the *Close* button in the Break List dialog box.
15. Leave Office Hours open for the next exercise.

APPOINTMENT SCHEDULING IN OFFICE HOURS

When setting up a patient visit, the first step is to select the provider for whom you are scheduling the appointment. Using Multi View, you can select the provider by clicking in the appointment grid column that displays the provider's name.

The next step is to select the date for the appointment by clicking the day in the calendar or using the arrows underneath the calendar to move to the desired date. There are also other methods you can use to find and select a date, which will be explained later in this chapter.

The third step is to enter the information in the New Appointment Entry dialog box. There are multiple ways to do this including the following:

- Click the Appointment List option on the Lists menu, and then click the New button, or
- Click the Appointment Entry button on the toolbar (first one on the left), or
- Double-click a time slot in the appointment grid.

Note: If, when attempting to enter an appointment in the following exercise, you receive the following error message: "The demonstration version of Office Hours has reached its Appointment Limit," you must go back and check that the end dates of the Break Entries in Procedure 3.4 are 3/8/2010.

Entering New Appointments

The New Appointment Entry dialog box (Figure 3.9) contains the following fields:

Chart. If the person for whom you are entering an appointment is an established patient, select the patient's chart number from the Chart field's list box. If the patient is new, press the F8 key to open the Patient/Guarantor dialog box, and enter demographic information for the new patient. (If you do not have time to add a new patient record, the program will allow you to skip the Chart field, key the person's name in the field beside the Chart field, and then go back later and complete the Patient/Guarantor dialog box.)

Home Phone and Cell Phone. Enter the phone numbers for the patient. If the appointment is being made for an established patient, the phone numbers automatically display. However, it is imperative to obtain or verify these phone numbers in case you need to contact the patient.

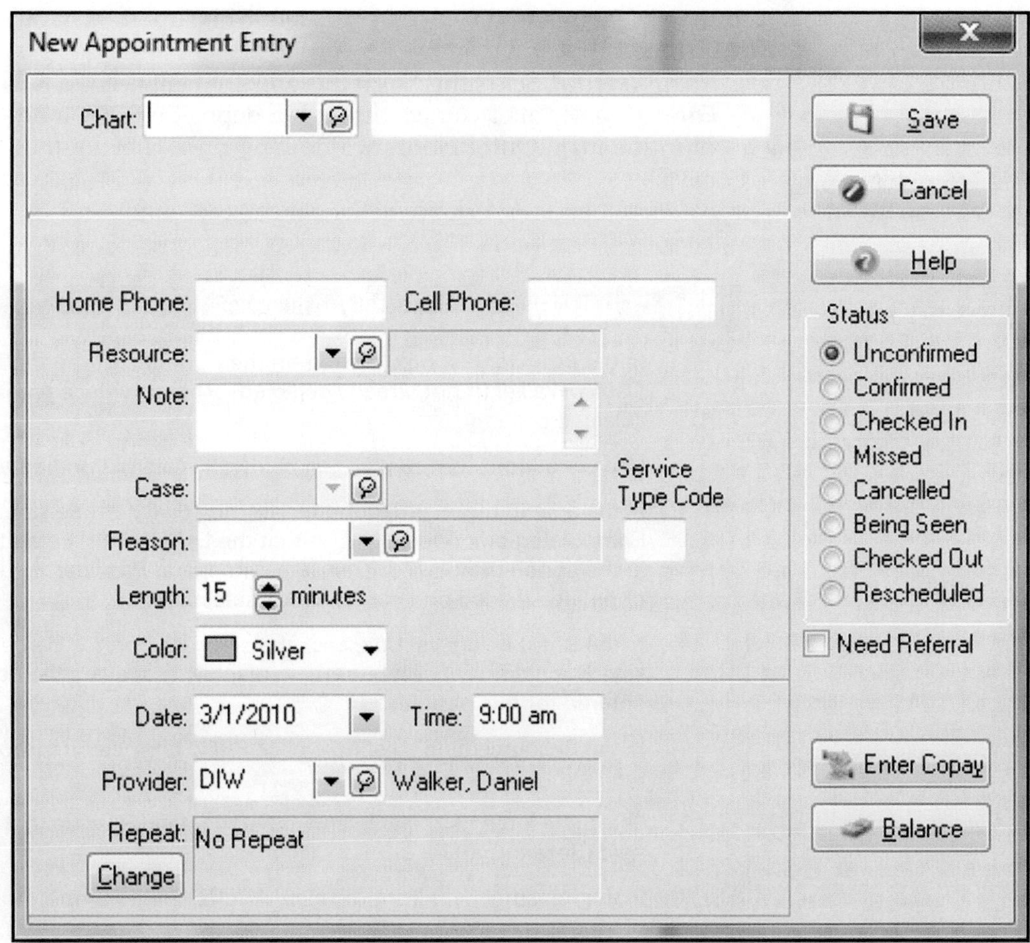

Figure 3.9 New Appointment Entry dialog box.

Resource. In this field's list box, click a resource needed for this appointment, such as Lab Room or Procedure Room. Keep in mind that this field can be left blank for many appointments.

Note. Enter any notes about the appointment in this field.

Case. The most recent Medisoft case number that pertains to this patient is displayed in this field. At this time, you can press the F8 key and enter insurance information for a new patient.

Reason. In the list box, click the appropriate reason for the visit. If necessary, you can press the F8 key, enter a new reason, and then select it from the Reason list box.

Length. Enter the amount of time needed for the visit, if it is different from the default value that displays.

Color. Set the color of the appointment.

Date. The date selected on the calendar in the main Office Hours window displays in this field. If necessary, you may enter a different date for the visit.

Time. The time slot selected in the appointment grid displays in this field. If necessary, you may enter a different time for the visit.

Provider. The provider code selected in the main Office Hours window displays in this field. You can change the provider by clicking a different code in the Provider list box.

Repeat/Change. The Repeat field indicates whether the appointment is scheduled to repeat. The default is No Repeat. You can click the Change button to open the Repeat Change dialog box and create a recurring appointment.

Status. This tracks appointment status. Once the appointment is made you can right-click on the appointment and select from the following: Unconfirmed, Confirmed, Checked In, Missed, Cancelled, Being Seen, Checked Out, and Reschedule. If you select Cancelled, the appointment is removed from the grid and any superbill attached to the appointment will also be deleted. The superbill number will be released and re-assigned.

Need Referral. Select this box if this appointment needs a referral.

Enter Copay. Enter copays through a deposit entry window. Also, create a copayment in the main Office Hours window by right-clicking the grid and selecting Enter Copay.

Balance. Check the balance of the patient's account.

PROCEDURE 3.5 ENTERING AN APPOINTMENT

1. In the Provider List box located on the right end of the toolbar, click the code for *Daniel Walker* (if not already selected). The provider's name displays beside the selected code.
2. Use the buttons that display just below the calendar to find and click *March 1, 2010.*
3. In the appointment grid, double-click the *10:00 AM* time slot. The New Appointment Entry dialog box opens. Notice that the Length field defaults to the length shown in the appointment grid. The Date, Time, and Provider fields are automatically populated, based on your previous selections.
4. In the Chart field's list box, click the code for *Charles Weber.* Then press the *Enter* key. The patient's phone numbers display, as well as the newest case previously entered for this patient.
5. In the Resource field's list box, click *PROC1.* Procedure Room 1 displays beside the field.
6. Leave the Note field blank, and leave the default value that displays in the Case field (Sore throat).
7. In the Reason field's list box, click *ACUTE.* Acute Symptoms displays beside the field.

8. The rest of the fields should be left alone. (Length should be 15, Color should be Silver, Date should be 3/1/2010, Time should be 10:00 AM, Provider should be Daniel Walker, and Status should be Unconfirmed.)
9. Click the *Save* button. The patient's name displays in the 10:00 AM time slot. In addition, information related to the patient and his appointment displays underneath the calendar.
10. Using the information provided in Table 3.1, schedule appointments for six more patients.
11. Leave Office Hours open for the next exercise.

TABLE 3.1 Scheduling Appointments for Six Patients

	William O'Connor	Cindy Wixen	Ronald Baxter	Jerry Silversmith	Peter Portman	Carlos Hernandez
Resource Code	PROC1	PROC2	PROC1	LAB	PROC2	PROC1
Case	Blood pressure recheck	Ankle sprain	Routine physical examination	Diabetic recheck	Earache	Sore throat
Reason Code	RECHECK	ACUTE	PHYS	RECHECK	ACUTE	ACUTE
Length	15 minutes	15 minutes	45 minutes	15 minutes	15 minutes	15 minutes
Date	3/1/2010	3/1/2010	3/1/2010	3/1/2010	3/1/2010	3/1/2010
Time	11:00 AM	10:00 AM	1:00 PM	3:30 PM	11:00 AM	10:30 AM
Provider	Daniel Berg	Roman Jagla	Emily Luther	Daniel Walker	Daniel Walker	Daniel Walker

Locating Available Time Slots

Many times, a patient will call the medical office asking to schedule an appointment on a particular day of the week or during a certain time of day. An easy way to locate available time slots in a provider's schedule is to access the Find Open Time dialog box (Figure 3.10). In this dialog box, you can specify search criteria such as the length of time required for the appointment, the start and end times, the desired day(s) of the week, and the reason (the codes you enter into the reason code list).

Another option includes searching in a specific provider's schedule versus all providers' schedules.

PROCEDURE 3.6 LOCATING AN AVAILABLE TIME SLOT

Cindy Wixen needs to schedule an appointment with Dr. Jagla. The best times for Cindy are on a Thursday or Friday during lunchtime, between 12:00 PM and 1:30 PM.

1. In the Office Hours window, click *Roman Jagla* in the Provider List box located on the toolbar.
2. Click *3/1/2010* on the calendar.
3. On the Edit menu, click *Find Open Time*. The Find Open Time dialog box displays.
4. In the Length field, leave the default value of *15*.
5. Change the Start Time field to *12:00 PM*.
6. Change the End Time field to *1:30 PM*.
7. Under Day of Week, click the *Thu* and *Fri* check boxes to select them.
8. Click the *Search* button. The next available time slot in Dr. Jagla's schedule that meets the search criteria, is selected (12:00 PM on Thursday, March 4).
9. Schedule an appointment in the selected time slot using the Resource code PROC1 and Reason Code FOLLOW. Associate the appointment with the ankle sprain case that is already set up in the system.
10. Leave Office Hours open for the next exercise.

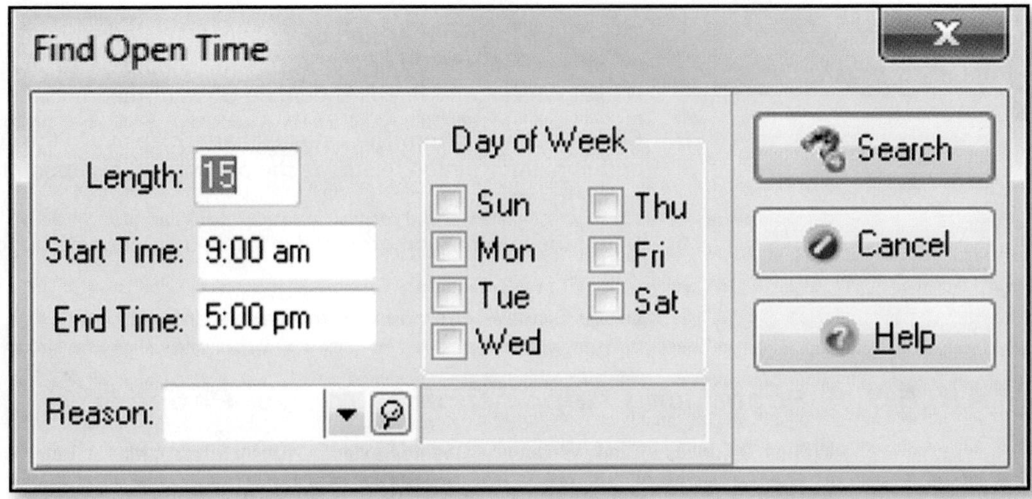

Figure 3.10
Find Open Time dialog box.

Finding and Editing Existing Appointments

Sometimes the information pertaining to an existing appointment needs to be changed. If you know the provider and the date of the appointment, first select them in the Office Hours window. Then, open the appointment record by double-clicking the time slot in the appointment grid where the patient's name displays. If you are unsure of the date, you can use the Appointment List dialog box (Figure 3.11) to search for an existing appointment and then edit it.

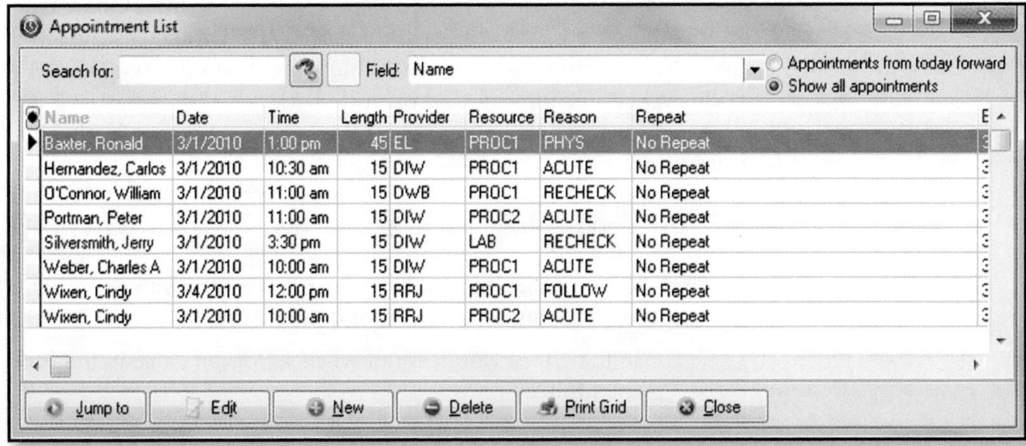

Name	Date	Time	Length	Provider	Resource	Reason	Repeat
Baxter, Ronald	3/1/2010	1:00 pm	45	EL	PROC1	PHYS	No Repeat
Hernandez, Carlos	3/1/2010	10:30 am	15	DIW	PROC1	ACUTE	No Repeat
O'Connor, William	3/1/2010	11:00 am	15	DWB	PROC1	RECHECK	No Repeat
Portman, Peter	3/1/2010	11:00 am	15	DIW	PROC2	ACUTE	No Repeat
Silversmith, Jerry	3/1/2010	3:30 pm	15	DIW	LAB	RECHECK	No Repeat
Weber, Charles A	3/1/2010	10:00 am	15	DIW	PROC1	ACUTE	No Repeat
Wixen, Cindy	3/4/2010	12:00 pm	15	RRJ	PROC1	FOLLOW	No Repeat
Wixen, Cindy	3/1/2010	10:00 am	15	RRJ	PROC2	ACUTE	No Repeat

Figure 3.11
Appointment List dialog box.

PROCEDURE 3.7 FINDING AND EDITING AN EXISTING APPOINTMENT

Cindy Wixen calls to verify the date and time of her follow-up appointment with Dr. Jagla. She also requests some extra time with Dr. Jagla to discuss alternative pain medications and physical therapy options.

1. Make sure that Dr. Jagla is the selected provider in the Office Hours window.
2. On the Lists menu, click *Appointment List*. The Appointment List dialog box opens.
3. In the upper-right corner of the dialog box, click the radio button *Show all appointments*. All appointments currently scheduled display in the Appointment List window.

4. Click the first button—*Locate* button—beside the Search for field. The Locate Appointment dialog box displays.
5. In the Field Value field, key *Wixen*.
6. Verify that *Name* is the value displayed under Fields.
7. Click the *First* button. The first record with the name Wixen is highlighted in the Appointment List window.
8. Click the next row in the window for Cindy Wixen with the 3/4/2010 date. Then, click the *Edit* button to access that appointment. The Edit Appointment dialog box displays.
9. Change the value in the Length field from 15 minutes to *30* minutes.
10. Click *Save* to close the Edit Appointment dialog box.
11. Click *Close* to close the Appointment List dialog box, but leave Office Hours open.

Creating Repeating Appointments

Many medical offices have patients that need to come in for blood tests or other lab work on a weekly or monthly basis. Patients generally find that coming in at routine times makes it easier to remember appointments. For example, Office Hours allows you to schedule repeating appointments on the same day of the week and the same time of day.

PROCEDURE 3.8 CREATING REPEATING APPOINTMENTS

In this exercise, you will schedule Mr. Silversmith for a repeating, 15-minute appointment for a blood glucose test.

1. In the main Office Hours window, select *Daniel Walker* as the provider and click *3/8/2010* in the calendar.
2. Double-click the *4:15 PM* time slot. The New Appointment Entry dialog box opens.
3. Click Mr. Silversmith's name in the Chart field's list box.
4. In the Resource field's list box, click *LAB*.
5. In the Reason field's list box, click *RECHECK*.
6. Verify that the appointment time length is 15 minutes, the date is 3/8/2010, the time is 4:15 PM, and the provider is Daniel Walker.
7. Click the *Change* button to open the Repeat Change dialog box.
8. Click the *Weekly* radio button in the Frequency column.
9. Leave the following default values unchanged: *1* in the Every Week(s) field, and the *M* (Monday) checkbox selected.
10. Click the down arrow beside the End on field to display a calendar. Then, click *3/29/2010*.
11. Click *OK*, and then click *Save*.

Rescheduling Appointments

Often patients discover that they are unable to keep a scheduled appointment and want to reschedule their appointment for a different time or on a different day. Rescheduling appointments is easily done by cutting and pasting entries in the appointment grid. You can also double-click an appointment in the grid to open the Edit Appointment dialog box and change the value in the Date field.

Another Way

After selecting a time slot, instead of using the Cut and Paste options on the Edit menu, you can right-click the appointment. This action displays a pop-up menu with the same Cut and Paste options.

PROCEDURE 3.9 RESCHEDULING APPOINTMENTS

1. Click *3/1/2010* in the calendar.
2. Locate and click the time slot where William O'Connor's name appears in Dr. Berg's schedule.
3. On the Edit menu, click *Cut.*
4. In the calendar, click the new appointment date of *3/3/2010.*
5. Click the new appointment time of *3:30 PM.*
6. On the Edit menu, click *Paste.* The appointment is moved from the original date and time to the new date and time.
7. Using similar steps as before, reschedule Ronald Baxter's appointment with Emily Luther, from 3/1/2010 at 1:00 PM to *3/5/2010* at *9:00 AM.* When finished, leave the Office Hours window open.

REPORTS AND FORMS IN OFFICE HOURS

On the Lists menu and Reports menu, a variety of reports and forms are available to print. One example is the Appointment List, which displays all the appointments for a specified time period. Individual pages are printed for each provider you select.

Printing Schedules

Printing provider schedules should be done each day at the beginning of the day, or prior to closing the medical office the previous night. The Appointment List is useful not only for the medical office assistants who may use it for patient check-in purposes, but also for the providers and medical staff who use it to manage their day-to-day activities. To print this report, the Appointment List option is clicked on the Reports menu.

As with other reports, the program gives you the choice of previewing the report on the computer screen, printing the report on a printer, or exporting the report to a file. You can also print a report for appointments that need a referral. This allows you to follow-up and make sure the necessary requirements have been met. After selecting one of these options and clicking the Start button, the Data Selection dialog box opens (Figure 3.12). Here, you can choose to print the report for just one provider or a range of providers. You can also select one day or a time period. If both Dates fields are blank, all appointments will be included on the report (up to 5 years old). Likewise, if both Providers fields are left blank, all of the providers' schedules will be printed. If the Print Blank Appointments checkbox is selected, any unassigned time slots will also be listed on the report.

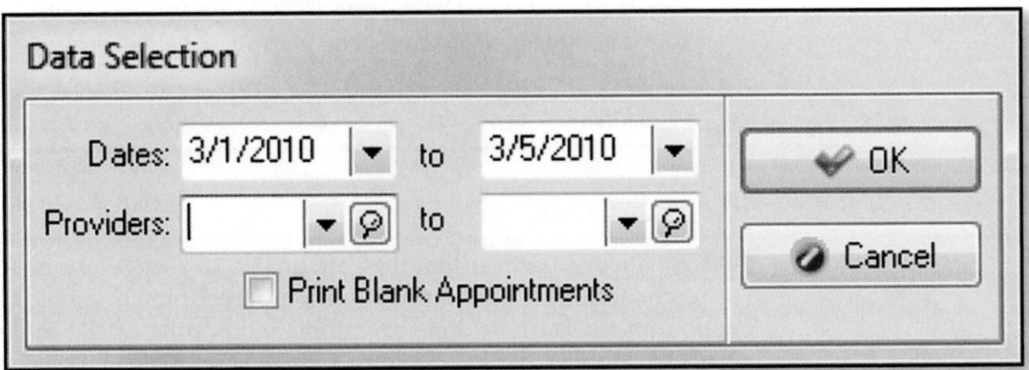

Figure 3.12 Data Selection dialog box when printing the Appointment List.

PROCEDURE 3.10 PRINTING THE APPOINTMENT LIST

1. On the Reports menu, click *Appointment List.* The Report Setup dialog box opens.
2. Click the radio button for *Print the report on the printer.*
3. Click the *Start* button. The Data Selection dialog box displays.
4. Enter *3/1/2010* to *3/5/2010* in the Dates fields.
5. Leave the Providers fields blank, and leave the Print Blank Appointments field unchecked.
6. Click *OK*, select a printer, and hand in the report to your instructor.
7. Leave Office Hours open for the next exercise.

Printing Superbills

You can print a superbill for each patient for whom you schedule an appointment. Remember, a superbill includes a list of procedures that may be performed by a provider, along with a list of possible, correlating diagnoses. A superbill printed in Office Hours also includes the patient's name, chart number, and appointment time. As such, superbills serve as worksheets for providers and are also used by office assistants when billing insurance companies for services rendered.

A superbill is often not printed until the patient checks in for his or her appointment. This is because the patient may not show up for the appointment. Or some of the patient's information may have changed and may need to be corrected before printing the superbill. However, some medical offices may choose to print the superbills for the current day's appointments all at one time.

You should *never* reprint superbills because each one has its own serial number. Reprinting superbills will cause the system to put new serial numbers on the forms, resulting in duplicate superbills for the same appointment. Duplicate superbills can cause problems when later entering transactions in Medisoft. Duplicates also make it difficult to track data accurately for reports.

To print superbills, the Print Superbills option on the Reports menu is clicked. This action causes the Open Report dialog box to display (Figure 3.13). Clicking the Superbills

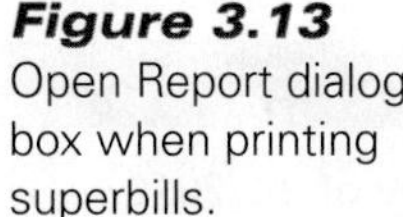

Figure 3.13 Open Report dialog box when printing superbills.

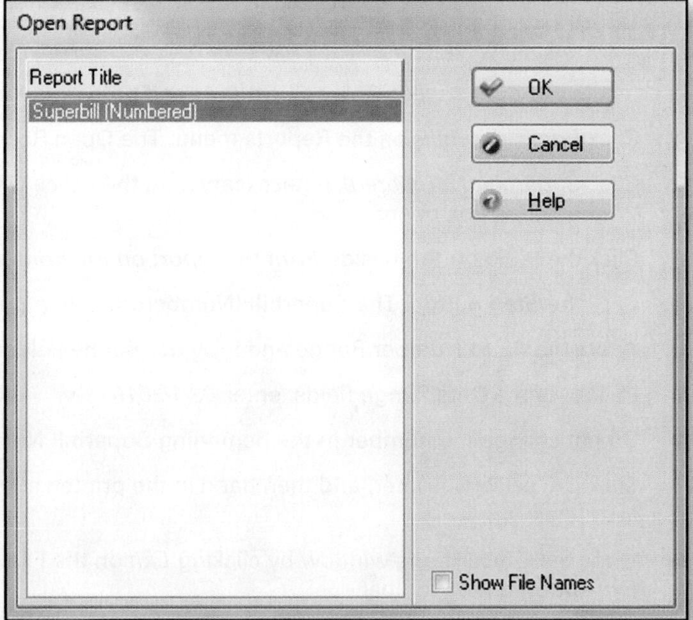

(Numbered) option and then clicking the OK button opens the Print Report Where dialog box. Normally, superbills should be printed on a printer (although you can preview on the computer screen and then print them directly from the Preview Report window).

Clicking the Start button in the Print Report Where dialog box causes the Superbill (Numbered) dialog box to open (Figure 3.14). It contains the following fields used to specify the desired data:

Chart Number Range. Click the chart number in this field's list boxes to select the first patient and the ending patient. To print a superbill for only one patient, select the same patient in both boxes.

Date Range. Enter the same date in both fields to print superbills for 1 day only. Or, enter beginning and end dates.

Provider Range. Click the same provider code in both list boxes, or select a range of providers.

Beginning Superbill Number. Medisoft automatically displays the next sequential number each time you print one or more superbills.

A quick way to print a superbill for one appointment is to right-click the specific appointment in the appointment grid. This causes a pop-up menu to display where you can click the Print Superbill option.

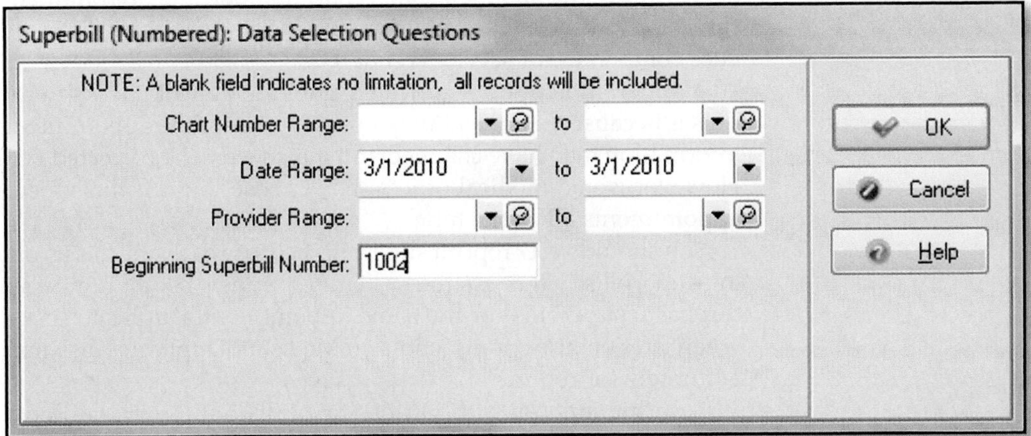

Figure 3.14
Superbill (Numbered) dialog box.

PROCEDURE 3.11 PRINTING SUPERBILLS

You are going to print superbills for all patients and providers for the day of 3/1/2010.

1. Click *Print Superbills* on the Reports menu. The Open Report dialog box displays.
2. Click *Superbill (Numbered)*, if necessary, and then click *OK*. The Print Report Where dialog box opens.
3. Click the radio button beside *Print the report on the printer.*
4. Click the *Start* button. The Superbill (Numbered) dialog box opens.
5. Leave the Chart Number Range and Provider Range fields blank.
6. In both of the Date Range fields, enter *03/1/2010.*
7. Do not change the number in the Beginning Superbill Number field.
8. Click *OK*, select a printer, and then hand in the printed superbills to your instructor.
9. Close the Office Hours window by clicking *Exit* on the File menu or by clicking the *Exit* button on the toolbar.

Using Terminology

Match the terms on the left with the definitions on the right.

_____ **1.** no-show
_____ **2.** cluster scheduling
_____ **3.** consultation appointment
_____ **4.** double-booking
_____ **5.** emergency appointment
_____ **6.** modified wave scheduling
_____ **7.** new patient appointment
_____ **8.** triage
_____ **9.** open office hours
_____ **10.** physical
_____ **11.** preoperative appointment
_____ **12.** resource
_____ **13.** routine appointment
_____ **14.** scheduling matrix
_____ **15.** stream scheduling
_____ **16.** time study
_____ **17.** walk-in
_____ **18.** wave scheduling

a. Process of prioritizing patients according to the severity of their conditions

b. Method in which patients are scheduled at regular intervals within a given hour

c. Method that schedules similar procedures together at the same time or same day of the week

d. Item in Office Hours, such as a room or piece of equipment, that can be associated with a particular patient's appointment or provider's activity

e. Office visit in which a patient or provider seeks the advice or opinion of another provider

f. Office visit requested by a patient that requires a quick response from the medical office staff and takes priority over other appointments

g. Office visit scheduled for someone being seen at the practice for the first time

h. Scheduling two patients in the same time slot for the same provider

i. Patient who does not show up for a scheduled appointment

j. Scheduling system in which patients are seen in the order they arrive at the medical office, with the exception that patients with a serious or life-threatening condition will be given priority

k. Routine examination to determine a patient's overall health

l. Data collected during a certain period to determine whether changes should be made to a system in current use

m. Pattern of working and nonworking hours for the medical office

n. Method in which a group of patients is scheduled at the top of the hour and seen in the order of arrival

o. Method in which each patient is scheduled in a predetermined time slot based on status and need; sometimes referred to as *individual scheduling*

p. Patient who arrives at the medical office without an appointment

q. Office visit scheduled for a patient prior to surgery

r. Office visit scheduled for an established patient to follow-up a previous diagnosis or treat new acute symptoms

Checking Your Understanding

1. When an emergency appointment is requested, what steps should the medical office staff take?
2. List the typical tasks performed before, during, and at the end of a patient's appointment.
3. How is a scheduling matrix helpful?
4. Explain the difference between wave scheduling and modified wave scheduling.
5. Name three of the defaults you can change in the Program Options dialog box, and explain how they affect the Office Hours program.
6. List the steps to schedule an appointment for a patient.
7. Explain one of the methods used to locate a patient's appointment quickly.
8. How do you create repeating appointments?
9. When rescheduling, how do you move an appointment from one time slot to another?
10. Explain why you should never reprint superbills.

Putting It into Practice

You will now enter information for seven more patients and create appointments for them. Perform the following steps:

1. Use the registration forms in Figures C.8 through C.14 in Appendix C and the case references in Table 3.2, to add seven patients and cases in the Medisoft program. Refer to Chapters 1 and 2, if needed. Dr. Berg is the assigned provider for all seven patients. No copayments are required by their insurance policies.
2. Use Office Hours and the information in Table 3.2 to schedule appointments for the seven new patients.
3. Print superbills for all patients and providers for the date of 03/02/2010.
4. Print an Appointment List for 03/02/2010 for Dr. Berg.
5. Before exiting Medisoft, backup your data as designated by your instructor.

TABLE 3.2 Scheduling Appointments for Seven Patients

	Ashuri Lee	Tonya McWilliams	Tim Butler	Carinna Grant	Vince Grant	Debbie Grant	Sammy Grant
Resource Code	PROC1	PROC2	PROC1	PROC2	PROC1	PROC2	PROC1
Case	Dermatitis	Swollen eye	Sore throat	Pink eye	Cold	Sore throat	Pink eye
Reason Code	ACUTE	ACUTE	ACUTE	ACUTE	ACUTE	ACUTE	ACUTE
Length	15 minutes	15 minutes	15 minutes	15 minutes	15 minutes	15 minutes	15 minutes
Date	3/2/2010	3/2/2010	3/2/2010	3/2/2010	3/2/2010	3/2/2010	3/2/2010
Time	9:00 AM	9:15 AM	9:30 AM	9:45 AM	10:00 AM	10:15 AM	10:30 AM
Provider	D. Berg	D. Berg	D. Berg	D. Berg	D. Berg	D. Berg	D. Berg

References

Adams DM: *Diagnosis: documentation and coding,* New York, 1997, McGraw Hill.
Flight M: *Law, liability, and ethics for medical office procedures,* ed 3, Albany, NY, 1998, Delmar.
Fordney MT: *Insurance handbook for the medical office,* ed 6, Philadelphia, 1999, Saunders–Elsevier.
HealthCare Consultants of America: Healthcare fraud and abuse, Augusta, Ga, 1997, The Consultants.
Holmes DL: *Practical guide to medical billing,* Springfield, Ill, 1997, US Department of Commerce.
Kuehn L: *Health information management: medical records process in group practice,* Englewood, Colo, 1997, Center for Research in Ambulatory Health Care Administration.
Moini J: *Glencoe medical assisting review: passing the CMA and RMA exams,* New York, 2001, Glencoe.
Redman B, editor: *Life and health insurance,* ed 4, Chicago, 1999, Dearborn Financial Institute.
Reid J: *A telemedicine primer: understanding the issues,* Billings, Mont, 1996, Artcraft Printers.
Rizzo C: *Uniform billing: a guide to claims processing,* Albany, NY, 2000, Delmar.
Ross A, Pavlock E, Williams S: *Ambulatory care management,* ed 3, Albany, NY, 1998, Delmar.
Rowell J: *Understanding health insurance: a guide to professional billing,* ed 5, Albany, NY, 2000, Delmar.

chapter 4

Medical Office Accounting Procedures

Objectives

1. Understand basic accounting principles and processes.
2. Explain how dates are used in Medisoft.
3. Enter charge transactions.
4. Enter and apply payments from patients.
5. Print walkout receipts.
6. Create, edit, and print insurance claims.
7. Enter and apply payments from insurance companies.
8. Print patient statements.
9. Print accounting reports, including day sheets, a practice analysis report, and patient ledgers.

Terminology

accounts payable: Money owed by a business for unpaid purchases

accounts receivable: Money owed to a business by others

accrual-basis accounting: Method in which revenues are recorded when services are performed and expenses are recorded when incurred, not when they are paid

assets: Items of value owned by a business

basic accounting equation: Formula that expresses how financial transactions affect a business (Assets = Liabilities + Owners' Equity)

cash-basis accounting: Method in which revenues and expenses are not recorded until they are actually paid

cash flow: Money coming into and going out of a business

cycle billing: System in which a portion of patient statements are prepared at regular time intervals throughout a month rather than all at once

day sheet: List of all transactions in chronological order for a given day or range of days

explanation of benefits (EOB): Report sent by an insurance carrier to a patient containing details on how benefits were paid

ledger: Report that shows a group of financial accounts with a detailed list of all the transactions related to each account

liabilities: Debts and other financial obligations of a business

once-a-month billing: System in which all patient statements are prepared once a month at the same time

owners' equity: Financial stake that the business owners, business partners, or shareholders have in a business

practice analysis: Report that shows the charges, payments, and adjustments made during a specified time period for procedures performed in a medical office

remittance advice (RA): Report sent from a payer to a practice, often electronically, showing how insurance benefits were paid for patients

statement: Document that shows the amount a patient owes to the medical office

The health care industry has changed significantly in the last 25 years. Computers play an important role in all aspects of the health care system, including financial record keeping. Although most medical offices today use computer programs to track their business transactions, it is still important to understand the main concepts on which all accounting systems are based.

BASIC ACCOUNTING PRINCIPLES

Although a medical office is in the business of helping people, its staff must still be mindful about keeping accurate and up-to-date financial records. Like other businesses, medical offices rely on accounting principles to determine **cash flow**—how much money is coming into and going out of the practice. Accounting is a system of recording all the business transactions made by the medical office and analyzing how those transactions affect the financial condition of the practice. The following **basic accounting equation** is the formula used in this process:

Assets = Liabilities + Owners' Equity

Assets are items of value owned by the medical office. Examples of assets include property (such as buildings and equipment), **accounts receivable**, (money owed to the practice by others for services rendered but not paid) and cash on hand. **Liabilities** are the debts and financial obligations of the medical office. Examples include bank loans, **accounts payable**, (money owed by the practice for unpaid purchases), taxes, and any staff wages (payroll) owed.

Owners' equity refers to the financial stake that the business owners, business partners, or shareholders have in the medical office. Normally, the owners' equity consists of the initial investment made to start the practice and the amount of profit or loss retained if the practice were sold today. Revenues (income) increase the owners' equity, and expenses decrease the owners' equity. There are two basic types of accounting systems used in medical offices. One method is **cash-basis accounting** in which revenues and expenses are not recorded until they are actually paid. The other method is **accrual-basis accounting**, in which revenues are recorded when services are performed, not when they are paid. Likewise, expenses are recorded when they are first incurred, not when they are paid.

For example, let us say that a physician performed a service for a patient in the month of March, but the practice was not paid for it by the insurance company until April. In cash-basis accounting, the revenue for the service performed would not be recorded until April when the payment was received. However, in accrual-basis accounting, the service would be recorded as income in March as an accounts receivable. Most offices use the accrual method.

Regardless of which accounting method is used, each transaction has a dual impact on the financial records. In other words, there is always a balancing effect for every transaction the medical office makes. Consider the following examples using accrual-basis accounting:

- The medical office buys some expensive equipment using credit. Assets (capital equipment) increase, but liabilities also increase because of the loan.
- The accrued electric bill is paid with cash from a checking account. The assets (cash) decrease, and the accounts payable liability also decreases.
- A patient pays an overdue charge. Assets equally increase and decrease. That is, cash increases and accounts receivable decreases.

Today, most medical offices use a computerized system to keep their financial records. Computer programs, such as Medisoft, provide a means to enter transactions and produce a variety of reports. Examples of these reports include the following:

- A **day sheet**, or daily journal, lists all transactions in chronological order for a given day or for a range of days.
- A **ledger** is a report that shows a group of financial accounts with a detailed list of all the transactions related to each account.
- Periodically, a **statement** is sent to each patient listing the amount owed to the medical office.
- A **practice analysis** is a report that shows the charges, payments, and adjustments made during a specified period for procedures performed in the medical office.

No matter what computer accounting program is used, the general concepts and skills you learn from using Medisoft can be transferred to other systems you may encounter.

HOW DATES ARE USED IN MEDISOFT

In any type of accounting system, manual or computerized, using accurate dates for financial transactions is critical. If dates are recorded incorrectly, then the reports and insurance claims based on that data will also be incorrect. To use Medisoft properly, it is important to understand how this program uses different types of dates.

Windows System Date

Computer operating systems, such as Microsoft Windows, have a system date. This date can be changed, although it is not normally necessary to do so. If your computer uses Windows Vista or Windows 7, you can click the time displayed in the bottom-right corner of the computer desktop. This action opens a pop-up calendar (Figure 4.1). If your computer uses Windows XP, you double-click the time, instead of clicking it once, to open the system date calendar. The calendar will look slightly different, depending on the version of Windows.

The Medisoft program uses the computer's system date to keep track of when you enter (create) financial transactions in Medisoft. In other words, Medisoft marks each medical charge or payment in its database with the date created.

Medisoft Program Date

The Medisoft program date appears in the bottom-right corner of the main Medisoft window. When Medisoft is opened, it automatically displays the same value for its program date as the Windows system date. So, if the system date is set to Mar. 2, 2010, the Medisoft program date will be the same.

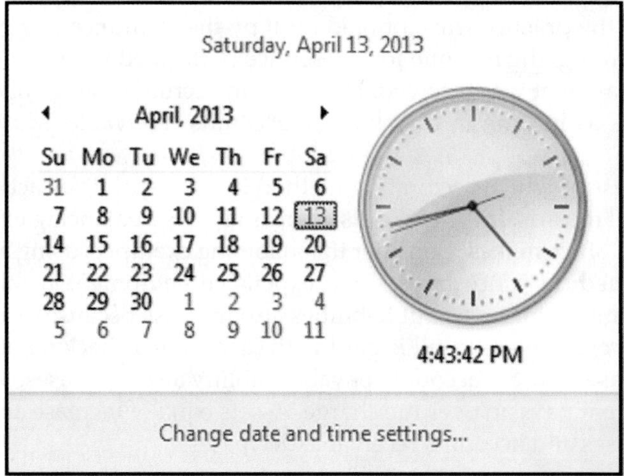

Figure 4.1
Windows system date.

Medisoft uses the program date as the default date in many of the software's dialog boxes. For example, in the Transaction Entry dialog box, you can accept the date that automatically displays when you enter transactions, or you can key a different date (Figure 4.2). It is important that you use the date when the transactions actually occurred. Otherwise, insurance claims and financial reports will be inaccurate. Think of a transaction date as the date of service because it represents when a medical service was performed or paid.

In a medical office setting, you may not be able to enter transactions into Medisoft on the same day they occur. For example, let us assume today is March 2, 2010 (Tuesday) and you have a large number of transactions that you need to enter into Medisoft that happened the previous day. To avoid having to change the default date multiple times in the Transaction Entry dialog box, you can temporarily change the Medisoft program date to March 1 before opening the dialog box. Then, after you finish entering the old transactions, you should change the Medisoft program date back to the current date (today).

The Medisoft program date is changed by clicking the date displayed in the bottom-right corner of the main Medisoft window, which opens a pop-up calendar (Figure 4.3).

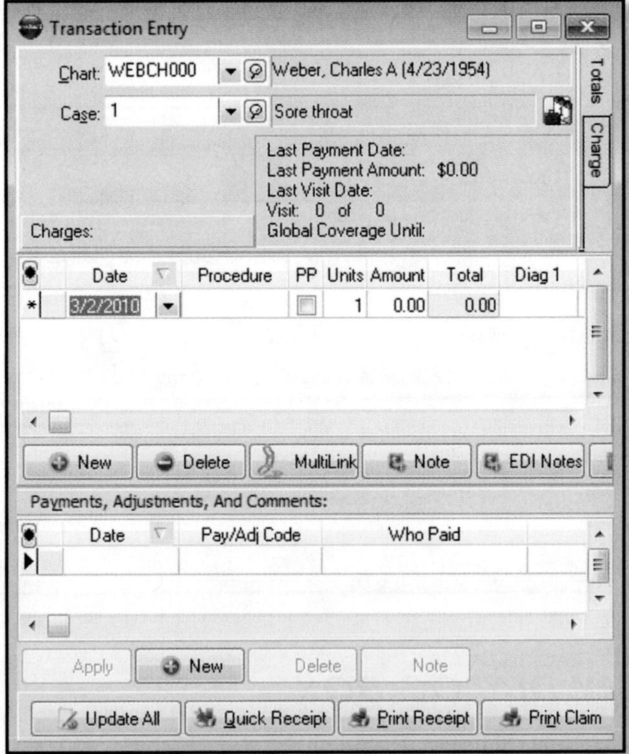

Figure 4.2
Portion of Transaction Entry dialog box showing Date fields.

Figure 4.3
Medisoft program date.

March, 2010

Sun	Mon	Tue	Wed	Thu	Fri	Sat
28	1	2	3	4	5	6
7	8	9	10	11	12	13
14	15	16	17	18	19	20
21	22	23	24	25	26	27
28	29	30	31	1	2	3
4	5	6	7	8	9	10

Today: 4/13/2013

You can click a different date or click Today to revert back to the current date. This calendar may look slightly different, depending on the version of Medisoft you are using.

To summarize, every Medisoft transaction has the following dates associated with it: (a) the date when you entered or created the transaction record in Medisoft (marked by Medisoft with the system date) and (b) the date when the transaction actually occurred (the date you used in the Transaction Entry dialog box)

Dates Used When Printing Reports

When printing reports in Medisoft, the program often displays a Search dialog box. A portion of one is shown in Figure 4.4. Look at the two sets of date range fields in Figure 4.4: Date Created and Date From. Date Created refers to the date when you entered or created the transactions in Medisoft (system date). Date From refers to the date when the transactions actually occurred—the date you used in the Transaction Entry dialog box (or Deposit dialog box). For the exercises in the textbook, it is best to leave the Date Created fields blank to force Medisoft to include all the system dates. If a default date automatically appears in a Date Created field, you can remove it by clicking the date to highlight it and then pressing the Delete key.

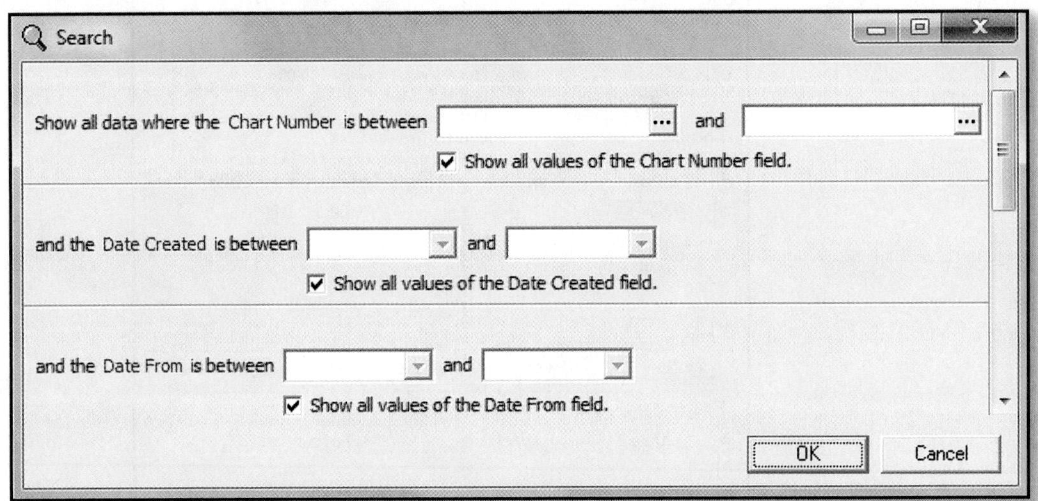

Figure 4.4
Date fields in a Search dialog box when printing reports.

TRANSACTION ENTRY DIALOG BOX

There are three types of transactions in Medisoft: (1) charges for services billed, (2) payments from patients and insurance carriers, and (3) adjustments. Charges entered in Medisoft stay active on ledger reports until they are paid. Transactions in Medisoft are usually tied to a specific case. As explained in Chapter 2, there are two main reasons for setting up a new case: when a patient is treated for a new and different condition and when a patient's insurance carrier changes.

The Transaction Entry dialog box (Figure 4.5) is used to enter all three types of transactions, so it is used often. You can open it by clicking the first button on the toolbar (far left) or by clicking Enter Transactions on the Activities menu. This dialog box has four main areas. The top area displays information about the specific patient and case combination you choose in the dialog box. The middle area, or Charges section, contains information about each charge associated with the selected patient and case. The next area below the Charges section is the Payment, Adjustments, and Comments section. At the bottom of the Transaction Entry dialog box is a row of buttons used to calculate totals, print receipts and claims, and save transactions. In addition, you can view statements for the patient. The View Statements button is part of BillFlash, an additional feature to which your clinic might subscribe.

Figure 4.5
Transaction Entry dialog box.

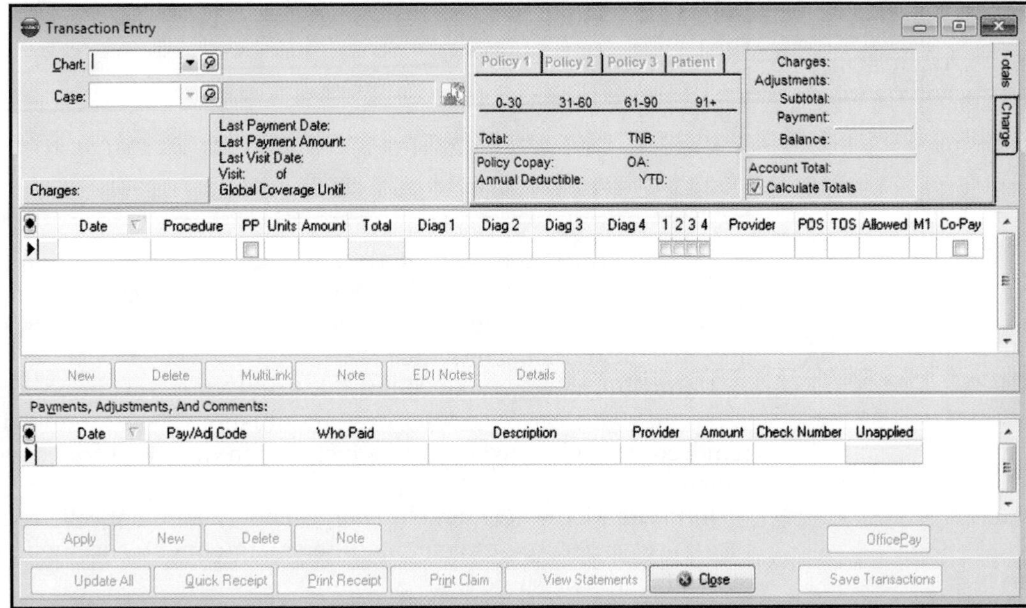

Patient and Account Information

After the Transaction Entry dialog box is opened, you must first select a patient by clicking a number in the Chart field's list box (upper-left corner of the dialog box). If the list of patients is long, you can type the first few letters of the patient's last name in the Chart field and then click the correct patient record in the list box. Next, the desired case in the Case field's list box should be clicked.

Just below and to the right of the Chart and Case fields, the system displays related patient, insurance, and account information (Figure 4.6). Down the right side of the dialog box are two tabs: Totals and Charge. Depending on which tab is clicked, the data displayed in the top area of the Transaction Entry dialog box will change.

Charge Transactions

Another Way
Before clicking the New button to enter a charge, you can change the Medisoft program date so that all charge entries default to the desired date. This will save data entry time if you have a lot of transactions to enter. Either click the date in the bottom-right corner of the main Medisoft window, or click Set Program Date on the File menu.

To enter a charge transaction, the New button at the bottom of the Charges section is clicked (Figure 4.7). The following fields are displayed in a column or grid format:

Date. The Medisoft program date automatically displays in this field when the New button is clicked. If the service procedure you are entering was not performed on the date displayed, then you can change the date by keying over it or clicking the arrow beside the Date field and selecting a different date.

Procedure. Click the appropriate Current Procedural Terminology (CPT) code in this field's list box. A code may be located faster by keying the first few digits in the field. If the desired code is not listed, you can add it by pressing the F8 key. Only one procedure code can be entered per line. If multiple procedures were performed during a visit, each one will require a separate line entry. The exception to this rule is a MultiLink code, which is a group of procedure codes associated with one particular activity.

Figure 4.6
Top section of the Transaction Entry dialog box.

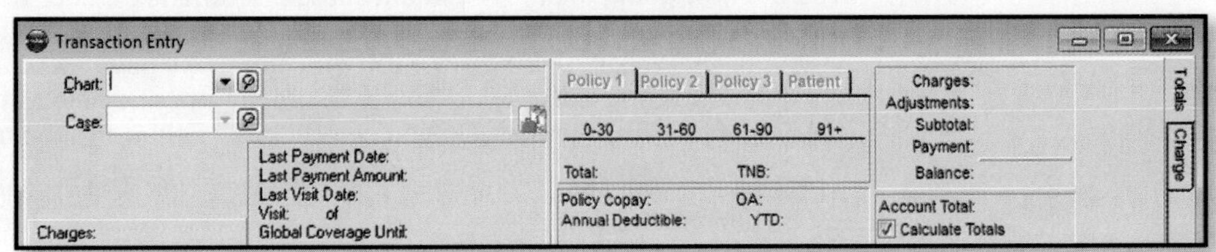

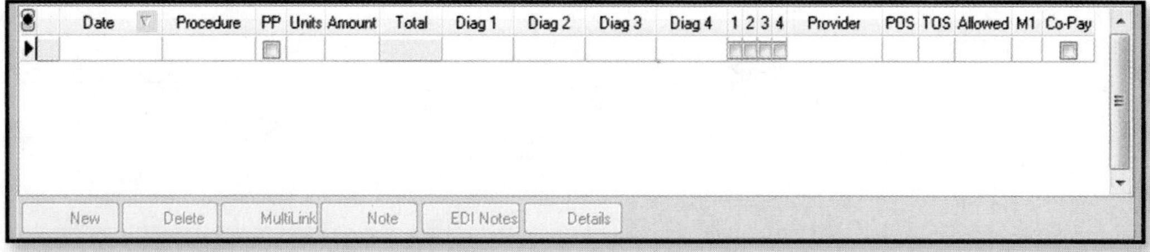

Figure 4.7 Charges section of the Transaction Entry dialog box.

PP. The Principle Procedure (PP) only displays if the option to suppress UB-04 fields is unchecked in the Program Options dialog box (accessed on the File menu). The UB-04 claim form is a special type of insurance form used by hospitals, skilled nursing facilities, and other institutional providers.

Units. Enter the number of times the procedure was performed. Typically, the unit is 1, but the value can be greater in some situations. For example, if four skin lesions were removed but only one lesion was included in the CPT code, a value of 4 units would be entered.

Amount. Medisoft enters the charge amount automatically based on the CPT code and insurance carrier. You can enter a different amount by clicking in the field and keying the amount.

Total. The total is calculated by the system, which multiplies the number of units by the amount.

Diag 1 to Diag 4. Medisoft allows you to enter up to four diagnosis codes, unless the quantity is increased using the Program Options dialog box.

1, 2, 3, and 4. These fields relate to the preceding diagnosis codes. Click the checkbox for each diagnosis that relates to the procedure performed. For example, if diagnoses 1 and 3 are related to the procedure, then click checkboxes 1 and 3 to select them.

Provider. The system automatically displays the patient's assigned provider in this field. If the patient was seen by another provider, then select that provider from the list box.

POS. This field is used for the Place of Service (POS) code, which represents where the procedure was performed. When this field is clicked, Medisoft enters a default code (which can be changed by keying a different value). All exercises in this textbook will use 11 to indicate Provider's Office.

TOS. A Type of Service (TOS) code is used to define the kind of service provided if the insurance carrier requires it. Default TOS codes can be set up in the Procedure/Payment/Adjustment dialog box. (Refer to Chapter 2 for more details.)

Allowed. The value in this field is the amount that the insurance carrier allows for the procedure. Allowed amounts can be entered in the Procedure/Payment/Adjustment dialog box when procedure and payment codes are initially set up in the system. However, keep in mind that an allowed amount may not be applicable, depending on the insurance carrier.

M1. This field is used to enter the modifier (if necessary) for the procedure code.

Co-Pay. If the code in the Procedure field requires a copayment, this checkbox should be check marked. (When setting up a code in the Procedure/Payment/Adjustment dialog box, you can click the Require Co-Pay checkbox in the General tab. This will cause Medisoft to display a checkmark in the Co-Pay field automatically when a charge associated with that procedure code is entered.)

PROCEDURE 4.1 ENTERING CHARGES FOR A PATIENT

You are now going to enter a patient charge for Charles Weber who was seen for a sore throat. The encounter form shown in **Figure C.15 in Appendix C** lists the charges for a visit with Dr. Walker on 3/1/2010. Each procedure will have a separate line charge, but the diagnosis code will stay the same. To move from one field to the next, you can press the Tab key or the Enter key. Or, you can click in a field using the mouse.

1. On the Activities menu, click *Enter Transactions.* The Transaction Entry dialog box opens.

2. In the Chart field's list box, click the code for *Charles Weber.* (Remember, to find a code in the list box quickly, you can key the first two or three letters of the patient's last name in the field.)
3. In the Case field's list box, click the case number associated with *Sore throat,* if not already selected. Information related to the chosen patient and case displays in the upper area of the Transaction Entry dialog box.
4. In the Charges area of the Transaction Entry dialog box, click the *New* button.
5. In the Date field, change the value to *3/1/2010.*
6. In the Procedure field, key *99213* (Office visit est pt, level 3), or click the number in the field's list box.
7. Press the *Tab* key or *Enter* key. The amount on file for the procedure ($48.00) automatically displays in the Amount field. Medisoft multiplies this amount by the number in the Units field (1) and displays the result in the Total field.
8. Leave the PP field unchecked, and leave the default value of *1* in the Units field.
9. In the Diag 1 field's list box, key *034.0* (Streptococcal sore throat), or click the number in the field's list box.
10. Press the *Tab* or *Enter* key. The 1 checkbox is automatically marked by the system. The Provider field should display the code *DIW,* and the POS field should display the code *11.*
11. Click the *Co-pay* checkbox to select it. Leave the rest of the fields blank or unchanged.
12. Click the *New* button in the Charges section of the dialog box. A second charge line displays. Some of the fields in the second charge line display the same values you entered in the first charge line.
13. In the Procedure field, key *87880* (Detection, Streptococcus A), or click the number in the field's list box.
14. Press the *Tab* or *Enter* key. The amount on file ($20.00) automatically displays. The screen should look similar to Figure 4.8 on the following page.
15. Click the *Save Transactions* button in the lower-right corner of the Transaction Entry dialog box. An Information box displays, warning you that this case requires a $20 copayment.
16. Click *OK.* (A payment amount will be entered during an exercise later in this chapter. Of course, in a real-life setting, copayments should only be entered in the system if they are actually received.) Notice that Medisoft updated the totals in the upper-right corner of the Transaction entry dialog box.
17. At the bottom of the dialog box, click the *Close* button.

PROCEDURE 4.2 ENTERING CHARGES FOR MULTIPLE PATIENTS

Using what you learned in the previous procedure, enter the following patient charges into the computer, making sure to save all your entries/changes. However, leave the Co-pay checkbox *un*checked for all charge entries.

1. Refer to the encounter form in **Figure C.16 in Appendix C** for William O'Connor. Enter a charge for the 3/3/2010 office visit with Dr. Berg to recheck his blood pressure.
2. Daniel Smith is a new patient. Carter Smith, his father and the guarantor, wants Daniel to have a routine physical examination. Use the patient registration

and encounter forms in **Figures C.17** and **C.18 in Appendix C** to complete the following steps:

a. Enter the guarantor Information first, the patient Information next, and finally, the case information into the system. Katherine Olsson is the assigned provider.

b. Schedule the patient for a 45-minute appointment on 3/3/2010 at 10:00 AM. Resource will be PROC1 and Reason will be PHYS.

c. Enter charges for the procedures performed on 3/3/2010: the office visit and a general health panel.

3. When finished entering and saving data, close the Transaction Entry dialog box.

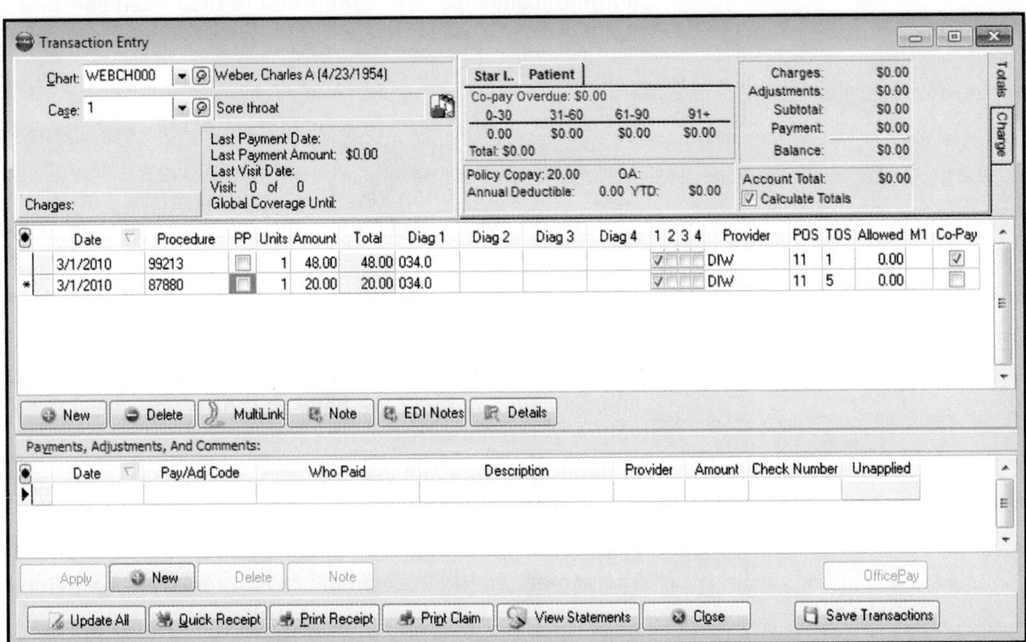

Figure 4.8 Completed charges for Mr. Weber.

To make changes to a saved charge transaction, the line that needs to be changed is first clicked to select it. Then you can make corrections to the existing charge. You can also enter additional charges for a particular case, if necessary. If a charge should not have been entered at all and needs to be deleted, you can click the appropriate line item to select the charge and then click the Delete button. However, be sure to use caution when deleting transactions because deleted data cannot be recovered. The following procedure provides steps for correcting data within the Transaction Entry dialog box.

PROCEDURE 4.3 CORRECTING TRANSACTION DATA

When the data for Daniel Smith was originally entered for his 3/3/10 visit (see Procedure 4.2), he was not charged for a handling fee for the use of an outside laboratory.

1. Open the Transaction Entry dialog box.
2. Select the chart and case numbers for Daniel Smith.
3. In the Charges area, click the *New* button.
4. Add a transaction for the procedure (99000) with the same diagnosis code used for the previous entries (V70.0).
5. Save the transaction, and close the dialog box.

Payment and Adjustment Transactions

Payments for services rendered come from two basic sources: patients or guarantors and insurance companies. There are two main ways to enter payment transactions in Medisoft: (1) in the Transaction Entry dialog box (Payments, Adjustments, and Comments area); and (2) in the Deposits dialog box (discussed later in this chapter).

If a patient makes a payment or copayment at the time of the office visit, that amount is usually entered in the Transaction Entry dialog box after the charges have been entered. If adjustments need to be made later on because of an overcharge or undercharge, those transactions can also be entered in the Transaction Entry dialog box. Following are the fields in the Payments, Adjustments, and Comments area of this dialog box as shown in Figure 4.9:

Date. The current date (Medisoft program date) is automatically entered by the system when the New button is clicked. If this date is different from the actual date when the payment was received, then change it by keying over the date or clicking the arrow beside the date field and selecting a different date.

Pay/Adj Code. Click the appropriate Payment/Adjustment code in the list box. (These codes were entered in Chapter 2.) If a new code needs to be entered, press the F8 key to open the Procedure/Payment/Adjustment dialog box.

Who Paid. This field is used to indicate who made the payment (patient, guarantor, or insurance carrier). After you enter a value in the Pay/Adj Code field and press the Tab or Enter key, Medisoft automatically displays the name stored in the patient's record. If necessary, a different name can be clicked in the Who Paid list box.

Description. If desired, additional information about the payment can be entered in this field.

Provider. Medisoft automatically displays the provider code in this field.

Amount. Enter the total amount paid. Medisoft will automatically subtract the payment amount entered from the charges.

Check Number. If a check was used to make the payment, enter the check number in this field.

Unapplied. This field shows the amount of money that has not yet been applied to the charge. (Applying payments is covered later in this chapter.)

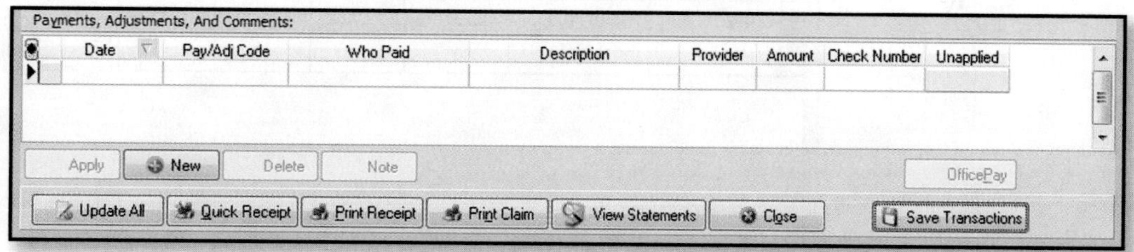

Figure 4.9 Payments, Adjustments, and Comments section of the Transaction Entry dialog box.

PROCEDURE 4.4 ENTERING A PATIENT PAYMENT

At the time of his visit on 3/1/2010 (for a sore throat), Charles Weber made a $20 copayment with a check. In this procedure, you will enter that transaction.

1. Open the Transaction Entry dialog box.
2. Select the chart and case numbers for Mr. Weber.
3. In the Payments, Adjustments, and Comments area, click the *New* button.
4. In the Date field, change the date to *3/1/2010.*
5. In the Pay/Adj field's list box, click *CHKCOPAY.* Then, press the *Tab* key or the *Enter* key. Mr. Weber's name appears in the Who Paid field, and DIW (the code for Dr. Walker) appears in the Provider field.

6. Leave Description field blank.
7. In the Amount field, key *20.00.* Then press *Tab* or *Enter.* The amount of $20 displays in the Unapplied field.
8. In the Check Number field, key *6723.*
9. Click the *Save Transactions* button. An Information box displays as a reminder about the required copayment.
10. Click *OK.* Notice that Medisoft updated the totals in the upper-right corner of the Transaction Entry dialog box.
11. Leave the Transaction Entry dialog box open for the next exercise.

After a payment transaction is entered, it needs to be applied to one or more charge transactions. You can choose to color-code payment transactions using the Program Options dialog box. For example, individual colors can be selected, or a set of default colors can be activated: red for unapplied payments, blue for partially applied payments, fuchsia (pink) for overapplied payments, and so on.

To apply payments, you must click the Apply button in the Payments, Adjustments, and Comments area of the Transaction Entry dialog box. This action opens the Apply Payment to Charges dialog box (Figure 4.10). In this dialog box, the Apply To Co-pay button is used to apply the payment to a required copayment amount. The Apply To Oldest button is used to apply the payment automatically to the oldest charge listed. Payment applications can also be made manually by keying amounts in the This Payment column for individual line items. The upper-right corner of this dialog box displays the unapplied amount for the current payment. As you apply the payment, the unapplied amount decreases.

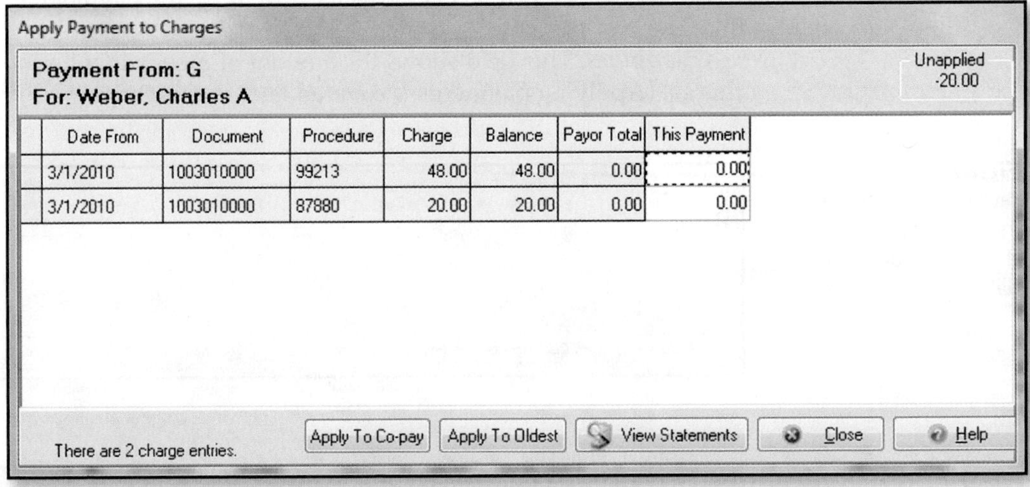

Figure 4.10
Apply Payments to Charges dialog box.

PROCEDURE 4.5 APPLYING A PATIENT'S PAYMENT

You will now apply the $20 copayment made by Mr. Weber. The Transaction Entry dialog box should still be open from the previous exercise (see Procedure 4.4).

1. In the Payments, Adjustments, and Comments area, click the *Apply* button. The Apply Payment to Charges dialog box opens.
2. Click the *Apply To* button. The $20.00 payment is applied to the procedure charge 99213, the Unapplied amount displayed in the upper-right corner changes to zero, and a pop-up message box displays with a message that this payment has been fully applied.

3. Click *OK* to close the pop-up message box. The Apply Payment to Charges dialog box should look like the one in Figure 4.11, with the exception of the tracking numbers in the Document column.
4. Click *Close* to close the Apply Payment to Charges dialog box. Notice that the Unapplied field is zero dollars.
5. Click the *Save Transactions* button, but do not close the Transaction Entry dialog box.

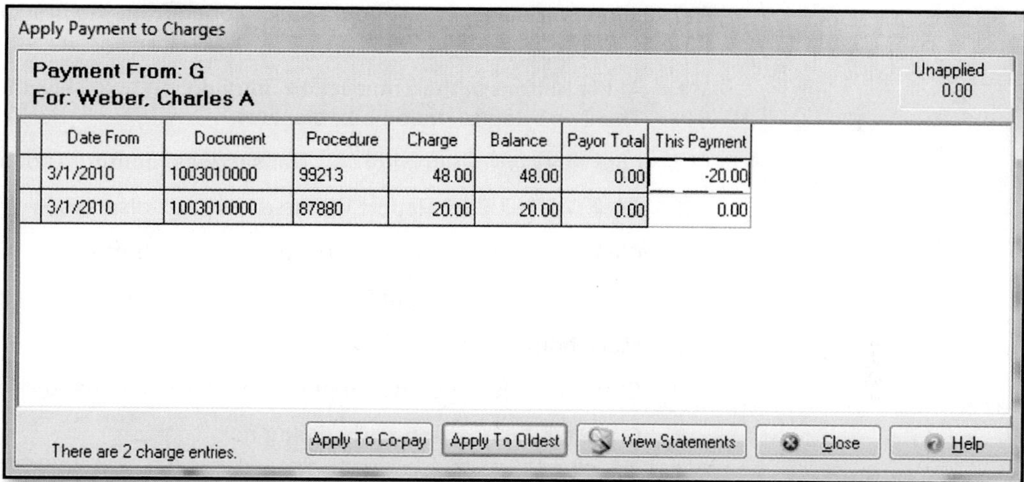

Figure 4.11
Mr. Weber's applied payment.

Walkout Receipts

If a patient makes a payment during an office visit and requests a receipt, a walkout receipt can be printed and given to the patient before he or she leaves. This task is easy to accomplish from the Transaction Entry dialog box, which has Quick Receipt and Print Receipt buttons at the bottom of the box. If the Quick Receipt button is clicked, then the system uses preferred user settings and skips some print options. If the Print Receipt button is clicked, several choices are displayed in the Open Report dialog box (Figure 4.12).

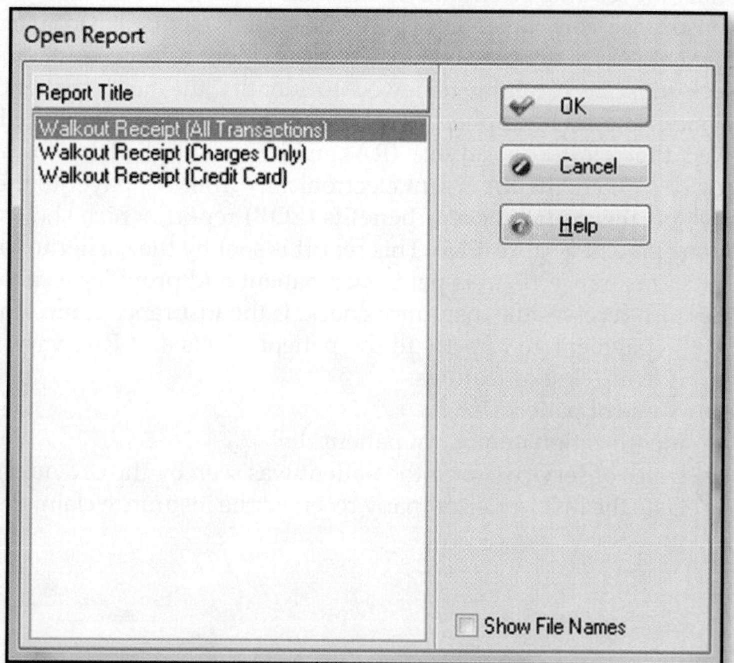

Figure 4.12
Open Report dialog box when printing a walkout receipt.

Walkout Receipt (All Transactions). This Walkout Receipt is the typical receipt printed because it lists all transactions (charges and payments).

Walkout Receipt (Charges Only). This Walkout Receipt lists only the charges to the patient for the day.

Walkout Receipt (Credit Card). This Walkout Receipt is similar to the All Transactions receipt but with the written authorization from the patient to bill his or her credit card.

PROCEDURE 4.6 PRINTING A WALKOUT RECEIPT

You will now print a receipt to give Mr. Weber for the $20 copayment he made. The Transaction Entry dialog box should still be open from the previous exercise (Procedure 4.5).

1. At the bottom of the Transaction Entry dialog box, click the *Print Receipt* button. The Open Report dialog box displays.
2. Click the *Walkout Receipt (All Transactions)* option, if not already selected.
3. Click *OK*. The Print Report Where dialog box displays.
4. Click the *Print the report on the printer* radio button.
5. Click *Start*. The Walkout Receipt (All Transactions) dialog box opens.
6. Make both dates *3/1/2010*.
7. Click *OK*. Select a printer to print the receipt, and hand it in to your instructor.
8. Close the Transaction Entry dialog box.

INSURANCE CLAIM MANAGEMENT

After entering charge transactions, health care claims must be generated and sent to insurance companies. Although claims can be printed on paper, most claims issued today are sent electronically. The CMS-1500 form displayed and described in Appendix B is the paper form approved by the National Uniform Claim Committee. This committee, led by the American Medical Association (AMA), decides the format and content of the CMS-1500 paper form and its electronic equivalent, the 837P. The 837P is the HIPAA standard format for sending electronic claims from providers to insurance carriers.

Insurance companies generally send their payments to a medical office as a batch payment versus separate checks for each patient or procedure. As a result, each insurance check must be carefully reviewed to identify the many patient accounts to which the payment should be applied. This process is usually accomplished by referring to a report called the **remittance advice (RA)**, which is supplied by the insurance carrier to the provider. Often, the RA is sent electronically from the payer to the practice. A variation of the RA is the **explanation of benefits (EOB)** report, which shows remittance information for one patient (Figure 4.13). This report is sent by the carrier to the patient.

If an insurance claim is paid, each patient and provider receives an EOB/RA. The provider also receives the insurance check. If the insurance claim was not assigned, the EOB and the payment go directly to the patient. EOBs and RAs vary, but they generally have the following similar features:

- Name of patient
- Identification number of patient
- Dates of service (when the patient was seen by the provider)
- Date the insurance company received the insurance claim and the date the claim was processed

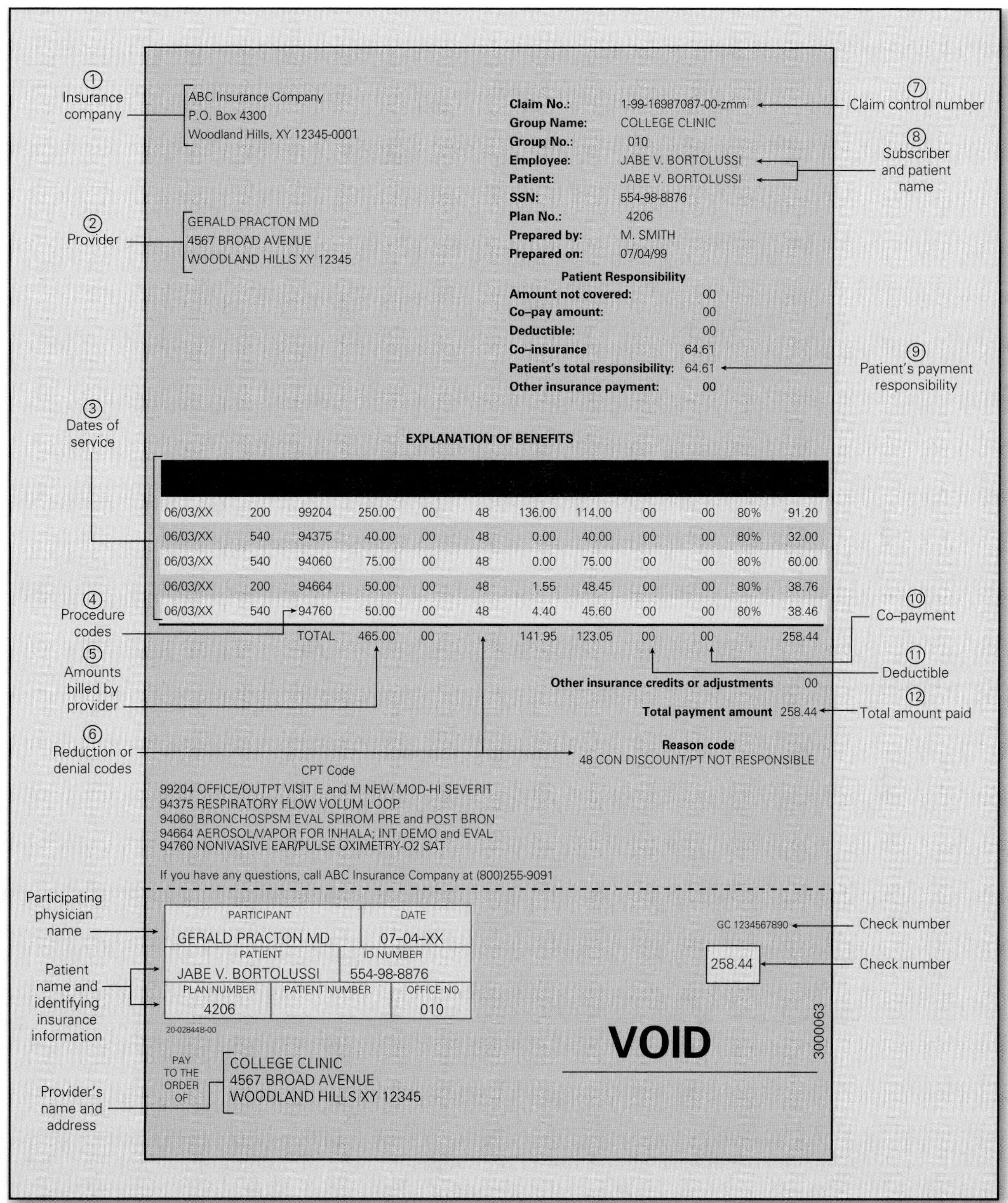

ABC Insurance Company
P.O. Box 4300
Woodland Hills, XY 12345-0001

Claim No.: 1-99-16987087-00-zmm
Group Name: COLLEGE CLINIC
Group No.: 010
Employee: JABE V. BORTOLUSSI
Patient: JABE V. BORTOLUSSI
SSN: 554-98-8876
Plan No.: 4206
Prepared by: M. SMITH
Prepared on: 07/04/99

GERALD PRACTON MD
4567 BROAD AVENUE
WOODLAND HILLS XY 12345

Patient Responsibility

Amount not covered: 00
Co-pay amount: 00
Deductible: 00
Co-insurance 64.61
Patient's total responsibility: 64.61
Other insurance payment: 00

EXPLANATION OF BENEFITS

06/03/XX	200	99204	250.00	00	48	136.00	114.00	00	00	80%	91.20
06/03/XX	540	94375	40.00	00	48	0.00	40.00	00	00	80%	32.00
06/03/XX	540	94060	75.00	00	48	0.00	75.00	00	00	80%	60.00
06/03/XX	200	94664	50.00	00	48	1.55	48.45	00	00	80%	38.76
06/03/XX	540	94760	50.00	00	48	4.40	45.60	00	00	80%	38.46
		TOTAL	465.00	00		141.95	123.05	00	00		258.44

Other insurance credits or adjustments 00

Total payment amount 258.44

Reason code
48 CON DISCOUNT/PT NOT RESPONSIBLE

CPT Code
99204 OFFICE/OUTPT VISIT E and M NEW MOD-HI SEVERIT
94375 RESPIRATORY FLOW VOLUM LOOP
94060 BRONCHOSPSM EVAL SPIROM PRE and POST BRON
94664 AEROSOL/VAPOR FOR INHALA; INT DEMO and EVAL
94760 NONIVASIVE EAR/PULSE OXIMETRY-O2 SAT

If you have any questions, call ABC Insurance Company at (800)255-9091

PARTICIPANT		DATE
GERALD PRACTON MD		07–04–XX
PATIENT	ID NUMBER	
JABE V. BORTOLUSSI	554-98-8876	
PLAN NUMBER	PATIENT NUMBER	OFFICE NO
4206		010

20-028448-00

GC 1234567890

258.44

VOID

3000063

PAY TO THE ORDER OF
COLLEGE CLINIC
4567 BROAD AVENUE
WOODLAND HILLS XY 12345

Figure 4.13 Explanation of benefits (EOB).
(Courtesy of Fordney MT: *Insurance handbook for the medical office,* ed 11, St Louis, 2010, Saunders–Elsevier.)

- Type of care (what services were provided for the patient)
- Amount charged by the provider, along with any provider reduction, medical necessity reduction, or maximum allowed (Generally, the provider reduction is the difference between what the provider charged and the maximum allowed. The maximum allowed is the contractual amount agreed on by the provider and the insurance company. For example, if the provider charges $58.00, but the maximum allowed is $52.20, then the provider reduction is $5.80.)
- The computation of the amount owed to the provider or patient (This computation includes any amount paid by other insurance companies, the patient's deductible, copayment, co-insurance, or other deductions.)
- Other information on the claim status, such as the plan's responsibility, noncovered services, and any additional notes

Note: It is important to read the notes because they are used to explain what was not allowed or why a claim was denied.

Whether submitted electronically or by paper, the medical office needs billing specialists to produce *clean* claims. Clean claims include all the information needed to receive payment. Even one error on a claim form can result in its rejection.

In Medisoft, the Claims Management dialog box allows you to create, edit, print/send, reprint, and delete claims (Figure 4.14). This dialog box is accessed by clicking Claim Management in the Activities menu or by clicking the Claim Management button on the toolbar.

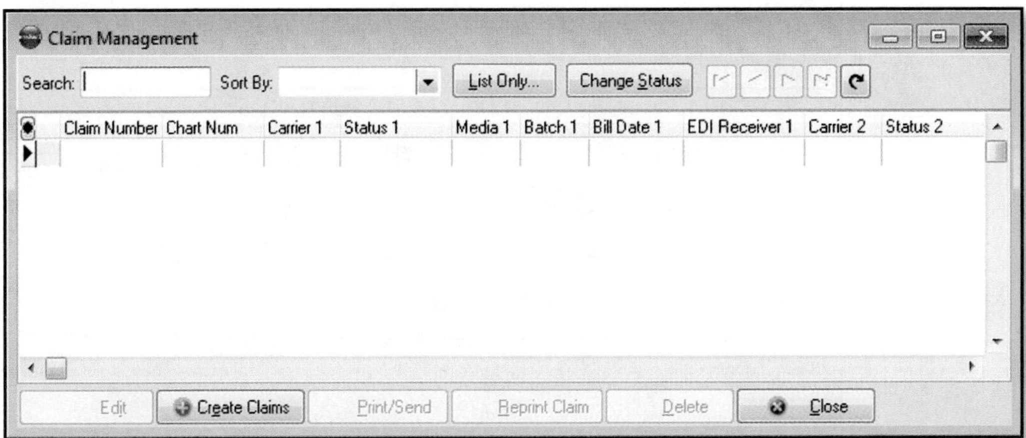

Figure 4.14
Claim Management dialog box.

Creating Claims

When the Create Claims button is clicked in the Claims Management dialog box, the Create Claims dialog box appears with the following fields (Figure 4.15):

Range of Transaction Dates and Chart Numbers. Enter the range of dates and range of patient chart numbers for which you want to create claims. If these fields are left blank, then all available claims will be created.

Select Transactions that Match. This set of fields should be left blank if you want all available claims to be created. Otherwise, you can enter single codes or enter multiple codes separated by commas. For example, to create claims for a specific insurance company, enter only that carrier's code in the Primary Insurance field. Or if you want to create claims related only to services that were performed at a certain type of place (e.g., inpatient hospital, laboratory), then the appropriate POS code can be entered in the Location field. The Provider radio buttons allow you to create claims for either the assigned provider or the attending provider.

Include Transactions If the Claim Total Is Greater Than (Enter Amount). Enter the minimum amount required for a claim to be created. Or leave this field blank to create claims with any total greater than zero.

PROCEDURE 4.7 CREATING CLAIM FORMS

1. Click *Claim Management* on the Activities menu. The Claim Management dialog box displays.
2. Click the *Create Claims* button. The Create Claims dialog box opens.
3. Leave the Assigned radio button selected and the rest of the fields blank.
4. Click the *Create* button. The Create Claims dialog box closes, and several claims appear in the Claim Management dialog box. (Make sure there is one each for Charles Weber, William O'Connor, and Daniel Smith.)
5. Click the *Close* button to close the dialog box.

Locating and Reviewing Claims

After claims are created, it is a good idea to review them for accuracy and any missing information. Reviewing claims helps ensure prompt payment for services and avoids claim rejections. There may be times when you need to review a single claim or a group of claims with common characteristics. In either case, you can quickly locate claims by using fields and buttons located at the top of the Claim Management dialog box (Figure 4.16).

The Search field and the Sort By field work together. First, click the item in the Sort By field's list box to indicate by which variable you want to sort all the claims displayed in the dialog box. Options include Chart Number, Claim Number, Date Created, and more. Next, in the Search field, key the first two or three characters of the item for which you are looking. For example, if you select Chart Number in the Sort By field, and then key *WE* in the Search field, the system will sort all the claims in order by patient chart number and then go to the first claim that has a chart number beginning with the letters *WE*.

Figure 4.15 Create Claims dialog box.

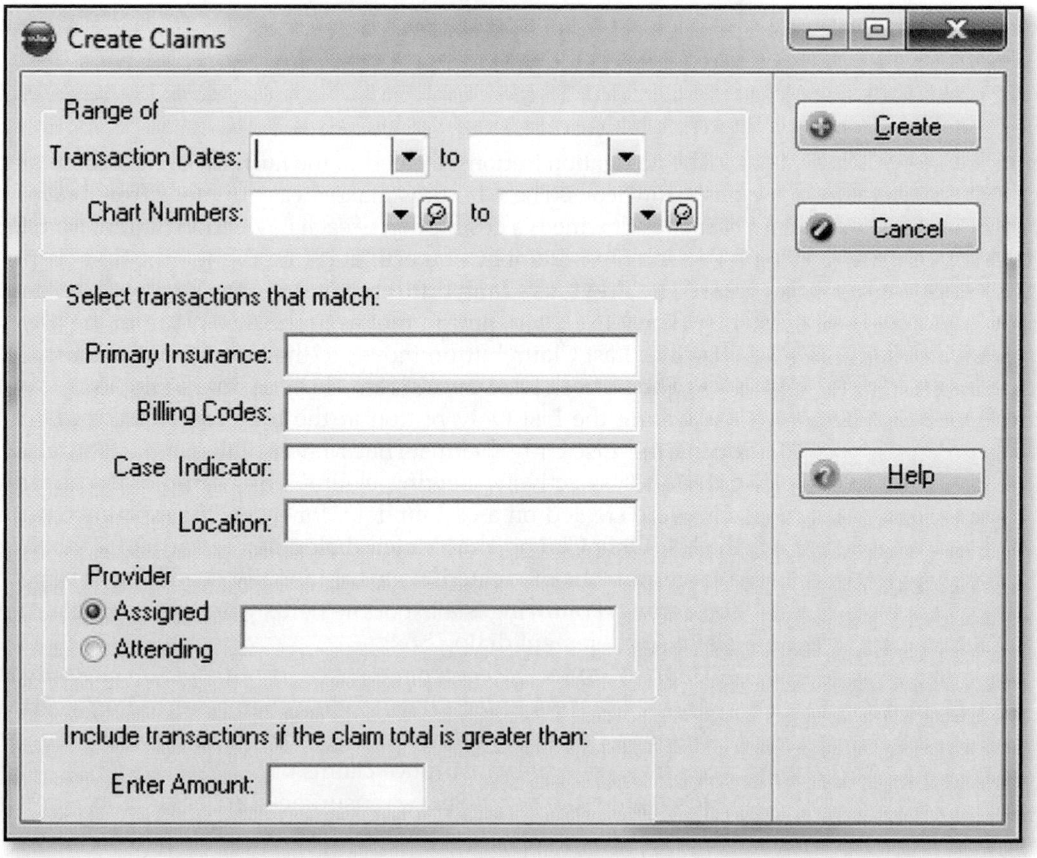

Create Claims

Range of
Transaction Dates: to
Chart Numbers: to

Select transactions that match:
Primary Insurance:
Billing Codes:
Case Indicator:
Location:
Provider
Assigned
Attending

Include transactions if the claim total is greater than:
Enter Amount:

Create
Cancel
Help

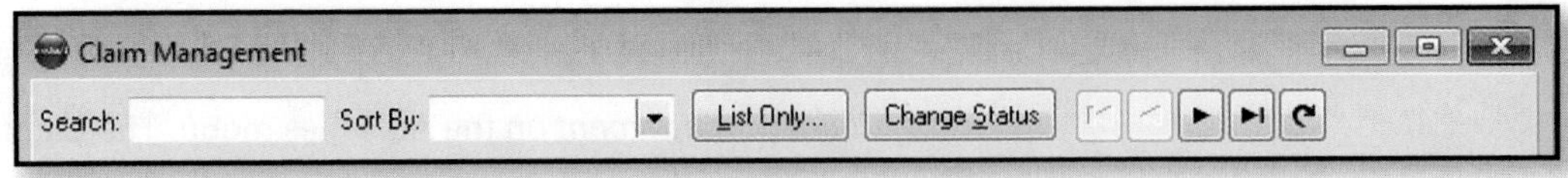

Figure 4.16 Search tools in the Claim Management dialog box.

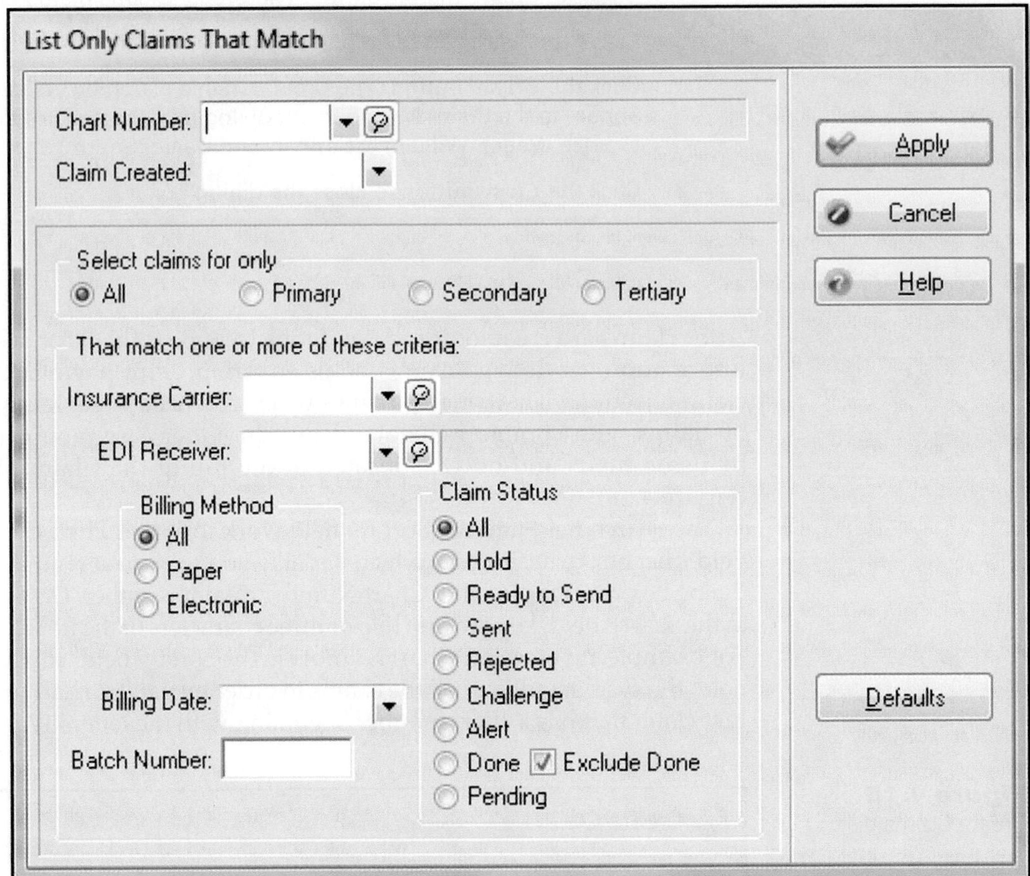

Figure 4.17 List Only Claims That Match dialog box.

The navigation buttons, located to the far right of the Search and Sort By fields, have various arrow icons. These buttons make it easy to move from one claim to another in the list of claims. Following is a description of each navigation button, from left to right (see Figure 4.16):

- The First Claim button activates (highlights) the first claim in the list.
- The Previous Claim button moves to the claim most recently activated.
- The Next Claim button moves to the next claim in the list.
- The Last Claim button moves to the last claim in the list.
- The Refresh Data button refreshes the data in the list.

Clicking the List Only button at the top-center of the Claim Management dialog box opens the List Only Claims That Match dialog box (Figure 4.17). Here you can set up criteria for selectively viewing claims. For example, if you only want to review claims that were created on a certain date, for a specific insurance carrier, you can do so. Using the List Only Claims That Match dialog box is particularly beneficial when working with a large number of created claims. Manually searching for specific claims could be time consuming. Following is a list of the fields you can use to filter the claims displayed in the Claim Management dialog box:

Chart Number. Select a patient's chart number to view only those patient's claims.

Claim Created. Enter a date to view claims created on a certain date.

Select Claims for Only. Choose to view claims for all insurance claims or for primary, secondary, or tertiary insurance claims only.

Insurance Carrier. Select an insurance carrier code to view all the claims for that particular carrier.

EDI Receiver. Select an EDI receiver to view all claims for that particular receiver. (As explained in Chapter 2, EDI is the exchange of information between computers.)

Billing Method. Choose whether you would like to view paper or electronic claims, or see both types (All).

Billing Date. Select a date to view claims that were billed that day.

Batch Number. Enter a specific batch number to see only those claims assigned to that batch.

Claim Status. Select the type of claim status you are searching to view those claims.

After selecting the desired filters, you must click the Apply button in the List Only Claims That Match dialog box. This action closes the dialog box, selects any claims with the specified criteria, and lists those claims in the Claims Management dialog box.

The Change Status button, at the top-center of the Claims Management dialog box, is used to change the status values in claims records. These values are displayed in the Status columns within the Claim Management dialog box's window. For example, you might wish to change a claim or group of claims from a Ready to Send status to a Hold status if some information needs to be verified or edited before sending the claim(s).

Editing Claims in the Claim Dialog Box

After reviewing an individual claim or group of claims, you may find that you need to make some changes before they are submitted for payment. Keep the following points in mind when editing claims:

- You cannot edit a claim if the corresponding patient record is open elsewhere in the system.
- Any changes you make to a claim will not affect the default settings in the patient's record. So, if you find that the same edits need to be made each time claims are created, the patient's default settings may need to be changed.

To edit a claim, activate it by clicking it in the Claim Management dialog box's window. An active record appears highlighted. Then click the Edit button at the bottom of the dialog box. This action opens the Claim dialog box for that record. The Claim dialog box has six tabs: Carrier 1, Carrier 2, Carrier 3, Transactions, Comment, and EDI Note. By default, the Carrier 1 tab displays when the dialog box is opened (Figure 4.18).

Carrier 1, Carrier 2, and Carrier 3 Tabs

The Carrier tabs correspond to the insurance plans (i.e., primary, secondary, and tertiary) being billed for a particular claim. So, in many cases, only the Carrier 1 tab will be used. The fields in all three of the Carrier tabs are similar:

Claim Status. As claims are processed, Medisoft changes the status. For example, after initially creating claims, the Ready to send radio button is selected by the system. If necessary, you can click a different radio button to change the claim's status, such as the Hold radio button to prevent a claim from being sent.

Billing Method. Two options are available for the billing method: Paper or Electronic. Click the appropriate radio button, if the desired option is not already selected.

Initial Billing Date. This field automatically displays the date when the claim was first submitted for payment.

Submission Count. This field indicates the number of times the claim has been submitted.

Billing Date. This field shows the most recent date the claim was billed.

Insurance. In the Carrier 1 tab, this field automatically displays the patient's primary insurance carrier. You can click the down arrow to select a different carrier. In the Carrier 2 and Carrier 3 tabs, this field pertains to the secondary and tertiary insurance carriers, respectively.

EDI Receiver. This field is only applicable if the claim is being sent electronically. If the appropriate receiver is not displayed, select it from the list box.

Frequency Type. When sending claims electronically, some insurance carriers require a frequency type. Following is a list of valid choices:

1: Original Claim
6: Corrected Claim (Adjustment of Prior Claim)

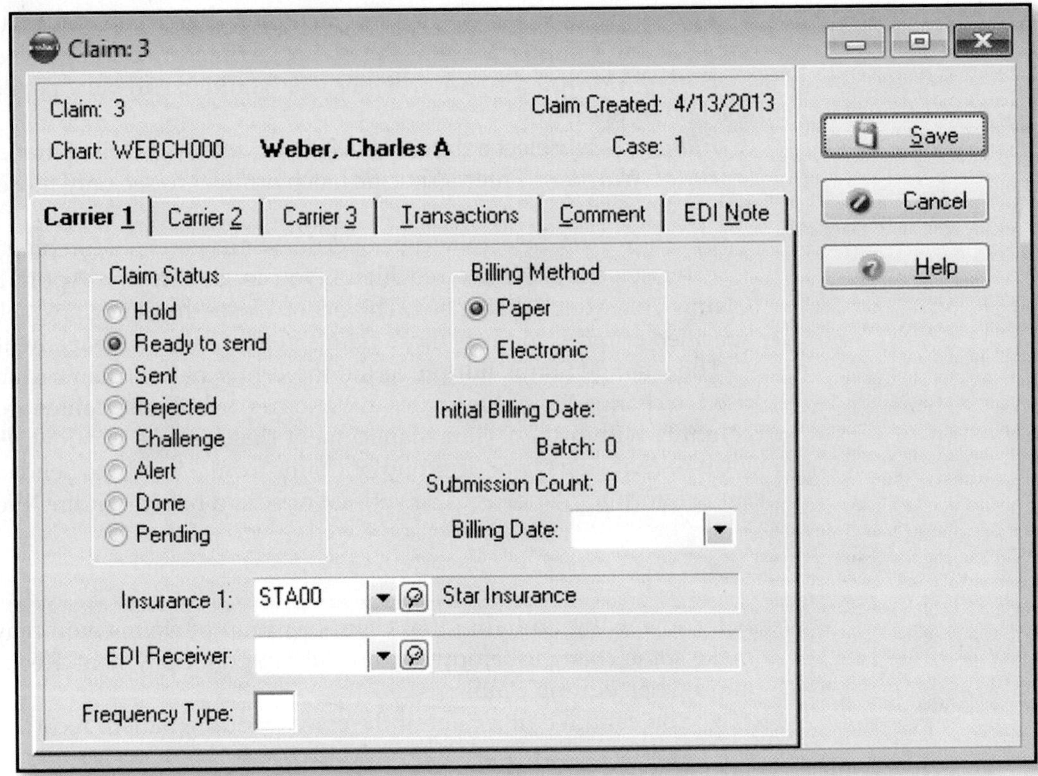

Figure 4.18 Claim dialog box with the Carrier 1 tab displayed.

7: Replacement of Prior Claim
8: Void/Cancellation of Prior Claim

Carrier 2 and 3 tabs are similar to the Carrier 1 tab except that neither Carrier 2 nor Carrier 3 has a Pending radio button in the Claim Status area; neither do they have a Frequency Type field.

Transactions Tab

The Transactions tab lists all the transactions related to the claim (Figure 4.19). The Ins 1 Resp, Ins 2 Resp, and Ins 3 Resp checkboxes indicate the insurance carrier(s) responsible for the claim. For example, if the Ins 1 Resp checkbox is marked, then the primary insurance carrier (identified in the Carrier 1 tab) will be responsible for the claim. The Ins 2 Resp and Ins 3 Resp checkboxes correspond to the secondary and tertiary carriers (see Carrier 2 and Carrier 3 tabs). At the bottom of the Transactions tab are three buttons:

Add. Click this button to add a transaction to the existing claim. You can add a transaction as long as that transaction is not already connected to another claim.

Split. To remove a single transaction from the claim and create a new claim for that transaction, click the transaction to highlight it, and then click the Split button. The system will ask you to confirm that you want to split the transaction. If you click the Yes button, a new claim will be added to the list displayed in the Claim Management dialog box's window.

Remove. Click this button to delete a selected transaction from the claim.

Comment Tab

Key any comments you might have about the claim in the Comment tab's window. These comments are for internal purposes, so they will not be transmitted to the insurance carrier.

EDI Note Tab

This tab allows you to edit EDI information that is or needs to be a part of a claim that will be filed electronically. Clicking this tab allows the user to edit specific EDI information before the claim is sent to a clearinghouse.

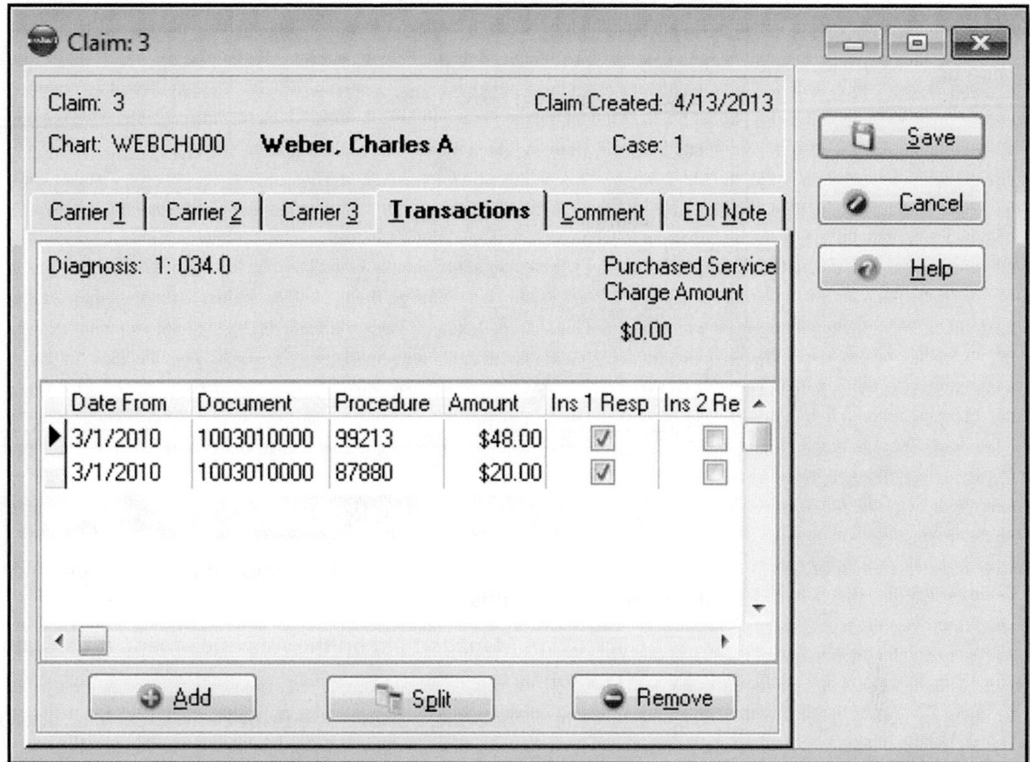

Figure 4.19
Claim dialog box with the Transactions tab displayed.

Submitting and Printing Claims

You can submit claims in paper form, or you can submit claims electronically through your computer. Electronic filing of claims is faster and less expensive than printing and mailing paper claims. A faster process also means that the medical office will get paid sooner.

Before claims can be billed electronically, certain items must initially be set up in Medisoft and in the Revenue Management program that automatically comes with Medisoft. This program is launched by clicking Revenue Management on Medisoft's Activities menu. The process for submitting claims electronically includes the following steps:

1. An EDI receiver is set up.
2. Claims are submitted to the EDI receiver, after which a claims response is sent to the medical office.
3. The EDI receiver forwards the claims to the insurance carrier(s).
4. Payments and RAs are sent to the medical office from the insurance carriers.

Many medical offices hire a clearinghouse company to check the claims for errors and missing data before they are submitted for payment. Clearinghouses first verify claim information. If problems are located, the medical office makes changes and resubmits the claims to the clearinghouse. The clearinghouse then transmits the claims to the insurance companies. This type of service can save the medical office a lot of time and also reduce the amount of claim rejections.

To print claims or to send them electronically, the Print/Send button in the Claim Management dialog box is clicked. This action opens the Print/Send Claims dialog box (Figure 4.20). The Paper radio button should be selected if you want to print paper claims. The Electronic radio button should be clicked if you want to send claims electronically using the Revenue Management feature. If you choose Electronic, then you will also need to select an EDI code in the Electronic Claim Receiver field. After the OK button is clicked, Medisoft will display the appropriate dialog boxes for the method you selected.

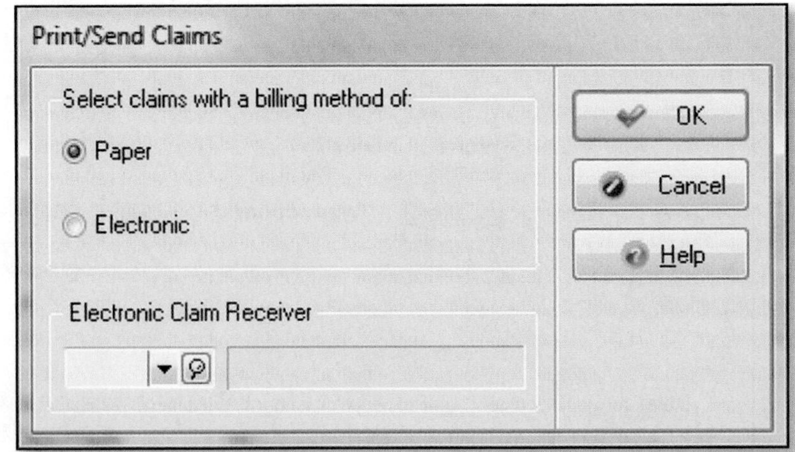

Figure 4.20 Print/Send Claims dialog box.

PROCEDURE 4.8 PRINTING CLAIMS

Because your computer is not set up to submit claims electronically, you will print claims on paper in this exercise.

1. Click *Claim Management* on the Activities menu. The Claim Management dialog box opens.
2. Click the *Print/Send* button. The Print/Send Claims dialog box displays.
3. Click the *Paper* radio button, if not already selected.
4. Click *OK*. The Open Report dialog box displays with a list of formats for printing claims, as shown in Figure 4.21. (Note: If you had selected the Electronic radio button in the Print/Send dialog box, a set of button options for sending claims and receiving reports would have been displayed instead of the Open Report dialog box.)
5. Click *Laser CMS (Primary) W/Form*, and then click *OK*. The Print Report Where dialog box appears.
6. Click the radio button for *Print the report on the printer*. Then click the *Start* button. A Data Selection Questions dialog box displays (Figure 4.22). Like many other data selection dialog boxes used to print reports in Medisoft, these fields filter the type of claims you want to print. If a field is left blank, the program will include all the available data. (Note: When submitting electronic claims, a similar data selection dialog box is displayed.)
7. Leave all the fields blank, and click *OK*. The Print dialog box displays.
8. Select a printer, and hand in the printed claims to your instructor.
9. Notice that the claims listed in the Claim Management dialog box now display Sent in the Status 1 column.
10. Click *Close* to close the Claim Management dialog box.

Applying Insurance Payments

Payments from insurance companies can be entered and applied through the Deposit List dialog box (Figure 4.23) using the RA report received. This dialog box is opened by clicking Enter Deposits/Payments on the Activities menu.

Deposits/Payments must be entered before they can be applied to patient accounts. After deposits/payments are saved, they display in the Deposit List dialog box's window. Various options are provided for viewing these entries. For example, if the Show All Deposits checkbox is selected, then all deposit entries will display. But if the Show Unapplied Only checkbox is selected, then only deposits with unapplied amounts will

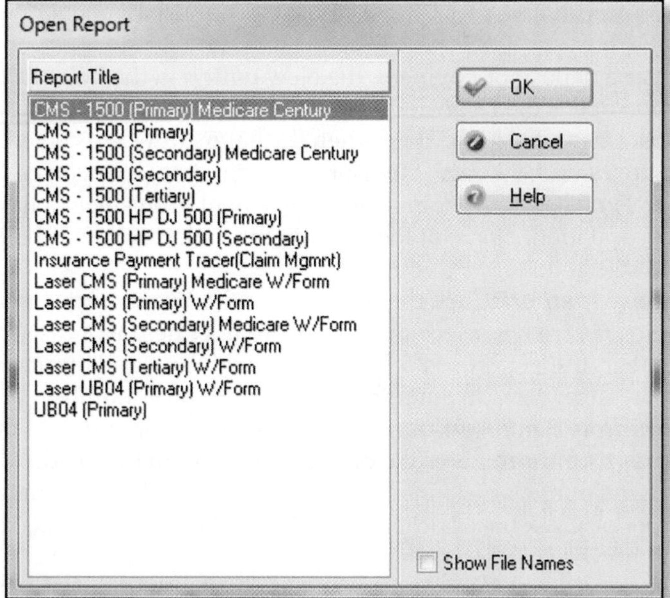
Open Report
Report Title
CMS - 1500 (Primary) Medicare Century
CMS - 1500 (Primary)
CMS - 1500 (Secondary) Medicare Century
CMS - 1500 (Secondary)
CMS - 1500 (Tertiary)
CMS - 1500 HP DJ 500 (Primary)
CMS - 1500 HP DJ 500 (Secondary)
Insurance Payment Tracer(Claim Mgmnt)
Laser CMS (Primary) Medicare W/Form
Laser CMS (Primary) W/Form
Laser CMS (Secondary) Medicare W/Form
Laser CMS (Secondary) W/Form
Laser CMS (Tertiary) W/Form
Laser UB04 (Primary) W/Form
UB04 (Primary)
OK
Cancel
Help
Show File Names

Figure 4.21 Open Report dialog box when printing claims.

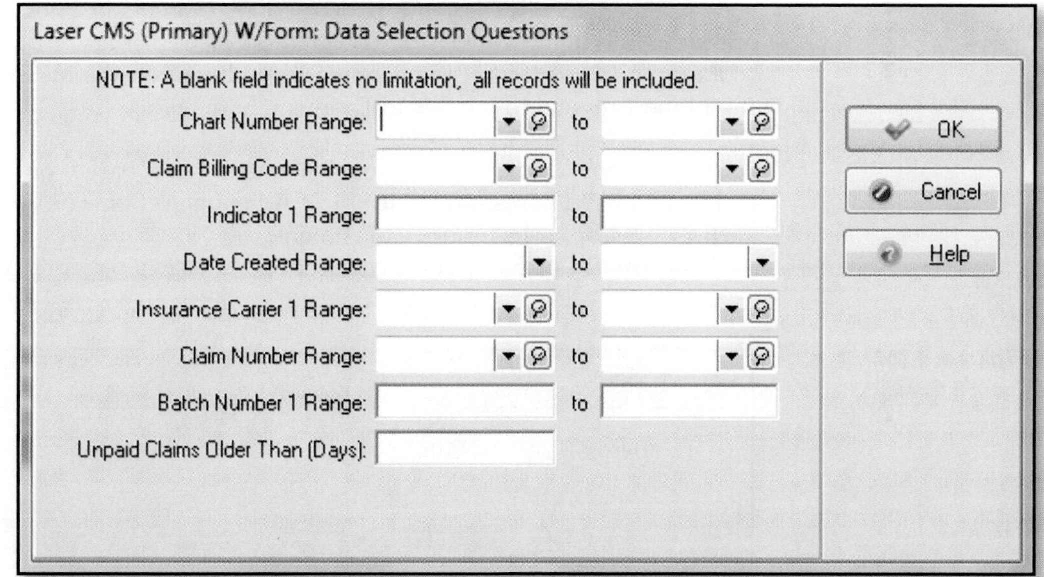
Laser CMS (Primary) W/Form: Data Selection Questions
NOTE: A blank field indicates no limitation, all records will be included.
Chart Number Range: to
Claim Billing Code Range: to
Indicator 1 Range: to
Date Created Range: to
Insurance Carrier 1 Range: to
Claim Number Range: to
Batch Number 1 Range: to
Unpaid Claims Older Than (Days):
OK
Cancel
Help

Figure 4.22 Data Selection Questions dialog box when printing claims.

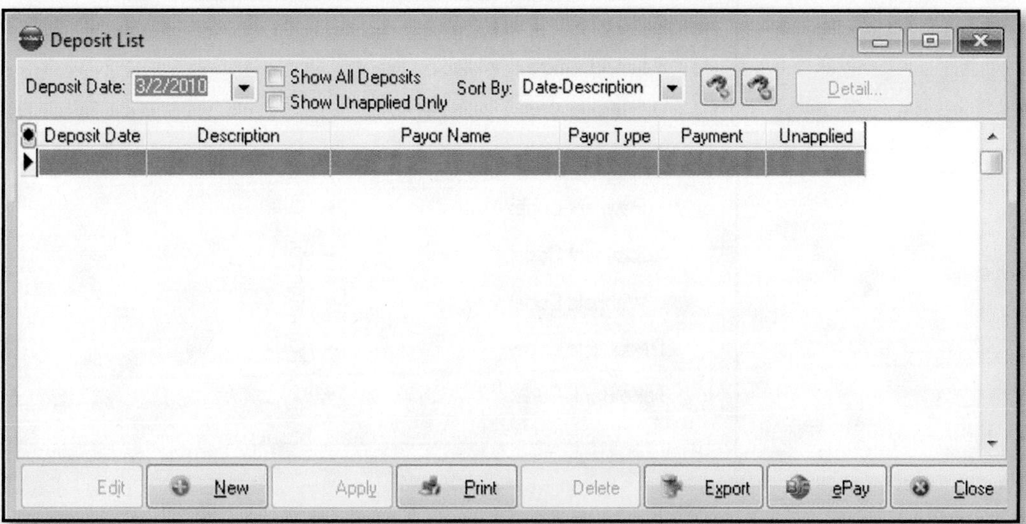

Figure 4.23 Deposit List dialog box.

display. You can also sort the list of deposits and payments by clicking an option in the Sort By list box.

To enter a deposit or payment, the New button in the Deposit List dialog box is clicked. This action opens the Deposit dialog box (Figure 4.24), which has the following fields:

Deposit Date. Enter the date when the payment was received. This field automatically defaults to the current date (Medisoft program date), but you can change it, if necessary.

Payor Type. Click the source of the payment in this field's list box (e.g., Patient, Insurance, or Capitation). Some of the fields in the dialog box will change, depending on which type you select.

Payment Method. Click the payment method used, (e.g., Check, Cash, Credit Card, or Electronic). If Check is selected, a Check Number field will display in which you can enter that number. If Electronic is selected, an electronic funds transfer (EFT) Tracer field will display in which you can enter the appropriate tracer number.

Description/Bank Number. Enter a payment description in this field.

Payment Amount. Enter the payment amount in this field.

Deposit Code. User-defined categories can be set up for this field, if desired, for sorting purposes. Click the appropriate code in this field's list box, if your office uses deposit codes. Otherwise, leave this field blank.

Insurance/Chart Number. This field displays differently, depending on the value selected in the Payor Type field. If an insurance payment is made, click the correct carrier code in this field's list box. If a patient payment is made, click the chart number of the appropriate patient.

Payment Code. Select the payment code based on the insurance, such as BCBSPAY for a Blue Cross and Blue Shield Payment. Some offices may use a general code such as INSPAY for Insurance Payment.

Adjustment Code. Select the adjustment code based on the insurance, such as BCBSADJ for Blue Cross and Blue Shield Adjustment. Some offices may use a general code such as INSADJ for Insurance Adjustment.

Copayment Code. Select the code that pertains to a patient's copayment.

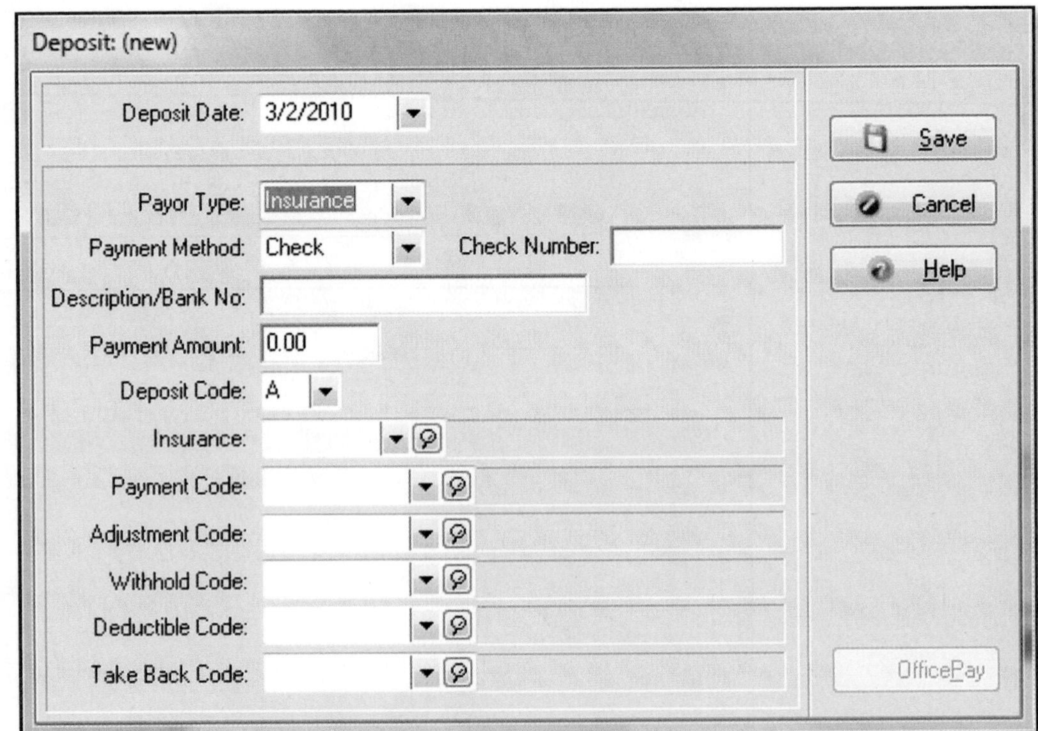

Figure 4.24
Deposit dialog box.

Note: The Copayment Code field is only used for patient payments. The Withhold Code, Deductible Code, and Take Back Code fields are used only for insurance deposits.

Withhold Code. Select the withhold code based on the insurance, such as BCBSWH for Blue Cross and Blue Shield Withhold. Some offices may use a general code such as INSWH for Insurance Withhold.

Deductible Code. Select the deductible code based on the insurance, such as BCBSDED for Blue Cross and Blue Shield Deductible. Some offices may use a general code such as INSDED for Insurance Deductible.

Take Back Code. Select the take back code based on the insurance, such as BCBSTB for Blue Cross and Blue Shield Take Back. Some offices may use a general code such as INSTB for Insurance Take Back.

After deposits and payments have been entered, the next step is to apply them to the transactions listed on the RA report. In the Deposit List window, click the entry you wish to apply (to highlight it). Then click the Apply button at the bottom of the dialog box to open the Apply Payment/Adjustments to Charges dialog box (Figure 4.25). The top part of the dialog box shows the payer information, the unapplied amount, and the patient (who you select from a list box). The middle area of the dialog box is a grid with columns where you apply the payments. At the bottom of the dialog box is a group of buttons and checkboxes. More details on various items in the Apply Payment/Adjustments to Charges dialog box are as follows:

For (patient). If the payment being applied was made by a patient, then his or her chart number and name will automatically display in this field. If the payment was made by an insurance carrier, click the patient's chart number in the list box.

Ins 1, Ins 2, Ins 3. The patient's insurance information automatically displays for reference.

List Only. If you want to see only certain transactions listed in the dialog box, click this button to select specific criteria.

View So Far. Click this button to display the payments and adjustments that you have already applied.

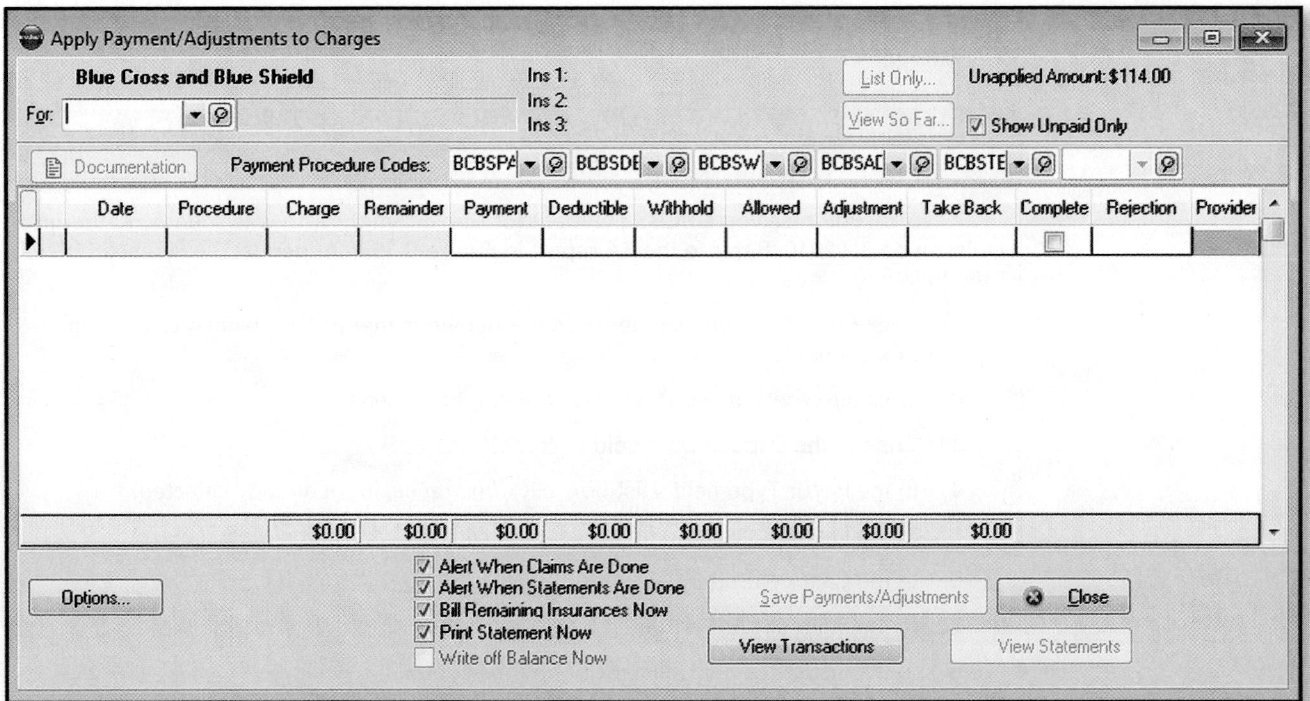

Figure 4.25 Apply Payment/Adjustments to Charges dialog box.

Unapplied Amount. This field displays the amount of the deposit that has not yet been applied.

Show Unpaid Only/Show Remainder Only. The name of this checkbox depends on whether you are entering an insurance or a patient payment. For insurance payments, selecting this checkbox displays unpaid transactions in the dialog box. For patient payments, selecting this checkbox displays transactions for which the patient is responsible for paying.

Documentation. Click this button to add a note about the selected transaction.

Payment Procedure Codes. These fields display the codes entered previously in the Deposit dialog box.

Payment. Enter the amount that you wish to apply to the transaction.

Deductible. If appropriate, enter the amount of the deductible provided in the RA report.

Withhold. If the insurance company has withheld payment in order to pay all at one time, then enter the withholding amount in this field.

Allowed. Enter the amount allowed by the insurance carrier.

Adjustment. This amount is calculated by Medisoft by subtracting the amount in the Allowed field from the amount in the Charge field.

Take Back. When the insurance company overpays, it will apply the overpayment to another transaction.

Complete. Medisoft enters a checkbox when the patient's responsibility is complete.

Rejection. If applicable, make a selection in the list box that reflects the rejection message from the RA report.

Provider. The assigned provider is listed in this field.

Options. If desired, this button can be clicked to change the default settings in the Program Options dialog box for patient payment application codes.

Save Payments/Adjustments. Click this button to save the payment or adjustment after you have verified that the applied entries are correct.

View Transactions. Click this button to open the Transaction Entry dialog box.

Close. Click this button to close the Apply Payment/Adjustment to Charges dialog box.

Checkboxes. Several checkboxes appear to the left of the Save Payment/Adjustment button. Clicking any one of these boxes will perform the description shown. For example, selecting the Print Statement Now checkbox allows you to print a patient statement after the payment entry is saved.

PROCEDURE 4.9 ENTERING AND APPLYING AN INSURANCE PAYMENT TO A SINGLE PATIENT ACCOUNT

On 3/15/10, you received a BCBS payment for Daniel Smith, who was seen by Katherine Olsson on 3/3/2010. Refer to the RA report in **Figure C.19 in Appendix C** as you complete the following steps.

1. Click *Enter Deposits/Payments* on the Activities menu. The Deposit List dialog box displays.
2. Click the *New* button. The Deposit dialog box opens.
3. Change the Deposit Date field to *3/15/2010.*
4. In the Payor Type field's list box, click *Insurance*, if not already selected.
5. In the Payment Method field's list box, click *Check*, if not already selected.
6. In the Check Number field, key *23455.*
7. In the Payment Amount field, key *114.00.*
8. In the Insurance field, click *BCBS* in the list box.

9. In the Payment Code field, click *BCBSPAY* in the list box.
10. In the Adjustment Code field, click *BCBSADJ* in the list box.
11. In the Withhold Code field, click *BCBSWH* in the list box.
12. A deductible code for BCBS is not on file; so you will have to add it first. Click in the Deductible Code field, and then press *F8* to open the Procedure/Payment/Adjustment dialog box; enter the following: Code 1, *BCBSDED*; Description, *Blue Cross/Shield deductible*; Code Type, *Deductible*. Be sure to save the new code. Then key or click *BCBSDED* if not already chosen in the Deposit dialog box's Deductible Code field.
13. In the Take Back Code field, click *BCBSTB* in the list box.
14. Click *Save* in the Deposit dialog box. (If the deposit entry does not display in the Deposit List dialog box's window, click the *Show All Deposits* checkbox.)
15. Click the *Blue Cross and Blue Shield* deposit entry in the window to highlight it.
16. Click the *Apply* button. The Apply Payment/Adjustments to Charges dialog box opens.
17. Click *Daniel Smith* in the For field's list box.
18. In the Payment field for procedure 99203, key *72.00*.
19. Press the *Tab* key three times to move to the Allowed field. Notice that the checkbox in the Complete column is marked by the system.
20. In the Allowed field for procedure 99203, key *72.00* (the maximum amount allowed by the insurance carrier).
21. Press the *Tab* key. Medisoft enters an adjustment (provider reduction) of $8.00 in the Adjustment field.
22. For procedure 80050, key *42.00* in both the Payment field and the Allowed field. Medisoft enters an adjustment of $3.00. Notice that the Unapplied Amount in the upper-right corner of the dialog box is now zero.
23. Click the *Print Statement Now* checkbox to deselect it.
24. Click the Save *Payments/Adjustments* button.
25. Then click *Close* (twice) to close both dialog boxes.
26. Open the Transaction Entry dialog box, select Daniel Smith's chart number and the appropriate case, and you will see the payment entries displayed.
27. Using what you learned in the preceding steps, enter and apply another insurance payment for a single patient. On 3/15/2010, you received a check from Medicare (MCARE) for William O'Connor. Use the RA shown in **Figure C.20 in Appendix C** and the following procedure codes: MCAREPAY, MCAREADJ, MCAREWH, MCAREDED, and MCARETB. Because MCAREDED is not on file, you will have to add it first to the Procedure/Payment/Adjustment dialog box. (These codes correspond to Medicare amounts for payment, adjustment, withhold adjustment, deductible, and take back adjustment.)
28. To save time when entering future insurance payments, open the Insurance Carrier List dialog box, click *Medicare* in the list, and then click the *Edit* button. In the Options and Codes tab of the Insurance Carrier dialog box, enter the codes *MCAREPAY, MCAREADJ, MCAREWH, MCAREDED,* and *MCARETB* in the fields designated for Default Payment Application Codes. Do the same thing for Blue Cross and Blue Shield, entering the codes *BCBSPAY, BCBSADJ, BCBSWH, BCBSDED,* and *BCBSTB*.

PROCEDURE 4.10 ENTERING AND APPLYING AN INSURANCE PAYMENT TO TWO PATIENTS' ACCOUNTS

You will now enter charges for two patients, Cindy Wixen and Ronald Baxter. Then you will enter a Blue Cross/Blue Shield insurance payment and apply it to both patients' accounts.

1. Enter the following charges for both patients using steps you learned in Procedure 4.1. Do not forget to save your entries!
    - Cindy Wixen was seen by Dr. Jagla on 3/1/2010 for an ankle sprain. Use the Encounter form in **Figure C.21 in Appendix C** to enter two charges.
    - Ronald Baxter was seen by Emily Luther on 3/5/2010 for a routine physical examination. Use the Encounter form in **Figure C.22 in Appendix C** to enter two charges.
2. Review the RA information in **Figure C.23 in Appendix C**.
3. Open the Deposit List dialog box and click *New*.
4. Change the Deposit Date field to *3/15/2010*.
5. Click *Insurance* in the Payor Type list box, if not already selected.
6. Click *Check* in the Payment Method list box, if not already selected.
7. Key *67890* in the Check Number field.
8. Key *182.40* in the Payment Amount field.
9. Click *BCBS* in the Insurance field's list box. The default payment codes on file in the Insurance Carrier dialog box are automatically entered in the rest of the fields.
10. Click the *Save* button.
11. Click the line in the Deposit List dialog box for the Blue Cross and Blue Shield payment you just entered.
12. Click the *Apply* button.
13. Click *Cindy Wixen* in the For list box.
14. Apply payment for the two transactions in the same manner used in Procedure 4.9.
15. Click the *Save Payments/Adjustments* button. In the upper-right corner of the dialog box, notice that there is still $96.00 unapplied.
16. Click *Ronald Baxter* in the For list box.
17. Apply payment for the two transactions.
18. Click the *Save Payments/Adjustments* button. The Unapplied Amount is now zero.
19. Close all dialog boxes.

PROCEDURE 4.11 ENTERING AND APPLYING INSURANCE PAYMENTS TO MULTIPLE PATIENTS' ACCOUNTS

Use what you learned in previous exercises to practice entering more payment and adjustment codes, charges, and insurance payments. You will apply two insurance companies' checks to multiple patients' accounts.

1. Open the Procedure/Payment/Adjustment List dialog box, and create five new payment/adjustment codes as follows:
    - Code 1 field: FMPAY; Description field: First Med payment; Code Type field: Insurance Payment.

- Code 1 field: FMADJ; Description field: First Med adjustment; Code Type field: Insurance Adjustment.
- Code 1 field: FMWH; Description field: First Med withhold; Code Type field: Insurance Withhold Adjustment.
- Code 1 field: FMDED; Description field: First Med deductible; Code Type field: Deductible.
- Code 1 field: FMTB; Description field: First Med take back; Code Type field: Insurance Take Back Adjustment.

2. Enter the new payment and adjustment codes as default codes in the Insurance Carrier dialog box for First Med (Options and Codes tab).
3. Enter the following patient charges:
   - Peter Portman was seen by Dr. Walker on 3/1/2010 for an earache. Use the encounter form in **Figure C.24 in Appendix C**. Because the diagnosis code on the form is not on file in Medisoft, you will need to add it by pressing F8 in the Diag 1 field (Transaction Entry dialog box).
   - Ashuri Lee was seen by Dr. Berg on 3/2/2010 for dermatitis. Use the encounter form in **Figure C.25 in Appendix C**.
   - Tonya McWilliams was seen by Dr. Berg on 3/2/2010 for a swollen eye. Use the encounter form in **Figure C.26 in Appendix C**.
   - Jerry Silversmith was seen by Dr. Walker on 3/1/2010 for a diabetic recheck. Use the encounter form in **Figure C.27 in Appendix C**.
   - Tim Butler was seen by Dr. Berg on 3/2/2010 for a sore throat. Use the encounter form in **Figure C.28 in Appendix C**.
4. Enter and apply payment information based on the following RA information:
   - Use the RA information for Blue Cross and Blue Shield in **Figure C.29 in Appendix C**. The check was received on 3/15/2010.
   - Use the RA for First Med in **Figure C.30 in Appendix C**. The check was received on 3/15/2010.

PATIENT STATEMENTS

A patient statement lists the amount the patient owes to the medical office and also includes the types of procedures that were performed at the time of his or her visit. A patient statement is sometimes sent to a patient who has insurance to notify the patient that the insurance company has been billed.

A regular system should be in place for mailing out patient statements. Some medical offices send statements immediately after providing treatment; others bill all patients on the same day each month. Most medical offices bill a patient every month until the bill is paid in full.

The two most common methods of billing patients are once-a-month billing and cycle billing. **Once-a-month billing** involves preparing all of the patients' statements to be mailed out at once, typically before the 25th of each month. This allows patients enough time to send out a payment. Because this method can be quite a burden for medical office personnel, some practices may choose to use cycle billing.

Cycle billing is used by most credit card companies and department stores. **Cycle billing** works on the concept of dividing up the statements to be sent at regular time intervals throughout a month, rather than all at once. This process helps spread out the work more evenly over time. How often you bill depends on the process and procedures in place at the medical office; it could be bi-monthly, weekly, or daily. For example, in a bi-monthly system, patients whose last names begin with one of the letters "A" through "M" could be prepared on the 15th of each month. Those whose last names start with "N" through "Z" could be prepared on the last day of the month. By spacing the billings, more time can be dedicated to each statement, which decreases the likelihood of errors.

Individual patient statements can be printed when applying payments. However, it may be more efficient to print a larger amount of statements at one time. Groups of statements can be processed in the following basic ways: clicking Patient Statements in the Reports menu or clicking Statement Management in the Activities menu. It is recommended that you choose either one method or the other, but not both. Keep in mind that printing statements via the Reports menu will not update the statement submission count that is tracked in the Medisoft program.

Using the Reports Menu to Print Statements

Using the Patient Statements option in the Reports menu is similar to printing many other reports and lists in Medisoft. Following is a brief list of the steps used:

1. Click the *Reports menu.*
2. Click *Patient Statements.*
3. Click the desired report format in the Open Report dialog box.
4. In the Print Report Where dialog box, click one of the three radio buttons: *Preview the report on the screen, Print the report on the printer,* or *Export the report to a file.* Then, click *Start.*
5. Enter or select the criteria for producing the statements in the Data Selection Questions dialog box (e.g., Chart Number Range, Guarantor Billing Code Range, Insurance Carrier Range, Date Range, Patient Indicator Match, and Statement Total Range). Then click *OK.*

Using the Statement Management Dialog Box

The Statement Management dialog box (Figure 4.26) is similar to the Claim Management dialog box. You first create the statements, after which Medisoft displays the statements in a searchable list format. You can view, edit, and print/send the statements from the same dialog box. The fields and buttons at the top of the Statement Management dialog box also operate in a similar manner to the ones in the Claim Management dialog box (Search and Sort By fields; List Only, Change Status, and navigation buttons). Unlike printing statements using the Reports menu, when you use the Statement Management dialog box to issue statements, Medisoft keeps track of the submission count.

When you click the Create Statements button in the Statement Management dialog box, the Create Statements dialog box displays with the following fields (Figure 4.27):

Transaction Dates. Enter the start and end dates for transactions that you want to print on the statements. Any transactions that fall within that date range will be included on the statements. If you leave these fields blank, all available transactions will print.

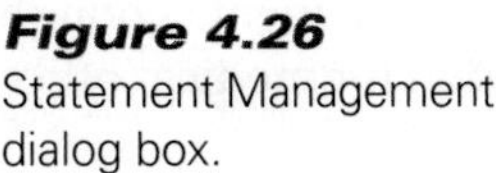

Figure 4.26
Statement Management dialog box.

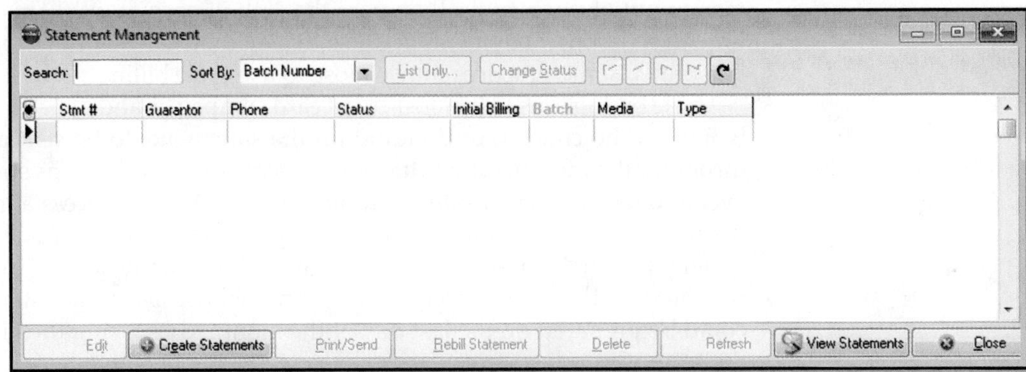

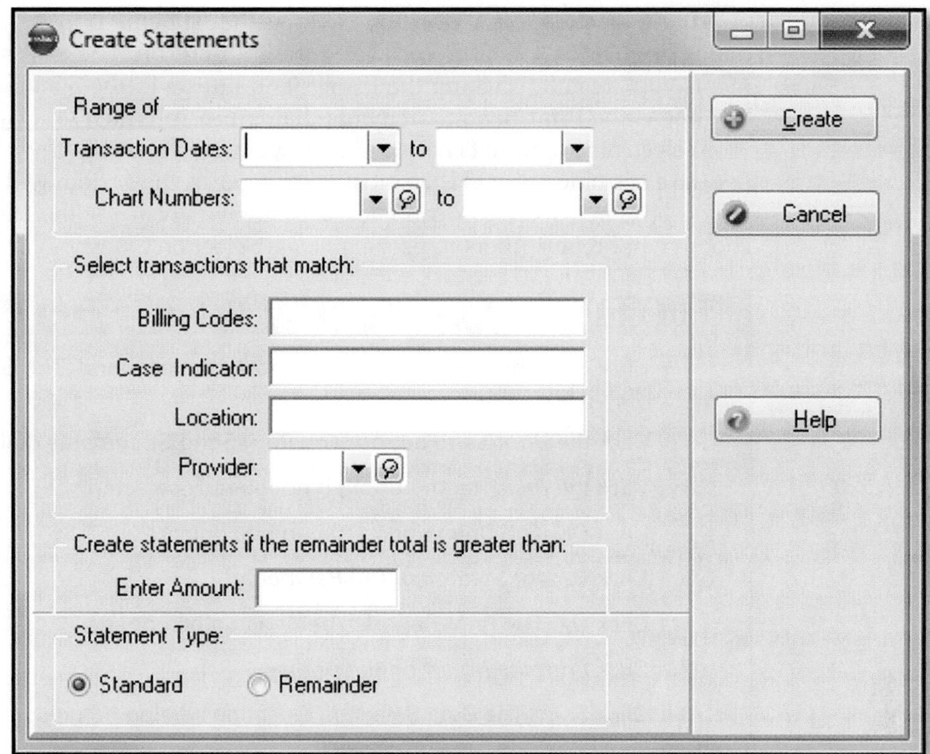

Figure 4.27 Create Statements dialog box.

Chart Numbers. Enter the patient chart number, or a range of chart numbers, for which you wish to create statements. Keep in mind that statements are only created for guarantors. So, for example, if a child's guarantor is his or her parent, then the transactions related to the child's record would appear on the parent's statement.

Select Transactions that Match. If you enter values in the Billing Codes, Case Indicator, Location, or Provider fields, the system will only create statements for transaction records with those codes. Leave the fields blank to include all codes.

Create Statements If the Remainder Total Is Greater Than. Enter the minimum outstanding balance for which you wish to create statements. The system will create statements for any accounts with balances greater than the amount entered in this field. If you leave this field blank, statements will be created for accounts with balances greater than zero.

Statement Type. Click the radio button for the type of statement you want to create—Standard or Remainder. Standard statements list all charge transactions, whether or not the insurance carrier has paid them. Remainder statements list only the charges that have been paid by insurance.

PROCEDURE 4.12 CREATING PATIENT STATEMENTS

1. Click *Statement Management* on the Activities menu. The Statement Management dialog box opens.
2. Click the *Create Statements* button. The Create Statements dialog box displays.
3. In the Enter Amount field, key *0.00*.
4. Click the *Standard* radio button for Statement Type, if not already selected. Leave the other fields blank.
5. Click the *Create* button. A message box displays indicating that statements have been created.
6. Click *OK*. A list of created statements appears in the Statement Management dialog box's window.
7. Close the dialog box.

Editing a statement is done by clicking that statement in the Statement Management dialog box window and then clicking the Edit button. The next step is to print the statements you created. Clicking the Print/Send button in the Statement Management dialog box opens the Print/Send Statements dialog box in which you can choose either a paper or an electronic option. (The medical office must be enrolled with a processing center to use the electronic option.) Like most other reports, the system will display an Open Report dialog box, in which you can click a particular form for the statements. Then you can choose what report filters to use (e.g., Data Selection Questions).

PROCEDURE 4.13 PRINTING PATIENT STATEMENTS

1. Click *Statement Management* in the Activities menu. The Statement Management dialog box opens.
2. Click the *Print/Send* button. The Print/Send Statements dialog box displays.
3. Click the *Paper* radio button, if not already selected.
4. Click *OK*. The Open Report dialog box opens.
5. Click *Patient Statement (All Payments).*
6. Click *OK*. The Print Report Where dialog box opens.
7. Click *Print the report on the printer.*
8. Click *Start*. The Data Selection Questions dialog box displays.
9. Leave all the fields unchanged.
10. Click *OK*, select a printer, and hand in the statements to your instructor.

ACCOUNTING REPORTS

The medical office manager and other administrative personnel use reports to analyze the practice's financial viability and cost-control measures. Three kinds of commonly used reports include day sheets, a practice analysis, and patient ledgers.

Day Sheets

Three different types of day sheets can be printed in Medisoft:

1. ***Patient Day Sheet.*** Reports all patients seen that day and all patient transactions for the day.
2. ***Procedure Day Sheet.*** Lists all procedures for the day.
3. ***Payment Day Sheet.*** Reports all transactions for a particular day.

All day sheets can be printed for a specific day or printed for a range of dates. Typically, the Patient Day Sheet is printed every day, whereas the other two reports are usually printed on an as-needed basis, such as weekly or monthly.

All three types of day sheets have similar Search dialog boxes used to filter data before printing the reports. To print a day sheet, click Day Sheets on the Reports menu. Then click the name of the day sheet you want to print. First, the Print Report Where dialog box displays. After choosing an option and clicking the Start button, a Search dialog box opens. Although the Search dialog box for each type of report may vary somewhat, they all operate the same way. That is, you choose ranges or specific codes to filter the data and create the report. Figure 4.28 shows the Search dialog box for the Procedure Day Sheet.

As explained previously in this chapter, two types of date ranges often seen when printing day sheets and other reports are Date From and Date Created. Date From refers to the date of service; that is, the actual date when a procedure was performed or a payment or adjustment was made. In other words, Date From is the date you used in the Date field(s) when entering charges, payments, and adjustments (Transaction Entry dialog box and Deposit dialog box).

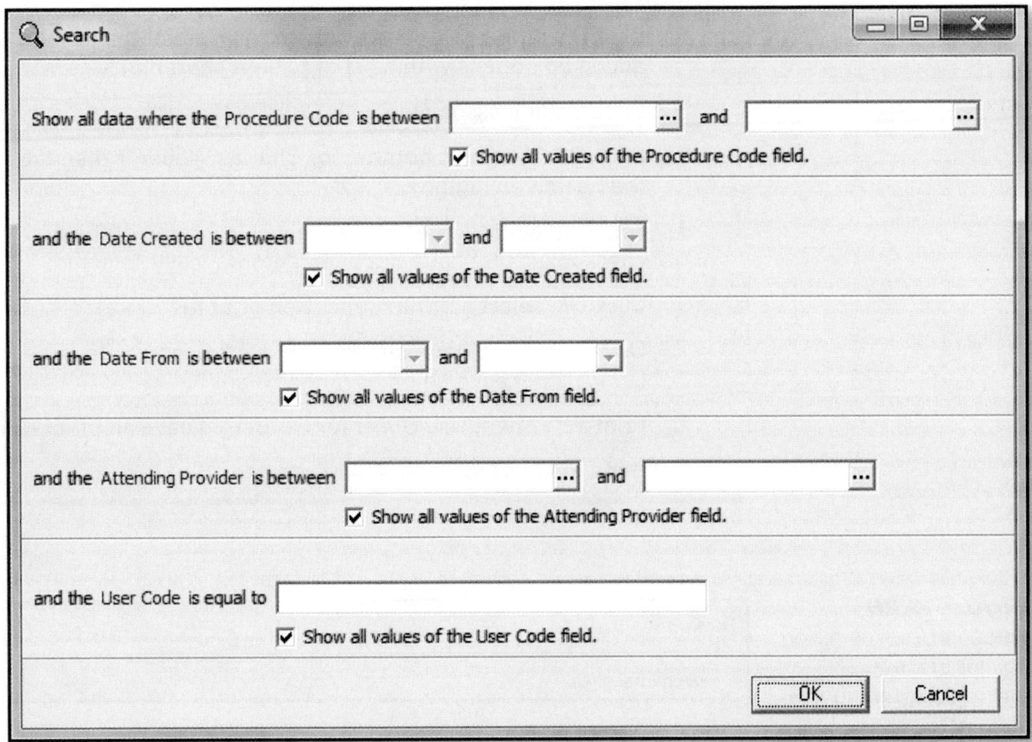

Figure 4.28
Search dialog box when printing the Procedure Day Sheet.

Date Created refers to the date when the transaction was saved or the report was created. Medisoft uses the Windows system date as the Date Created. As a result, this date is tracked behind the scenes by Medisoft and is not affected by changing the Medisoft program date.

Following is an example to help clarify the difference between Date From and Date Created. Suppose today is Monday, June 8, and you need to enter charges for services performed the previous Friday, June 5. In the Transaction Entry dialog box, you should backdate the transactions, using June 5. However, the Windows system date when you input or created the entries, June 8, is tracked by Medisoft as the Date Created.

By default, the system selects the Show all values checkboxes for most or all the fields in a Search dialog box. You can easily override these default settings by keying in specific values in the appropriate fields. Some fields have a button beside them with three dots. Clicking this button opens a Lookup dialog box with a searchable list. Figure 4.29 shows a portion of the Lookup dialog box for Procedure/Payment/Adjustment codes. If you click a specific line in a Lookup dialog box and then click OK, Medisoft will insert the selected value in the Search dialog box.

PROCEDURE 4.14 PRINTING PATIENT DAY SHEETS

In this exercise, you will print each of the three types of day sheets.

1. Click *Day Sheets* on the Reports menu. A submenu displays with the three types of day sheets.
2. Click *Patient Day Sheet*. The Print Report Where dialog box opens.
3. Click the radio button for *Print the report on the printer.*
4. Click *Start*. The Search dialog box displays.
5. Click in the second field associated with chart numbers, located at the top of the dialog box (upper-right corner). The system deselects the Show all values of the Chart Number field checkbox and activates the field.

6. Click the button with three dots to the right of the second field's box. A Lookup dialog box opens with a list of patient chart numbers.
7. Click the line associated with *Charles Weber.*
8. Click *OK.* The chart number for Charles Weber is inserted in the second field of the Search dialog box.
9. Leave all other ranges blank. That is, click any of the other Show all values checkboxes that have not been automatically selected.
10. Click *OK,* select a printer, and then print the report.
11. Using what you have learned, print a Procedure Day Sheet for code 99213 for Dr. Walker. Leave all other ranges blank.
12. Print a Payment Day Sheet for Dr. Berg. Leave all other ranges blank.
13. Hand in your reports to your instructor.

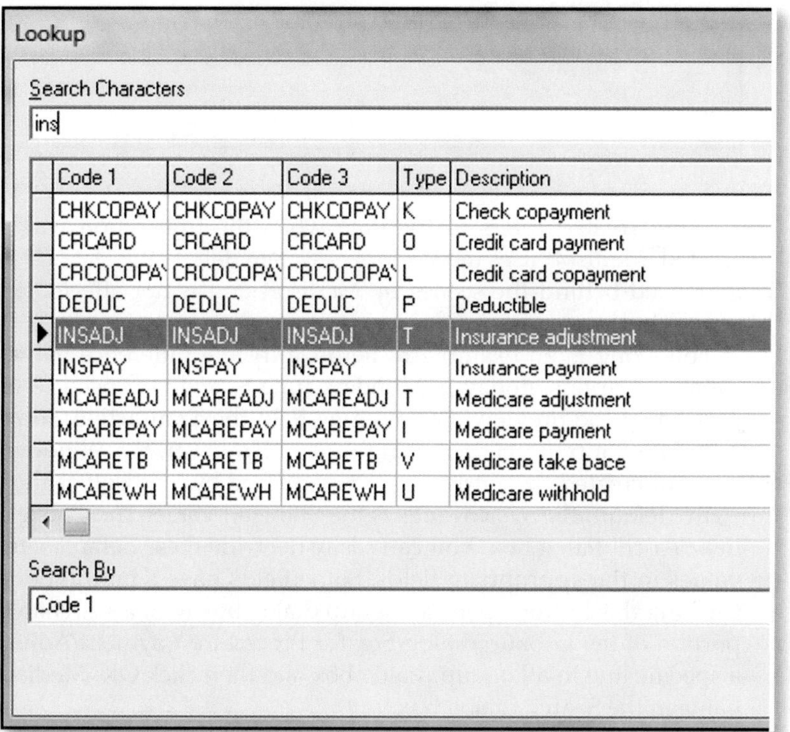

Figure 4.29
Portion of Lookup dialog box for Procedure/ Payment/Adjustment codes.

Practice Analysis Report

The Practice Analysis Report provides the total count of all procedures performed at the medical office. The manager can use this report to determine the number of procedures being billed and may even use it to determine inventory levels. It is usually printed at the end of the month. The Practice Analysis Report is useful to determine what procedures are being ordered and how often they are performed. In other words, this report does not give any patient details. Instead, it gives a summarized report of the medical office's completed procedures, which can be used for profit analysis. Many of the data selection ranges for the Practice Analysis Report are similar to other accounting reports.

PROCEDURE 4.15 PRINTING A PRACTICE ANALYSIS REPORT

1. On the Reports menu, click *Analysis Reports.* A submenu displays.
2. Click *Practice Analysis.* The Print Report Where dialog box opens.
3. If necessary, click the radio button for *Preview the report on the screen.*
4. Click *Start.* The Search dialog box displays.
5. Leave all the fields blank and click *OK.* The Print Preview window displays the report.
6. Click the *Print* button in the upper-left corner of the window.
7. Select a printer and hand in the report to your instructor.

Patient Ledger

The Patient Ledger shows transaction information grouped by patient and by date. This report lists detailed transaction history information about the patient, including all financial activity and totals for charges and payments. You also have the capability to print the report for one patient, a range of patients, or all patients. Data selection ranges are similar to other accounting reports you have printed.

PROCEDURE 4.16 PRINTING PATIENT LEDGERS

1. Click *Patient Ledger* on the Reports menu. The Print Report Where dialog box displays.
2. If necessary, click the radio button for *Preview the report on the screen.*
3. Click *Start.* The Search dialog box displays.
4. In the Chart Number fields, enter the chart number for Charles Weber in the first field and Cindy Wixen in the second field.
5. Click *OK.* The Print Preview window displays the report.
6. Click the *Print* button in the upper-left corner of the window.
7. Select a printer and hand in the report to your instructor.

Using Terminology

Match the terms on the left with the definitions on the right.

_____ **1.** owners' equity
_____ **2.** ledger
_____ **3.** day sheet
_____ **4.** assets
_____ **5.** cash flow
_____ **6.** cycle billing
_____ **7.** accounts payable
_____ **8.** remittance advice (RA)
_____ **9.** liabilities
_____ **10.** once-a-month billing
_____ **11.** accounts receivable
_____ **12.** accrual-basis accounting
_____ **13.** explanation of benefits (EOB)
_____ **14.** statement
_____ **15.** practice analysis
_____ **16.** cash-basis accounting
_____ **17.** basic accounting equation

a. Formula that expresses how financial transactions affect a business
b. Money owed by a business for unpaid purchases
c. Report that shows the charges, payments, and adjustments made during a specified time period for procedures performed in a medical office
d. Money owed to a business by others
e. Method in which revenues are recorded when services are performed and expenses are recorded when incurred, not when they are paid
f. Report sent by an insurance carrier to a patient containing details on how benefits were paid
g. Items of value owned by a business
h. Method in which revenues and expenses are not recorded until they are actually paid
i. Money coming into and going out of a business
j. Financial stake that the business owners, business partners, or shareholders have in a business
k. List of all transactions in chronological order for a given day or range of days
l. System in which a portion of patient statements are prepared at regular time intervals throughout a month rather than all at once
m. Report that shows a group of financial accounts with a detailed list of all the transactions related to each account
n. Debts and other financial obligations of a business
o. System in which all patient statements are prepared once a month at the same time
p. Report sent from a payer to a practice, often electronically, showing how insurance benefits were paid for patients
q. Document that shows the amount a patient owes to the medical office

Checking Your Understanding

1. Explain the three components of the basic accounting equation.
2. What is the difference between Date From fields and Date Created fields when printing Medisoft reports?
3. Explain how charges are entered in Medisoft.
4. After entering a patient payment and saving the transaction, what else must you do?
5. Where in Medisoft can you print a walkout receipt?
6. What is the process used to create insurance claims?
7. List the information needed to enter a payment from an insurance company.
8. Which method of printing patient statements updates the statement submission count tracked in Medisoft?
9. What are the three types of day sheets and when are they typically printed?

Putting It into Practice

Complete the following exercise that uses all the knowledge you have gained so far, and then review the terminology and chapter concepts before moving on to the next chapter.

1. Enter information in Medisoft for the following patients using the registration forms in Appendix C. Dr. Jagla is the assigned provider for each patient.
    - For David Simpson, use Figure C.31 in Appendix C.
    - For Melissa Jones, use Figure C.32 in Appendix C.
    - For Anne Potter, use Figure C.33 in Appendix C.
    - For Richard Potter, use Figure C.34 in Appendix C.
    - For Michael Ruha, use Figure C.35 in Appendix C.
2. The patients entered in step 1 need to be scheduled for an appointment on 3/9/2010 with Dr. Jagla: David Simpson for a forearm injury, Melissa Jones for contact dermatitis, Anne Potter for a well-woman examination, Richard Potter for a routine physical examination, and Michael Ruha for a well-child examination.
3. Enter the charges for these patients using the encounter forms in Appendix C (see Figures C.36 through C.40). You may have to add some of the diagnosis and procedure codes in Medisoft.
4. Print a Patient Day Sheet report for 3/9/2010 for these five patients.
5. Create and print insurance claims for these five patients.
6. Enter and apply the payments for these patients, received from their insurance carriers on 3/22/2010. Use the RA information shown in Appendix C (see Figures C.41 and C.42).
7. Print Patient Statements for these patients.
8. Hand in all printouts to your instructor. Before exiting Medisoft, back up your data as designated by your instructor.

References

Adams DM: *Diagnosis: documentation and coding,* New York, 1997, McGraw Hill.
Flight M: *Law, liability, and ethics for medical office procedures,* ed 3, Albany, NY, 1998, Delmar.
Fordney MT: *Insurance handbook for the medical office,* ed 11, Philadelphia, 2010, Saunders–Elsevier.
HealthCare Consultants of America: *Health care fraud and abuse,* Augusta, Ga, 1997, The Consultants.
Holmes DL: *Practical guide to medical billing,* Springfield, Ill, 1997, US Department of Commerce.
Kuehn L: *Health information management: medical records process in group practice,* Englewood, Colo, 1997, Center for Research in Ambulatory Health Care Administration.
Moini J: *Glencoe medical assisting review: passing the CMA and RMA exams,* New York, 2001, Glencoe.
Redman B, editor: *Life and health insurance,* ed 4, Chicago, 1999, Dearborn Financial Institute.
Reid J: *A telemedicine primer: understanding the issues,* Billings, Mont, 1996, Artcraft Printers.
Rizzo C: *Uniform billing: a guide to claims processing,* Albany, NY, 2000, Delmar.
Ross A, Pavlock E, Williams S: *Ambulatory care management,* ed 3, Albany, NY, 1998, Delmar.
Rowell J: *Understanding health insurance: a guide to professional billing,* ed 5, Albany, NY, 2000, Delmar.

chapter 5

Collection in the Medical Office

Objectives

1. Explain ways to manage and reduce collections problems.
2. Describe methods used to collect overdue patient accounts.
3. Add tickler items to a collections list.
4. Print patient collection letters and a Collection Tracer Report.
5. Describe the steps used to make adjustments and write-offs in Medisoft.

Terminology

aging report: Printout that shows unpaid charges as current or delinquent, based on the number of days they have *aged* (been outstanding)

collection: Process of obtaining payment for services rendered, usually involving accounts that are past due an extended period

collection agency: Organization that acts as a third party to collect unpaid debts

collection letter: Correspondence sent to a patient to remind him or her of an overdue payment

collection list: Tool used to follow-up on unpaid accounts by creating reminders

Collection Tracer Report: Feature that tracks the quantities and dates of collection letters sent

payment plan: Agreement that allows a patient to pay a specified dollar amount at regular time intervals to reduce his or her debt; may include interest and late fees

sliding fee scale: System of charging for services based on the patient's income and family size

tickler: Time-sensitive reminder note added to a collection list

write-off: Accounts receivable item that is uncollectable and therefore recorded as a loss or expense in the financial records; also called a *bad debt*

Overall, the word **collection** has a negative connotation, but this meaning does not always accurately portray this important element of a well-run medical office. Collection can simply mean the process of obtaining payment for services rendered. However, in many medical offices, collection refers to patients' accounts that are past due for an extended period of time. These accounts may require additional efforts to secure payment. This chapter reviews the collection process and explains how to use Medisoft to complete various collection-related activities.

WAYS TO MANAGE AND REDUCE COLLECTIONS PROBLEMS

Although many patients promptly pay their bills, there are multiple explanations why some bills are not paid on time. Reasons may include absentmindedness, job loss, other financial problems, service complaints, and inadequate or no insurance. For instance, in difficult economic times, when unemployment is high, patients may find it hard to pay their bills, even though they may want to.

Another source of past-due accounts is related to unpaid insurance claims. Problems may be due to inadequate or incorrect information submitted, causing a carrier to contest a claim. Unfortunately, insurance companies are not always quick to notify medical offices about issues with claims. These delays, plus the additional time it takes a medical office to resubmit claims, can affect the financial stability of a medical office.

Fortunately, there are tools in Medisoft that can help you limit the impact of delayed payments. Features, such as insurance eligibility verification, aging reports, and the ability to create patient payment plans, allow you to address collection issues before they become larger problems. It is also important to make sure patients understand and agree to the medical office's financial policies before services are rendered.

Communicating Financial Policies

Almost all medical offices have policies related to the patient's responsibility and the ways in which payments may be made. Usually, patients (or their guarantors) are asked to read and sign a document that outlines the medical office's financial policies. In addition to this document, the medical office most likely has an internal policy for its staff that outlines the process and steps for collecting payments. Following are examples of topics often addressed within the financial policy document given to patients:

- In the event that the insurance carrier does not pay in full for the medical services performed, the patient (or guarantor) is responsible for paying the balance.
- If the patient's insurance plan requires a referral before seeing a specialist, it is usually the patient's responsibility to obtain that referral.
- Copayments are expected at the time of service.
- If the patient has no insurance, some offices require full payment up front.
- Forms of payment accepted may be indicated, such as cash, personal checks, or types of credit cards.
- A late fee may be added to a patient's account if payment is not made within a certain amount of time. Also, a service fee is frequently charged to a patient account if a personal check is returned by the bank due to insufficient funds (also referred to as a *bounced check*).
- Some medical offices reserve the right to charge for missed appointments or visits cancelled less than 24 hours before the appointment time.

Verifying Patients' Insurance Eligibility

Many collection problems can be avoided if each patient's insurance eligibility is verified prior to appointments. Medisoft's Eligibility Verification feature is an optional, fee-based service in which a medical office can enroll. This service allows you to check insurance coverage via the Internet.

Eligibility verification inquiries can be made from two places within Medisoft. You can click F10 on the toolbar, or you can open Office Hours Professional and right-click a patient's name in the appointment grid. In either of these scenarios, right-clicking causes a pop-up menu to display. When you click the Eligibility Verification option on the pop-up menu, the Eligibility Verification Results dialog box opens (Figure 5.1). The next step is to click the Verify button, which opens the Real-Time Eligibility Verification window with the patient's information. When the Verify button is clicked, Medisoft makes the inquiry, and the result displays in the window. Remember, this feature is an optional, fee-based service, and, as such, you will not be able to access it in your student program.

You can access verification results for previous inquiries or redo an inquiry by clicking Eligibility Verification on the Activities menu and then clicking the View Results option on the submenu that displays. When the Eligibility Verification Results dialog box opens (see Figure 5.1), click the inquiry you wish to redo and then click the Verify button. Keep in mind that records only appear in the Eligibility Verification Results dialog box after one or more inquiries have been made.

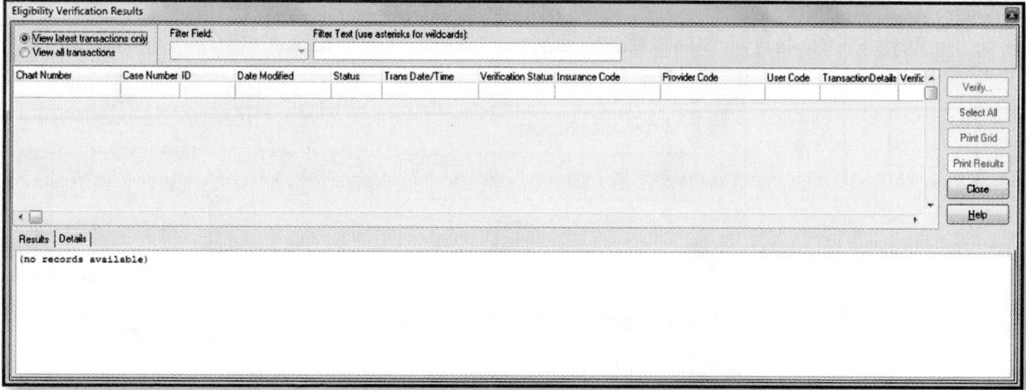

Figure 5.1
Eligibility Verification Results dialog box.

Printing Aging Reports

One way to anticipate and avoid collection problems is to print one or more aging reports on a regular basis. In Medisoft, you can create an **aging report** for both patients and insurance carriers. These reports show the status of each account; that is, whether an account is current or past due. By pinpointing potential issues early, aging reports help limit the need to do write-offs. A **write-off** is an uncollectable accounts receivable item (also called a *bad debt*) that is recorded in the financial records as a loss or expense.

In general, aging reports show the amounts of money owed to the practice based on the length of time those amounts have been owed. An account balance is listed by age in the following default columns: 0–30, 31–60, 61–90, and 91+ days. The number of days in these aging columns can be changed by opening the Program Options dialog box (File menu) and clicking the Aging Reports tab.

Keep in mind that Medisoft calculates the age of transaction or claim amounts based on the date when you run a report (Windows system date). So, for example, if you printed a Patient Aging Report on April 27, 2013 and $48 was charged on February 15, 2010, then that amount would be included in the past 91+ days column by default (Figure 5.2).

The Patient Remainder Aging Report and the Patient Remainder Aging Detail Report list the age and print past-due balances for which the patient is responsible. In other words, these reports show only the amounts that remain after the insurance portions have been paid. Consequently, no charges will display on these reports until all related insurance payments have been applied and marked completed.

Insurance aging reports print the age of claims for primary, secondary, or tertiary carriers. The older a claim becomes, the less likely it is to be paid. Insurance aging reports should be printed every month. Outstanding claims should be followed up with insurance carriers as dictated by the medical office's collection policies. As with patient aging reports, the Aging Reports tab in the Program Options dialog box allows you to change the default number of days in the aging columns.

To print an aging report, the Aging Reports option is clicked on the Reports menu. This action displays a submenu shown in Figure 5.3. Whenever an aging report is selected,

Figure 5.2
Patient Aging Report.

Elsevier Clinic

Patient Aging by Date of Service

As of April 27, 2013

Chart	Name		Current 0 - 30	Past 31 - 60	Past 61 - 90	Past 91 ---->	Total Balance
SMIDA000	**Daniel Smith**					10.00	10.00
Last Pmt: -114.00	On:3/15/2010	(555)253-2345					
WEBCH000	**Charles A Weber**					48.00	48.00
Last Pmt: -20.00	On:3/1/2010	(555)555-2352					
Report Aging Totals			$0.00	$0.00	$0.00	$58.00	$58.00
Percent of Aging Total			0.0 %	0.0 %	0.0 %	100.0 %	100.0 %

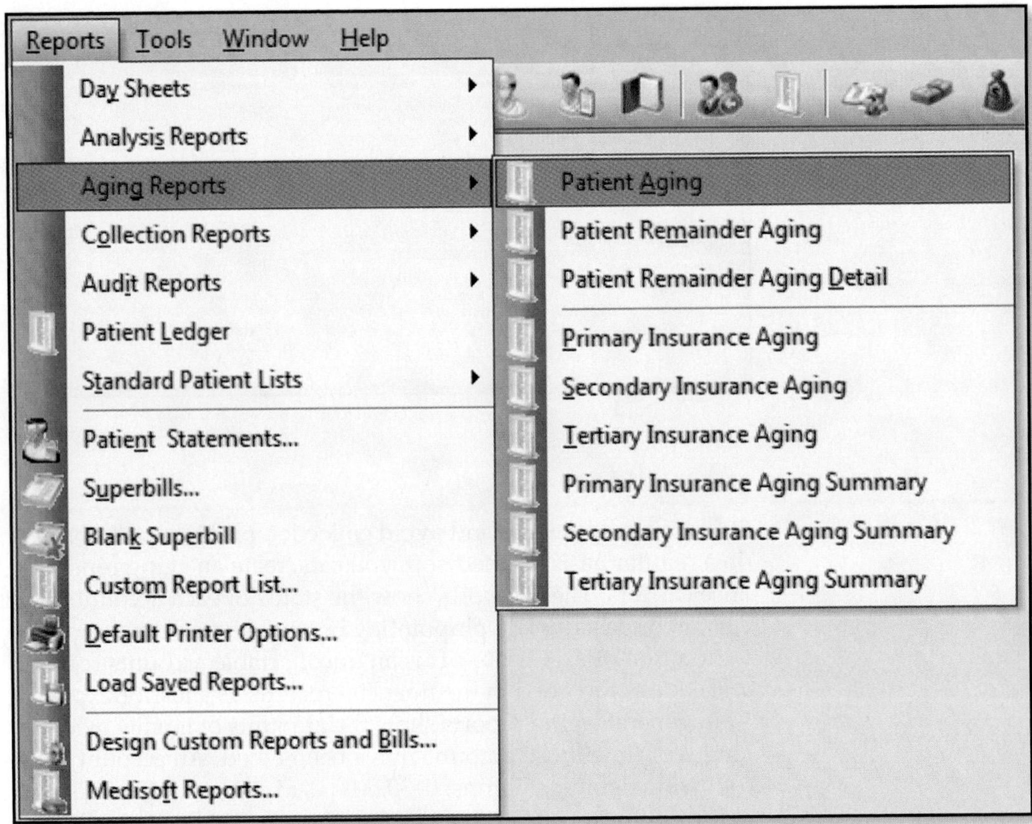

Figure 5.3 Aging Reports submenu.

Medisoft displays a Print Report Where dialog box followed by a Search dialog box. The fields in the Search dialog box are used as filters to select the desired data for a report. These fields vary, depending on the type of report you are printing. For example, Figure 5.4 shows the Search dialog box when printing the Patient Aging Report.

Filters in the two Patient Remainder Aging reports include Chart Number Range, Billing Code Range, and Patient Indicator Range. For the Insurance Aging reports, filters include Insurance Carrier Code Range, Billing Date Range, and Attending Provider Range. As a default, the Show All Values checkboxes in aging reports are automatically selected (see Figure 5.4) for an example. However, you can choose to enter specific codes or ranges of values. Also, notice that beside some fields there is a button with three dots. You can click this button to open a Lookup dialog box that contains a searchable list of corresponding codes.

PROCEDURE 5.1 PRINTING AGING REPORTS

In this exercise, you will print both a Patient Aging Report and a Primary Insurance Aging Report.

1. On the Reports menu, click or point to the *Aging Reports* option. A submenu displays with a list of reports.
2. Click *Patient Aging.* The Print Report Where dialog box displays.
3. Click the radio button for *Print the report on the printer.*
4. Click the *Start* button. A Search dialog box opens with the Show All Values checkboxes selected.
5. Leave all the fields unchanged, and click *OK.*
6. Select a printer, and click *OK.*
7. Using the preceding steps, print a Primary Insurance Aging Report. Hand in both reports to your instructor.

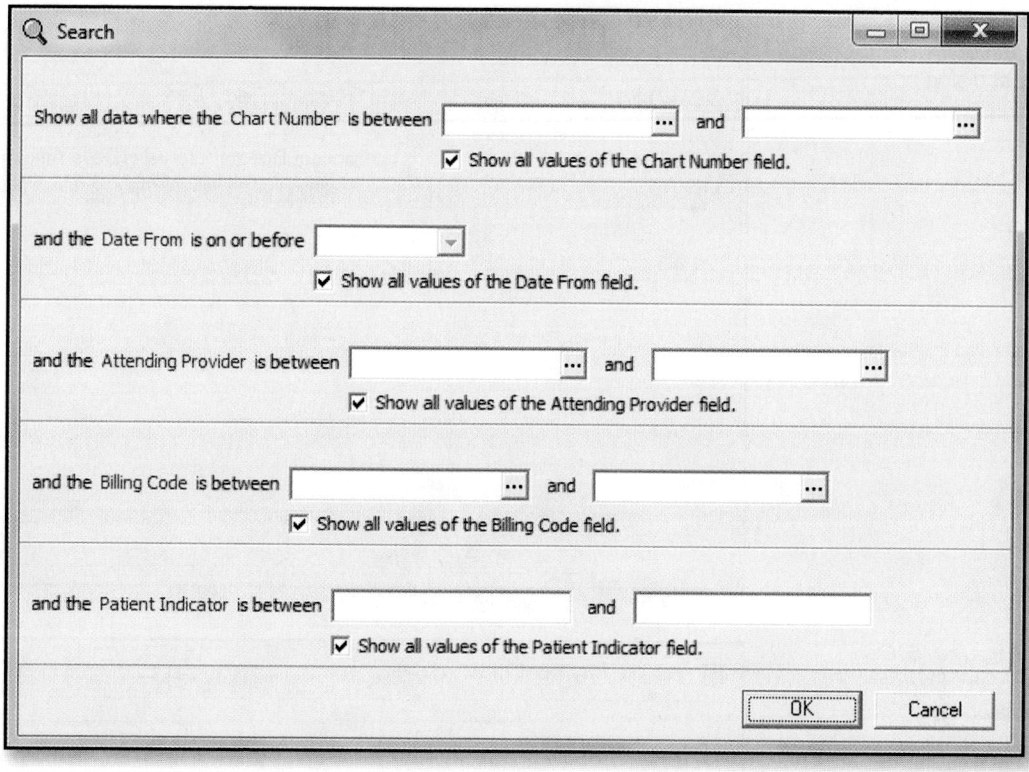

Figure 5.4
Search dialog box for the Patient Aging Report.

Search

Show all data where the Chart Number is between [ ] and [ ]
☑ Show all values of the Chart Number field.

and the Date From is on or before [ ]
☑ Show all values of the Date From field.

and the Attending Provider is between [ ] and [ ]
☑ Show all values of the Attending Provider field.

and the Billing Code is between [ ] and [ ]
☑ Show all values of the Billing Code field.

and the Patient Indicator is between [ ] and [ ]
☑ Show all values of the Patient Indicator field.

OK Cancel

Creating Patient Payment Plans

The reasons for not paying a medical bill are numerous: the loss of a job, the loss of insurance, a major unexpected expense for the home, or car repairs, and so on. The majority of patients who have outstanding medical bills want to pay them, but they may need assistance to do so. A method used by some medical clinics is a **sliding fee scale.** This system allows for a reduced payment, based on the patient's income and family size. The income is usually verified through payment stubs or income tax forms. Services are then billed to the patient at the discounted rate. However, certain requirements are involved in the use of a sliding fee scale. For more information, visit the government Web site of the Health Resources and Services Administration at http://bphc.hrsa.gov/technicalassistance/taresources/slidingrequirements.html.

Another option that a medical office can use is to work out a **payment plan** with the patient. Such a plan usually allows a patient to pay a set dollar amount at a specific time interval (e.g., every 30 days) until the bill is completely paid. Potential service charges and late fees also need to be discussed with the patient when establishing a payment plan.

One or more payment plans can be set up in Medisoft by clicking the Patient Payment Plan option in the Lists menu (Advanced or Network Professional versions only). This action opens the Patient Payment Plan List dialog box (Figure 5.5). Next, the New button is clicked to open the Patient Payment Plan dialog box (Figure 5.6). After a plan is set up, its code needs to be entered in the patient's record (Payment Plan tab in the Patient/Guarantor dialog box). Following is a description of the fields in the Patient Payment Plan dialog box:

Code. Up to three characters can be used to identify a payment plan.
Inactive. This field should only be check marked if the code is no longer active.
Description. Enter a brief description of the payment plan.
First Payment Due. Enter the day of the month when the first payment is due.
Due Every. Enter the number of days between each payment.
Amount Due. Enter the amount due for each payment in the plan.

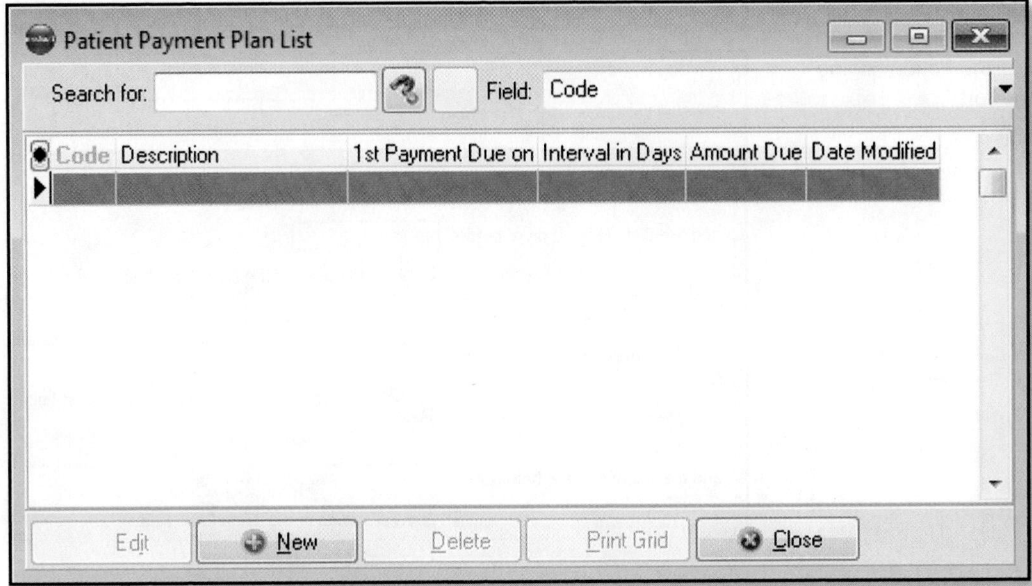

Figure 5.5
Patient Payment Plan List dialog box.

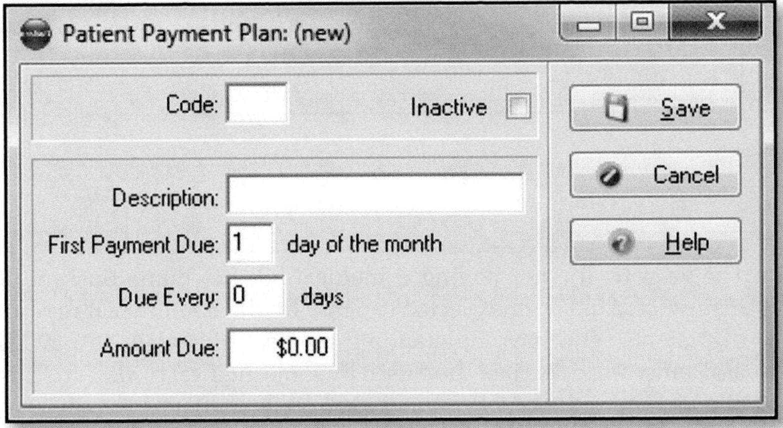

Figure 5.6
Patient Payment Plan dialog box.

PROCEDURE 5.2 CREATING AND ASSIGNING A PAYMENT PLAN CODE

Due to financial problems, Mr. Weber was unable to pay his insurance premiums. The claim for Mr. Weber's visit was denied because his insurance coverage lapsed. The balance due on his account is $48.00. Dr. Walker agrees to allow the patient to pay for services based on a plan that requires a payment of $16 every month until the bill is fully paid.

1. On the Lists menu, click *Patient Payment Plan*. The Patient Payment Plan List dialog box opens.
2. Click the *New* button. The Patient Payment Plan dialog box displays.
3. In the Code field, key *W16*.
4. In the Description field, key *$16 Every 30 Days*.
5. In the First Payment Due field, key *1* if this value is not already displayed.
6. In the Due Every field, key *30*.
7. In the Amount Due field, key *16.00*.
8. Click *Save*. The Patient Payment Plan dialog box closes, and the new entry displays in the Patient Payment Plan list.

9. Click *Close*.
10. On the Lists menu, click *Patient/Guarantors and Cases*. The Patient List dialog box opens.
11. Click the record for *Charles Weber*, and then click *Edit Patient*.
12. Click the *Payment Plan* tab.
13. In the Payment Code field, key *W16*. The rest of the fields are automatically completed.
14. Click *Save* to update the patient's record.
15. Click *Close* to close the Patient List dialog box.

COLLECTION METHODS FOR OVERDUE ACCOUNTS

Often, the routine act of mailing out patient statements will be enough to remind and encourage patients to pay any outstanding amounts. However, if no response is received, then it may become necessary to attempt collecting overdue balances by other means. Frequently used methods involve telephone calls, collection letters, and collection agencies. Most medical offices have an established policy or timeline that outlines when calls are made and letters are sent.

As with all other tasks in a medical office, it is important to be both professional and kind when collecting money from patients. You should also be aware of behaviors that are considered illegal or unethical. The Fair Debt Collection Practices Act (FDCPA) is a federal law that regulates the manner in which debts are collected. Its purpose is to protect consumers from harassment and unfair debt collection practices. Some states may also have laws regarding collection practices. For more information on the FDCPA, visit the Federal Trade Commission's Web site at www.ftc.gov/os/statutes/fdcpajump.shtm.

Making Telephone Calls

A telephone call is the most personal way to address overdue account balances because it allows both parties to discuss the situation and hopefully come to a successful resolution. Following are some general rules that should be observed when making collection calls:

- Call only between 8 AM and 9 PM.
- Ask to speak only with the person who is financially responsible for the account.
- Be friendly with a positive attitude.
- Ask the patient or guarantor to commit to pay the bill in some manner; for example, a specified amount by a certain date.
- Do not allow yourself to get hostile or upset, even if the patient does.
- Keep a record of when you called and what was said.
- Do not make repeated telephone calls.
- Do not be deceptive, make threats, or use profane language.

Sending Collection Letters

If sending a statement and making a telephone call does not lead to the payment of an overdue account, sending a collection letter is usually the next step. A **collection letter** is a useful means of communication when a patient or guarantor cannot be reached by telephone. A collection letter can be sent by regular mail, or it can be sent by certified mail that requires the recipient to sign for the letter. Regardless of the mailing method, the letter should include the following information:

- Medical office's desire to provide the best possible treatment and care for the patient
- Amount that is overdue with a description, such as $20 copayment

- Who to call at the medical office to set up payment arrangements
- Acceptable forms of payment, such as credit card, cash, or check
- Where to send the payment, if mailing
- Place for a signature and date to indicate who sent the letter and when it was sent

Collection letters are often sent more than one time to patients who continue not to pay their accounts. Each time another collection letter is sent, the message may be changed to reflect the urgency of the circumstances or to point out the amount of time the account has been past due. For examples of collection letters, visit the Web site of Collection Agency Services, Inc., at www.collectionagencyservices.net/collectionletters/sample collectionletters.html.

Using Collection Agencies

When telephone calls and collection letters fail to produce results, the medical office has two more options: (1) to write off the amount in the financial records, or (2) to refer the amount to a collection agency. A **collection agency** is a third party, which means it has no affiliation with the medical practice. A collection agency will attempt to collect the payment for the medical office in exchange for a flat fee or a percentage of the amount collected.

When an overdue account is sent to a collection agency, the medical office ceases all attempts to contact the patient for payment; the agency is now responsible for contacting the patient. If the patient sends a payment to the medical office, the collection agency should be notified immediately.

COLLECTION LIST DIALOG BOX

After printing aging reports to identify which accounts are overdue, you can use a **collection list** to help manage the medical office's collection efforts. In Medisoft, the Collection List dialog box is used to create one or more tickler items (Advanced or Network Professional versions). A **tickler** is a time-sensitive reminder or note that singles out an account requiring special attention, such as a collection telephone call or letter. Your office's collection policy will provide guidelines for deciding when and for whom ticklers should be added to the Collection List.

To create a tickler, the Collection List option is clicked on the Activities menu. This action opens the Collection List dialog box (Figure 5.7). It displays buttons along the bottom for adding, editing, printing, and deleting ticklers. There is also a Reassign button to associate one or more ticklers with a different account. After ticklers have been added, they are listed in the window portion of the dialog box in grid-like columns.

Along the top of the Collection List dialog box are fields and buttons used to locate or sort the list of tickler items in the window.

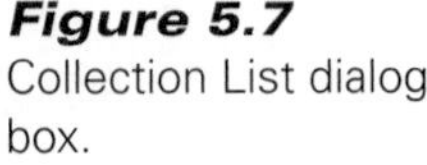

Figure 5.7
Collection List dialog box.

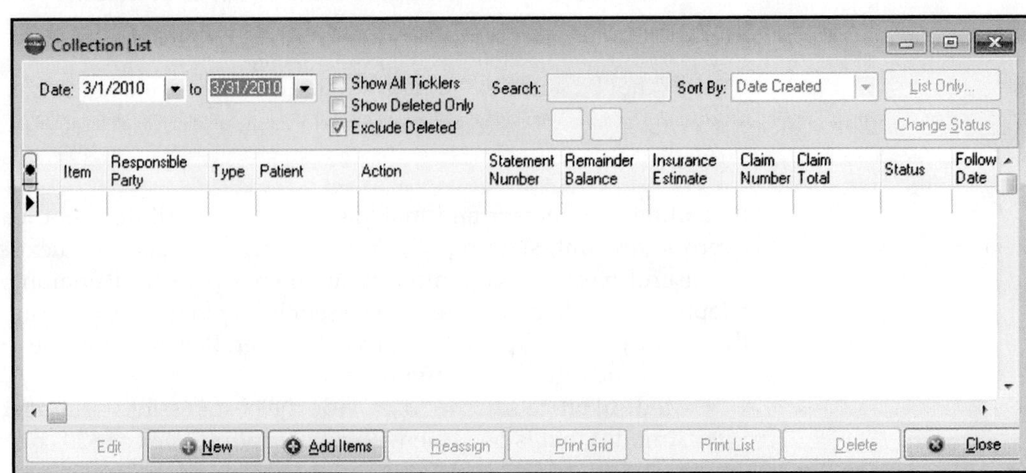

Date. By default, the current date displays in both Date fields, and only those tickler items due on this date are listed in the window. However, you can enter or select a different date or range of dates.

Show All Ticklers. If this checkbox is selected, the Date fields become unavailable and all tickler items display in the window.

Show Deleted Only. Only previously deleted ticklers display in the window if this checkbox is selected.

Exclude Deleted. Previously deleted ticklers do not display in the window if this checkbox is selected.

Search and Sort By. Use these two fields to locate a particular tickler item quickly. First, click an option in the Sort By list box by which to sort the list of ticklers. The choices are Balance, Claim Total, Date Created, Date Deleted, Date Resolved, Follow Up Date, Insurance Estimate, Item Number, or Patient. Next, in the Search field, key the first few characters related to the chosen Sort By option. For example, if you clicked Patient in the Sort By field and then keyed SMI in the Search field, the first tickler with a patient chart number starting with SMI will appear highlighted in the list.

List Only. Click this button to open the List Only Ticklers That Match dialog box, allowing you to select and view a group of tickler items containing specific information.

Change Status. Click this button to open the Change Status/Follow Up Dates dialog box, allowing you to change the status or date for one tickler item or a group of ticklers.

Adding a Single Tickler Item

Keep in mind that before you can add tickler items, a case must be created for the patient. In the Collection List dialog box, you can add a single tickler by clicking the New button. This action opens the Tickler Item dialog box (Figure 5.8). There are two tabs in this dialog box: Tickler and Office Notes. The Office Notes tab contains a large window in which you can key various notes about the particular tickler. For example, you might use this tab to enter notes about a telephone call with the patient about his or her overdue account. The

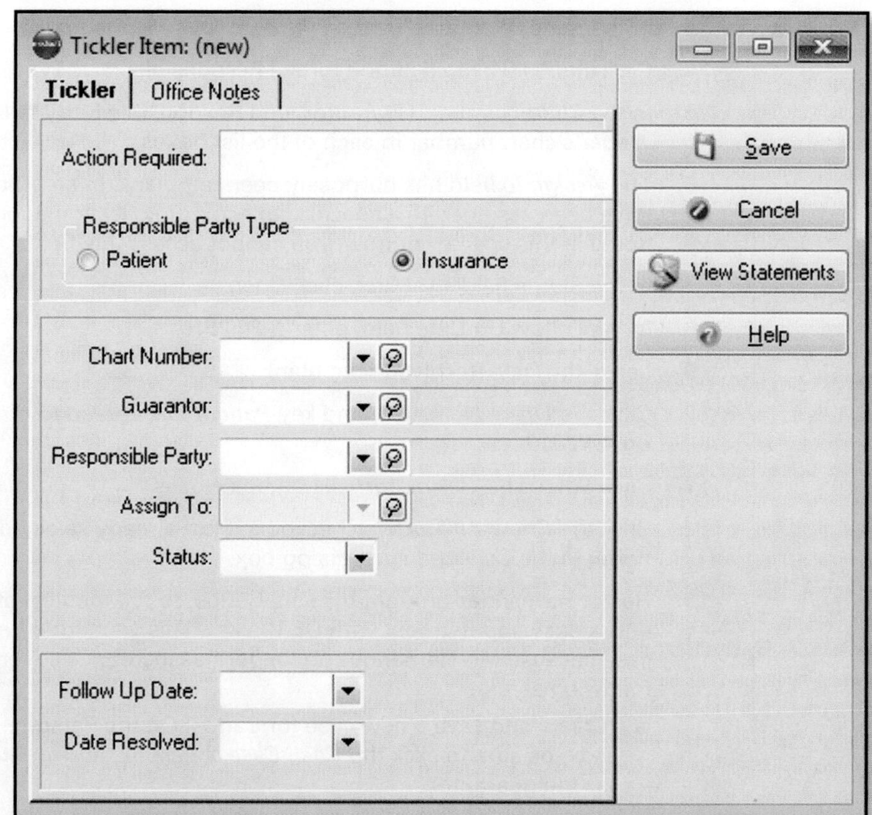

Figure 5.8 Tickler Item dialog box with Tickler tab displayed.

Tickler tab displays by default when the Tickler Item dialog box is opened. Please note for Medisoft version 17 and 18 the View Statements button is below the Cancel button. The fields in this tab are as follows:

Action Required. Key the action required to resolve the situation, for example, "Call patient about overdue bill."

Responsible Party Type. Click the radio button for the type of entity responsible for resolving this tickler item, the patient or the insurance carrier.

Chart Number. Key the patient's chart number, or click the appropriate number in the list box.

Guarantor. If applicable, key the guarantor's number or click it in the list box.

Responsible Party. The options in this field's list box correspond to the radio button previously chosen for Responsible Party Type. If Patient was chosen, patient chart numbers will display in the list box. If Insurance was chosen, insurance carrier codes will display in the list box.

Assign To. Click the down arrow to select the employee who is responsible for following up on this tickler item.

Status. In this field's list box, click one of three options: Open, Resolved, or Deleted.

Follow Up Date. Enter the date when this tickler should be followed up. If Open was previously chosen in the Status field, the current date automatically displays.

Date Resolved. When appropriate, enter the date when this tickler was resolved. If Resolved was chosen in the Status field, the current date automatically displays.

PROCEDURE 5.3 CREATING NEW TICKLER ITEMS

According to Mr. Weber's payment plan, the first $16 is due on the first day of the next month. In this exercise, you will add a tickler item to remind yourself to send Mr. Weber a copy of the signed payment agreement. You will also create a new tickler for an overdue "cash case" for another patient.

1. Click *Collection List* on the Activities menu. The Collection List dialog box opens.
2. Click *New*. The Tickler Item dialog box opens with the Tickler tab displayed.
3. In the Action Required field, key *Mail copy of signed payment agreement.*
4. Click the *Patient* radio button for the Responsible Party Type, if not already selected.
5. In the Chart Number, Guarantor, and Responsible Party fields, click Charles Weber's chart number in each of the list boxes.
6. The *Assign To* field has purposely been left blank. In an office, this account would have been assigned to a specific collector or collection agency that would be noted in this space. For now, you cannot access this field.
7. In the Status field's list box, click *Open*.
8. In the Follow Up Date field, enter *3/25/2010*.
9. Leave the Date Resolved field blank.
10. Click the *Office Notes* tab, and key *Patient has agreed to make his first payment on 4/1/2010.*
11. Click *Save*. The Tickler Item dialog box closes.
12. Click the *Show All Ticklers* checkbox, if not already selected, to display the new tickler in the Collection List dialog box.
13. Hector Hernandez brought his son, Carlos, to the medical office and requested an emergency appointment with Dr. Walker. This visit, for a hand injury, is a cash case because Mr. Hernandez no longer has insurance coverage. Complete the following steps:
    a. Create and save a new case for Carlos. On the Personal tab of the Case dialog box, be sure to click the *Cash Case* checkbox, and identify Hector Hernandez as the guarantor.

b. Enter and save a charge transaction for this case, using the date *3/5/2010*. The procedure code is *99213* for the office visit. The diagnosis code is *959.4* for the hand injury.

c. Mr. Hernandez promised to pay his bill the following week, but no payment was received. Create a new tickler to send a follow-up letter to Mr. Hernandez on 3/15/2010.

14. Click *Close* to close the Collection List dialog box.

Adding a Group of Tickler Items

Although clicking the New button in the Collection List dialog box lets you add a single tickler, clicking the Add Items button allows you to create tickler items for multiple patients or insurance companies based on the criteria you choose. Do not worry about accidentally creating duplicate tickler items. Medisoft will not create a new tickler if one is already on file for a particular patient, guarantor, and claim or statement number, which also has an open status.

When you click the Add Items button in the Collection List dialog box or, optionally, when you click Add Collection List Items on the Activities menu, the Add Collection List Items dialog box opens (Figure 5.9).

At the top of the dialog box are two radio buttons on which all ticklers created will be based: Statements or Claims. Depending on which of these two buttons you click, other fields in the dialog box will change or become active or inactive. For example, if you choose Claims, four radio buttons related to the type of insurance carriers will become active, allowing you to choose All, Primary, Secondary, or Tertiary carriers. In the Range of fields, you can select a range of insurance codes if the ticklers are to be based on claims, or a range of patient chart numbers if the ticklers are to be based on statements.

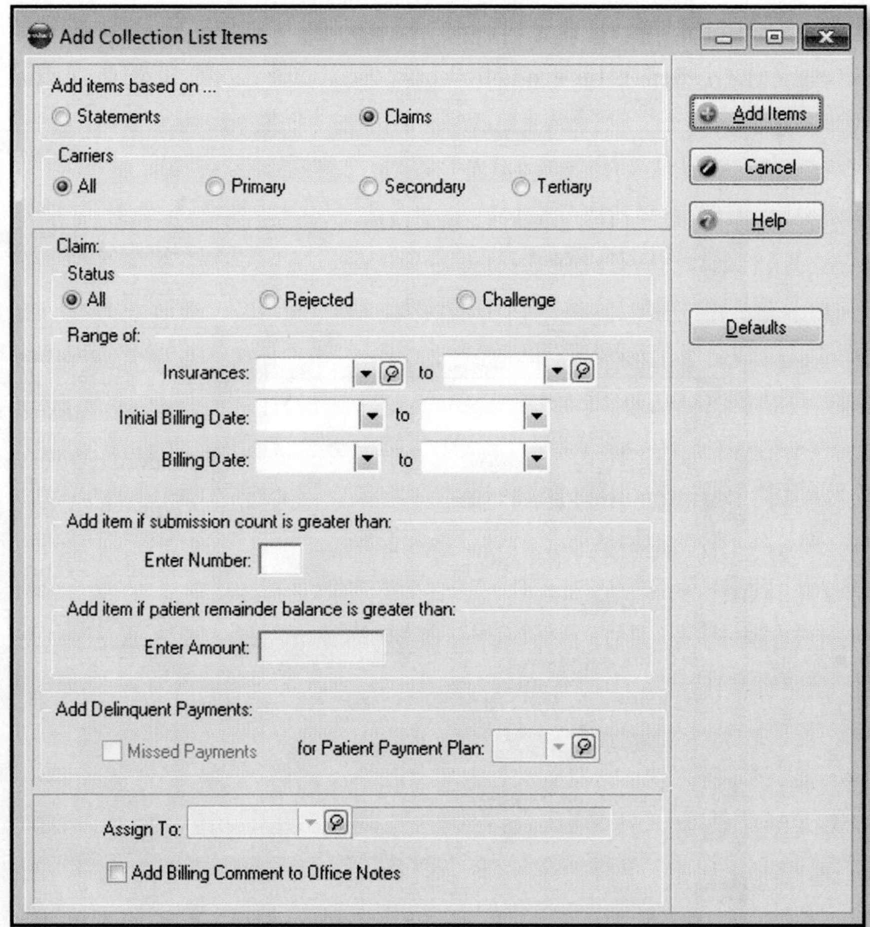

Figure 5.9 Add Collection List Items dialog box.

PROCEDURE 5.4 USING THE ADD COLLECTION LIST ITEMS FEATURE

1. Open the Collection List dialog box.
2. Click the *Add Items* button. The Add Collection List Items dialog box opens.
3. If not already selected, click the *Claims* radio button to base all ticklers on claims previously created.
4. Leave the rest of the fields blank or with their current default values.
5. Click *Add Items.* A confirm dialog box opens asking if you want to add more collection list items. Click *No*, and the *Add Collection List Items* dialog box closes, and a new tickler appears in the Collection List dialog box's window. Had there been other overdue claims, multiple ticklers would have displayed.
6. Click *Close* to close the Collection List dialog box.

COLLECTION REPORTS

Medisoft has a series of reports to assist you with the collections process. These are listed on a submenu accessed by clicking or pointing to the Collection Reports option on the Reports menu (Figure 5.10). Following is a brief description of each type of collection report (Medisoft Advanced or Network Professional versions):

- *Patient Collection Report.* Print this report to see what transactions have not been paid. Report data is based on previously generated statements (marked with a Sent status in the Statement Management dialog box).
- *Insurance Collection Reports.* All three of these reports are similar except they each pertain to a particular insurance level: primary, secondary, or tertiary. Insurance Collection Reports provide transaction information from previously generated insurance claims, including outstanding amounts.
- *Patient Collection Letters.* This menu selection allows you to print a Collection Letter Report for evaluation purposes before generating the actual letters. Before collection

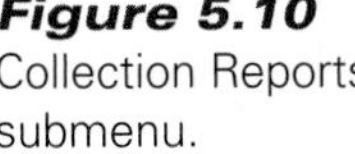

Figure 5.10 Collection Reports submenu.

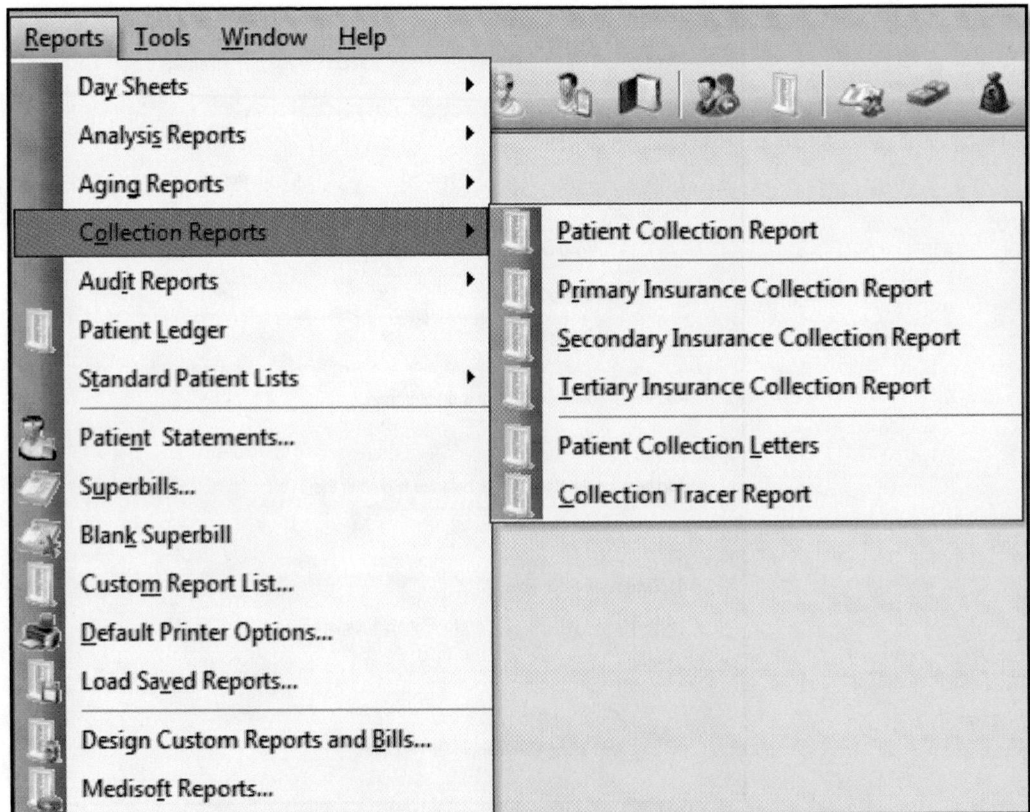

letters can be produced, there must be at least one tickler item (in the Collection List dialog box) for which the patient or guarantor is the entity responsible for payment.

- **Collection Tracer Report.** Each time collection letters are printed, Medisoft keeps track of how many letters have been created and when they were produced. You can print the Collection Tracer Report to review this tracking information.

All of the collection reports display the Print Report Where dialog box when they are first clicked on the Collection Reports submenu. Next, depending on the report, either a Search dialog box or a Data Selection Questions dialog box displays. Both types of dialog boxes provide various filters used to select the desired report data. For example, Figure 5.11 shows the Data Selection Questions dialog box for the Collection Letter Report, which is also used to print collection letters.

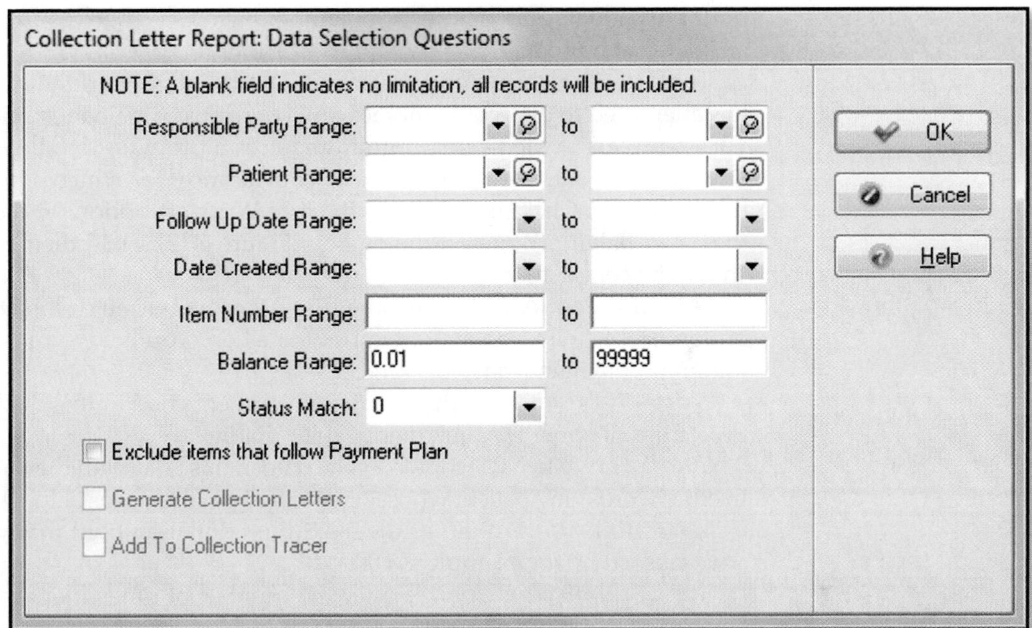

Figure 5.11 Data Selection Questions dialog box for the Collection Letter Report.

PROCEDURE 5.5 PRINTING A COLLECTION LETTER

1. Click or point to the *Collection Reports* option on the Reports menu. The Collection Reports submenu displays.
2. Click *Patient Collection Letters.* The Print Report Where dialog box opens.
3. Click the radio button for *Print the report on the printer.*
4. Click the *Start* button. The Data Selection Questions dialog box opens.
5. Leave all the Range fields blank to include all available records.
6. Click the down arrow beside the Status Match field to see the three options: Open, Resolved, and Deleted. Choose *0 Open* (the value that displays in this field by default).
7. Click the checkbox for *Exclude items that follow Payment Plan,* to select it. The Generate Collection Letters option is now available.
8. Click the checkbox for *Generate Collection Letters.* The checkbox for Add To Collection Tracer is automatically selected as well.
9. Click the *OK* button.
10. Select a printer, and click *OK* to print the Collection Letter Report.
11. When asked if you want to print collection letters, click *Yes.* The Open Report dialog box opens.

12. Click *Collection Letter*, if not already highlighted. Then click *OK*. The Print Report Where dialog box displays.
13. Click the radio button for *Print the report on the printer*. Then click *Start*.
14. Select a printer, and click *OK* to print the collection letter.

PATIENT ACCOUNT WRITE-OFFS

Patient account adjustments can be made in the Payments, Adjustments, and Comments area (lower third) of the Transaction Entry dialog box. For example, if a patient overpays, an adjustment should be entered to refund him or her the overpaid amount. Medisoft also has an adjustment feature that allows you to write off small remainder balances for multiple patients at one time. A remainder balance is the amount still owed by the patient after the insurance carrier has paid its portion.

To avoid fraud, remainder balances should only be written off after the medical office has attempted to collect the monies and confirmed the financial circumstances of patients. For example, the Medicare program requires a provider to follow a series of steps before any amounts, such as copayments or coinsurance, for which a patient is responsible, can be written off. Clicking the Small Balance Write-off option on the Activities menu opens the Small Balance Write-off dialog box (Figure 5.12). First, the fields on the left-hand side should be completed:

Patient Selection. Choose either the All radio button or the Delinquent Patients radio button. Delinquent patients are those for whom you have set up a payment plan, but no minimum payments have been received.

Write-off Code. Click the desired adjustment code in this field's list box (set up in the Procedure / Payment / Adjustment Codes dialog box).

Cutoff Date. Medisoft compares the date in this field with the patients' last payment date. In other words, any patient whose most recent payment was before this date will be included.

Maximum Amount. Enter the maximum dollar amount that you want to write off for any transaction; for example, $5.00.

Stmt Submission Count. Enter the number of times that a statement should be sent before a balance is written off.

Next, clicking the Apply button at the bottom of the dialog box signals Medisoft to select patients based on the criteria entered. This data is then displayed in the Write-off Preview List on the right side of the dialog box. (Clicking the Clear button removes the values from the fields above the button, as well as the items in the Write-off Preview List window.) Options on the right side of the dialog box allow you to narrow the list further before clicking the Write-off button to perform the actual write-offs.

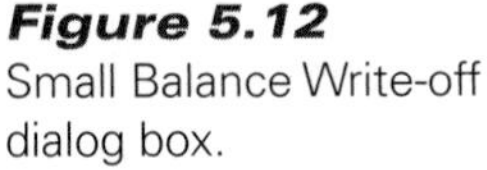

Figure 5.12
Small Balance Write-off dialog box.

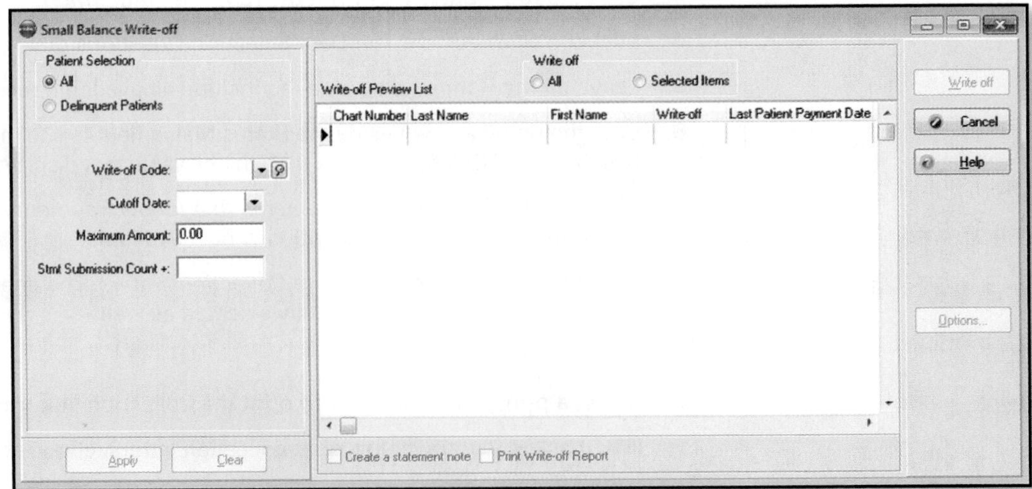

Using Terminology

Match the terms on the left with the definitions on the right.

_____ **1.** tickler
_____ **2.** collection agency
_____ **3.** collection list
_____ **4.** collection letter
_____ **5.** payment plan
_____ **6.** sliding fee scale
_____ **7.** collection
_____ **8.** Collection Tracer Report
_____ **9.** write-off
_____ **10.** aging report

a. Accounts receivable item that is uncollectable and therefore recorded as a loss or expense in the financial records
b. Correspondence sent to a patient to remind them of an overdue payment
c. Feature that tracks the quantities and dates of collection letters sent
d. Printout that shows unpaid charges as current or delinquent, based on the number of days they have been outstanding
e. Time-sensitive reminder note added to a collection list
f. Tool used to follow up on unpaid accounts by creating reminders
g. Process of obtaining payment for services rendered, usually involving accounts that are past due an extended period
h. Agreement that allows a patient to pay a specified dollar amount at regular time intervals to reduce his or her debt
i. Organization that will act as a third party to collect unpaid debts
j. System of charging for services based on the patient's income and family size

Checking Your Understanding

1. Explain how to create and apply a patient payment plan.
2. List the general rules in making collection telephone calls. What would you do if a patient got hostile?
3. How does the process of adding a single tickler item to the Collections List differ from the process used to add a group of ticklers at one time?
4. Describe two types of collection reports available in Medisoft.
5. What is the process used to write-off small balances for multiple patient accounts?

Putting It into Practice

1. Enter information in Medisoft for the following patients, using the registration forms in Appendix C. Dr. Walker is the assigned provider for each patient.
   - For Ben Kenner, use Figure C.43 in Appendix C.
   - For Ewan Daniels, use Figure C.44 in Appendix C.
   - For Jean Franks, use Figure C.45 in Appendix C.
2. Create cases, and enter the 3/10/2010 charges for these patients using the encounter forms in Figures C.46 through C.48 in Appendix C. Take note that the insurance policy for Ewan Daniels (Star Insurance) requires a $20 copayment per visit. Also, you may have to add a new procedure code.
3. Create and print insurance claims for these three patients.
4. Enter and apply insurance payments, which were received from their carriers on 3/17/2010, for these three patients. Use the RA information shown in Figures C.49 and C.50 in Appendix C.
5. Print a Patient Aging Report and a Primary Insurance Aging Report. Notice the following: Ewan Daniels did not pay his $20 copayment at the time of his visit. In addition, Medicare has not sent a payment for Jean Franks.
6. Create and print statements for these patients.
7. You have investigated the claim for Jean Franks and resolved the issue; payment should be forthcoming. However, Ewan Daniels has not paid his outstanding amount. Enter a tickler in the Collection List to remind you to send a collection letter.
8. Print a Collection Letter for Ewan Daniels.
9. Before exiting Medisoft, backup your data as designated by your instructor.

References

Adams DM: *Diagnosis: documentation and coding,* New York, 1997, McGraw Hill.
Flight M: *Law, liability, and ethics for medical office procedures,* ed 3, Albany, NY, 1998, Delmar.
Fordney MT: *Insurance handbook for the medical office,* ed 11, Philadelphia, 2010, Saunders–Elsevier.
HealthCare Consultants of America: *Health care fraud and abuse,* Augusta, Ga, 1997, The Consultants.
Holmes DL: *Practical guide to medical billing,* Springfield, Ill, 1997, US Department of Commerce.
Kuehn L: *Health information management: medical records process in group practice,* Englewood, Colo, 1997, Center for Research in Ambulatory Health Care Administration.
Moini J: *Glencoe medical assisting review: passing the CMA and RMA exams,* New York, 2001, Glencoe.
Proctor D, Young A: *Kinn's the medical assistant: an applied learning approach,* ed 10, St Louis, 2007, Saunders–Elsevier.
Redman B, editor: *Life and health insurance,* ed 4, Chicago, 1999, Dearborn Financial Institute.
Reid J: *A telemedicine primer: understanding the issues,* Billings, Mont, 1996, Artcraft Printers.
Rizzo C: *Uniform billing: a guide to claims processing,* Albany, NY, 2000, Delmar.
Ross A, Pavlock E, Williams S: *Ambulatory care management,* ed 3, Albany, NY, 1998, Delmar.
Rowell J: *Understanding health insurance: a guide to professional billing,* ed 5, Albany, NY, 2000, Delmar.

chapter 6

The Electronic Medical Office

Objectives

1. Name some benefits and difficulties in using telemedicine.
2. List the primary functions of electronic health records (EHRs).
3. Explain how voice recognition technology can benefit a medical office.
4. Create patient notes using Medisoft's Final Draft word processor.
5. Modify an existing Medisoft report using the Report Designer tool.
6. Describe how settings in the Program Options dialog box affect Medisoft's operations.

Terminology

e-health: Broad term used to describe the exchange of information and services in the health care industry by means of the Internet and other electronic technologies

electronic health record (EHR): Electronic version of a patient's medical records

e-prescribing: Using the Internet to send providers' medical prescriptions to patients' local pharmacies

Final Draft: Medisoft's word processor

information technology (IT): Use of computers, the Internet, and other electronic or digital resources to locate, process, transmit, and store data

patient notes: Information recorded in the patient's record about conditions and treatments

Report Designer: Medisoft tool that allows you to modify existing reports and to create new ones

risk management: Process of identifying practices that may put the medical office at risk and correcting those practices

telemedicine: Use of telecommunications technology to provide types of medical care that do not require a patient to physically visit a provider

voice recognition: Process that transforms spoken language into digital information that a computer can use

As a medical office assistant, you should be aware of the various ways in which information technology may affect your job, as well as those who practice medicine in a medical office setting. **Information technology (IT)** refers to the use of computers, the Internet, and other electronic or digital resources to locate, process, transmit, and store data. The Internet is a worldwide system of computer networks that are linked together. The number of people using the Internet is growing every day.

Computer software, such as Medisoft, has many features to run a medical office easily and more efficiently, including the ability to transmit claims and receive remittance via the Internet. This chapter provides examples of how IT is impacting the health care industry and then describes some Medisoft tools you can use to broaden your IT skills and knowledge.

E-HEALTH AND TELEMEDICINE

The word **e-health** (sometimes called *telehealth*) is a broad term used to describe various forms of IT communications used in the health care industry. E-health includes a wide range of electronic services that have increased the quality, quantity, and efficiency of health care. Closely associated with e-health is telemedicine. **Telemedicine** is the use of telecommunication and IT technologies to provide types of medical care that do not require a patient to physically visit a provider. Although the words *e-health* and *telemedicine* are sometimes used interchangeably, keep in mind that different organizations may define and interpret these two terms somewhat differently.

E-health or telemedicine may use the telephone, the Internet, and other computer networks such as local intranets. An *intra*net is generally a more private and secured connection than the Internet. An intranet is used internally by many companies and organizations to transmit information primarily to authorized personnel. Outside access to a company's local intranet is available by permission only.

Telemedicine reduces the amount of travel and time required by patients to physically visit medical providers and to handle other health-related transactions. Providers can also use telemedicine to reach out to people who otherwise would have limited or no access to health care. As a result, telemedicine has significantly changed the way medical clinics do business. Following are a few examples of how patients may use e-health or telemedicine technology without leaving their homes:

- Purchase medical supplies.
- Check the status of or order prescription refills.
- Set up, reschedule, or cancel appointments.
- Become more knowledgeable about a disease, condition, and treatment options before visiting a provider.
- Talk to or participate in an online chat with medical personnel about questions related to symptoms, treatments, and medicines. Keep in mind that the assumption of risk is usually considered too great for a medical office to provide diagnostic services over the telephone without seeing a patient. **Risk management** is the process of identifying and defining practices that may put the medical office in jeopardy and correcting those risky practices. To find out more about risk management, visit the following Web sites:
    - ECRI Institute at www.ecri.org/
    - Harvard's Risk Management Foundation at www.rmf.harvard.edu/

Some of the many things that medical providers may use e-health or telemedicine technology to perform include the following:

- Order drug prescriptions at local retail pharmacies or mail-order pharmacies for patients, a process called **e-prescribing**. Ordering prescriptions electronically also gives the provider an opportunity to access informational databases about drugs that are available, potential negative interactions with other drugs the patient is using, prescription instructions, and so on. E-prescribing helps the medical office avoid costly lawsuits that could result from prescription mistakes, such as the pharmacist misreading the provider's prescription.
- Consult with other medical providers and specialists. One example is sending a patient's magnetic resonance image (MRI) for review by a leading radiologist in a different city. Another example is participating in a videoconference with other medical professionals.
- Remotely monitor a patient's progress or medical status.
- Perform or direct certain medical procedures. For example, the U.S. Department of Defense is actively developing and implementing telesurgery techniques, during which a surgeon can operate on a patient from a distance. The actual surgery is performed by robotic arms that the surgeon can control or by giving instructions to another surgeon who is physically on site with the patient.

One drawback to telemedicine is reimbursement and billing. Insurance carriers may reimburse for some telemedicine services but not all. Another difficulty in telemedicine is licensure. Each provider has to be licensed in the state in which he or she practices medicine.

For example, a provider in Wisconsin cannot practice medicine in Minnesota until he or she has filed the proper papers and obtained approval from the state of Minnesota. Because telemedicine has no physical boundaries, it raises the issue of jurisdiction. The question becomes whether providers licensed in a different state from the one where the patient was diagnosed must also be licensed in the patient's state. As a result, the relevant state medical board(s) should be consulted about licensure requirements before telemedicine is used across state lines.

As e-health and telemedicine technologies and services continue to grow, you can be sure they will affect your career at some point. For additional information on this subject, visit the following Web sites:

- American Telemedicine Association: www.americantelemed.org/
- Centers for Medicare and Medicaid Services: www.cms.hhs.gov/telehealth
- Certification Commission for Health Information Technology: www.cchit.org/
- Cleveland Clinic, Resources for Patients: http://my.clevelandclinic.org/heart/guide.aspx
- Healthcare Information and Management Systems Society: www.himss.org/
- U.S. Department of Health and Human Services: Health Resources and Services Information, www.hrsa.gov/healthit/

ELECTRONIC HEALTH RECORDS

An **electronic health record (EHR)** is an electronic version of a patient's medical record. All of the patient's data, such as demographic information, medications, vital signs, and laboratory test results, are connected and brought together through the use of information technology. EHRs have been used in various degrees for several decades and, over time, have had many names including electronic medical record, computerized medical record, computer-based patient record, and many others.

EHRs enable medical professionals to provide medical services more proficiently, both in the medical office and by means of various telemedicine technologies. For example, a typical complaint of providers and nursing staff in the past has been the lack of access to medical records. Sometimes, paper-based medical records have been misfiled or simply lost. EHRs are stored in what is commonly called a *data repository*. Authorized personnel can access the data for each patient's visit and see how well the patient is performing with certain medications and other treatments. An EHR gives a more complete picture by allowing the provider to analyze all of the data, included in the patient's medical record.

For more information about EHRs and their general benefits, visit the Web site of the Centers for Medicare and Medicaid Services at www.cms.hhs.gov/ehealthrecords/. The Institute of Medicine (IOM) also provides a list of the core functions of EHRs in its 2003 report, *Key Capabilities of an Electronic Health Record System* (http://www.iom.edu/Reports.aspx):

- *Health information and data.* EHRs include information and data concerning diagnoses, allergies, laboratory test results, demographic information, and patient histories.
- *Result management.* Having test results available at the time they are completed is important in treating critical cases. EHRs can provide the medical staff with the information needed to make quick and accurate decisions.
- *Order management.* Order management through EHRs can benefit the patient and provider. Reducing errors of dosage, type of drug, and interactions can save the life of a patient. (Electronic prescriptions are discussed later in this chapter.)
- *Decision support.* Reminders to have certain examinations, vaccinations, or laboratory tests performed help physicians provide the best care to their patients.
- *Electronic communication and connectivity.* Communication between all parties involved in the patient's health is one of the benefits of EHRs. A provider can communicate with the pharmacist or with the patient through e-mail.
- *Patient support.* Monitoring certain chronic illnesses can be tracked in the EHR.
- *Administrative processes and reporting.* Medisoft is an example of this category in which scheduling and prior authorizations can all be performed.

- *Reporting and population health.* Reporting to public health agencies can be performed through the EHR with fewer errors; using the EHR is not as time consuming as other data gathering.

Working with patient information in any capacity requires confidentiality and knowledge of the legislation passed by Congress in 1996: the Health Insurance Portability and Accountability Act (HIPAA). This law ensures the security and privacy of health information and helps decrease fraud in health insurance. To learn more about HIPAA, visit the Web site of the U.S. Department of Health and Human Services at www.hhs.gov/ocr/privacy/. The fourth document in the HIPAA Security Series, *Security Standards: Technical Safeguards*, provides guidelines for protecting electronic records. This document can be downloaded at www.hhs.gov/ocr/privacy/hipaa/administrative/securityrule/techsafeguards.pdf.

VOICE RECOGNITION FOR MEDICAL DICTATION

Over the years, the practice of dictating **patient notes** has evolved from speaking into a tape recorder and later transcribing (typing) those recordings to using computer technology to document notes about a patient's condition and treatment. Patient notes become part of a person's medical record. You can view samples of handwritten patient notes at the Web site of the United States Medical Licensing Examination®.

Voice recognition, also called *speech recognition*, transforms spoken language into digital information that a computer can use. The provider dictates, or speaks, into a microphone attached to a computer with voice recognition software. The computer then interprets the provider's dictation into written form.

Medical office assistant duties may include transcription duties. Medical transcriptionists (MTs) have expertise in medical language and health care. They often edit dictated material for grammar and clarity. Other options may include using an online service such as World Wide Dictation (www.worldwidedictation.com/) for medical dictation needs.

ADDITIONAL MEDISOFT TOOLS AND OPTIONS

The following sections offers a brief introduction to some additional tools and options that can help you use Medisoft more effectively. These features include a word processor, a program used to modify and create reports, and a series of options that controls various Medisoft operations.

Final Draft

Final Draft is Medisoft's word processing program. With it, you can enter notes, narratives, and letters. You can also insert patient accounting information from the main Medisoft program into Final Draft to create customized letters. For example, if you were writing a letter to an insurance company justifying the cost of a procedure, that letter could be attached to the patient's record.

Content created in Final Draft can be sent (exported) to other word processors. In addition, text from other word processors, such as Microsoft Word, can be pulled into (imported) into Final Draft. Make sure that any letter you plan to import and attach to the patient's record is saved as either a Plain Text file (.txt file name extension) or a Rich Text Format file (.rtf file name extension).

Final Draft has its own window, menu bar, and toolbar (Figure 6.1). You can access Final Draft from the main Medisoft window in three different ways:

- Click the Patient Notes option on the Tools menu.
- Click the Edit Patient Notes in Final Draft button on the toolbar.
- Click the Final Draft option on the Activities menu.

The Final Draft menu bar and toolbar both operate in a manner similar to the menu bar and toolbar in the main Medisoft window. Final Draft provides formatting capabilities

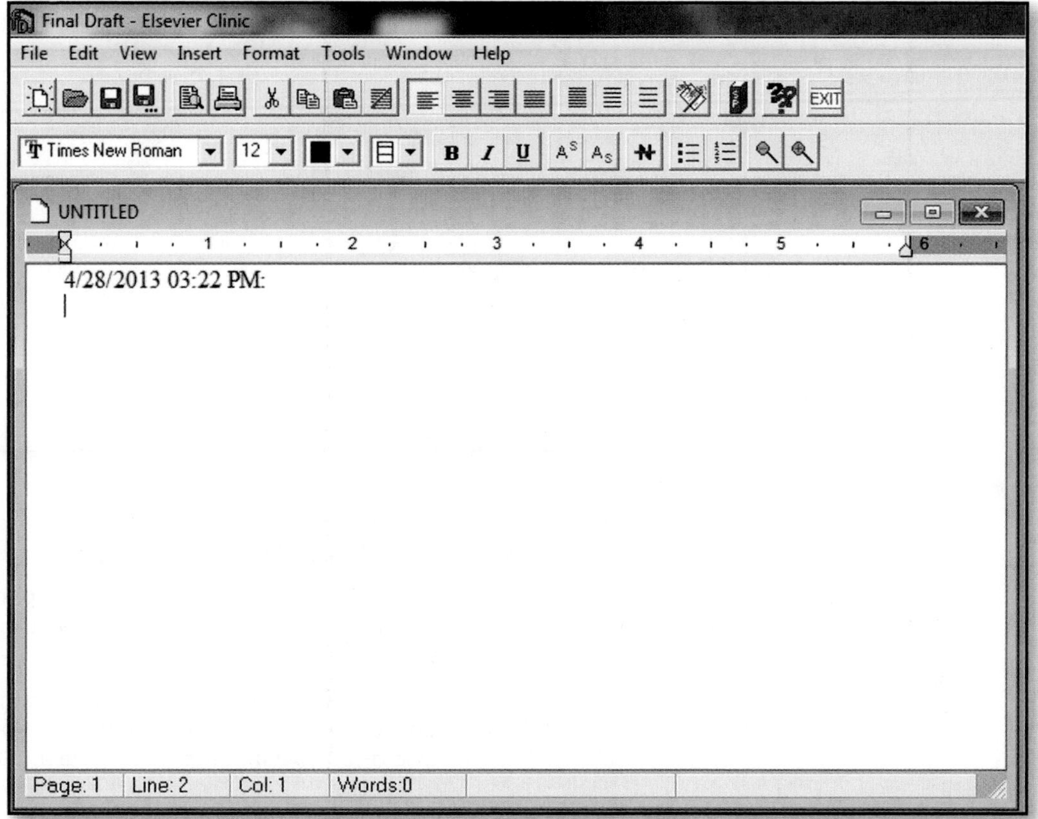

Figure 6.1
Final Draft menu bar, toolbar, and an untitled document window are displayed.

such as bolding text, changing the size of the text font, and changing the color of the font. You can also add bullet points, change how the text aligns (such as centering text), define the paper size and orientation, and set up document margins and paragraph parameters. As with other word processors, Final Draft allows you to move, copy, paste, delete, and spell-check text.

When you first open Final Draft, a new, untitled document window displays in which you can key text (see Figure 6.1). However, before you initially begin using Final Draft, you may want to modify default options by clicking Program Options on Final Draft's File menu. This action opens the Program Options dialog box (Figure 6.2). Following is a description of this dialog box's fields:

Default Font. In the Name, Size, and Color fields, you can specify the default font style, font size, and font color. Final Draft will use these settings each time you create a new document. However, you can always change these items for any particular document by using the Final Draft toolbar.

Default Author. The name of the person entered in this field will appear as the author in Final Draft's Document Information dialog box (accessed by clicking the Document Information option on the File menu).

Show Balloon Hints. When this field is check-marked, the name of a toolbar button will display when you *rest* the mouse pointer on the button's icon.

Autosave Every...Minutes. The number entered in this field represents how many minutes will elapse before the program automatically saves an active document. For example, entering 5 would cause Final Draft to save the document text automatically every 5 minutes.

Any time you open a new document window (by clicking the New Document option on the File menu), you can set defaults for that particular document. For example, on the Format menu there are Font, Paragraph, and Page Layout options that open dialog boxes used to change the appearance of the document.

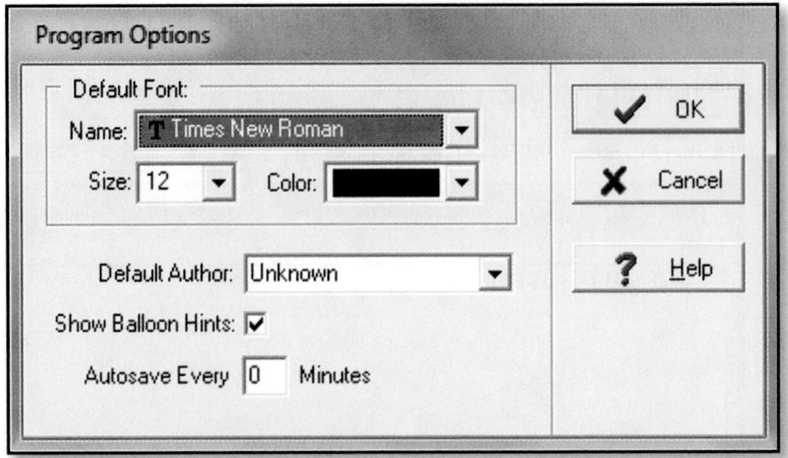

Figure 6.2
Final Draft's Program Options dialog box.

PROCEDURE 6.1 ENTERING NOTES USING FINAL DRAFT

In this exercise, you will create and save notes that reflect telephone calls you made this morning to patients. Like most word processors, you can use the Delete key or the Backspace key in Final Draft to remove typing mistakes.

1. With the main Medisoft window open, click *Final Draft* on the Activities menu. The Final Draft window opens with the Final Draft menu bar and toolbar. An untitled document also displays with the current date and time.
2. Leave the current date and time that displays in the document window unchanged.
3. Where the cursor is blinking, key the following text, inserting your initials in place of XX: *Notified patient of his lab results, XX.*
4. On the Final Draft's File menu, click *Save Document.* The Save Document As dialog box displays.
5 In the File Name field, key *CharlesWeber,* without a space between Charles and Weber.
6. In the Save As field, click *Note*, if not already selected.
7. Click the *Save* button. The Document Information dialog box displays.
8. In the Title field, key *CharlesWeber*, if it is not already displayed in this field.
9. In the Author field, key your initials.
10. In the Subject field, key *Lab results notification.*
11. Click *OK.* The document is renamed from "Untitled" to "CharlesWeber."
12. On the File menu, click *Close Document.* The document window closes, but the main Final Draft window remains open.
13. On the File menu, click *New Document.* A new, untitled document window opens.
14. Repeat steps 3 through 12 to enter a note for Anne Potter: *Notified patient of her lab results, XX.* (Insert the current date and time using the Date or Time option on the Insert menu.)
15. On the File menu, click *Open Document.* The Open Document dialog box displays.
16. Click the *Notes* radio button, if not already selected. The two files you created and saved should display in the dialog box's window.
17. Click *Cancel.* Then click the *Exit* button on the toolbar to close the Final Draft program.

Report Designer

Medisoft's **Report Designer** can be used to modify existing Medisoft reports and bills, as well as create new custom versions. If you click Design Custom Reports and Bills on the Reports menu, the Report Designer window will open with its own menu bar and toolbar (Figure 6.3). These features operate similar to the menu bar and toolbar in the main Medisoft window.

Medisoft already has a number of existing formats and styles for reports, superbills, claim forms, collection letters, lists, and statements from which to choose. The best way to get familiar with how the Report Designer works is to modify an existing report. (Creating custom reports from scratch is a more time-consuming and complex process.) It is always a good idea to save an existing format under a different name before modifying the report. That way, you will have access to both versions of the report or form, in case you need the original format in the future.

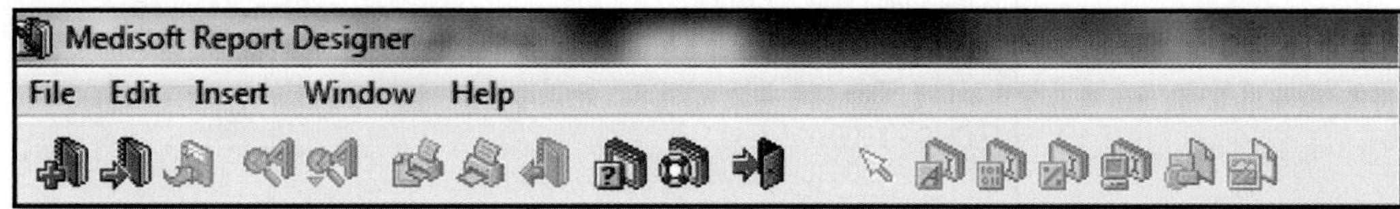

Figure 6.3 Report Designer menu bar and toolbar.

PROCEDURE 6.2 MODIFYING AN EXISTING REPORT

In this exercise, you will create a copy of the report titled Superbill (Numbered) and modify it.

1. On the Reports menu, click *Design Custom Reports and Bills.* The Report Designer window opens with its menu bar and toolbar displayed.
2. On the Report Designer's File menu, click *Open Report.* The Open Report dialog box displays (Figure 6.4). On the right side of the dialog box, under Show Report Style, the All radio button is selected by default. Correspondingly, on the left side of the dialog box, a list of all existing reports display under Report Title.
3. Click the *Superbill* radio button. The title Superbill (Numbered) displays, and all other titles related to other types of forms or reports disappear from the dialog box's window. Because this is the only superbill listed, it is automatically highlighted.
4. Click *OK.* A format grid for this superbill displays (Figure 6.5).
5. On the File menu, click *Save As.* The dialog box displays.
6. In the Report Title field, key *Superbill [Your Name],* for example, Superbill Tom Smith. Click *OK*; the original format is stored, and the new name displays at the top of the format grid.
7. Scroll down the window until you see [ECG] in the middle column of the window.
8. Click *[ECG].* A group of handles display as dots around the border of the text field to show that it has been selected.
9. Double-click the selected text field. The Text Properties dialog box displays (Figure 6.6).
10. In the Text field, change the wording to *ECG, complete.*
11. Click *OK.* The Text Properties field closes and the modified text field displays.
12. On the File menu, click *Save.* The changes you made are saved.
13. On the File menu, click *Close.* The format grid of the modified report closes.
14. On the File menu, click *Exit.* The Report Designer window closes.
15. Print a superbill for one of the patients using the modified report format, and hand it in to your instructor.

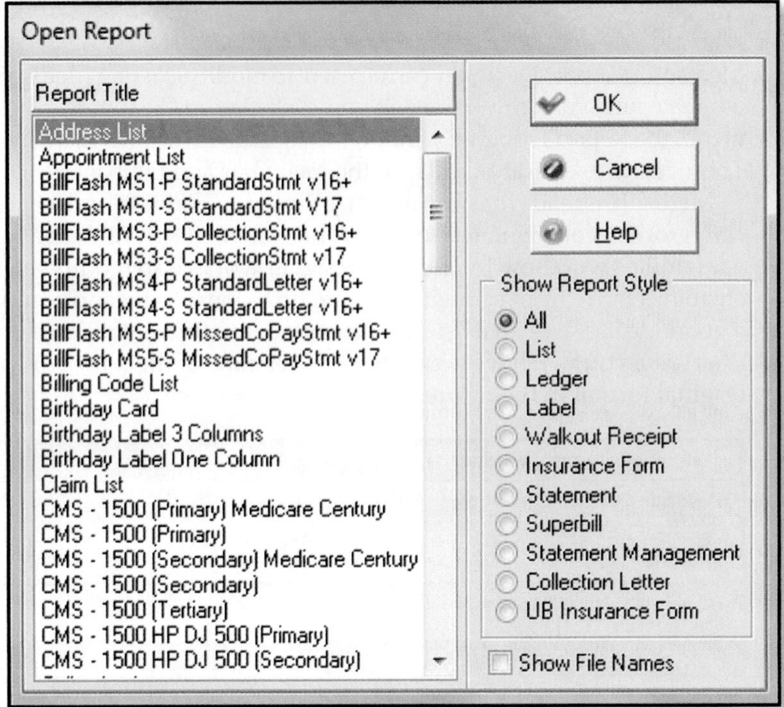

Figure 6.4 Open Report dialog box in Report Designer.

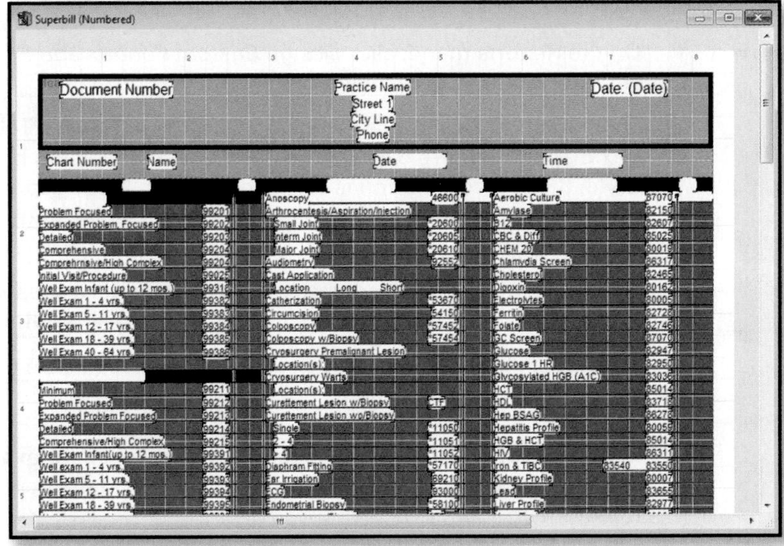

Figure 6.5 Format grid for the superbill.

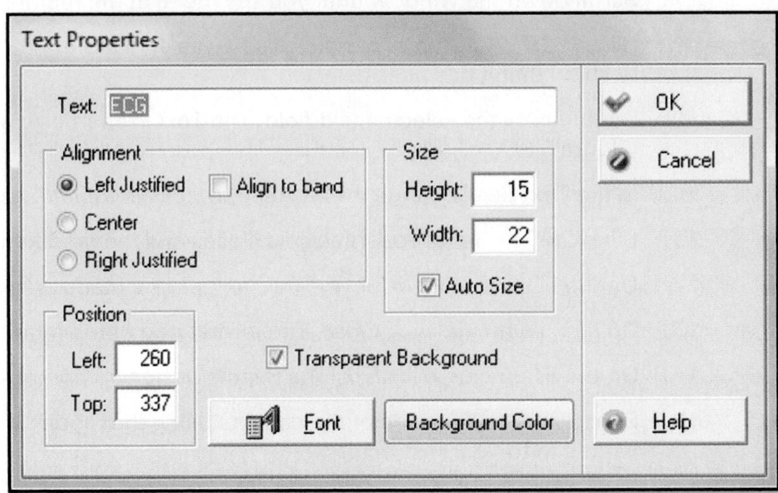

Figure 6.6 Text Properties dialog box.

Program Options Dialog Box

The Program Options dialog box allows you to define conditions that affect fields and processes throughout the Medisoft program. Initially, Medisoft provides default options when the program is installed. However, these options can be changed later when needed or desired. Many of the options provided are often easier to understand and evaluate after you have become familiar with the primary components and functions of Medisoft.

The Program Options dialog box (Figure 6.7) is accessed by clicking Program Options on the File menu. This dialog box contains nine tabs with many fields. (Enable HL7 Triggers is a feature new to Medisoft version 17.) Select this checkbox if you use Communications Manager to transmit information to other medical applications.) Following is a brief description of each tab:

- *General.* This tab includes fields for miscellaneous, backup, and account alert settings. A few examples include displaying a backup reminder when exiting Medisoft, having certain dialog boxes automatically display when Medisoft is opened, choosing when patient remainder balances are calculated, and deciding the circumstances when you wish patient account alerts to display.
- *Data Entry.* As its name implies, this tab contains fields that affect the way information is entered in Medisoft. In addition to global settings, which apply to data entry throughout the program, there are also patient, transaction, and EDI data entry options.
- *Payment Application.* This tab's fields affect the operations used by the program when payments are applied. You can also set up default codes for small balance write-offs.
- *Aging Reports.* The fields in this tab are used to change the Patient Aging and the Insurance Aging reports. For example, you can alter the number of days in the reports' aging columns.
- *HIPAA.* The options in this tab are used to help prevent unauthorized people from accessing patient information. There is also an option that alerts you when codes not compliant with HIPAA are entered or selected.
- *Color Coding.* This tab is used to assign certain colors to particular types of transactions and patients.
- *Billing.* The fields in the Billing tab affect the information that appears on Statements and Claims.

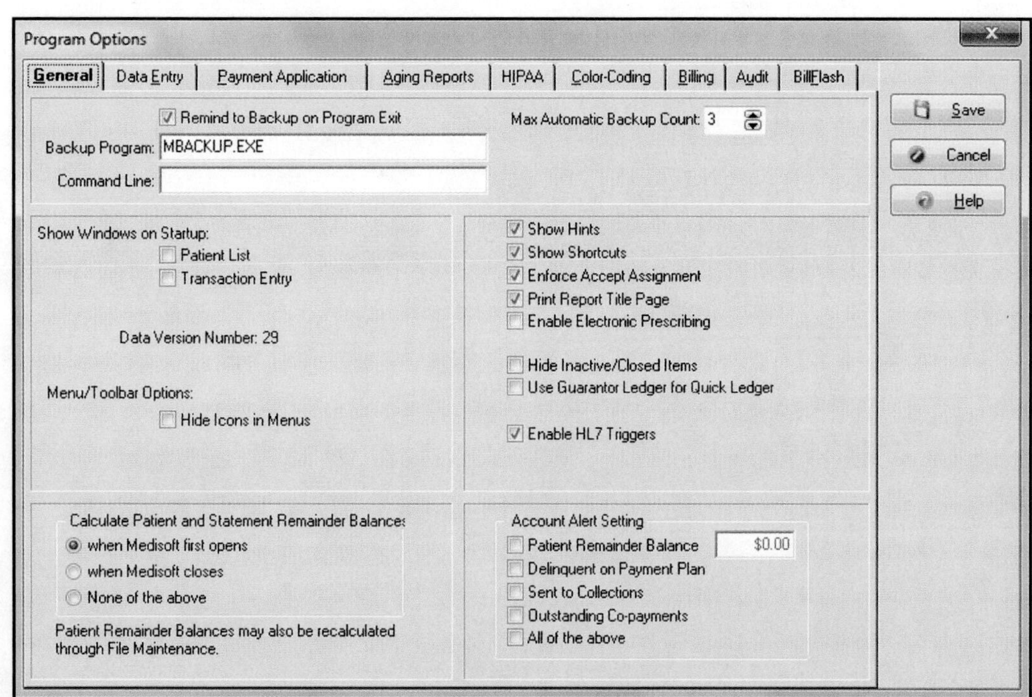

Figure 6.7
Program Options dialog box with General tab displayed.

- *Audit.* The Audit tab works in conjunction with a tool called the Audit Generator—a feature used to print the Data Audit Report. This report is used to examine information for accuracy.
- *BillFlash.* Use this tab to decide what information is included in BillFlash statements.

PROCEDURE 6.3 EXPLORING PROGRAM OPTIONS

In this exercise, you will use Medisoft's Help feature to explore the various types of program options available. Do not change any options unless your instructor tells you to do so.

1. On the File menu, click *Program Options.* The Program Options dialog box opens with the General tab displayed.
2. In the dialog box, click the *Help* button. Medisoft's Help window opens with the topic Program Options displayed.
3. In the Help window, click on the various links related to the Program Options dialog box. As you do this, click each tab in the Program Options dialog box to view the associated fields.
4. When finished, close the Help window by clicking the red button with an *X* in the upper-right corner. Then, click the *Cancel* button in the Program Options dialog box to close it.

Using Terminology

Match the terms on the left with the definitions on the right.

_____ **1.** information technology (IT)
_____ **2.** e-health
_____ **3.** risk management
_____ **4.** e-prescribing
_____ **5.** Final Draft
_____ **6.** patient notes
_____ **7.** electronic health record (EHR)
_____ **8.** voice recognition
_____ **9.** Report Designer
_____ **10.** telemedicine

a. Electronic version of a patient's medical records
b. Medisoft tool that allows you to modify existing reports and to create new ones
c. Process that transforms spoken language into digital information that a computer can use
d. Using the Internet to send providers' medical prescriptions to patients' local pharmacies
e. Medisoft's word processor
f. Use of computers, the Internet, and other electronic and digital resources to locate, process, transmit, and store data
g. Process of identifying practices that may put the medical office at risk and correcting those practices
h. Broad term used to describe the exchange of information and services in the health care industry by means of the Internet and other electronic technologies
i. Use of telecommunications technology to provide types of medical care that do not require a patient to physically visit a provider
j. Information recorded in the patient's record about conditions and treatments

Checking Your Understanding

1. What are some benefits and difficulties in using telemedicine?
2. According to the IOM, what are the core functions of EHRs?
3. How can voice recognition technology benefit a medical office?
4. What are the general steps used to enter patient notes in Final Draft?
5. Why is it a good idea to save a copy of a Medisoft report before changing it with the Report Designer?
6. Summarize the general purpose of each tab in the Program Options dialog box.

Putting It into Practice

1. Use Final Draft to create and save a form letter to inform patients with Star Insurance that the practice will no longer accept this insurance after the end of the year.
2. Use the Report Designer to open a report or form, save a copy of it, and then change it. Access Medisoft's Help feature to obtain additional guidelines for using the Report Designer. Use what you learn to experiment with various Report Designer tools.
3. Before exiting Medisoft, backup your data as designated by your instructor.

References

Adams DM: *Diagnosis: documentation and coding,* New York, 1997, McGraw Hill.
Flight M: *Law, liability, and ethics for medical office procedures,* ed 3, Albany, NY, 1998, Delmar.
Fordney MT: *Insurance handbook for the medical office,* ed 11, Philadelphia, 2010, Saunders–Elsevier.
Gillay CZ, Sullivan PL: *Windows 2000 professional concepts and examples,* Wilsonville, Ore, 2001, Franklin, Beedle & Associates.
HealthCare Consultants of America: *Health care fraud and abuse,* Augusta, Ga, 1997, The Consultants.
Holmes DL: *Practical guide to medical billing,* Springfield, Ill, 1997, US Department of Commerce.
Kuehn L: *Health information management: medical records process in group practice,* Englewood, Colo, 1997, Center for Research in Ambulatory Health Care Administration.
Moini J: *Glencoe medical assisting review: passing the CMA and RMA exams,* New York, 2001, Glencoe.
Redman B, editor: *Life and health insurance,* ed 4, Chicago, 1999, Dearborn Financial Institute.
Reid J: *A telemedicine primer: understanding the issues,* Billings, Mont, 1996, Artcraft Printers.
Rizzo C: *Uniform billing: a guide to claims processing,* Albany, NY, 2000, Delmar.
Ross A, Pavlock E, Williams S: *Ambulatory care management,* ed 3, Albany, NY, 1998, Delmar.
Rowell J: *Understanding health insurance: a guide to professional billing,* ed 5, Albany, NY, 2000, Delmar.

appendix A

Day-by-Day Simulations (2 Weeks)

This 2-week simulation will take everything you have learned throughout the book, and you will use these skills in a simulated medical office environment. Feel free to go back to the chapters to refresh your memory on how to complete a specific task. Each simulation expands on what you have previously learned.

As you complete each day of the simulation, you will gather all of your printed materials for that day and then turn them in as directed by your instructor. Remember to print everything requested in these daily simulations. Each day will have approximately 10 simulations, including entering new patients, setting up and editing appointments, canceling appointments, entering charges for patients, creating claim forms for insurance companies, recording payments from patients and insurance companies, printing statements, and many other tasks inherent to a medical office.

Note: All required forms (e.g., registration and encounter forms) are located in Appendix C of this text. We have chosen to start the simulation on Monday, February 4, 2013. Simply click the date in the bottom-right corner of the screen, and change that date to the date you are working on in the simulation. You will need to change that date for each new day of the simulation; if you exit out of the program, you will need to change the date to the day you left off when you get back into the program and begin working again. Finally, this new practice is different from the one you created in the previous chapters; thus you will use different sets of diagnoses and procedure codes, and charges may vary from what you input previously. The point to remember is that each insurance company negotiates a different contract and a different allowed charge for each provider.

WEEK ONE

Day One (Monday, 02/04/2013)

Use a date on a Monday of the current year.

1. Congratulations! Today is your first day as the newest employee of the Goode Medical Clinic and William B. Goode, MD. Your first duties are to meet with the office manager, Betty Goode, to learn the name of the practice and to receive important identification, Social Security numbers, and other insurance identification numbers for the physician and medical practice. You will be spending the entire morning setting up the practice using the Medisoft Office Management computer software. In the afternoon, the first five patients are scheduled to arrive.
2. Your first task is to input the new practice information into the Medisoft program. The following sections detail how to input the practice information. Click *File* in the upper

left corner of the Medisoft window, then click on *New Practice*. A new window will open, asking for a Practice or Doctor's name to identify this data. In the first box, you will key *Goode (Your Name)* medical clinic. The second box will ask you to specify the path for the data. It should show *c:\Medidata*. Make sure it is the drive where your program is loaded, then type *Goode (Your Name)* and click *Create*. Answer *Yes* when it asks if you want to create a new directory with that name. In this way, your instructor can distinguish your submission from a fellow classmate's work.

Note: Anytime XX appears, you will need to provide that information by creating it.

Practice Information

1. Name of Practice: Goode Medical Clinic
2. Address: 1612 Southwest Blvd., St. Paul, MN 55100
3. Telephone and Fax Numbers: (555) 456-7689–office, (555) 456-7690–fax
4. Type: Medical
5. Tax ID Number: 23-XX-12345
6. Practice Type: Group
7. Entity Type: Non-person

Provider Information

1. Name: William B. Goode, MD
2. This textbook will refer to this provider as *Dr. Bill.*
3. Address and Telephone Number: These are the same as for the practice.

License Information

1. Social Security Number: 123-XX-1234
2. Tax ID Number: Use the Practice Tax ID number
3. State License: 98XX76
4. Signature on File: Yes; Signature Date: 01/01/2010; Medicare Participating: Yes
5. Entity Type: Person

Default PINS

1. Commercial Insurance: Use the provider's SSN, 123-XX-1234
2. Medicare Number: 123457XX6
3. BCBS Number: 567XX
4. UPIN: 7890XX976
5. NPI: 54123XX678

Insurance Company Information

Input the information for each of the following insurance carriers.

1. BCBS of MN
   1355 Insurance Carrier Loop
   Minneapolis, MN 55401
   (763) 555-0426; (763) 555-0445 (fax)

   Signature on File: On the Options and Codes tab, ensure these boxes are checked to indicate signatures are on file for the patient, insured, and physician.

2. Medicare, Part B
   Wisconsin Physicians Service
   4502 Wisconsin Ave.
   Milwaukee, WI 53201
   (414) 555-0943; (414) 555-0944 (fax)

   Signature on File: Ensure these boxes are checked to indicate signatures are on file for the patient, insured, and physician.

3. First Med EGHP Claims
   1324 Insurance Carrier Loop
   Minneapolis, MN 55401
   (763) 345-9124; (763) 345-8356 (fax)

   Signature on File: Ensure these boxes are checked to indicate signatures are on file for the patient, insured, and physician.

Transactional and Diagnosis Code Information

You will now need to enter the procedure, financial transaction, and diagnosis codes.

When you are entering the procedure codes under the General Tab, also enter 11 for the Place of Service code, click the Amounts Tab and input the charge amount, and then click to the Allowed Amounts tab and enter the amounts indicated in the next section for each of the indicated insurance companies.

Note: The procedure type will be Procedure-Charge.

New Patient Office Visit Levels

Code	Description	Charge Amount	First Med	Medicare	BCBS
99201	Level 1: New	$ 40.00	$ 36.00	$ 31.20	$ 36.00
99202	Level 2: New	$ 60.00	$ 56.00	$ 52.10	$ 56.00
99203	Level 3: New	$ 80.00	$ 76.00	$ 68.60	$ 76.00
99204	Level 4: New	$100.00	$ 96.00	$ 86.20	$ 96.00
99205	Level 5: New	$150.00	$116.00	$110.00	$116.00

The following example (99201) is how you will need to enter the code into Medisoft.

General Tab: Enter description, code, procedure-charge, and 11 for place of service.
Amounts Tab: Enter $40.00 for Charge Amount (In A only).
Allowed Amounts: First Med: $36.00, Medicare: $31.20, BCBS: $36.00.

Established Patient Office Visit Levels

Code	Description	Charge Amount	First Med	Medicare	BCBS
99211	Level 1: Est	$ 30.00	$26.00	$18.20	$26.00
99212	Level 2: Est	$ 38.00	$33.00	$22.80	$33.00
99213	Level 3: Est	$ 48.00	$46.00	$28.60	$46.00
99214	Level 4: Est	$ 60.00	$56.00	$46.20	$56.00
99215	Level 5: Est	$110.00	$96.00	$82.40	$96.00

Other Procedure Codes

Code	Description	Charge Amount	First Med	Medicare	BCBS
93000	ECG	$ 50.00	$27.00	$18.00	$27.00
81001	UA	$ 78.00	$43.00	$34.00	$43.00
85023	CBC-Man	$120.00	$50.00	$43.00	$50.00

CBC-Man, Complete blood count–manual; *ECG*, electrocardiogram; *UA*, urinalysis.

Preventative Medicine Codes

Code	Description	Charge Amount	First Med	Medicare	BCBS
99385	New 18-39 YR	$85.00	$36.00	$34.00	$36.00
99395	Est 18-39 YR	$75.00	$41.00	$37.00	$41.00
99386	New 40-64 YR	$85.00	$31.50	$29.00	$31.50
99396	Est 40-64 YR	$75.00	$46.00	$32.00	$46.00

Financial Transactional Codes

Code	Description/Code Type
INSPAY	Insurance Payment
PTCASH	Patient Cash Payment
PTCHECK	Patient Check Payment
INSADJ	Insurance Adjustment
INSWH	Insurance Withhold Adjustment
INSDED	Deductible
INSTB	Insurance Take Back Adjustment
COPAYCASH	Cash Copayment
COPAYCHK	Check Copayment

Note: No charges for these codes are needed because they are description codes used for financial purposes.

Enter the following codes for BCBS. Input the same type of information for Medicare and First Med. For example, input MCAREPAY for a Medicare payment and FMPAY for First Med Payment.

Code	Code Type	Description
BCBSPAY	Insurance Payment	BCBS Payment
BCBSADJ	Insurance Adjustment	BCBS Adjustment
BCBSWH	Insurance Withhold Adjustment	BCBS Withhold
BCBSTB	Insurance Take Back Adjustment	BCBS Take Back

PROCEDURE A.1

Perform the following procedure to input default codes for the individual insurance carriers.

1. Enter *Insurance Carriers* from the Lists Menu.
2. Double-click *Blue Cross and Blue Shield of MN.*
3. Click *Options and codes* tab.
4. Click the drop-down menu for the Payment field.

5. Select *BCBSPAY* from the drop-down menu.
6. Repeat steps 4 and 5 for each of the categories. For the Deductible field, select *INSDED*.
7. Click *Save*.
8. Repeat steps 1 through 7 for the remaining two insurance carriers, Medicare and First Med.
9. Click *Close* when finished with all insurance carriers.

Diagnosis Codes

Enter the following diagnosis codes for the Goode Clinic.

Diagnosis Code	Description	Code 1
Circulatory System		
794.31	ECG, EKG, nonspecific	794.31
790.4	Elevated LDH, nonspecific	790.4
796.2	Elevated BP w/o hypertension diagnosis	796.2
786.59	Chest pain discomfort	786.59
428.0	CHF	428.0
401.1	Hypertension, benign	401.1
401.0	Hypertension, malignant	401.0
401.9	Hypertension, unspecified	401.9
Digestive System		
794.8	Liver function study	794.8
792.1	Stool contents	792.1
569.0	Anal/rectal polyps	569.0
578.1	Blood in stool	578.1
Endocrine/Metabolic Disorders		
272.0	Hypercholesterolemia, pure	272.0
272.1	Hyperglyceridemia, pure	272.1
272.2	Hyperlipidemia, mixed	272.2
276.7	Hyperpotassemia	276.7
Neoplasm, Benign		
211.3	Colon	211.3
216.9	Skin, site unspecified	216.9
Nervous Disorders		
314.00	ADD	314.00
314.01	ADD with hyperactivity	314.01
Blood/Blood-Forming Organs		
790.6	Blood chemistry	790.6
280.9	Iron deficiency	280.9
Examination, Vaccination		
V70.3	School, camp, insurance examination	V70.3
V72.3	Gynecologic examination	V72.3
V70.0	Routine general examination	V70.0
V76.12	Breast screen	V76.12
V06.1	DTP	V06.1
V04.8	Influenza	V04.8
V06.5	Tetanus-diphtheria (Td)	V06.5
Musculoskeletal Disorders		
716.90	Arthritis, NOS	716.90
847.0	Neck strain	847.0
Skin		
692.9	Contact dermatitis, NOS	692.9

ADD, Attention deficit disorder; *BP,* blood pressure; *CHF,* congestive heart failure; *DTP,* diphtheria, pertussis, and tetanus; *ECG/EKG,* electrocardiogram; *LDH,* lactate dehydrogenase; *NOS,* not otherwise specified; *w/o,* without.

Resource and Reason Codes

You will now enter the following Resource and Reason codes for Dr. Bill.

Resource Code	Description
ROOM1	Exam Room 1
ROOM2	Exam Room 2
ROOM3	Exam Room 3
CAST	Casting/Ortho Room
LAB	Lab Room
ECG	ECG/EKG Room
LUNCH	Lunch Room
INJECT	Injection Room

Reason Code	Description	Default Length
FOLLOWUP	Follow-Up Appointment	15 minutes
CHECKBP	Blood Pressure Check	15 minutes
INIT	Initial Visit	30 minutes
WELLWMAN	Well-Woman Examination	60 minutes
PHYS	Physical/Ins/School Examination	30 minutes
CHECKGLU	Blood Glucose Check	15 minutes
URGENT	Urgent or Acute Visit	30 minutes
INJECTIO	Influenza or Allergy Shots	15 minutes
ROUTINE	Routine Office Visit	15 minutes

You have now entered the required information needed to start your practice. You can start entering patients who will be seen in the afternoon.

1. You have opened up the clinic and are ready to welcome your patients for the afternoon. Enter the following five patients into the Office Hours schedule: Raymond Cross at 1:00 PM for 30 minutes (physical), (555) 555-1234; Debra Jackson at 1:30 PM for 60 minutes (well-woman examination), (555) 555-6789; Tiffany Carter at 3:00 PM for 15 minutes (routine–contact dermatitis), (555) 555-4795; Robert Jones at 3:30 PM for 30 minutes (Check BP–hypertension, you will need to adjust the length of the visit), (555) 555-4567; and Alex Neumann at 4:00 PM for 15 minutes (Routine–neck strain), (555) 555-9235. If the reason code is not already entered, then press F8 to make a new one. You are only scheduling the patients now and will enter the rest of their information into the system when they arrive for their appointments.
2. Print a schedule.
3. Your first patient arrives, and you greet him, "Good afternoon, Mr. Cross." Mr. Cross is a new patient (see the registration form in Appendix C). Enter Mr. Cross into the computer, and notify Dr. Bill's medical assistant of his arrival. His case will be a physical.
4. Ms. Debra Jackson arrives for her 1:30 PM appointment. Have her fill out the registration form, and copy her insurance card. She has a copay of $10.00 for this visit. Give her a receipt for the copayment (paid with cash), and record this payment when you enter the charges for today's visit.
5. You receive a phone call for a new patient named Cindy Mann who wants to be seen as soon as possible. She has not been feeling well the past week. Find an appointment time for tomorrow with Dr. Bill. You find an available spot for 9:00 AM. Make sure you obtain her home and work telephone numbers, if possible, and remind her to bring her insurance card. When you enter the appointment code, enter the resource as ROOM1 and the reason as Urgent.

6. Mr. Cross is finished with his appointment and brings his encounter form to you. You need to make a follow-up appointment 1 week from today for his blood test results and enter the charges for today's visit in Medisoft (see encounter form in Appendix C).
7. Ms. Tiffany Carter arrives for her appointment. She has written a check (number 1045) for a copay of $10.00. Notify the medical assistant of her arrival.
8. Robert Jones calls to see if he can reschedule his appointment for tomorrow afternoon. Reschedule Mr. Jones for tomorrow at 2:00 PM. When you enter the appointment, use ROOM1 as the resource and CHECKBP as the reason. Extend the appointment time to 30 minutes.
9. Ms. Jackson is finished with her appointment and brings her encounter form to you. You need to enter the charges for her visit and make sure you credit her copay. Print a receipt for this patient.
10. Alex Neumann calls and says he has an emergency to attend to and would like to reschedule his appointment for Wednesday at the same time (4:00 PM). Check the schedule, and make the appointment. Resource, ROOM1; Reason, ROUTINE
11. Ms. Carter is finished with her appointment, and the doctor would like to see Ms. Carter in 1 week. Make an appointment for Ms. Carter 1 week from now and around the same time. Enter the charges for today's visit into the computer. Also, credit her account for her $10.00 copay. Resource, ROOM2; Reason, FOLLOWUP
12. Confirm that all patients have been seen and that you have received all encounter forms for today's visits. You should have entered charges for the three patients who were seen.
13. Print out tomorrow's schedule.
14. Print today's insurance claim forms.
15. Print out a Patient, Procedure, and Payment Day Sheet. Hand in your materials to your instructor.

Note: Remember, when you enter the patients, you will create cases based on the reason they are being seen. In addition, remember to schedule the patients around Dr. Bill's 1-hour lunch from 12:00 PM to 1:00 PM. Create this recurring lunch break for Dr. Bill. The workday for Dr. Bill is from 9:00 AM to 5:00 PM and Saturdays from 10:00 AM to 2:00 PM.

Day Two (Tuesday, 02/05/2013) Remember to change the date!

Remember to change the date in the bottom right corner.

1. Start your day by confirming that all medical charts are given to the correct staff person. If not, you will need to pull the charts unless they are new patients.
2. Your answering service has notified you that five new patients with various conditions would like to be seen today. You write down their names, phone numbers, and chief complaints from the service. You call each of them to schedule the following appointments for today:
   a. Curtis Gorge, 10:00 AM, coughing for 1 week, (555) 555-2716 (15 minutes). Resource, ROOM1; Reason, ROUTINE
   b. Lynn Stone, 10:30 AM, no energy, (555) 555-6419 (15 minutes). Resource, ROOM2; Reason, ROUTINE

c. Dylan Hill, 11:00 AM, physical, (555) 555-5678 (60 minutes). Resource, ROOM1; Reason, PHYS. Increase length to 60 minutes.

d. Nancy Hutton, 1:00 PM, well-woman examination, (555) 555-8826. Resource, ROOM1; Reason, WELLWMAN

e. Sammy Paul, 3:00 PM, earache, (555) 555-2203 (15 minutes). Resource, ROOM2; Reason, ROUTINE

3. Print encounter forms (superbills) for the five patients entered in step 2, plus the two patients scheduled yesterday.

4. Ms. Mann arrives for her 9:00 AM appointment. She fills out the registration form and gives you her insurance card to photocopy. There is no copay. Notify the medical assistant of her arrival. After she has been seen by the physician, Ms. Mann leaves and gives you her encounter form. Enter the charges for today's visit.

5. Mr. Gorge arrives for his 10:00 AM appointment. Enter this patient into the computer. He is complaining of a cough for the past week and receives a chest x-ray. Using the encounter form, enter the charge and record the payment from the patient of $50.00 (check number 2903). He also requests a receipt because he has no insurance; print a receipt for him.

6. Ms. Stone arrives for her 10:30 AM appointment. Enter her into Medisoft. After the doctor examines her, he orders blood work to check for anemia. A follow-up appointment (15 minutes) is made for this Friday at 9:00 AM. Resource, ROOM1; Reason, ROUTINE. Enter charges.

7. Mr. Hill arrives for his physical appointment. Enter him into Medisoft. The medical records from Mr. Hill's previous clinic indicate that he has an iron deficiency and is receiving vitamin B12 injections and a prescription for ascorbic acid (500 mg). Dr. Bill wants him to come back every third week of the month for vitamin B12 injections. Because his injections are up to date, his next injection will be given at the next appointment. Set up the regularly scheduled appointments 1 year in advance (he prefers morning hours). In addition, enter the charges using the encounter form.

8. Ms. Hutton arrives for her 1:00 PM appointment. She is a new patient and needs to complete the patient registration form. According to her insurance card, she has a $20.00 copay. Enter her patient information, as well as her charges and payment for this visit into Medisoft. Print a receipt for the $20.00 cash copay.

9. Robert Jones arrives for his 2:00 PM appointment. You notice that he seems pale and is having difficulty breathing. You ask him if he is having any pain. He says, "Yes, in my shoulders and chin." You immediately bring him to an examination room and notify the doctor of his symptoms. Dr. Bill orders an electrocardiogram (ECG). The ECG notes acute anterior left ventricular infarction. An ambulance is called right away. Mr. Jones is transported to the local hospital. The encounter form indicates a Level 3 visit, and an ECG is performed on the patient. Enter those charges and the patient into Medisoft.

10. Sammy Paul arrives with his mother. Enter him into the system, as well as Sammy's father, John Paul, who is the guarantor. Sammy is prescribed an antibiotic for an ear infection. Enter the charges.

11. Print insurance claims for today, and confirm that all patients seen today have been entered into the computer.

12. Print a current Patient List using the Print Grid button from the Patient List.

13. Print Procedure, Payment, and Patient Day Sheets.

Day Three (Wednesday, 02/06/2013) Did you forget to change the date?

Remember to change the date.

1. Your clinic manager wants you to block off time in the schedule for a staff meeting every Wednesday beginning this week. The meeting will be from 9:00 AM to 10:00 AM. If any patients are scheduled during that time, you should reschedule them.
2. Sara Tschida calls to schedule an appointment today at 11:00 AM for a well-woman examination. Her telephone number is (555) 555-3636. Resource, ROOM1; Reason, WELLWMAN
3. Danny Smith, a walk-in, is crying when he comes in with his parents. He apparently shoved a penny up his right nostril. The child and mother are ushered back to the examination room. For your records, document this visit into the appointment schedule as an office visit at the time they arrived in the office. In addition, obtain all information from the father, and print an encounter form. The father, Doug Smith, is the guarantor on this account for Danny. Resource, ROOM2; Reason, ROUTINE
4. Sara Tschida calls back to reschedule her appointment, originally scheduled for today at 11:00 AM, to tomorrow at the same time.
5. As Danny Smith leaves, his mother gives you the encounter form and needs to schedule a follow-up visit in 2 days. Make an appointment for 10:00 AM on Friday. Enter the charges for Danny. Resource, ROOM1; Reason, FOLLOWUP
6. Enter the following four patients for tomorrow, and print their encounter forms:
    a. Lynn Taylor, 9:00 AM, new patient, arthritis, (555) 555-5562. Resource, ROOM1; Reason, INIT
    b. Tiffany Carter, 9:30 AM, established, dermatitis is getting worse, (555) 555-4795. Resource, ROOM2; Reason, FOLLOWUP
    c. Adam Burns, 2:15 PM, new patient, headaches, (555) 555-8323. Resource, ROOM1; Reason, INIT
    d. Robert Jones, 3:30 PM, established, follow-up heart attack, (555) 555-4567. Resource, ROOM2; Reason, FOLLOWUP
7. Print your insurance claims for the day.
8. Print tomorrow's schedule.
9. Print Procedure, Payment, and Patient Day Sheets.

Day Four (Thursday, 02/07/2013) See! You remembered to change the date!

1. Your first week is almost over, and the doctor has noticed how professional and efficient you are in your position. Good job!
2. The mail today brings insurance payments for charges from your Monday and Tuesday's patients. Use the explanation of benefits (EOBs) in Appendix C, and enter those payments.

3. Mike Johnson walks in asking to be seen by a doctor to discuss his hypertension and diabetes. Typically, you would not be able to see a new patient on a walk-in basis, but you do have openings. Ask the doctor if you can schedule him for an appointment today. It is approved, so you schedule him for 10:00 AM (Resource, ROOM1; Reason, INIT) and have him fill out a registration form. Enter the new patient information, and print an encounter form for Mr. Johnson.
4. Your first scheduled patient, Lynn Taylor, arrives. She has an appointment regarding her arthritis. Have her fill out a registration form. As she is leaving, she brings the encounter form to you and says, "Goodbye." Enter the charges using her encounter form.
5. Ms. Carter arrives for her appointment at 9:30 AM (15 minutes). Notify the medical assistant. The laundry detergent Ms. Carter used yesterday might have caused her contact dermatitis. The inflammation is quite severe. The doctor has told her to switch detergents and monitor the skin condition. He orders a dose of Prednisone, 60 mg/day for 12 days. She is to make a follow-up appointment in 1 week unless the condition worsens. Enter the appointment and today's charges into Medisoft.
6. Mr. Johnson's blood sugar has not been controlled, and his blood pressure is high. Dr. Bill has ordered blood tests for blood glucose levels and increases his Atenolol to 100 mg. Dr. Bill requests you schedule a follow-up visit in 1 week for Mr. Johnson. Enter the charges for today's visit from the encounter form. Note that Mr. Johnson has two diagnoses for his visit today. Diabetes should be the primary diagnosis.
7. Ms. Sara Tschida arrives for her appointment. She is being seen for a well-woman examination. She is a new patient and should complete the registration form. Enter the new patient information, and print an encounter form. Sara is a Cash Pay Patient and pays her charges in full with check number 4324 as she leaves the office. Enter the charges and payment for today's visit from the encounter form.
8. Adam Burns arrives for his appointment. He is a new patient and is asked to complete the registration form. After he is taken to the examination room and upon checking his vital signs, the medical assistant discovers a reading of 160/120 mm Hg, which is high. After waiting 10 minutes, his blood pressure is 158/122 mm Hg in the right arm and 164/130 mm Hg in the left arm. The medical assistant reports these readings to Dr. Bill. On examination, the doctor prescribes Atenolol, 50 mg/day, and requests to see him tomorrow. Enter the charges for today's visit, and schedule the appointment for tomorrow at 1:00 PM. Resource, ROOM1; Reason, FOLLOWUP
9. Print out Friday's schedule, and make sure all of the medical charts have been pulled. If some of the charts are not there, you will need to pull or locate them for tomorrow.
10. Your final patient, Robert Jones, arrives for the day. He looks better than he did on Tuesday. He is carrying nitroglycerin tablets and is seeing a dietitian for his eating habits. Another ECG is ordered for today, and the results are normal. Enter the charges using the encounter form.
11. Print your insurance claims for the day.
12. Print any necessary encounter forms based on Friday's schedule.
13. Print Procedure, Payment, and Patient Day Sheets.

Note: Insurance payments do not usually arrive this quickly; however, this is a simulation and we wanted you to experience the routine in a medical office as it happens on a day-to-day basis.

Day Five (Friday, 02/08/2013) Don't forget to change me!

1. Your mail brings three payments from insurance companies and patients for Tuesday, Wednesday, and Thursday's visits. (See Appendix C for the three EOBs, and enter them into the computer.)
2. Ms. Stone arrives for her appointment. She has anemia and receives a B12 injection today. See the encounter form for today's charges. Schedule a follow-up visit for next week on Wednesday, first available time slot.
3. Debra Jackson has switched insurance companies. She no longer has BCBS and now has First Med Insurance. This insurance takes effect the first of the month. She has no outstanding balance. She gives you the information over the phone; the next time she comes in, you will need to get two copies of her insurance card. You will add a reminder to her account using Final Draft to get two copies of the insurance card.
4. Steve Nelson, a new patient, calls to ask for an appointment today to follow-up on an emergency department visit. He can be seen at 9:30 AM today; his phone number is (555) 555-4545.
5. Mr. Nelson arrives for his 9:30 AM appointment. He was in a car accident, and you need to put this information in the computer. His primary insurance, BCBS, will not cover medical care related to the car accident. His car insurance, State Farm, will cover his medical expenses. Add State Farm as a new insurance carrier under Steve Nelson's account. The address for Claims is: State Farm Insurance Company of MN, 3489 Walkahead Rd., St. Paul, MN, 55100. The phone number to follow-up the claims is (555) 555-6026. Be sure to put the first date of the accident as 02/03/2013, and enter the auto accident under the Condition tab of the new case for Mr. Nelson. After Mr. Nelson has been seen by the physician, enter the charges from the encounter form.
6. Danny Smith arrives for his follow-up visit. His nose is swollen, but he is doing much better. After he is done with the physician, enter the charges for today's visit into Medisoft.
7. Adam Burns arrives for his appointment. His blood pressure has improved slightly with a consistent reading of 154/92 mm Hg. Dr. Bill is concerned about the readings and increases the Atenolol to 100 mg and requests to see him tomorrow when the clinic opens at 10:00 AM. Use the encounter form to enter the charges for today.
8. Raymond Cross calls to make an appointment for next Friday at 9:00 AM with Dr. Bill. Make the appointment in the Medisoft system for Mr. Cross.
9. Print out insurance claim forms.
10. Print Procedure, Payment, and Patient Day Sheets.

Day Six (Saturday, 02/09/2013) Remember me? Your date!

1. Insurance and patient payments arrive in the mail for Friday's visits. The remittance advice is from Blue Cross Blue Shield for patients Stone, Smith, and Burns. Enter the payments as listed in **Figures C.93.1, C.93.2,** and **C.93.3 in Appendix C**.
2. An insurance payment arrives from State Farm Insurance for Steve Nelson. Enter the payment into Medisoft, and apply it to his account. (See **Figure C.94 in Appendix C**.)

3. Adam Burns arrives for his 10:00 AM appointment. His blood pressure has dropped to 130/88 mm Hg. Dr. Bill is pleased to see that the medication is beginning to work and does not adjust the dosage at this time. He wants to see Adam for a follow-up appointment in 1 week. Schedule an appointment for Mr. Burns for next Friday at the same time. Mr. Burns is told to call the office if he begins feeling lightheaded or faint. Enter the charges from the encounter form.
4. Print next week's schedule.
5. Print a Patient List Report for the practice.
6. Print a Practice Analysis Report.
7. Print a Patient Ledger Report.
8. Print Procedure, Payment, and Patient Day Sheets.
9. Hand in all materials from this week-long simulation to your instructor.

WEEK TWO

Day Seven (Monday 02/11/2013) Meet you in the bottom right corner!

1. Open the office and transfer the phones. You take appointments from the following new patients:
   a. Addison Brown (vertigo), (555) 555-8865, Monday at 1:15 PM
   b. Cody Rose (carpal tunnel syndrome), (555) 555-9364, Tuesday at 9:00 AM
   c. Karen London (head cold), (555) 555-4321, Wednesday at 10:00 AM
   d. Matt Johnson (bronchitis), (555) 555-5431, Thursday at 3:00 PM
2. Print an encounter form (superbill) for each of the patients this week.
3. Print a schedule for today because the schedule has changed from Saturday.
4. Ms. Carter arrives for her 1-week follow-up appointment. Her contact dermatitis is greatly improved since stopping the use of the new detergent. The doctor would still like to see her again in 1 week for a follow-up visit. Make an appointment for her for next Monday. Ms. Carter advises you that she will be changing employment at the end of the month. She will bring her new insurance information to you as soon as she receives it. Make a note of this impending change in her record.
5. Addison Brown arrives for her appointment. Enter the patient information found on the registration form. Note that Ms. Brown is a cash patient because she has no insurance. Enter the charges from the encounter form. The total charges of $100.00 are the responsibility of Ms. Brown. Make payment arrangements for $25.00 per week. Enter the payment plan in Medisoft.
6. Print tomorrow's schedule.
7. Print Procedure, Payment, and Patient Day Sheets.
8. Hand in all forms to your instructor.

Day Eight (Tuesday 02/12/2013) It should be a habit by now!

1. Today, you have a new doctor, Dr. Jagla, who previously worked with Dr. Bill. Enter Dr. Jagla's information as outlined:

Name:	Roman Roland Jagla, MD
Address:	Same as the clinic
Signature on File:	Check box
State License Number:	124054
Specialty:	General practice
Entity Type:	Person
SSN:	100-11-1222
Medicare:	111555332
BCBS:	43329
Commercial:	01253
UPIN:	1087654
NPI:	3456789012

2. Schedule the following new patients to see Dr. Jagla: Louise Brooks (arthritis) at 1:00 PM and Tim Camon (physical) at 2:00 PM.
3. Print encounter forms for Louise Brooks and Tim Camon.
4. Print a new schedule for both Dr. Bill and Dr. Jagla.
5. Print a Patient List for the practice.
6. Cody Rose arrives for his appointment. He needs some help filling out the registration form because of his carpal tunnel syndrome. Enter his information into the system; the description for the case is carpal tunnel syndrome.
7. Enter the charges for Cody Rose from the encounter form.
8. Louise Brooks arrives for her appointment with Dr. Jagla at 1:00 PM. Enter her into the system.
9. Ms. Brooks is finished with Dr. Jagla and returns to your desk with her encounter form. Dr. Jagla did not specify a follow-up date, so Ms. Brooks is told to call and make an appointment as needed. Enter the charges from the encounter form. Make sure that the provider for Ms. Brooks is Dr. Jagla.
10. At 2:00 PM, Tim Camon arrives for his physical. After he has completed the patient registration form, enter him into the system. Notify the medical assistant of Mr. Camon's arrival.
11. Tim Camon drops the completed encounter form on your desk as he leaves. Enter his charges, and make sure that the provider for Mr. Camon is Dr. Jagla.
12. Print Procedure, Payment, and Patient Day Sheets.
13. Hand in all printed material to your instructor.

Day Nine (Wednesday 02/13/2013) After Friday, I won't nag you!

1. Ms. Stone arrives for her follow-up appointment and is shown to an examination room by the medical assistant.
2. The doctor drops the encounter form on your desk as he escorts Ms. Stone to the door. Enter the charges for Ms. Stone's appointment.
3. Karen London, a new patient for Dr. Bill, arrives for her appointment. Enter her into the Medisoft system. Enter the description on the case as head cold.
4. Enter Ms. London's charges into Medisoft using the completed encounter form.

5. Payment arrives for Monday's patient Tiffany Carter. Enter the payment into Medisoft.
6. The first payment for Addison Brown arrives in the mail. It is a personal check, number 2263, for the agreed-on payment amount of $25.00. Apply this payment to Ms. Brown's account.
7. Print tomorrow's schedule.
8. Print Procedure, Payment, and Patient Day Sheets.
9. Hand all your printed work in to your instructor.

Day Ten (Thursday 02/14/2013) Quick! What's the date?

1. Two insurance payments have arrived in the mail. The first payment is from First Med for patients Louise Brooks and Tim Camon seen on Tuesday by Dr. Jagla.
2. The second payment is from BCBS for Cody Rose who also saw Dr. Bill on Tuesday.
3. Enter these two payments into Medisoft.
4. Mike Johnson arrives for his follow-up appointment for hypertension. He seems to be in a good mood and states that he is feeling much better. Enter the charges for Mr. Johnson's follow-up visit as listed on the encounter form.
5. Matt Johnson, a new patient, arrives for his 3:00 PM appointment with Dr. Bill. Enter the patient and insurance information into Medisoft. The description for the case will be bronchitis.
6. Enter Matt Johnson's charges into Medisoft as they are listed on the encounter form.
7. Print Procedure, Payment, and Patient Day Sheets, and hand them in to your instructor.

Day Eleven (Friday 02/15/2013) It's been a great 2 weeks!

1. Payments arrive today from BCBS. The check is payment for patients seen on Wednesday and Thursday.
2. Enter these payments into Medisoft.
3. Raymond Cross has missed his 9:00 AM appointment with Dr. Bill. Using Final Draft, make a notation in his record that he missed this appointment. Write a short letter to Mr. Cross advising him that he has missed his appointment and would he please call at his earliest convenience to reschedule the appointment. Print the copy of the letter for Dr. Bill to sign.
4. Peter Pearson calls to schedule an appointment for 11:15 AM on Monday morning. He is a new patient. He wants his hearing to be checked.
5. Print Claim forms.
6. Print Patient Statements.
7. Print a Patient List.
8. Print a Provider List.
9. Print a Diagnosis List.
10. Print a Procedure/Payments/Adjustment Code list.
11. Print Procedure, Payment, and Patient Day Sheets.
12. Hand in everything printed to your instructor, including the letter to Mr. Cross.

Congratulations! You have successfully completed all of the work required for the 2-week day-by-day simulation. You have gained a better understanding of how a medical clinic operates, even though you only performed administrative duties for 11 days. Many clinics operate at a much faster pace and will require you to make quick and fair decisions when dealing with patients, staff, and providers. By completing this simulation, you will have a better understanding of how a computerized medical office works, and you can transfer those skills to other computerized applications. These skills will make you a valuable member of the office staff. Good luck in your future career within the health care field.

appendix B

Centers for Medicare and Medicaid Services (CMS)-1500 Step-by-Step Instructions

Appendix B will take you step by step through the CMS-1500 form (Figure B.1). These are guidelines, and, if you have any questions, contact the insurance company.

Box 1, Payer Type. This is a required box. Indicate the type of payer with an X. If this is a workers' compensation claim, mark *Other*. If you do not know the right box to mark, call your payer. If you mark the wrong box, the claim will be rejected.

Box 1a, Insured's ID Number. This is a required box. The patient's identification (ID) number will be entered into this field and is used by the insurance company to confirm benefits.

Box 2, Patient Name. This is a required box. Enter the name as last name/first name/middle initial, and remember to spell the patient's name exactly as it appears on the insurance card.

Box 3, Patient Birth Date and Gender. This is a required box. Enter the required information as 10/03/1974. Enter X for the correct gender. If this box is left blank, the claim could be rejected.

Box 4, Insured's Name. Enter the insured's name. This field may be left blank only if the insured's name is the patient. Use this box when the patient is not the policyholder.

Box 5, Patient Address. This is a required box. Enter the patient's address and telephone number in this box. Remember to make sure that the address and phone number match the information on file with the payer; otherwise, the claim will be rejected.

Box 6, Patient Relationship to Insured. This is a required box. Mark an X next to how the patient is related to the policyholder. Claims are rejected without this information.

Box 7, Insured's Address. This is a required box if Box 4 is completed and if the insured has a different address than the patient. Enter *Same* if both patient and insured live at the same address.

Box 8, Reserve for NUCC Use. Reserve this space for NUCC Use. Do not fill in this box.

Box 9, Other Insured's Name. This is used to indicate a secondary policy. Enter the required information for the secondary insurance into Boxes 9a through 9d. This includes the policy number of the secondary insurance; the other insured's birth date and gender; the employer's name or school name; and the insurance plan (e.g., Medigap).

Box 10, Is Patient's Condition Related To. This is a required box. Insurance companies are determining if the medical care reported on the claim form is necessary because of a current or former work-related incident, an auto accident and state (place) of occurrence, or any other type of accident. This box will help insurance companies that are responsible for covering this care.

DRAFT - NOT FOR OFFICIAL USE

HEALTH INSURANCE CLAIM FORM

APPROVED BY NATIONAL UNIFOR MCLAIM COMMITTEE (NUCC) 02/12

PICA | PICA

CARRIER

1. MEDICARE (Medicare#) MEDICAID (Medicaid#) TRICARE (ID#DoD#) CHAMPVA (Member ID#) GROUP HEALTH PLAN (ID#) FECA BLK LUNG (ID#) OTHER (ID#)

1a. INSURED'S I.D. NUMBER (For Program in Item 1)

2. PATIENT'S NAME (Last Name, First Name, Middle Initial)

3. PATIENT'S BIRTH DATE MM DD YY SEX M F

4. INSURED'S NAME (Last Name, First Name, Middle Initial)

5. PATIENT'S ADDRESS (No., Street)

6. PATIENT RELATIONSHIP TO INSURED Self Spouse Child Other

7. INSURED'S ADDRESS (No., Street)

CITY STATE

8. RESERVED FOR NUCC USE

CITY STATE

ZIP CODE TELEPHONE (Include Area Code) ( )

ZIP CODE TELEPHONE (Include Area Code) ( )

9. OTHER INSURED'S NAME (Last Name, First Name, Middle Initial)

10. IS PATIENT'S CONDITION RELATED TO:

11. INSURED'S POLICY GROUP OR FECA NUMBER

a. OTHER INSURED'S POLICY OR GROUP NUMBER

a. EMPLOYMENT? (Current or Previous) YES NO

a. INSURED'S DATE OF BIRTH MM DD YY SEX M F

b. RESERVED FOR NUCC USE

b. AUTO ACCIDENT? YES NO PLACE (State)

b. OTHER CLAIM ID (Designated by NUCC)

c. RESERVED FOR NUCC USE

c. OTHER ACCIDENT? YES NO

c. INSURANCE PLAN NAME OR PROGRAM NAME

d. INSURANCE PLAN NAME OR PROGRAM NAME

10d. CLAIM CODES (Designated by NUCC)

d. IS THERE ANOTHER HEALTH BENEFIT PLAN? YES NO *If yes*, complete items 9, 9a, and 9d.

READ BACK OF FORM BEFORE COMPLETING & SIGNING THIS FORM.

12. PATIENT'S OR AUTHORIZED PERSON'S SIGNATUREI authorize the release of any medical or other information necessary to process this claim. I also request payment of government benefits either to myself or to the party who accepts assignment below.

SIGNED ______ DATE ______

13. INSURED'S OR AUTHORIZED PERSON'S SIGNATURE I authorize payment of medical benefits to the undersigned physician or supplier for services described below.

SIGNED ______

PATIENT AND INSURED INFORMATION

14. DATE OF CURRENT: ILLNESS, INJURY, or PREGNANCY(LMP) MM DD YY QUAL.

15. OTHER DATE QUAL. MM DD YY

16. DATES PATIENT UNABLE TO WORK IN CURRENT OCCUPATION FROM MM DD YY TO MM DD YY

17. NAME OF REFERRING PROVIDER OR OTHER SOURCE

17a. 17b. NPI

18. HOSPITALIZATION DATES RELATED TO CURRENT SERVICES FROM MM DD YY TO MM DD YY

19. ADDITIONAL CLAIM INFORMATION (Designated by NUCC)

20. OUTSIDE LAB? YES NO $ CHARGES

21. DIAGNOSIS OR NATURE OF ILLNESS OR INJURY Relate A-L to service line below (24E) ICD Ind.

A. B. C. D.
E. F. G. H.
I. J. K. L.

22. RESUBMISSION CODE ORIGINAL REF. NO.

23. PRIOR AUTHORIZATION NUMBER

	24. A. DATE(S) OF SERVICE From MM DD YY To MM DD YY	B. PLACE OF SERVICE	C. EMG	D. PROCEDURES, SERVICES, OR SUPPLIES (Explain Unusual Circumstances) CPT/HCPCS MODIFIER	E. DIAGNOSIS POINTER	F. $ CHARGES	G. DAYS OR UNITS	H. EPSDT Family Plan	I. ID. QUAL.	J. RENDERING PROVIDER ID. #
1									NPI	
2									NPI	
3									NPI	
4									NPI	
5									NPI	
6									NPI	

PHYSICIAN OR SUPPLIER INFORMATION

25. FEDERAL TAX I.D. NUMBER SSN EIN

26. PATIENT'S ACCOUNT NO.

27. ACCEPT ASSIGNMENT? (For govt. claims, see back) YES NO

28. TOTAL CHARGE $

29. AMOUNT PAID $

30. Rsvd for NUCC Use $

31. SIGNATURE OF PHYSICIAN OR SUPPLIER INCLUDING DEGREES OR CREDENTIALS (I certify that the statements on the reverse apply to this bill and are made a part thereof.)

SIGNED DATE

32. SERVICE FACILITY LOCATION INFORMATION

a. NPI b.

33. BILLING PROVIDER INFO & PH # ( )

a. NPI b.

NUCC Instruction Manual available at: www.nucc.org *PLEASE PRINT OR TYPE* OMB APPROVAL PENDING

Figure B.1 Copy of the CMS-1500 (02-12) Health Insurance Claim Form.

Box 11, Insured's Policy, Group, or FECA Number. Enter the policy, group, or FECA number in this box. The number can be found on the patient's insurance card. If no number is listed or you are unable to find the number, call the insurance company and ask them for the number.

Enter the patient's date of birth and gender, employer's name or school name, and insurance plan name. Answer the question, "Are you covered by another health benefit plan?" Boxes 11a through 11d are required when the patient is not the policyholder listed in Box 4.

Box 12, Release of Information. The signature of the patient, the parent of the minor, or a legal guardian may sign a release of information statement. If the patient has signed a consent form, enter *Signature on File*.

Box 13, Assignment of Benefits. If the patient signs in this box, the payment for the claim will be sent directly to the provider. If no signature is provided, the payment is sent directly to the patient. If the patient has signed a consent form, enter *Signature on File*.

Box 14, Date of Current Illness. This is a required box for accidents, injuries, and pregnancy claims. Accidents and injuries require you to fill in Box 21 with where and how the accident or injury occurred.

Box 15, Date of Other Illness. Insurance companies use this box to determine patterns or preexisting conditions for statistical purposes. Remember to give the date of the first illness and not the date of the current illness.

Box 16, Dates Unable to Work. The provider will enter dates the patient is unable to work. This box is primarily used for workers' compensation plans.

Box 17, Name of Referring Physician or Other Source. Enter the complete name of the referring physician. As of May 23, 2007, Box 17a is not to be reported, but 17b must be reported when a service was ordered or referred by a physician.

Box 18, Hospitalization Dates. Enter the dates of the hospital stay by the patient. *From* is the admission date and *To* is the discharge date.

Box 19, Additional Claim Information. The insurance companies reserve this box for a variety of information.

Box 20, Outside Lab. Mark with an *X* whether an outside laboratory performed any services entered in Box 24D. The provider will pay the laboratory, and the provider bills the insurance company for reimbursement.

Box 21, Diagnosis Information. This is a required box. Enter the diagnosis codes of the illness or injury for the claim. These codes will relate to Box 24.

Box 22, Resubmission Code. Enter the resubmission code and original reference number given by Medicaid.

Box 23, Prior Authorization. Insurance companies may provide the medical office with a prior authorization number. Enter that number exactly as given to you by the insurance company. Be sure to follow the specific insurance company's requirements for their prior authorization.

Box 24, Procedures, Services, or Supplies (including dates of service and charges). This is a required box. A maximum of six items may be listed per claim. The following 10 items are needed to complete the claim:

1. *24A, Date of Service:* Enter both from and to dates.
2. *24B, Place of Service:* Enter the place of service code as required by the insurance company. Example of a place of service code is 11, referring to office.
3. *24C, EMG:* EMG stands for Emergency and if service was rendered in a hospital emergency room. Enter *Y* for yes or leave blank for no.
4. *24D, Procedures, Services, or Supplies:* Using the current procedure codes, enter the CPT code and appropriate modifier. Only two modifiers per procedure code are available, although some insurance companies will accept three modifiers per procedure code if the claim is sent electronically. If more modifiers are needed than the insurance company will accept, enter modifier *–99* in Box 24D and enter the remaining modifiers in Box 19.
5. *24E, Diagnosis Pointer:* Enter the line number from Box 21 to link the diagnosis code to the procedure code. This is used to ensure medical necessity.

6. *24F, Charges:* Enter the charge for the procedure code on this line. If the provider is paid under a capitation plan, all the charges amounts are 0 dollars. The claim is filed for tracking purposes.
7. *24G, Days or Units:* Enter the appropriate number of days or units in the box. If only one visit, service, or procedure has occurred, enter the number *1*.
8. *24H, EPSDT Family Plan:* The Early Periodic Screening and Diagnostic Testing (EPS-DT) is only for Medicaid. Medicare requires this field to be left blank.
9. *24I, ID Qual:* If the provider does not have an NPI number, enter *IC* in this box to report a non-NPI number being reported.
10. *24J, Rendering Provider ID Number:* Enter the provider's NPI number in the white shaded area of the box.

Box 25, Federal Tax ID Number. This is a required box. Enter the provider's tax ID number, which may be a Social Security number or federal employer ID number.

Box 26, Patient's Account Number. This is a required box. Enter the patient's account number given to the patient from the medical office. This enables the insurance company to link together other claims by the patient.

Box 27, Accept Assignment. This is a required box. This box indicates whether the provider is willing to accept assignment. This is different from Box 12 where the patient gives permission to accept assignment. A *Yes* in this field indicates the provider is willing to accept assignment, and payment will be mailed to the medical office. A *No* in this field indicates the provider is not willing to accept assignment, and the payment is sent to the patient. Because it is harder to receive payment from the patient directly, it is always beneficial to accept assignment.

Box 28, Total Charge. Enter the charges by adding the total of column 24F.

Box 29, Amount Paid. Enter the payments or co-payments made by the patient into this box.

Box 30, Balance Due. Subtract the amount paid (Box 29) from the total charges (Box 28) to arrive at the balance due.

Box 31, Signature of Physician or Supplier. This is a required box. The provider's signature and date the claim was filed are entered in this box. Only if the provider has given you written permission can you type the provider's name in this box. Another item to be aware of is that the insurance company will send claims received through edits. The insurance company computer will check to see if the ID numbers listed in Box 24K and Box 33 match the name entered in the box. The edit will also check to see if contractual filing requirements were met by checking the date service was rendered and the claim was filed.

Box 32, Service Facility Location Information. This box identifies laboratories, radiology, hospitals, and other medical service centers. If services rendered in Box 24D were not performed at the patient's home or the medical office (e.g., emergency department), the address of where the services were performed needs to be entered in this box.

Box 33, Physician's Billing Name, Address, Zip Code. This is a required box. Enter the name, address, zip code, and phone number. The provider's NPI number is reported in Box 33a. Box 33b is not to be reported.

appendix C

Patient Data

Patient Registration Information

Account # : ______
Insurance # : ______
Co-Payment: $ ______

Please PRINT AND complete ALL sections below!

PATIENT'S PERSONAL INFORMATION Marital Status ☐ Single ☒ Married ☐ Divorced ☐ Widowed Sex: ☐ Male ☐ Female

Name: Weber (last name) Charles (first name) A (initial)

Street address: 2340 Port Field St. (Apt # ____) City: St. Paul State: MN Zip: 55100

Home phone: (555) 555-2352 Work phone: (555) 222-2222 Social Security # 432 - XX - 0009

Date of Birth: 4 (month) / 23 (day) / 1954 (year)

Employer / Name of School Central Lakes Warehouse ☐ Full Time ☐ Part Time

PATIENT'S / RESPONSIBLE PARTY INFORMATION

Responsible party: Self Date of Birth: ______

Relationship to Patient: ☒ Self ☐ Spouse ☐ Other ______ Social Security # ____-____-____

Responsible party's home phone: (____) ______

Address: ______ (Apt # ____) City: ______ State: ______ Zip: ______

Employer's name: Central Lakes Warehouse Phone number: (555) 222-2222

Address: 5555 Warehouse Circle City: Fridley State: MN Zip: 55112

Name of Parent/Guardian: ______

PATIENT'S INSURANCE INFORMATION Please present insurance cards to receptionist.

PRIMARY insurance company's name: Star Insurance

Insurance address: 45 Country Farm Lane City: Woodsfield State: MN Zip: 55432

Name of insured: ______ Date of Birth: ______ Relationship to insured: ☒ Self ☐ Spouse ☐ Other ☐ Child

Insurance ID number: SI-938102 Group number: ______

Does your insurance cover medication? ______

EMERGENCY CONTACT

Name of person not living with you: Sarah Weber Relationship: Sister

Address: ______ City: ______ State: ______ Zip: ______

Phone number: (555) 555-1234

Assignment of Benefits • Financial Agreement

I hereby give lifetime authorization for payment of insurance benefits to be made directly to ______, and any assisting physicians, for services rendered. I understand that I am financially responsible for all charges whether or not they are covered by insurance. In the event of default, I agree to pay all costs of collection, and reasonable attorney's fees. I hereby authorize this healthcare provider to release all information necessary to secure the payment of benefits.
I further agree that a photocopy of this agreement shall be as valid as the original.

Date: XX/XX/XXXX Your Signature: Charles A. Weber

FORM # 58-8423 • BIBBERO SYSTEMS, INC.• PETALUMA, CA.• TO ORDER CALL TOLL FREE :800-BIBBERO (800-242-2376) • FAX (800) 242-9330 (REV.7/94)

Figure C.1 Registration form for Charles Weber (Chapter 1).

Patient Registration Information

Account # :
Insurance # :
Co-Payment: $

Please PRINT AND complete ALL sections below!

PATIENT'S PERSONAL INFORMATION Marital Status ☒ Single ☐ Married ☐ Divorced ☐ Widowed Sex: ☒ Male ☐ Female

Name: Hernandez (last name) Carlos (first name) (initial)

Street address: 20 Fawn Hill Road (Apt #) City: St. Paul State: MN Zip: 55100

Home phone: (555) 422-1122 Work phone: ( ) Social Security # 794 - XX - 9998

Date of Birth: 12 (month) / 20 (day) / 2003 (year)

Employer / Name of School High Ridge Elementary School ☐ Full Time ☐ Part Time

PATIENT'S / RESPONSIBLE PARTY INFORMATION

Responsible party: Hector Hernandez Date of Birth: 8/16/1975

Relationship to Patient: ☐ Self ☐ Spouse ☒ Other Father Social Security # 103 - XX - 8077

Responsible party's home phone: (555) 422-1122

Address: 20 Fawn Hill Road (Apt #) City: St. Paul State: MN Zip: 55100

Employer's name: Lakeview Plaza Associates Phone number: (555) 262-9817

Address: 10 First Street City: Minneapolis State: MN Zip: 55200

Name of Parent/Guardian:

PATIENT'S INSURANCE INFORMATION Please present insurance cards to receptionist.

PRIMARY insurance company's name: Star Insurance

Insurance address: 45 Country Farm Lane City: Woodsfield State: MN Zip: 55432

Name of insured: Date of Birth: Relationship to insured: ☐ Self ☐ Spouse ☐ Other ☒ Child

Insurance ID number: SI-203918 Group number:

Does your insurance cover medication?

EMERGENCY CONTACT

Name of person not living with you: Same as responsible party Relationship:

Address: City: State: Zip:

Phone number: (555) 555-1234

Assignment of Benefits • Financial Agreement

I hereby give lifetime authorization for payment of insurance benefits to be made directly to ____________ ,and any assisting physicians, for services rendered. I understand that I am financially responsible for all charges whether or not they are covered by insurance. In the event of default, I agree to pay all costs of collection, and reasonable attorney's fees. I hereby authorize this healthcare provider to release all information necessary to secure the payment of benefits.
I further agree that a photocopy of this agreement shall be as valid as the original.

Date: XX/XX/XXXX Your Signature: Hector Hernandez

FORM # 58-8423 • BIBBERO SYSTEMS, INC.• PETALUMA, CA.• TO ORDER CALL TOLL FREE :800-BIBBERO (800-242-2376) • FAX (800) 242-9330 (REV.7/94)

Figure C.2 Registration form for Carlos Hernandez (Chapter 1).

Patient Registration Information

Account # : ______
Insurance # : ______
Co-Payment: $ ______

Please PRINT AND complete ALL sections below!

PATIENT'S PERSONAL INFORMATION Marital Status ☒ Single ☐ Married ☐ Divorced ☐ Widowed Sex: ☒ Male ☐ Female

Name: D'Connor (last name) William (first name) ______ (initial)

Street address: 789 Hansen Ave (Apt # ____) City: St. Paul State: MN Zip: 55100

Home phone: (555) 696-9999 Work phone: (____) ______ Social Security # 777 - XX - 1234

Date of Birth: 10 (month) / 08 (day) / 1945 (year)

Employer / Name of School ______ ☐ Full Time ☐ Part Time

PATIENT'S / RESPONSIBLE PARTY INFORMATION

Responsible party: Self Date of Birth: ______

Relationship to Patient: ☒ Self ☐ Spouse ☐ Other ______ Social Security # ____-____-____

Responsible party's home phone: (____) ______

Address: ______ (Apt # ____) City: ______ State: ______ Zip: ______

Employer's name: Retired Phone number: (____) ______

Address: ______ City: ______ State: ______ Zip: ______

Name of Parent/Guardian: ______

PATIENT'S INSURANCE INFORMATION Please present insurance cards to receptionist.

PRIMARY insurance company's name: Medicare

Insurance address: 233 N. Michigan Ave. City: Chicago State: IL Zip: 60601

Name of insured: William D'Connor Date of Birth: 10/8/35 Relationship to insured: ☒ Self ☐ Spouse ☐ Other ☐ Child

Insurance ID number: 777XX1234A Group number: ______

Does your insurance cover medication? Yes

EMERGENCY CONTACT

Name of person not living with you: Debbie D'Connor Relationship: Sister

Address: 123 Second Street City: Duluth State: MN Zip: 55802

Phone number: (555) 232-1111

Assignment of Benefits • Financial Agreement

I hereby give lifetime authorization for payment of insurance benefits to be made directly to Your Name Clinic ,and any assisting physicians, for services rendered. I understand that I am financially responsible for all charges whether or not they are covered by insurance. In the event of default, I agree to pay all costs of collection, and reasonable attorney's fees. I hereby authorize this healthcare provider to release all information necessary to secure the payment of benefits.

I further agree that a photocopy of this agreement shall be as valid as the original.

Date: XX/XX/XXXX Your Signature: William D'Connor

FORM # 58-8423 • BIBBERO SYSTEMS, INC.• PETALUMA, CA.• TO ORDER CALL TOLL FREE :800-BIBBERO (800-242-2376) • FAX (800) 242-9330 (REV.7/94)

Figure C.3 Registration form for William O'Connor (Chapter 1).

Patient Registration Information

Account # :
Insurance # :
Co-Payment: $

Please PRINT AND complete ALL sections below!

PATIENT'S PERSONAL INFORMATION Marital Status ☐ Single ☒ Married ☐ Divorced ☐ Widowed Sex: ☐ Male ☒ Female

Name: Wixen (last name) Cindy (first name) ____ (initial)

Street address: 900 Hudson River Rd. (Apt # ____) City: St. Paul State: MN Zip: 55100

Home phone: (555) 636-9032 Work phone: (555) 789-4388 Social Security # 123 - XX - 9876

Date of Birth: 3 (month) / 12 (day) / 1976 (year)

Employer / Name of School Home Products, Inc. ☐ Full Time ☒ Part Time

PATIENT'S / RESPONSIBLE PARTY INFORMATION

Responsible party: Henry Wixen Date of Birth: 11/22/73

Relationship to Patient: ☐ Self ☒ Spouse ☐ Other ____ Social Security # 845 - XX - 3823

Responsible party's home phone: (555) 636-9032

Address: 900 Hudson River Rd, (Apt # ____) City: St. Paul State: MN Zip: 55100

Employer's name: Custom Fittings, Inc. Phone number: (555) 838-7832

Address: 987 Industrial Avenue City: St. Paul State: MN Zip: 55100

Name of Parent/Guardian:

PATIENT'S INSURANCE INFORMATION Please present insurance cards to receptionist.

PRIMARY insurance company's name: Blue Cross/ Blue Shield

Insurance address: XXXX Blue Cross Road City: Eagan State: MN Zip: 55122

Name of insured: Henry Wixen/Cindy Wixen Date of Birth: ____ Relationship to insured: ☐ Self ☒ Spouse ☐ Other ☐ Child

Insurance ID number: 845XX3823 Group number: EU125-XL

Does your insurance cover medication? Yes

EMERGENCY CONTACT

Name of person not living with you: Henry Wixen Relationship: Husband

Address: See above City: ____ State: ____ Zip: ____

Phone number: (555) 123-3432

Assignment of Benefits • Financial Agreement

I hereby give lifetime authorization for payment of insurance benefits to be made directly to Your Name Clinic ,and any assisting physicians, for services rendered. I understand that I am financially responsible for all charges whether or not they are covered by insurance. In the event of default, I agree to pay all costs of collection, and reasonable attorney's fees. I hereby authorize this healthcare provider to release all information necessary to secure the payment of benefits.
I further agree that a photocopy of this agreement shall be as valid as the original.

Date: XX/XX/XXXX Your Signature: Cindy Wixen

FORM # 58-8423 • BIBBERO SYSTEMS, INC.• PETALUMA, CA.• TO ORDER CALL TOLL FREE :800-BIBBERO (800-242-2376) • FAX (800) 242-9330 (REV.7/94)

Figure C.4 Registration form for Cindy Wixen (Chapter 1).

Patient Registration Information

Account # : ______
Insurance # : ______
Co-Payment: $ ______

Please PRINT AND complete ALL sections below!

PATIENT'S PERSONAL INFORMATION Marital Status ❑ Single ❑ Married ☒ Divorced ❑ Widowed Sex: ☒ Male ❑ Female

Name: Baxter (last name) Ronald (first name) ______ (initial)

Street address: 2300 Anoka Drive (Apt # ______) City: St. Paul State: MN Zip: 55100

Home phone: (555) 555-5323 Work phone: (555) 253-1832 Social Security # 321 - XX - 3456

Date of Birth: 07 / 02 / 1968 (month / day / year)

Employer / Name of School Donald's Burgers ☒ Full Time ❑ Part Time

PATIENT'S / RESPONSIBLE PARTY INFORMATION

Responsible party: Self Date of Birth: ______

Relationship to Patient: ☒ Self ❑ Spouse ❑ Other ______ Social Security # ___-___-___

Responsible party's home phone: (___) ______

Address: ______ (Apt # ___) City: ______ State: ______ Zip: ______

Employer's name: Donald's Burgers Phone number: (555) 789-3823

Address: 98 Old Mac Road City: Minneapolis State: MN Zip: 55111

Name of Parent/Guardian: ______

PATIENT'S INSURANCE INFORMATION Please present insurance cards to receptionist.

PRIMARY insurance company's name: Blue Cross and Blue Shield

Insurance address: XXXX Blue Cross Road City: Eagan State: MN Zip: 55122

Name of insured: Ronald Baxter Date of Birth: 07/02/68 Relationship to insured: ☒ Self ☐ Spouse ☐ Other ☐ Child

Insurance ID number: 321XX3456 Group number: ZA-873-BA

Does your insurance cover medication? ______

EMERGENCY CONTACT

Name of person not living with you: Diane Baxter Relationship: Mother

Address: 58 Winding Lane City: Edina State: MN Zip: 55200

Phone number: (555) 434-4322

Assignment of Benefits • Financial Agreement

I hereby give lifetime authorization for payment of insurance benefits to be made directly to Your Name Clinic ,and any assisting physicians, for services rendered. I understand that I am financially responsible for all charges whether or not they are covered by insurance. In the event of default, I agree to pay all costs of collection, and reasonable attorney's fees. I hereby authorize this healthcare provider to release all information necessary to secure the payment of benefits.

I further agree that a photocopy of this agreement shall be as valid as the original.

Date: XX/XX/XXXX Your Signature: Ronald Baxter

FORM # 58-8423 • BIBBERO SYSTEMS, INC.• PETALUMA, CA.• TO ORDER CALL TOLL FREE :800-BIBBERO (800-242-2376) • FAX (800) 242-9330 (REV.7/94)

Figure C.5 Registration form for Ronald Baxter (Chapter 1).

Patient Registration Information

Account # :
Insurance # :
Co-Payment: $

Please PRINT AND complete ALL sections below!

PATIENT'S PERSONAL INFORMATION Marital Status ☒ Single ☐ Married ☐ Divorced ☐ Widowed Sex: ☒ Male ☐ Female

Name: Silversmith (last name) Jerry (first name) ____ (initial)

Street address: 6834 Portland Ave. (Apt # ____) City: St. Paul State: MN Zip: 55100

Home phone: (555) 631-0932 Work phone: (555) 544-1239 Social Security # 987 - XX - 1987

Date of Birth: 07 (month) / 01 (day) / 1976 (year)

Employer / Name of School Dyer's Industries ☒ Full Time ☐ Part Time

PATIENT'S / RESPONSIBLE PARTY INFORMATION

Responsible party: Self Date of Birth:

Relationship to Patient: ☒ Self ☐ Spouse ☐ Other Social Security # ____ - ____ - ____

Responsible party's home phone: (____)

Address: (Apt # ____) City: State: Zip:

Employer's name: Dyer's Industries Phone number: (555) 544-1239

Address: 123 Washington Street City: St. Paul State: MN Zip: 55100

Name of Parent/Guardian:

PATIENT'S INSURANCE INFORMATION Please present insurance cards to receptionist.

PRIMARY insurance company's name: First Med

Insurance address: 1 Medical Blvd. City: Detroit State: MI Zip: 48226

Name of insured: Jerry Silversmith Date of Birth: 1/1/76 Relationship to insured: ☒ Self ☐ Spouse ☐ Other ☐ Child

Insurance ID number: 987XX1987 Group number: DI-2341

Does your insurance cover medication? Yes

EMERGENCY CONTACT

Name of person not living with you: Emily Silversmith Relationship: Mother

Address: 482 Southlawn Avenue City: Washington State: DC Zip: 55555

Phone number: (555) 293-8234

Assignment of Benefits • Financial Agreement

I hereby give lifetime authorization for payment of insurance benefits to be made directly to Your Name Clinic ,and any assisting physicians, for services rendered. I understand that I am financially responsible for all charges whether or not they are covered by insurance. In the event of default, I agree to pay all costs of collection, and reasonable attorney's fees. I hereby authorize this healthcare provider to release all information necessary to secure the payment of benefits.

I further agree that a photocopy of this agreement shall be as valid as the original.

Date: XX/XX/XXXX Your Signature: Jerry Silversmith

FORM # 58-8423 • BIBBERO SYSTEMS, INC.• PETALUMA, CA.• TO ORDER CALL TOLL FREE :800-BIBBERO (800-242-2376) • FAX (800) 242-9330 (REV.7/94)

Figure C.6 Registration form for Jerry Silversmith (Chapter 2).

Patient Registration Information

Account # :
Insurance # :
Co-Payment: $

Please PRINT AND complete ALL sections below!

PATIENT'S PERSONAL INFORMATION Marital Status ☒ Single ☐ Married ☐ Divorced ☐ Widowed Sex: ☒ Male ☐ Female

Name: Portman (last name) Peter (first name) (initial)

Street address: 712 Carter Avenue (Apt #) City: St. Paul State: MN Zip: 55100

Home phone: (555) 414-9872 Work phone: ( ) Social Security # 834 - XX - 1233

Date of Birth: 8 (month) / 01 (day) / 1993 (year)

Employer / Name of School Carter High School ☒ Full Time ☐ Part Time

PATIENT'S / RESPONSIBLE PARTY INFORMATION

Responsible party: Paul Portman Date of Birth: 7/15/1963

Relationship to Patient: ☐ Self ☐ Spouse ☒ Other father Social Security # 678 - XX - 3455

Responsible party's home phone: ( ) See above

Address: (Apt #) City: State: Zip:

Employer's name: State College of Minnesota Phone number: (555) 312-6434

Address: 1 State Street City: St. Paul State: MN Zip: 55100

Name of Parent/Guardian: Paul and Mary Portman

PATIENT'S INSURANCE INFORMATION Please present insurance cards to receptionist.

PRIMARY insurance company's name: Blue Cross/ Blue Shield

Insurance address: XXXX Blue Cross Rd. City: Eagan State: MN Zip: 55122

Name of insured: Paul Portman Date of Birth: 1/1/93 Relationship to insured: ☐ Self ☐ Spouse ☐ Other ☒ Child

Insurance ID number: RTS 678XX3455 Group number: UT-4324-XA

Does your insurance cover medication? Yes

EMERGENCY CONTACT

Name of person not living with you: Paul and Mary Portman Relationship: Parents

Address: 712 Carter Avenue City: St. Paul State: MN Zip: 55100

Phone number: (555) 414-9872

Assignment of Benefits • Financial Agreement

I hereby give lifetime authorization for payment of insurance benefits to be made directly to Your Name Clinic ,and any assisting physicians, for services rendered. I understand that I am financially responsible for all charges whether or not they are covered by insurance. In the event of default, I agree to pay all costs of collection, and reasonable attorney's fees. I hereby authorize this healthcare provider to release all information necessary to secure the payment of benefits.
I further agree that a photocopy of this agreement shall be as valid as the original.

Date: XX/XX/XXXX Your Signature: Paul Portman

FORM # 58-8423 • BIBBERO SYSTEMS, INC.• PETALUMA, CA.• TO ORDER CALL TOLL FREE :800-BIBBERO (800-242-2376) • FAX (800) 242-9330 (REV.7/94)

Figure C.7 Registration form for Peter Portman (Chapter 2).

Patient Registration Information

Account # :
Insurance # :
Co-Payment: $

Please PRINT AND complete ALL sections below!

PATIENT'S PERSONAL INFORMATION Marital Status ☐ Single ☒ Married ☐ Divorced ☐ Widowed Sex: ☐ Male ☒ Female

Name: Lee (last name) Ashuri (first name) (initial)

Street address: 988 Marshall Avenue (Apt #) City: Minneapolis State: MN Zip: 55111

Home phone: (555) 838-1123 Work phone: (555) 353-9877 Social Security # 012 - XX - 3828

Date of Birth: 11 (month) / 12 (day) / 1963 (year)

Employer / Name of School Pinewood Gardens ☒ Full Time ☐ Part Time

PATIENT'S / RESPONSIBLE PARTY INFORMATION

Responsible party: James Lee Date of Birth:

Relationship to Patient: ☐ Self ☒ Spouse ☐ Other Social Security # 822 - XX - 3482

Responsible party's home phone: (555) 838-1123

Address: See above (Apt #) City: State: Zip:

Employer's name: Software Enterprises Phone number: (555) 732-0344

Address: 651 Enterprise Street City: St. Paul State: MN Zip: 55100

Name of Parent/Guardian:

PATIENT'S INSURANCE INFORMATION Please present insurance cards to receptionist.

PRIMARY insurance company's name: Blue Cross and Blue Shield

Insurance address: XXXX Blue Cross Rd. City: Eagan State: MN Zip: 55122

Name of insured: James Lee Date of Birth: Relationship to insured: ☐ Self ☒ Spouse ☐ Other ☐ Child

Insurance ID number: 822XX3482 Group number: OP-8432-RT

Does your insurance cover medication? Yes

EMERGENCY CONTACT

Name of person not living with you: James Lee Relationship: husband

Address: 988 Marshall Avenue City: Minneapolis State: MN Zip: 55111

Phone number: (555) 352-5323

Assignment of Benefits • Financial Agreement

I hereby give lifetime authorization for payment of insurance benefits to be made directly to Your Name Clinic ,and any assisting physicians, for services rendered. I understand that I am financially responsible for all charges whether or not they are covered by insurance. In the event of default, I agree to pay all costs of collection, and reasonable attorney's fees. I hereby authorize this healthcare provider to release all information necessary to secure the payment of benefits.
I further agree that a photocopy of this agreement shall be as valid as the original.

Date: XX/XX/XXXX Your Signature: Ashuri Lee

FORM # 58-8423 • BIBBERO SYSTEMS, INC.• PETALUMA, CA.• TO ORDER CALL TOLL FREE :800-BIBBERO (800-242-2376) • FAX (800) 242-9330 (REV.7/94)

Figure C.8 Registration form for Ashuri Lee (Chapter 3).

Patient Registration Information

Account # : ____
Insurance # : ____
Co-Payment: $ ____

Please PRINT AND complete ALL sections below!

PATIENT'S PERSONAL INFORMATION Marital Status ☒ Single ☐ Married ☐ Divorced ☐ Widowed Sex: ☐ Male ☒ Female

Name: McWilliams (last name) Tonya (first name) ____ (initial)

Street address: 321 Hamline Lane (Apt # ____) City: St. Paul State: MN Zip: 55100

Home phone: (555) 638-0001 Work phone: (____) ____ Social Security # 222 - XX - 1186

Date of Birth: 04 (month) / 12 (day) / 74 (year)

Employer / Name of School State College of Minnesota ☒ Full Time ☐ Part Time

PATIENT'S / RESPONSIBLE PARTY INFORMATION

Responsible party: Self Date of Birth: ____

Relationship to Patient: ☒ Self ☐ Spouse ☐ Other ____ Social Security # ____-____-____

Responsible party's home phone: (____) See above

Address: ____ (Apt # ____) City: ____ State: ____ Zip: ____

Employer's name: State College of Minnesota Phone number: (555) 312-6412

Address: 1 State Street City: St. Paul State: MN Zip: 55100

Name of Parent/Guardian: ____

PATIENT'S INSURANCE INFORMATION Please present insurance cards to receptionist.

PRIMARY insurance company's name: Blue Cross/ Blue Shield

Insurance address: XXXX Blue Cross Road City: Eagan State: MN Zip: 55122

Name of insured: Self Date of Birth: ____ Relationship to insured: ☒ Self ☐ Spouse ☐ Other ☐ Child

Insurance ID number: 222XX1186 Group number: UT-4324-XA

Does your insurance cover medication? Yes

EMERGENCY CONTACT

Name of person not living with you: Ben McWilliams Relationship: father

Address: 35 Centre Street City: Minneapolis State: MN Zip: 55111

Phone number: (555) 544-5833

Assignment of Benefits • Financial Agreement

I hereby give lifetime authorization for payment of insurance benefits to be made directly to Your Name Clinic ,and any assisting physicians, for services rendered. I understand that I am financially responsible for all charges whether or not they are covered by insurance. In the event of default, I agree to pay all costs of collection, and reasonable attorney's fees. I hereby authorize this healthcare provider to release all information necessary to secure the payment of benefits.

I further agree that a photocopy of this agreement shall be as valid as the original.

Date: XX/XX/XXXX Your Signature: Tonya McWilliams

FORM # 58-8423 • BIBBERO SYSTEMS, INC.• PETALUMA, CA.• TO ORDER CALL TOLL FREE :800-BIBBERO (800-242-2376) • FAX (800) 242-9330 (REV.7/94)

Figure C.9 Registration form for Tonya McWilliams (Chapter 3).

Patient Registration Information

Account # : ____
Insurance # : ____
Co-Payment: $ ____

Please PRINT AND complete ALL sections below!

PATIENT'S PERSONAL INFORMATION Marital Status ☒ Single ☐ Married ☐ Divorced ☐ Widowed Sex: ☒ Male ☐ Female

Name: Butler (last name) Tim (first name) ____ (initial)

Street address: TRS Plaza (Apt # ____) City: St. Paul State: MN Zip: 55100

Home phone: (555) 352-7424 Work phone: (555) 555-2003 Social Security # 020 - XX - 0030

Date of Birth: 4 / 27 / 68 (month / day / year)

Employer / Name of School TRS Partners ☐ Full Time ☐ Part Time

PATIENT'S / RESPONSIBLE PARTY INFORMATION

Responsible party: Tim Butler (self) Date of Birth: ____

Relationship to Patient: ☒ Self ☐ Spouse ☐ Other ____ Social Security # ____-____-____

Responsible party's home phone: (____) ____

Address: ____ (Apt # ____) City: ____ State: ____ Zip: ____

Employer's name: TRS Partners Phone number: (555) 555-2003

Address: TRS Plaza City: St. Paul State: MN Zip: 55100

Name of Parent/Guardian: ____

PATIENT'S INSURANCE INFORMATION Please present insurance cards to receptionist.

PRIMARY insurance company's name: First Med

Insurance address: 1 Medical Blvd. City: Detroit State: MI Zip: 48226

Name of insured: Self Date of Birth: ____ Relationship to insured: ☒ Self ☐ Spouse ☐ Other ☐ Child

Insurance ID number: 020XX0030 Group number: TRS-0800

Does your insurance cover medication? Yes

EMERGENCY CONTACT

Name of person not living with you: Kim Butler Relationship: Mother

Address: 5 Mapleshade Drive City: Minneapolis State: MN Zip: 55111

Phone number: (555) 453-4474

Assignment of Benefits • Financial Agreement

I hereby give lifetime authorization for payment of insurance benefits to be made directly to Your Name Clinic ,and any assisting physicians, for services rendered. I understand that I am financially responsible for all charges whether or not they are covered by insurance. In the event of default, I agree to pay all costs of collection, and reasonable attorney's fees. I hereby authorize this healthcare provider to release all information necessary to secure the payment of benefits.

I further agree that a photocopy of this agreement shall be as valid as the original.

Date: XX/XX/XXXX Your Signature: Tim Butler

FORM # 58-8423 • BIBBERO SYSTEMS, INC.• PETALUMA, CA.• TO ORDER CALL TOLL FREE :800-BIBBERO (800-242-2376) • FAX (800) 242-9330 (REV.7/94)

Figure C.10 Registration form for Tim Butler (Chapter 3).

Patient Registration Information

Account # :
Insurance # :
Co-Payment: $

Please PRINT AND complete ALL sections below!

PATIENT'S PERSONAL INFORMATION Marital Status ☐ Single ☒ Married ☐ Divorced ☐ Widowed Sex: ☐ Male ☒ Female

Name: Grant (last name) Carinna (first name) (initial)

Street address: 988 Madison Ave. (Apt #) City: St. Paul State: MN Zip: 55100

Home phone: (555) 631-9342 Work phone: (555) 472-2348 Social Security # 453 - XX - 0234

Date of Birth: 2 (month) / 17 (day) / 1970 (year)

Employer / Name of School St. Paul Daycare ☒ Full Time ☐ Part Time

PATIENT'S / RESPONSIBLE PARTY INFORMATION

Responsible party: Vince Grant Date of Birth: 5/19/1966

Relationship to Patient: ☐ Self ☒ Spouse ☐ Other Social Security # 093 - XX - 8532

Responsible party's home phone: ( ) See above

Address: See above (Apt #) City: State: Zip:

Employer's name: Grant Corporation Phone number: (555) 248-8348

Address: 120 Walnut Street City: St. Paul State: MN Zip: 55100

Name of Parent/Guardian:

PATIENT'S INSURANCE INFORMATION Please present insurance cards to receptionist.

PRIMARY insurance company's name: Blue Cross/Blue Shield

Insurance address: XXX Blue Cross Blvd. City: Eagan State: MN Zip: 55122

Name of insured: Vince Grant Date of Birth: 5/19/66 Relationship to insured: ☐ Self ☒ Spouse ☐ Other ☐ Child

Insurance ID number: 093XX8532 Group number: GC-8342-EP

Does your insurance cover medication? Yes

EMERGENCY CONTACT

Name of person not living with you: Vince Grant Relationship: Spouse

Address: 120 Walnut Street City: St. Paul State: MN Zip: 55100

Phone number: (555) 248-8348

Assignment of Benefits • Financial Agreement

I hereby give lifetime authorization for payment of insurance benefits to be made directly to Your Name Clinic ,and any assisting physicians, for services rendered. I understand that I am financially responsible for all charges whether or not they are covered by insurance. In the event of default, I agree to pay all costs of collection, and reasonable attorney's fees. I hereby authorize this healthcare provider to release all information necessary to secure the payment of benefits.

I further agree that a photocopy of this agreement shall be as valid as the original.

Date: XX/XX/XXXX Your Signature: Carinna Grant

FORM # 58-8423 • BIBBERO SYSTEMS, INC.• PETALUMA, CA.• TO ORDER CALL TOLL FREE :800-BIBBERO (800-242-2376) • FAX (800) 242-9330 (REV.7/94)

Figure C.11 Registration form for Carinna Grant (Chapter 3).

Patient Registration Information

Account # : ______
Insurance # : ______
Co-Payment: $ ______

Please PRINT AND complete ALL sections below!

PATIENT'S PERSONAL INFORMATION Marital Status ❑ Single ☒ Married ❑ Divorced ❑ Widowed Sex: ☒ Male ❑ Female

Name: Grant (last name) Vince (first name) ____ (initial)

Street address: 988 Madison Avenue (Apt # ____) City: St. Paul State: MN Zip: 55100

Home phone: (555) 631-9342 Work phone: (555) 248-8348 Social Security # 093 - XX - 8532

Date of Birth: 5 / 19 / 1966 (month / day / year)

Employer / Name of School Grant Corporation ☒ Full Time ❑ Part Time

PATIENT'S / RESPONSIBLE PARTY INFORMATION

Responsible party: Self Date of Birth: ______

Relationship to Patient: ☒ Self ❑ Spouse ❑ Other ______ Social Security # ____-____-____

Responsible party's home phone: (____) See above

Address: See above (Apt # ____) City: ______ State: ______ Zip: ______

Employer's name: Grant Corporation Phone number:(555) 248-8348

Address: 120 Walnut Street City: St. Paul State: MN Zip: 55100

Name of Parent/Guardian: ______

PATIENT'S INSURANCE INFORMATION Please present insurance cards to receptionist.

PRIMARY insurance company's name: Blue Cross/Blue Shield

Insurance address: XXX Blue Cross Blvd. City: Eagan State: MN Zip: 55122

Name of insured: Vince Grant Date of Birth: 5/19/66 Relationship to insured: ☒ Self ☐ Spouse ☐ Other ☐ Child

Insurance ID number: 093XX8532 Group number: GC-8342-EP

Does your insurance cover medication? Yes

EMERGENCY CONTACT

Name of person not living with you: Carinna Grant Relationship: Spouse

Address: See above City: ______ State: ______ Zip: ______

Phone number: (555) 631-9342/(555) 472-2348

Assignment of Benefits • Financial Agreement

I hereby give lifetime authorization for payment of insurance benefits to be made directly to Your Name Clinic ,and any assisting physicians, for services rendered. I understand that I am financially responsible for all charges whether or not they are covered by insurance. In the event of default, I agree to pay all costs of collection, and reasonable attorney's fees. I hereby authorize this healthcare provider to release all information necessary to secure the payment of benefits.

I further agree that a photocopy of this agreement shall be as valid as the original.

Date: XX/XX/XXXX Your Signature: Vince Grant

FORM # 58-8423 • BIBBERO SYSTEMS, INC.• PETALUMA, CA.• TO ORDER CALL TOLL FREE :800-BIBBERO (800-242-2376) • FAX (800) 242-9330 (REV.7/94)

Figure C.12 Registration form for Vince Grant (Chapter 3).

Patient Registration Information

Account # : ______
Insurance # : ______
Co-Payment: $ ______

Please PRINT AND complete ALL sections below!

PATIENT'S PERSONAL INFORMATION Marital Status ☒ Single ☐ Married ☐ Divorced ☐ Widowed Sex: ☐ Male ☒ Female

Name: Grant (last name) Debbie (first name) ______ (initial)

Street address: 988 Madison Avenue (Apt # ____) City: St. Paul State: MN Zip: 55100

Home phone: (555) 631-9342 Work phone: (____) ______ Social Security # 377 - XX - 1234

Date of Birth: 5 / 8 / 2003 (month / day / year)

Employer / Name of School First Street Elemenatry School ☒ Full Time ☐ Part Time

PATIENT'S / RESPONSIBLE PARTY INFORMATION

Responsible party: Vince Grant Date of Birth: 5/19/66

Relationship to Patient: ☐ Self ☐ Spouse ☒ Other Parent Social Security # 093 - XX - 8532

Responsible party's home phone: (____) See above

Address: ______ (Apt # ____) City: ______ State: ______ Zip: ______

Employer's name: Grant Corporation Phone number: (555) 248-8348

Address: 120 Walnut Street City: St. Paul State: MN Zip: 55100

Name of Parent/Guardian: Vince and Carinna Grant

PATIENT'S INSURANCE INFORMATION Please present insurance cards to receptionist.

PRIMARY insurance company's name: Blue Cross/Blue Shield

Insurance address: XXX Blue Cross Blvd. City: Eagan State: MN Zip: 55122

Name of insured: Vince Grant Date of Birth: 5/19/66 Relationship to insured: ☐ Self ☐ Spouse ☐ Other ☒ Child

Insurance ID number: 093XX8532 Group number: GC-8342-EP

Does your insurance cover medication? Yes

EMERGENCY CONTACT

Name of person not living with you: Carinna Grant Relationship: Mother

Address: See above City: ______ State: ______ Zip: ______

Phone number: (555) 631-9342/ (555) 472-3457 wk.

Assignment of Benefits • Financial Agreement

I hereby give lifetime authorization for payment of insurance benefits to be made directly to Your Name Clinic ,and any assisting physicians, for services rendered. I understand that I am financially responsible for all charges whether or not they are covered by insurance. In the event of default, I agree to pay all costs of collection, and reasonable attorney's fees. I hereby authorize this healthcare provider to release all information necessary to secure the payment of benefits.
I further agree that a photocopy of this agreement shall be as valid as the original.

Date: XX/XX/XXXX Your Signature: Carinna Grant

FORM # 58-8423 • BIBBERO SYSTEMS, INC.• PETALUMA, CA.• TO ORDER CALL TOLL FREE :800-BIBBERO (800-242-2376) • FAX (800) 242-9330 (REV.7/94)

Figure C.13 Registration form for Debbie Grant (Chapter 3).

Patient Registration Information

Account # : ______
Insurance # : ______
Co-Payment: $ ______

Please PRINT AND complete ALL sections below!

PATIENT'S PERSONAL INFORMATION Marital Status ☒ Single ☐ Married ☐ Divorced ☐ Widowed Sex: ☒ Male ☐ Female

Name: Grant (last name) Sammy (first name) ______ (initial)

Street address: 988 Madison Ave. (Apt # ____) City: St. Paul State: MN Zip: 55100

Home phone: (555) 631-9342 Work phone: (____) ______ Social Security # 773 - XX - 4321

Date of Birth: 12 (month) / 24 (day) / 2007 (year)

Employer / Name of School n/a ☐ Full Time ☐ Part Time

PATIENT'S / RESPONSIBLE PARTY INFORMATION

Responsible party: Vince Grant Date of Birth: 5/19/66

Relationship to Patient: ☐ Self ☐ Spouse ☒ Other Parent Social Security # 093 - XX - 8532

Responsible party's home phone: (____) See above

Address: See above (Apt # ____) City: ______ State: ______ Zip: ______

Employer's name: Grant Corporation Phone number:(555) 248-8348

Address: 120 Walnut Street City: St. Paul State: MN Zip: 55100

Name of Parent/Guardian: Vince and Carinna Grant

PATIENT'S INSURANCE INFORMATION Please present insurance cards to receptionist.

PRIMARY insurance company's name: Blue Cross/Blue Shield

Insurance address: XXX Blue Cross Blvd. City: Eagan State: MN Zip: 55122

Name of insured: Vince Grant Date of Birth: 5/19/66 Relationship to insured: ☐ Self ☐ Spouse ☐ Other ☒ Child

Insurance ID number: 093XX8532 Group number: GC-8342-EP

Does your insurance cover medication? Yes

EMERGENCY CONTACT

Name of person not living with you: Carinna Grant Relationship: Mother

Address: See above City: ______ State: ______ Zip: ______

Phone number: (555) 631-9342/ (555) 472-3457

Assignment of Benefits • Financial Agreement

I hereby give lifetime authorization for payment of insurance benefits to be made directly to Your Name Clinic ,and any assisting physicians, for services rendered. I understand that I am financially responsible for all charges whether or not they are covered by insurance. In the event of default, I agree to pay all costs of collection, and reasonable attorney's fees. I hereby authorize this healthcare provider to release all information necessary to secure the payment of benefits.

I further agree that a photocopy of this agreement shall be as valid as the original.

Date: XX/XX/XXXX Your Signature: Carinna Grant

FORM # 58-8423 • BIBBERO SYSTEMS, INC.• PETALUMA, CA.• TO ORDER CALL TOLL FREE :800-BIBBERO (800-242-2376) • FAX (800) 242-9330 (REV.7/94)

Figure C.14 Registration form for Sammy Grant (Chapter 3).

Goode Medical Clinic
1234 Larsen Avenue
Saint Paul, Minnesota 55316

Phone: (555) 555-1234
Fax: (555) 555-5678

PATIENT NAME	CHART #	DATE		
Charles Weber		*3/1/2010*	☐ MEDI-MEDI ☐ SELF PAY ☐ MEDICARE	☐ MEDICAL ☐ PRIVATE ☐ HMO____

☐	CPT/Md	DESCRIPTION	FEE
	OFFICE VISIT - NEW PATIENT		
	99202	Focused Ex.	
	99203	Detailed Ex.	
	99204	Comprehensive Ex.	
	99205	Complex Ex.	
	OFFICE VISIT - ESTABLISHED PATIENT		
	99212	Focused Ex.	
√	99213	Expanded Ex.	*$48.00*
	99214	Detailed Ex.	
	99215	Complex Ex.	
	PREVENTATIVE MEDICINE - NEW PATIENT		
	99381	< 1 year old	
	99382	1-4 year old	
	99383	5-11 year old	
	99384	12-17 year old	
	99385	18-39 year old	
	99386	40-64 year old	
	99387	65 + year old	
	PREVENTATIVE MEDICINE - ESTABLISHED PATIENT		
	99391	< 1 year old	
	99392	1-4 year old	
	99393	5-11 year old	
	99394	12-17 year old	
	99395	18-39 year old	
	99396	40-64 year old	
	99397	65 + year old	

☐	CPT/Md	DESCRIPTION	FEE
	LAB STUDIES		
	36415	Venipucture	
	81000	Urinalysis	
	81003	- w/o Micro	
	84703	HCG (Urine, Pregnancy)	
	82948	Glucose	
	82270	Hemoccult	
	85025	CBC -diff.	
	85018	Hemoglobin	
	88174	Pap Smear	
	87210	KOH/ Saline Wet Mount	
	87430	Strep Antigen	
	87070	Throat Culture	
	80053	Chem profile	
	80061	Lipid profile	
	82465	Cholesterol	
	99000	Handling fee	
	X-RAY		
	70210	Sinuses	
	70360	Neck Soft Tissue	
	71010	CXR (PA only)	
	71020	Chest 2V	
	72040	C-Spine 2V	
	72100	Lumbrosacral	
	73030	Shoulder 2V	
	73070	Elbow 2V	
	73120	Hand 2V	
	73560	Knee 2V	
	73620	Foot 2V	
	74000	KUB	

☐	CPT/Md	DESCRIPTION	FEE
	PROCEDURES		
	92551	Audiometry	
	29705	Cast Removal Full Arm/Leg	
	2900__	Casting (by location)	
	92567	Ear Check	
	69210	Ear Wax Rem. 1 2	
	93000	EKG	
	93005	EKG tracing only	
	93010	EKG Int. and Rep	
	11750	Excision Nail	
	94375	Respiratory Flow Volume	
	93224	Holter up to 48 hours	
	10060	I & D Abscess Simple	
	10061	I & D Abscess Comp.	
	94761	Oximetry w/Exercise	
	94726	Plethysmography	
	94760	Pulse Oximetry	
	11100	Skin Bx	
	94010	Spirometry	
	99173	Visual Acuity	
	17110	Wart destruction up to 14	
	17111	Wart destruction 15 lesions +	
	11042	Wound Debrid.	

☐	CPT/Md	DESCRIPTION	FEE
	INJECTIONS		
	90655	Influenza 6-35 months	
	90656	Influenza 3 years +	
	90732	Pneumoccal	
	J0295	Ampicillin, 1.5 gr	
	J2001	Liocaine for IV infusion 10mg	
	J1885	Toradol 15mg	
	90720	DTP - HIB	
	90746	HEP B - HIB	
	90707	MMR	
	86580	PPD	
	90732	Pneumovax	
	90716	Varicella	
	82607	Vitamin B12 Inj.	
	90712	Polio oral use (OPV)	
	90713	Polio injection (IPV)	
	90714	Td preservative free 7 yrs +	
	90718	Td 7 years +	
	95115	Allergy inj., single	
	95117	Allergy inj., multiple	
	OTHER		
√	*87880*	*Detection Strep A*	*$20.00*

DIAGNOSTIC CODES (ICD-9-CM)

☐	Code	Description	☐	Code	Description	☐	Code	Description	☐	Code	Description
	789.0__	Abdominal Pain		564.0	Constipation		784.0	Headache		782.1	Rash or ezanthem
	682.__	Abscess/Cellulitis		692.6	Contact dermatitis due to plants		414.9	Heart Dis., Coronary		714.0	Rheumatoid Arthritis
	995.3	Allergic Reaction		692.9	Contact dermatitis, NOS		599.70	Hematuria		V70.0	Routine general exam
	331	Alzheimer's		V25.09	Contraceptive management		455.6	Hemorrhoids		V76.10	Screen, breast
	285.__	Anemia, other & unspec		923.10	Contusion, forearm		573.3	Hepatitus, NOS		V76.2	Screen, cervix
	280.9	Anemia-iron deficiency		434.91	CVA		V03.81	HIB		V76.44	Screen, prosate
	281.0	Anemia-pernicious		266.2	Deficiency, folic acid B12		V65.44	HIV counseling		V76.47	Screen, vagina
	285.9	Anemia-unspecified		311	Depression		401.1	Hypertension, benign		216.5	Sebaceous cyst
	413.9	Angina, pectoris, oyher/unspecified		250.01	Diabetes, type I, juvenile type		401.9	Hypertension, unspecified		706.2	Sebaceous cyst
	300.00	Anxiety state, NOS		787.91	Diarrhea		401.0	Hypertension, malignant		786.05	Shortness of Breath
	300.4	Anxiety reaction		780.4	Dizziness		V04.81	Influenza		701.9	Skin tag
	716.90	Arthritis, NOS		V06.1	DTP		271.3	Lactose intolerance		845.00	Strain, ankle
	493.20	Asthma; chronic obstruction		V06.3	DTP + polio		573.9	Liver Disease		307.81	Tension headache
	493.00	Asthma; extrinic		536.8	Dyspepsia		724.5	Low Back Pain		V06.5	Tetanus - distheria (Td)
	493.10	Asthma; intrinsic		788.1	Dysuria		346.9	Migraine		305.1	Tobacco dependence
	493.90	Asthmas; unspecified		782.3	Edema		V06.4	MMR		788.41	Urinary frequency
	427.31	Atrial fibulation		530.81	Esophageal reflux		278.01	Obesity/Morbid		599.0	Urinary tract infection, NOS
	724.5	Backache, unspecified		530.11	Esophagitis reflux		715.90	Osteoarthritis		V05.3	Viral hepatitis
	790.6	Blood chemistry		530.10	Esophagitis, unspecified		719.43	Pain in joint, forearm		368.40	Visual field defect, unspecified
	E906.3	Cat bite		780.6	Fever		625.4	PMS		V20.2	Well Child Exam
	786.50	Chest Pain		789.07	Generalized abdominal pain		486	Pneumonia			
	428.0	CHF		V72.3	Gynecological examiniation		V25.01	Prescription of oral contraceptivess			

DIAGNOSIS: (IF NOT CHECKED ABOVE)		RECEIVED BY:	TODAY'S FEE	*$68.00*
034.0 Strep Throat		☐ CASH	AMOUNT RECEIVED	*$20.00*
PROCEDURES: (IF NOT CHECKED ABOVE)	RETURN APPOINTMENT INFORMATION:	☐ CREDIT CARD		
	(DAYS) (WKS.) (MOS.) (PRN)	☒ CHECK # *6723*	BALANCE	*$48.00*

Figure C.15 Encounter form (Superbill) for Charles Weber (Chapter 4).

Goode Medical Clinic
1234 Larsen Avenue
Saint Paul, Minnesota 55316

Phone: (555) 555-1234
Fax: (555) 555-5678

PATIENT NAME	CHART #	DATE		
William O'Connor		*3/3/2010*	☐ MEDI-MEDI ☐ SELF PAY ☐ MEDICARE	☐ MEDICAL ☐ PRIVATE ☐ HMO__________

✓	CPT/Md	DESCRIPTION	FEE	✓	CPT/Md	DESCRIPTION	FEE	✓	CPT/Md	DESCRIPTION	FEE	✓	CPT/Md	DESCRIPTION	FEE
OFFICE VISIT - NEW PATIENT				**LAB STUDIES**				**PROCEDURES**				**INJECTIONS**			
	99202	Focused Ex.			36415	Venipucture			92551	Audiometry			90655	Influenza 6-35 months	
	99203	Detailed Ex.			81000	Urinalysis			29705	Cast Removal Full Arm/Leg			90656	Influenza 3 years +	
	99204	Comprehensive Ex.			81003	- w/o Micro			2900__	Casting (by location)			90732	Pneumoccal	
	99205	Complex Ex.			84703	HCG (Urine, Pregnancy)			92567	Ear Check			J0295	Ampicillin, 1.5 gr	
OFFICE VISIT - ESTABLISHED PATIENT					82948	Glucose			69210	Ear Wax Rem. 1 2			J2001	Licocaine for IV infusion 10mg	
	99212	Focused Ex.			82270	Hemoccult			93000	EKG			J1885	Toradol 15mg	
✓	99213	Expanded Ex.	*$48.00*		85025	CBC -diff.			93005	EKG tracing only			90720	DTP - HIB	
	99214	Detailed Ex.			85018	Hemoglobin			93010	EKG Int. and Rep			90746	HEP B - HIB	
	99215	Complex Ex.			88174	Pap Smear			11750	Excision Nail			90707	MMR	
PREVENTATIVE MEDICINE - NEW PATIENT					87210	KOH/ Saline Wet Mount			94375	Respiratory Flow Volume			86580	PPD	
	99381	< 1 year old			87430	Strep Antigen			93224	Holter up to 48 hours			90732	Pneumovax	
	99382	1-4 year old			87070	Throat Culture			10060	I & D Abscess Simple			90716	Varicella	
	99383	5-11 year old			80053	Chem profile			10061	I & D Abscess Comp.			82607	Vitamin B12 Inj.	
	99384	12-17 year old			80061	Lipid profile			94761	Oximetry w/Exercise			90712	Polio oral use (OPV)	
	99385	18-39 year old			82465	Cholesterol			94726	Plethysmography			90713	Polio injection (IPV)	
	99386	40-64 year old			99000	Handling fee			94760	Pulse Oximetry			90714	Td preservative free 7 yrs +	
	99387	65 + year old		**X-RAY**					11100	Skin Bx			90718	Td 7 years +	
PREVENTATIVE MEDICINE - ESTABLISHED PATIENT					70210	Sinuses			94010	Spirometry			95115	Allergy inj., single	
	99391	< 1 year old			70360	Neck Soft Tissue			99173	Visual Acuity			95117	Allergy inj., multiple	
	99392	1-4 year old			71010	CXR (PA only)			17110	Wart destruction up to 14					
	99393	5-11 year old			71020	Chest 2V			17111	Wart destruction 15 lesions +					
	99394	12-17 year old			72040	C-Spine 2V			11042	Wound Debrid.		**OTHER**			
	99395	18-39 year old			72100	Lumbrosacral									
	99396	40-64 year old			73030	Shoulder 2V									
	99397	65 + year old			73070	Elbow 2V									
					73120	Hand 2V									
					73560	Knee 2V									
					73620	Foot 2V									
					74000	KUB									

DIAGNOSTIC CODES (ICD-9-CM)											
	789.0__	Abdominal Pain		564.0	Constipation		784.0	Headache		782.1	Rash or ezanthem
	682.__	Abscess/Cellulitis		692.6	Contact dermatitis due to plants		414.9	Heart Dis., Coronary		714.0	Rheumatoid Arthritis
	995.3	Allergic Reaction		692.9	Contact dermatitis, NOS		599.70	Hematuria		V70.0	Routine general exam
	331	Alzheimer's		V25.09	Contraceptive management		455.6	Hemorrhoids		V76.10	Screen, breast
	285.__	Anemia, other & unspec		923.10	Contusion, forearm		573.3	Hepatitus, NOS		V76.2	Screen, cervix
	280.9	Anemia-iron deficiency		434.91	CVA		V03.81	HIB		V76.44	Screen, prosate
	281.0	Anemia-pernicious		266.2	Deficiency, folic acid B12		V65.44	HIV counseling		V76.47	Screen, vagina
	285.9	Anemia-unspecified		311	Depression		401.1	Hypertension, benign		216.5	Sebaceous cyst
	413.9	Angina, pectoris, oyher/unspecified		250.01	Diabetes, type I, juvenile type	✓	401.9	Hypertension, unspecified		706.2	Sebaceous cyst
	300.00	Anxiety state, NOS		787.91	Diarrhea		401.0	Hypertension, malignant		786.05	Shortness of Breath
	300.4	Anxiety reaction		780.4	Dizziness		V04.81	Influenza		701.9	Skin tag
	716.90	Arthritis, NOS		V06.1	DTP		271.3	Lactose intolerance		845.00	Strain, ankle
	493.20	Asthma; chronic obstruction		V06.3	DTP + polio		573.9	Liver Disease		307.81	Tension headache
	493.00	Asthma; extrinic		536.8	Dyspepsia		724.5	Low Back Pain		V06.5	Tetanus - distheria (Td)
	493.10	Asthma; intrinsic		788.1	Dysuria		346.9	Migraine		305.1	Tobacco dependence
	493.90	Asthmas; unspecified		782.3	Edema		V06.4	MMR		788.41	Urinary frequency
	427.31	Atrial fibulation		530.81	Esophageal reflux		278.01	Obesity/Morbid		599.0	Unrinary tract infection, NOS
	724.5	Backache, unspecified		530.11	Esophagitis reflux		715.90	Osteoarthritis		V05.3	Viral hepatitis
	790.6	Blood chemistry		530.10	Esophagitis, unspecified		719.43	Pain in joint, forearm		368.40	Visual field defect, unspecified
	E906.3	Cat bite		780.6	Fever		625.4	PMS		V20.2	Well Child Exam
	786.50	Chest Pain		789.07	Generalized abdominal pain		486	Pneumonia			
	428.0	CHF		V72.3	Gynecological examiniation		V25.01	Prescription of oral contraceptivess			

DIAGNOSIS: (IF NOT CHECKED ABOVE)		RECEIVED BY:	TODAY'S FEE	*$48.00*
PROCEDURES: (IF NOT CHECKED ABOVE)	RETURN APPOINTMENT INFORMATION: (DAYS) (WKS.) (MOS.) (PRN)	☐ CASH ☐ CREDIT CARD ☐ CHECK # ________	AMOUNT RECEIVED	———
			BALANCE	*$48.00*

Figure C.16 Encounter form (Superbill) for William O'Connor (Chapter 4).

Patient Registration Information

Account # :
Insurance # :
Co-Payment: $

Please PRINT AND complete ALL sections below!

PATIENT'S PERSONAL INFORMATION Marital Status ☒ Single ☐ Married ☐ Divorced ☐ Widowed Sex: ☒ Male ☐ Female

Name: Smith (last name) Daniel (first name) (initial)

Street address: 4500 Birch Avenue (Apt #) City: St. Paul State: MN Zip: 55100

Home phone: (555) 253-2345 Work phone: ( ) Social Security # 901 - XX - 2345

Date of Birth: 2 (month) / 7 (day) / 1995 (year)

Employer / Name of School Southend High School ☒ Full Time ☐ Part Time

PATIENT'S / RESPONSIBLE PARTY INFORMATION

Responsible party: Carter Smith Date of Birth: 3/27/50

Relationship to Patient: ☐ Self ☐ Spouse ☒ Other parent Social Security # 456 - XX - 7890

Responsible party's home phone: ( ) See above

Address: (Apt #) City: State: Zip:

Employer's name: Smith Brothers Phone number: (555) 618-6789

Address: 89 Orange Street City: St. Paul State: MN Zip: 55100

Name of Parent/Guardian: Carter and Angela Smith

PATIENT'S INSURANCE INFORMATION Please present insurance cards to receptionist.

PRIMARY insurance company's name: Blue Cross/Blue Shield

Insurance address: XXX Blue Cross Blvd. City: Eagan State: MN Zip: 55122

Name of insured: Carter Smith Date of Birth: 3/27/50 Relationship to insured: ☐ Self ☐ Spouse ☐ Other ☒ Child

Insurance ID number: 456XX7890 Group number: DS-3456-SB

Does your insurance cover medication? Yes

EMERGENCY CONTACT

Name of person not living with you: Carter Smith Relationship: father

Address: See above City: State: Zip:

Phone number: (555) 253-2345/(555) 618-6789 work

Assignment of Benefits • Financial Agreement

I hereby give lifetime authorization for payment of insurance benefits to be made directly to Your Name Clinic ,and any assisting physicians, for services rendered. I understand that I am financially responsible for all charges whether or not they are covered by insurance. In the event of default, I agree to pay all costs of collection, and reasonable attorney's fees. I hereby authorize this healthcare provider to release all information necessary to secure the payment of benefits.

I further agree that a photocopy of this agreement shall be as valid as the original.

Date: XX/XX/XXXX Your Signature: Carter Smith

FORM # 58-8423 • BIBBERO SYSTEMS, INC.• PETALUMA, CA.• TO ORDER CALL TOLL FREE :800-BIBBERO (800-242-2376) • FAX (800) 242-9330 (REV.7/94)

Figure C.17 Registration form for Daniel Smith (Chapter 4).

Goode Medical Clinic
1234 Larsen Avenue
Saint Paul, Minnesota 55316

Phone: (555) 555-1234
Fax: (555) 555-5678

PATIENT NAME	CHART #	DATE		
Daniel Smith		*3/3/2010*	☐ MEDI-MEDI ☐ SELF PAY ☐ MEDICARE	☐ MEDICAL ☐ PRIVATE ☐ HMO_____

☐	CPT/Md	DESCRIPTION	FEE	☐	CPT/Md	DESCRIPTION	FEE	☐	CPT/Md	DESCRIPTION	FEE	☐	CPT/Md	DESCRIPTION	FEE
OFFICE VISIT - NEW PATIENT				**LAB STUDIES**				**PROCEDURES**				**INJECTIONS**			
	99202	Focused Ex.			36415	Venipucture			92551	Audiometry			90655	Influenza 6-35 months	
✓	99203	Detailed Ex.	*$80.00*		81000	Urinalysis			29705	Cast Removal Full Arm/Leg			90656	Influenza 3 years +	
	99204	Comprehensive Ex.			81003	- w/o Micro			2900__	Casting (by location)			90732	Pneumoccal	
	99205	Complex Ex.			84703	HCG (Urine, Pregnancy)			92567	Ear Check			J0295	Ampicillin, 1.5 gr	
OFFICE VISIT - ESTABLISHED PATIENT					82948	Glucose			69210	Ear Wax Rem. 1 2			J2001	Liocaine for IV infusion 10mg	
	99212	Focused Ex.			82270	Hemoccult			93000	EKG			J1885	Toradol 15mg	
	99213	Expanded Ex.			85025	CBC -diff.			93005	EKG tracing only			90720	DTP - HIB	
	99214	Detailed Ex.			85018	Hemoglobin			93010	EKG Int. and Rep			90746	HEP B - HIB	
	99215	Complex Ex.			88174	Pap Smear			11750	Excision Nail			90707	MMR	
PREVENTATIVE MEDICINE - NEW PATIENT					87210	KOH/ Saline Wet Mount			94375	Respiratory Flow Volume			86580	PPD	
	99381	< 1 year old			87430	Strep Antigen			93224	Holter up to 48 hours			90732	Pneumovax	
	99382	1-4 year old			87070	Throat Culture			10060	I & D Abscess Simple			90716	Varicella	
	99383	5-11 year old			80053	Chem profile			10061	I & D Abscess Comp.			82607	Vitamin B12 Inj.	
	99384	12-17 year old			80061	Lipid profile			94761	Oximetry w/Exercise			90712	Polio oral use (OPV)	
	99385	18-39 year old			82465	Cholesterol			94726	Plethysmography			90713	Polio injection (IPV)	
	99386	40-64 year old			99000	Handling fee			94760	Pulse Oximetry			90714	Td preservative free 7 yrs +	
	99387	65 + year old		**X-RAY**					11100	Skin Bx			90718	Td 7 years +	
PREVENTATIVE MEDICINE - ESTABLISHED PATIENT					70210	Sinuses			94010	Spirometry			95115	Allergy inj., single	
	99391	< 1 year old			70360	Neck Soft Tissue			99173	Visual Acuity			95117	Allergy inj., multiple	
	99392	1-4 year old			71010	CXR (PA only)			17110	Wart destruction up to 14					
	99393	5-11 year old			71020	Chest 2V			17111	Wart destruction 15 lesions +					
	99394	12-17 year old			72040	C-Spine 2V			11042	Wound Debrid.		**OTHER**			
	99395	18-39 year old			72100	Lumbrosacral						✓	*80050*	*Gen Health Panel*	*$45.00*
	99396	40-64 year old			73030	Shoulder 2V									
	99397	65 + year old			73070	Elbow 2V									
					73120	Hand 2V									
					73560	Knee 2V									
					73620	Foot 2V									
					74000	KUB									

DIAGNOSTIC CODES (ICD-9-CM)

☐	Code	Description	☐	Code	Description	☐	Code	Description	☐	Code	Description
	789.0__	Abdominal Pain		564.0	Constipation		784.0	Headache		782.1	Rash or ezanthem
	682.__	Abscess/Cellulitis		692.6	Contact dermatitis due to plants		414.9	Heart Dis., Coronary		714.0	Rheumatoid Arthritis
	995.3	Allergic Reaction		692.9	Contact dermatitis, NOS		599.70	Hematuria	✓	V70.0	Routine general exam
	331	Alzheimer's		V25.09	Contraceptive management		455.6	Hemorrhoids		V76.10	Screen, breast
	285.__	Anemia, other & unspec		923.10	Contusion, forearm		573.3	Hepatitus, NOS		V76.2	Screen, cervix
	280.9	Anemia-iron deficiency		434.91	CVA		V03.81	HIB		V76.44	Screen, prosate
	281.0	Anemia-pernicious		266.2	Deficiency, folic acid B12		V65.44	HIV counseling		V76.47	Screen, vagina
	285.9	Anemia-unspecified		311	Depression		401.1	Hypertension, benign		216.5	Sebaceous cyst
	413.9	Angina, pectoris, oyher/unspecified		250.01	Diabetes, type I, juvenile type		401.9	Hypertension, unspecified		706.2	Sebaceous cyst
	300.00	Anxiety state, NOS		787.91	Diarrhea		401.0	Hypertension, malignant		786.05	Shortness of Breath
	300.4	Anxiety reaction		780.4	Dizziness		V04.81	Influenza		701.9	Skin tag
	716.90	Arthritis, NOS		V06.1	DTP		271.3	Lactose intolerance		845.00	Strain, ankle
	493.20	Asthma; chronic obstruction		V06.3	DTP + polio		573.9	Liver Disease		307.81	Tension headache
	493.00	Asthma; extrinic		536.8	Dyspepsia		724.5	Low Back Pain		V06.5	Tetanus - distheria (Td)
	493.10	Asthma; intrinsic		788.1	Dysuria		346.9	Migraine		305.1	Tobacco dependence
	493.90	Asthmas; unspecified		782.3	Edema		V06.4	MMR		788.41	Urinary frequency
	427.31	Atrial fibulation		530.81	Esophageal reflux		278.01	Obesity/Morbid		599.0	Unrinary tract infection, NOS
	724.5	Backache, unspecified		530.11	Esophagitis reflux		715.90	Osteoarthritis		V05.3	Viral hepatitis
	790.6	Blood chemistry		530.10	Esophagitis, unspecified		719.43	Pain in joint, forearm		368.40	Visual field defect, unspecified
	E906.3	Cat bite		780.6	Fever		625.4	PMS		V20.2	Well Child Exam
	786.50	Chest Pain		789.07	Generalized abdominal pain		486	Pneumonia			
	428.0	CHF		V72.3	Gynecological examiniation		V25.01	Prescription of oral contraceptivess			

DIAGNOSIS: (IF NOT CHECKED ABOVE)		RECEIVED BY:	TODAY'S FEE	*$125.00*
		☐ CASH	AMOUNT RECEIVED	———
PROCEDURES: (IF NOT CHECKED ABOVE)	RETURN APPOINTMENT INFORMATION: (DAYS) (WKS.) (MOS.) (PRN)	☐ CREDIT CARD ☐ CHECK # ________	BALANCE	*$125.00*

Figure C.18 Encounter form (Superbill) for Daniel Smith (Chapter 4).

BCBS of MN
1355 Insurance Carrier Loop
Minneapolis, MN 55111
(763)555-0426

Remittance advice

Elsevier Clinic
1234 College Avenue
St. Paul, MN 55316

Page: 1 of 1
Date: XX/XX/XX
Group Practice ID#: 593XX
Check number: 23455

Patient name	DOS	Procedure code	Units	Total charge	Allowable	Provider responsibility	Co-pay	Amount paid
Smith, Daniel	03/03/2010	99203	1	80.00	72.00	8.00		72.00
	03/03/2010	80050	1	45.00	42.00	3.00		42.00

Total charges $125.00 Total provider responsibility $11.00 Total co-pay 0 Total paid $114.00

Figure C.19 Remittance Advice—Blue Cross and Blue Shield for Daniel Smith (Chapter 4).

Medicare
233 N. Michigan Ave.
Chicago, IL 60601
(555)555-1000

Remittance advice

Elsevier Clinic
1234 College Avenue
St. Paul, MN 55316

Page: 1 of 1
Date: XX/XX/XX
Group Practice ID#: 593XX
Check number: 12345

Patient name	DOS	Procedure code	Units	Total charge	Allowable	Provider responsibility	Co-pay	Amount paid
O'Connor, William	03/03/2010	99213	1	48.00	38.40	9.60		38.40

Total charges $48.00 Total provider responsibility $9.60 Total co-pay 0 Total paid $38.40

Figure C.20 Remittance Advice—Medicare for William O'Connor (Chapter 4).

Goode Medical Clinic
1234 Larsen Avenue
Saint Paul, Minnesota 55316

Phone: (555) 555-1234
Fax: (555) 555-5678

PATIENT NAME	CHART #	DATE		
Cindy Wixen		3/1/2010	☐ MEDI-MEDI ☐ SELF PAY ☐ MEDICARE	☐ MEDICAL ☐ PRIVATE ☐ HMO____

✓	CPT/Md	DESCRIPTION	FEE	✓	CPT/Md	DESCRIPTION	FEE	✓	CPT/Md	DESCRIPTION	FEE	✓	CPT/Md	DESCRIPTION	FEE
OFFICE VISIT - NEW PATIENT				**LAB STUDIES**				**PROCEDURES**				**INJECTIONS**			
	99202	Focused Ex.			36415	Venipucture			92551	Audiometry			90655	Influenza 6-35 months	
	99203	Detailed Ex.			81000	Urinalysis			29705	Cast Removal Full Arm/Leg			90656	Influenza 3 years +	
	99204	Comprehensive Ex.			81003	- w/o Micro			2900__	Casting (by location)			90732	Pneumoccal	
	99205	Complex Ex.			84703	HCG (Urine, Pregnancy)			92567	Ear Check			J0295	Ampicillin, 1.5 gr	
OFFICE VISIT - ESTABLISHED PATIENT					82948	Glucose			69210	Ear Wax Rem. 1 2			J2001	Liocaine for IV infusion 10mg	
	99212	Focused Ex.			82270	Hemoccult			93000	EKG			J1885	Toradol 15mg	
√	99213	Expanded Ex.	$48.00		85025	CBC -diff.			93005	EKG tracing only			90720	DTP - HIB	
	99214	Detailed Ex.			85018	Hemoglobin			93010	EKG Int. and Rep			90746	HEP B - HIB	
	99215	Complex Ex.			88174	Pap Smear			11750	Excision Nail			90707	MMR	
PREVENTATIVE MEDICINE - NEW PATIENT					87210	KOH/ Saline Wet Mount			94375	Respiratory Flow Volume			86580	PPD	
	99381	< 1 year old			87430	Strep Antigen			93224	Holter up to 48 hours			90732	Pneumovax	
	99382	1-4 year old			87070	Throat Culture			10060	I & D Abscess Simple			90716	Varicella	
	99383	5-11 year old			80053	Chem profile			10061	I & D Abscess Comp.			82607	Vitamin B12 Inj.	
	99384	12-17 year old			80061	Lipid profile			94761	Oximetry w/Exercise			90712	Polio oral use (OPV)	
	99385	18-39 year old			82465	Cholesterol			94726	Plethysmography			90713	Polio injection (IPV)	
	99386	40-64 year old			99000	Handling fee			94760	Pulse Oximetry			90714	Td preservative free 7 yrs +	
	99387	65 + year old		**X-RAY**					11100	Skin Bx			90718	Td 7 years +	
PREVENTATIVE MEDICINE - ESTABLISHED PATIENT					70210	Sinuses			94010	Spirometry			95115	Allergy inj., single	
	99391	< 1 year old			70360	Neck Soft Tissue			99173	Visual Acuity			95117	Allergy inj., multiple	
	99392	1-4 year old			71010	CXR (PA only)			17110	Wart destruction up to 14					
	99393	5-11 year old			71020	Chest 2V			17111	Wart destruction 15 lesions +					
	99394	12-17 year old			72040	C-Spine 2V			11042	Wound Debrid.		**OTHER**			
	99395	18-39 year old			72100	Lumbrosacral						√	73610	X-ray Complete Ankle	$60.00
	99396	40-64 year old			73030	Shoulder 2V									
	99397	65 + year old			73070	Elbow 2V									
					73120	Hand 2V									
					73560	Knee 2V									
					73620	Foot 2V									
					74000	KUB									

DIAGNOSTIC CODES (ICD-9-CM)

✓	Code	Description	✓	Code	Description	✓	Code	Description	✓	Code	Description
	789.0__	Abdominal Pain		564.0	Constipation		784.0	Headache		782.1	Rash or ezanthem
	682.__	Abscess/Cellulitis		692.6	Contact dermatitis due to plants		414.9	Heart Dis., Coronary		714.0	Rheumatoid Arthritis
	995.3	Allergic Reaction		692.9	Contact dermatitis, NOS		599.70	Hematuria		V70.0	Routine general exam
	331	Alzheimer's		V25.09	Contraceptive management		455.6	Hemorrhoids		V76.10	Screen, breast
	285.__	Anemia, other & unspec		923.10	Contusion, forearm		573.3	Hepatitus, NOS		V76.2	Screen, cervix
	280.9	Anemia-iron deficiency		434.91	CVA		V03.81	HIB		V76.44	Screen, prosate
	281.0	Anemia-pernicious		266.2	Deficiency, folic acid B12		V65.44	HIV counseling		V76.47	Screen, vagina
	285.9	Anemia-unspecified		311	Depression		401.1	Hypertension, benign		216.5	Sebaceous cyst
	413.9	Angina, pectoris, oyher/unspecified		250.01	Diabetes, type I, juvenile type		401.9	Hypertension, unspecified		706.2	Sebaceous cyst
	300.00	Anxiety state, NOS		787.91	Diarrhea		401.0	Hypertension, malignant		786.05	Shortness of Breath
	300.4	Anxiety reaction		780.4	Dizziness		V04.81	Influenza		701.9	Skin tag
	716.90	Arthritis, NOS		V06.1	DTP		271.3	Lactose intolerance	√	845.00	Strain, ankle
	493.20	Asthma; chronic obstruction		V06.3	DTP + polio		573.9	Liver Disease		307.81	Tension headache
	493.00	Asthma; extrinic		536.8	Dyspepsia		724.5	Low Back Pain		V06.5	Tetanus - distheria (Td)
	493.10	Asthma; intrinsic		788.1	Dysuria		346.9	Migraine		305.1	Tobacco dependence
	493.90	Asthmas; unspecified		782.3	Edema		V06.4	MMR		788.41	Urinary frequency
	427.31	Atrial fibulation		530.81	Esophageal reflux		278.01	Obesity/Morbid		599.0	Unrinary tract infection, NOS
	724.5	Backache, unspecified		530.11	Esophagitis reflux		715.90	Osteoarthritis		V05.3	Viral hepatitis
	790.6	Blood chemistry		530.10	Esophagitis, unspecified		719.43	Pain in joint, forearm		368.40	Visual field defect, unspecified
	E906.3	Cat bite		780.6	Fever		625.4	PMS		V20.2	Well Child Exam
	786.50	Chest Pain		789.07	Generalized abdominal pain		486	Pneumonia			
	428.0	CHF		V72.3	Gynecological examiniation		V25.01	Prescription of oral contraceptivess			

DIAGNOSIS: (IF NOT CHECKED ABOVE)		RECEIVED BY:	TODAY'S FEE	$108.00
		☐ CASH	AMOUNT RECEIVED	—
PROCEDURES: (IF NOT CHECKED ABOVE)	RETURN APPOINTMENT INFORMATION: (DAYS) (WKS.) (MOS.) (PRN)	☐ CREDIT CARD ☐ CHECK # ________	BALANCE	$108.00

Figure C.21 Encounter form (Superbill) for Cindy Wixen (Chapter 4).

Goode Medical Clinic
1234 Larsen Avenue
Saint Paul, Minnesota 55316

Phone: (555) 555-1234
Fax: (555) 555-5678

PATIENT NAME	CHART #	DATE		
Ronald Baxter		*3/5/2010*	☐ MEDI-MEDI ☐ SELF PAY ☐ MEDICARE	☐ MEDICAL ☐ PRIVATE ☐ HMO____

✓	CPT/Md	DESCRIPTION	FEE	✓	CPT/Md	DESCRIPTION	FEE	✓	CPT/Md	DESCRIPTION	FEE	✓	CPT/Md	DESCRIPTION	FEE
OFFICE VISIT - NEW PATIENT				LAB STUDIES				PROCEDURES				INJECTIONS			
	99202	Focused Ex.			36415	Venipucture			92551	Audiometry			90655	Influenza 6-35 months	
	99203	Detailed Ex.			81000	Urinalysis			29705	Cast Removal Full Arm/Leg			90656	Influenza 3 years +	
	99204	Comprehensive Ex.			81003	- w/o Micro			2900__	Casting (by location)			90732	Pneumoccal	
	99205	Complex Ex.			84703	HCG (Urine, Pregnancy)			92567	Ear Check			J0295	Ampicillin, 1.5 gr	
OFFICE VISIT - ESTABLISHED PATIENT					82948	Glucose			69210	Ear Wax Rem. 1 2			J2001	Liocaine for IV infusion 10mg	
	99212	Focused Ex.			82270	Hemoccult			93000	EKG			J1885	Toradol 15mg	
	99213	Expanded Ex.			85025	CBC -diff.			93005	EKG tracing only			90720	DTP - HIB	
	99214	Detailed Ex.			85018	Hemoglobin			93010	EKG Int. and Rep			90746	HEP B - HIB	
	99215	Complex Ex.			88174	Pap Smear			11750	Excision Nail			90707	MMR	
PREVENTATIVE MEDICINE - NEW PATIENT					87210	KOH/ Saline Wet Mount			94375	Respiratory Flow Volume			86580	PPD	
	99381	< 1 year old			87430	Strep Antigen			93224	Holter up to 48 hours			90732	Pneumovax	
	99382	1-4 year old			87070	Throat Culture			10060	I & D Abscess Simple			90716	Varicella	
	99383	5-11 year old			80053	Chem profile			10061	I & D Abscess Comp.			82607	Vitamin B12 Inj.	
	99384	12-17 year old			80061	Lipid profile			94761	Oximetry w/Exercise			90712	Polio oral use (OPV)	
	99385	18-39 year old			82465	Cholesterol			94726	Plethysmography			90713	Polio injection (IPV)	
	99386	40-64 year old			99000	Handling fee			94760	Pulse Oximetry			90714	Td preservative free 7 yrs +	
	99387	65 + year old		X-RAY					11100	Skin Bx			90718	Td 7 years +	
PREVENTATIVE MEDICINE - ESTABLISHED PATIENT					70210	Sinuses			94010	Spirometry			95115	Allergy inj., single	
	99391	< 1 year old			70360	Neck Soft Tissue			99173	Visual Acuity			95117	Allergy inj., multiple	
	99392	1-4 year old			71010	CXR (PA only)			17110	Wart destruction up to 14					
	99393	5-11 year old			71020	Chest 2V			17111	Wart destruction 15 lesions +					
	99394	12-17 year old			72040	C-Spine 2V			11042	Wound Debrid.		OTHER			
	99395	18-39 year old			72100	Lumbrosacral									
✓	99396	40-64 year old	*$75.00*		73030	Shoulder 2V									
	99397	65 + year old			73070	Elbow 2V									
✓	*80050*	*Gen Health Panel*	*$45.00*		73120	Hand 2V									
					73560	Knee 2V									
					73620	Foot 2V									
					74000	KUB									

DIAGNOSTIC CODES (ICD-9-CM)

✓	Code	Description	✓	Code	Description	✓	Code	Description	✓	Code	Description
	789.0__	Abdominal Pain		564.0	Constipation		784.0	Headache		782.1	Rash or ezanthem
	682.__	Abscess/Cellulitis		692.6	Contact dermatitis due to plants		414.9	Heart Dis., Coronary		714.0	Rheumatoid Arthritis
	995.3	Allergic Reaction		692.9	Contact dermatitis, NOS		599.70	Hematuria	✓	V70.0	Routine general exam
	331	Alzheimer's		V25.09	Contraceptive management		455.6	Hemorrhoids		V76.10	Screen, breast
	285.__	Anemia, other & unspec		923.10	Contusion, forearm		573.3	Hepatitus, NOS		V76.2	Screen, cervix
	280.9	Anemia-iron deficiency		434.91	CVA		V03.81	HIB		V76.44	Screen, prosate
	281.0	Anemia-pernicious		266.2	Deficiency, folic acid B12		V65.44	HIV counseling		V76.47	Screen, vagina
	285.9	Anemia-unspecified		311	Depression		401.1	Hypertension, benign		216.5	Sebaceous cyst
	413.9	Angina, pectoris, oyher/unspecified		250.01	Diabetes, type I, juvenile type		401.9	Hypertension, unspecified		706.2	Sebaceous cyst
	300.00	Anxiety state, NOS		787.91	Diarrhea		401.0	Hypertension, malignant		786.05	Shortness of Breath
	300.4	Anxiety reaction		780.4	Dizziness		V04.81	Influenza		701.9	Skin tag
	716.90	Arthritis, NOS		V06.1	DTP		271.3	Lactose intolerance		845.00	Strain, ankle
	493.20	Asthma; chronic obstruction		V06.3	DTP + polio		573.9	Liver Disease		307.81	Tension headache
	493.00	Asthma; extrinic		536.8	Dyspepsia		724.5	Low Back Pain		V06.5	Tetanus - distheria (Td)
	493.10	Asthma; intrinsic		788.1	Dysuria		346.9	Migraine		305.1	Tobacco dependence
	493.90	Asthmas; unspecified		782.3	Edema		V06.4	MMR		788.41	Urinary frequency
	427.31	Atrial fibulation		530.81	Esophageal reflux		278.01	Obesity/Morbid		599.0	Unrinary tract infection, NOS
	724.5	Backache, unspecified		530.11	Esophagitis reflux		715.90	Osteoarthritis		V05.3	Viral hepatitis
	790.6	Blood chemistry		530.10	Esophagitis, unspecified		719.43	Pain in joint, forearm		368.40	Visual field defect, unspecified
	E906.3	Cat bite		780.6	Fever		625.4	PMS		V20.2	Well Child Exam
	786.50	Chest Pain		789.07	Generalized abdominal pain		486	Pneumonia			
	428.0	CHF		V72.3	Gynecological examiniation		V25.01	Prescription of oral contraceptivess			

DIAGNOSIS: (IF NOT CHECKED ABOVE)		RECEIVED BY:	TODAY'S FEE	*$120.00*
		☐ CASH	AMOUNT RECEIVED	——
PROCEDURES: (IF NOT CHECKED ABOVE)	RETURN APPOINTMENT INFORMATION: (DAYS) (WKS.) (MOS.) (PRN)	☐ CREDIT CARD ☐ CHECK # ________	BALANCE	*$120.00*

Figure C.22 Encounter form (Superbill) for Ronald Baxter (Chapter 4).

BCBS of MN
1355 Insurance Carrier Loop
Minneapolis, MN 55111
(763)555-0426

Remittance advice

Elsevier Clinic
1234 College Avenue
St. Paul, MN 55316

Page: 1 of 1
Date: XX/XX/XX
Group Practice ID#: 593XX
Check number: 67890

Patient name	DOS	Procedure code	Units	Total charge	Allowable	Provider responsibility	Co-pay	Amount paid
Wixen, Cindy	03/01/2010	99213	1	48.00	38.40	9.60		38.40
	03/01/2010	73610	1	60.00	48.00	12.00		48.00
Baxter, Ronald	03/05/2010	99396	1	75.00	60.00	15.00		60.00
	03/05/2010	80050	1	45.00	36.00	9.00		36.00

Total charges $228.00 Total provider responsibility $45.60 Total co-pay 0 Total paid $182.40

Figure C.23 Remittance Advice—Blue Cross and Blue Shield for patients Wixen and Baxter (Chapter 4).

Goode Medical Clinic

1234 Larsen Avenue
Saint Paul, Minnesota 55316

Phone: (555) 555-1234
Fax: (555) 555-5678

PATIENT NAME	CHART #	DATE		
Peter Portman		*3/1/2010*	☐ MEDI-MEDI ☐ SELF PAY ☐ MEDICARE	☐ MEDICAL ☐ PRIVATE ☐ HMO____

☐	CPT/Md	DESCRIPTION	FEE	☐	CPT/Md	DESCRIPTION	FEE	☐	CPT/Md	DESCRIPTION	FEE	☐	CPT/Md	DESCRIPTION	FEE
	OFFICE VISIT - NEW PATIENT				**LAB STUDIES**				**PROCEDURES**				**INJECTIONS**		
	99202	Focused Ex.			36415	Venipucture			92551	Audiometry			90655	Influenza 6-35 months	
	99203	Detailed Ex.			81000	Urinalysis			29705	Cast Removal Full Arm/Leg			90656	Influenza 3 years +	
	99204	Comprehensive Ex.			81003	- w/o Micro			2900__	Casting (by location)			90732	Pneumoccal	
	99205	Complex Ex.			84703	HCG (Urine, Pregnancy)			92567	Ear Check			J0295	Ampicillin, 1.5 gr	
	OFFICE VISIT - ESTABLISHED PATIENT				82948	Glucose			69210	Ear Wax Rem. 1 2			J2001	Liocaine for IV infusion 10mg	
	99212	Focused Ex.			82270	Hemoccult			93000	EKG			J1885	Toradol 15mg	
✓	99213	Expanded Ex.	*$48.00*		85025	CBC -diff.			93005	EKG tracing only			90720	DTP - HIB	
	99214	Detailed Ex.			85018	Hemoglobin			93010	EKG Int. and Rep			90746	HEP B - HIB	
	99215	Complex Ex.			88174	Pap Smear			11750	Excision Nail			90707	MMR	
	PREVENTATIVE MEDICINE - NEW PATIENT				87210	KOH/ Saline Wet Mount			94375	Respiratory Flow Volume			86580	PPD	
	99381	< 1 year old			87430	Strep Antigen			93224	Holter up to 48 hours			90732	Pneumovax	
	99382	1-4 year old			87070	Throat Culture			10060	I & D Abscess Simple			90716	Varicella	
	99383	5-11 year old			80053	Chem profile			10061	I & D Abscess Comp.			82607	Vitamin B12 Inj.	
	99384	12-17 year old			80061	Lipid profile			94761	Oximetry w/Exercise			90712	Polio oral use (OPV)	
	99385	18-39 year old			82465	Cholesterol			94726	Plethysmography			90713	Polio injection (IPV)	
	99386	40-64 year old			99000	Handling fee			94760	Pulse Oximetry			90714	Td preservative free 7 yrs +	
	99387	65 + year old			**X-RAY**				11100	Skin Bx			90718	Td 7 years +	
	PREVENTATIVE MEDICINE - ESTABLISHED PATIENT				70210	Sinuses			94010	Spirometry			95115	Allergy inj., single	
	99391	< 1 year old			70360	Neck Soft Tissue			99173	Visual Acuity			95117	Allergy inj., multiple	
	99392	1-4 year old			71010	CXR (PA only)			17110	Wart destruction up to 14					
	99393	5-11 year old			71020	Chest 2V			17111	Wart destruction 15 lesions +					
	99394	12-17 year old			72040	C-Spine 2V			11042	Wound Debrid.			**OTHER**		
	99395	18-39 year old			72100	Lumbrosacral									
	99396	40-64 year old			73030	Shoulder 2V									
	99397	65 + year old			73070	Elbow 2V									
					73120	Hand 2V									
					73560	Knee 2V									
					73620	Foot 2V									
					74000	KUB									

DIAGNOSTIC CODES (ICD-9-CM)

Code	Description	Code	Description	Code	Description	Code	Description
789.0__	Abdominal Pain	564.0	Constipation	784.0	Headache	782.1	Rash or ezanthem
682.__	Abscess/Cellulitis	692.6	Contact dermatitis due to plants	414.9	Heart Dis., Coronary	714.0	Rheumatoid Arthritis
995.3	Allergic Reaction	692.9	Contact dermatitis, NOS	599.70	Hematuria	V70.0	Routine general exam
331	Alzheimer's	V25.09	Contraceptive management	455.6	Hemorrhoids	V76.10	Screen, breast
285.__	Anemia, other & unspec	923.10	Contusion, forearm	573.3	Hepatitus, NOS	V76.2	Screen, cervix
280.9	Anemia-iron deficiency	434.91	CVA	V03.81	HIB	V76.44	Screen, prosate
281.0	Anemia-pernicious	266.2	Deficiency, folic acid B12	V65.44	HIV counseling	V76.47	Screen, vagina
285.9	Anemia-unspecified	311	Depression	401.1	Hypertension, benign	216.5	Sebaceous cyst
413.9	Angina, pectoris, oyher/unspecified	250.01	Diabetes, type I, juvenile type	401.9	Hypertension, unspecified	706.2	Sebaceous cyst
300.00	Anxiety state, NOS	787.91	Diarrhea	401.0	Hypertension, malignant	786.05	Shortness of Breath
300.4	Anxiety reaction	780.4	Dizziness	V04.81	Influenza	701.9	Skin tag
716.90	Arthritis, NOS	V06.1	DTP	271.3	Lactose intolerance	845.00	Strain, ankle
493.20	Asthma; chronic obstruction	V06.3	DTP + polio	573.9	Liver Disease	307.81	Tension headache
493.00	Asthma; extrinic	536.8	Dyspepsia	724.5	Low Back Pain	V06.5	Tetanus - distheria (Td)
493.10	Asthma; intrinsic	788.1	Dysuria	346.9	Migraine	305.1	Tobacco dependence
493.90	Asthmas; unspecified	782.3	Edema	V06.4	MMR	788.41	Urinary frequency
427.31	Atrial fibulation	530.81	Esophageal reflux	278.01	Obesity/Morbid	599.0	Unrinary tract infection, NOS
724.5	Backache, unspecified	530.11	Esophagitis reflux	715.90	Osteoarthritis	V05.3	Viral hepatitis
790.6	Blood chemistry	530.10	Esophagitis, unspecified	719.43	Pain in joint, forearm	368.40	Visual field defect, unspecified
E906.3	Cat bite	780.6	Fever	625.4	PMS	V20.2	Well Child Exam
786.50	Chest Pain	789.07	Generalized abdominal pain	486	Pneumonia		
428.0	CHF	V72.3	Gynecological examiniation	V25.01	Prescription of oral contraceptivess		

DIAGNOSIS: (IF NOT CHECKED ABOVE)		RECEIVED BY:	TODAY'S FEE	*$48.00*
382.00 Acute Ear Infection		☐ CASH	AMOUNT RECEIVED	——
PROCEDURES: (IF NOT CHECKED ABOVE)	RETURN APPOINTMENT INFORMATION:	☐ CREDIT CARD		
	(DAYS) (WKS.) (MOS.) (PRN)	☐ CHECK # ________	BALANCE	*$48.00*

Figure C.24 Encounter form (Superbill) for Peter Portman (Chapter 4).

Goode Medical Clinic
1234 Larsen Avenue
Saint Paul, Minnesota 55316

Phone: (555) 555-1234
Fax: (555) 555-5678

PATIENT NAME	CHART #	DATE	☐ MEDI-MEDI ☐ SELF PAY ☐ MEDICARE	☐ MEDICAL ☐ PRIVATE ☐ HMO______
Ashuri Lee		*3/2/2010*		

☐	CPT/Md	DESCRIPTION	FEE	☐	CPT/Md	DESCRIPTION	FEE	☐	CPT/Md	DESCRIPTION	FEE	☐	CPT/Md	DESCRIPTION	FEE
OFFICE VISIT - NEW PATIENT				**LAB STUDIES**				**PROCEDURES**				**INJECTIONS**			
	99202	Focused Ex.			36415	Venipucture			92551	Audiometry			90655	Influenza 6-35 months	
	99203	Detailed Ex.			81000	Urinalysis			29705	Cast Removal Full Arm/Leg			90656	Influenza 3 years +	
	99204	Comprehensive Ex.			81003	- w/o Micro			2900__	Casting (by location)			90732	Pneumoccal	
	99205	Complex Ex.			84703	HCG (Urine, Pregnancy)			92567	Ear Check			J0295	Ampicillin, 1.5 gr	
OFFICE VISIT - ESTABLISHED PATIENT					82948	Glucose			69210	Ear Wax Rem. 1 2			J2001	Liocaine for IV infusion 10mg	
	99212	Focused Ex.			82270	Hemoccult			93000	EKG			J1885	Toradol 15mg	
✓	99213	Expanded Ex.	*$48.00*		85025	CBC -diff.			93005	EKG tracing only			90720	DTP - HIB	
	99214	Detailed Ex.			85018	Hemoglobin			93010	EKG Int. and Rep			90746	HEP B - HIB	
	99215	Complex Ex.			88174	Pap Smear			11750	Excision Nail			90707	MMR	
PREVENTATIVE MEDICINE - NEW PATIENT					87210	KOH/ Saline Wet Mount			94375	Respiratory Flow Volume			86580	PPD	
	99381	< 1 year old			87430	Strep Antigen			93224	Holter up to 48 hours			90732	Pneumovax	
	99382	1-4 year old			87070	Throat Culture			10060	I & D Abscess Simple			90716	Varicella	
	99383	5-11 year old			80053	Chem profile			10061	I & D Abscess Comp.			82607	Vitamin B12 Inj.	
	99384	12-17 year old			80061	Lipid profile			94761	Oximetry w/Exercise			90712	Polio oral use (OPV)	
	99385	18-39 year old			82465	Cholesterol			94726	Plethysmography			90713	Polio injection (IPV)	
	99386	40-64 year old			99000	Handling fee			94760	Pulse Oximetry			90714	Td preservative free 7 yrs +	
	99387	65 + year old		**X-RAY**					11100	Skin Bx			90718	Td 7 years +	
PREVENTATIVE MEDICINE - ESTABLISHED PATIENT					70210	Sinuses			94010	Spirometry			95115	Allergy inj., single	
	99391	< 1 year old			70360	Neck Soft Tissue			99173	Visual Acuity			95117	Allergy inj., multiple	
	99392	1-4 year old			71010	CXR (PA only)			17110	Wart destruction up to 14					
	99393	5-11 year old			71020	Chest 2V			17111	Wart destruction 15 lesions +					
	99394	12-17 year old			72040	C-Spine 2V			11042	Wound Debrid.		**OTHER**			
	99395	18-39 year old			72100	Lumbrosacral									
	99396	40-64 year old			73030	Shoulder 2V									
	99397	65 + year old			73070	Elbow 2V									
					73120	Hand 2V									
					73560	Knee 2V									
					73620	Foot 2V									
					74000	KUB									

DIAGNOSTIC CODES (ICD-9-CM)

☐	Code	Description	☐	Code	Description	☐	Code	Description	☐	Code	Description
	789.0__	Abdominal Pain		564.0	Constipation		784.0	Headache		782.1	Rash or ezanthem
	682.__	Abscess/Cellulitis		692.6	Contact dermatitis due to plants		414.9	Heart Dis., Coronary		714.0	Rheumatoid Arthritis
	995.3	Allergic Reaction		692.9	Contact dermatitis, NOS		599.70	Hematuria		V70.0	Routine general exam
	331	Alzheimer's		V25.09	Contraceptive management		455.6	Hemorrhoids		V76.10	Screen, breast
	285.__	Anemia, other & unspec		923.10	Contusion, forearm		573.3	Hepatitus, NOS		V76.2	Screen, cervix
	280.9	Anemia-iron deficiency		434.91	CVA		V03.81	HIB		V76.44	Screen, prosate
	281.0	Anemia-pernicious		266.2	Deficiency, folic acid B12		V65.44	HIV counseling		V76.47	Screen, vagina
	285.9	Anemia-unspecified		311	Depression		401.1	Hypertension, benign		216.5	Sebaceous cyst
	413.9	Angina, pectoris, oyher/unspecified		250.01	Diabetes, type I, juvenile type		401.9	Hypertension, unspecified		706.2	Sebaceous cyst
	300.00	Anxiety state, NOS		787.91	Diarrhea		401.0	Hypertension, malignant		786.05	Shortness of Breath
	300.4	Anxiety reaction		780.4	Dizziness		V04.81	Influenza		701.9	Skin tag
	716.90	Arthritis, NOS		V06.1	DTP		271.3	Lactose intolerance		845.00	Strain, ankle
	493.20	Asthma; chronic obstruction		V06.3	DTP + polio		573.9	Liver Disease		307.81	Tension headache
	493.00	Asthma; extrinic		536.8	Dyspepsia		724.5	Low Back Pain		V06.5	Tetanus - distheria (Td)
	493.10	Asthma; intrinsic		788.1	Dysuria		346.9	Migraine		305.1	Tobacco dependence
	493.90	Asthmas; unspecified		782.3	Edema		V06.4	MMR		788.41	Urinary frequency
	427.31	Atrial fibulation		530.81	Esophageal reflux		278.01	Obesity/Morbid		599.0	Unrinary tract infection, NOS
	724.5	Backache, unspecified		530.11	Esophagitis reflux		715.90	Osteoarthritis		V05.3	Viral hepatitis
	790.6	Blood chemistry		530.10	Esophagitis, unspecified		719.43	Pain in joint, forearm		368.40	Visual field defect, unspecified
	E906.3	Cat bite		780.6	Fever		625.4	PMS		V20.2	Well Child Exam
	786.50	Chest Pain		789.07	Generalized abdominal pain		486	Pneumonia			
	428.0	CHF		V72.3	Gynecological examiniation		V25.01	Prescription of oral contraceptivess			

DIAGNOSIS: (IF NOT CHECKED ABOVE)		RECEIVED BY:	TODAY'S FEE	*$48.00*
692.9 Dermatitis		☐ CASH	AMOUNT RECEIVED	——
PROCEDURES: (IF NOT CHECKED ABOVE)	RETURN APPOINTMENT INFORMATION: (DAYS) (WKS.) (MOS.) (PRN)	☐ CREDIT CARD ☐ CHECK #______	BALANCE	*$48.00*

Figure C.25 Encounter form (Superbill) for Ashuri Lee (Chapter 4).

Goode Medical Clinic

1234 Larsen Avenue
Saint Paul, Minnesota 55316

Phone: (555) 555-1234
Fax: (555) 555-5678

PATIENT NAME	CHART #	DATE		
Tonya McWilliams		*3/2/2010*	☐ MEDI-MEDI ☐ SELF PAY ☐ MEDICARE	☐ MEDICAL ☐ PRIVATE ☐ HMO_____

✓	CPT/Md	DESCRIPTION	FEE	✓	CPT/Md	DESCRIPTION	FEE	✓	CPT/Md	DESCRIPTION	FEE	✓	CPT/Md	DESCRIPTION	FEE
OFFICE VISIT - NEW PATIENT				**LAB STUDIES**				**PROCEDURES**				**INJECTIONS**			
	99202	Focused Ex.			36415	Venipucture			92551	Audiometry			90655	Influenza 6-35 months	
	99203	Detailed Ex.			81000	Urinalysis			29705	Cast Removal Full Arm/Leg			90656	Influenza 3 years +	
	99204	Comprehensive Ex.			81003	- w/o Micro			2900__	Casting (by location)			90732	Pneumoccal	
	99205	Complex Ex.			84703	HCG (Urine, Pregnancy)			92567	Ear Check			J0295	Ampicillin, 1.5 gr	
OFFICE VISIT - ESTABLISHED PATIENT					82948	Glucose			69210	Ear Wax Rem. 1 2			J2001	Liocaine for IV infusion 10mg	
	99212	Focused Ex.			82270	Hemoccult			93000	EKG			J1885	Toradol 15mg	
✓	99213	Expanded Ex.	*$48.00*		85025	CBC -diff.			93005	EKG tracing only			90720	DTP - HIB	
	99214	Detailed Ex.			85018	Hemoglobin			93010	EKG Int. and Rep			90746	HEP B - HIB	
	99215	Complex Ex.			88174	Pap Smear			11750	Excision Nail			90707	MMR	
PREVENTATIVE MEDICINE - NEW PATIENT					87210	KOH/ Saline Wet Mount			94375	Respiratory Flow Volume			86580	PPD	
	99381	< 1 year old			87430	Strep Antigen			93224	Holter up to 48 hours			90732	Pneumovax	
	99382	1-4 year old			87070	Throat Culture			10060	I & D Abscess Simple			90716	Varicella	
	99383	5-11 year old			80053	Chem profile			10061	I & D Abscess Comp.			82607	Vitamin B12 Inj.	
	99384	12-17 year old			80061	Lipid profile			94761	Oximetry w/Exercise			90712	Polio oral use (OPV)	
	99385	18-39 year old			82465	Cholesterol			94726	Plethysmography			90713	Polio injection (IPV)	
	99386	40-64 year old			99000	Handling fee			94760	Pulse Oximetry			90714	Td preservative free 7 yrs +	
	99387	65 + year old		**X-RAY**					11100	Skin Bx			90718	Td 7 years +	
PREVENTATIVE MEDICINE - ESTABLISHED PATIENT					70210	Sinuses			94010	Spirometry			95115	Allergy inj., single	
	99391	< 1 year old			70360	Neck Soft Tissue			99173	Visual Acuity			95117	Allergy inj., multiple	
	99392	1-4 year old			71010	CXR (PA only)			17110	Wart destruction up to 14					
	99393	5-11 year old			71020	Chest 2V			17111	Wart destruction 15 lesions +					
	99394	12-17 year old			72040	C-Spine 2V			11042	Wound Debrid.		**OTHER**			
	99395	18-39 year old			72100	Lumbrosacral									
	99396	40-64 year old			73030	Shoulder 2V									
	99397	65 + year old			73070	Elbow 2V									
					73120	Hand 2V									
					73560	Knee 2V									
					73620	Foot 2V									
					74000	KUB									

DIAGNOSTIC CODES (ICD-9-CM)

✓	Code	Description	✓	Code	Description	✓	Code	Description	✓	Code	Description
	789.0__	Abdominal Pain		564.0	Constipation		784.0	Headache		782.1	Rash or ezanthem
	682.__	Abscess/Cellulitis		692.6	Contact dermatitis due to plants		414.9	Heart Dis., Coronary		714.0	Rheumatoid Arthritis
	995.3	Allergic Reaction		692.9	Contact dermatitis, NOS		599.70	Hematuria		V70.0	Routine general exam
	331	Alzheimer's		V25.09	Contraceptive management		455.6	Hemorrhoids		V76.10	Screen, breast
	285.__	Anemia, other & unspec		923.10	Contusion, forearm		573.3	Hepatitus, NOS		V76.2	Screen, cervix
	280.9	Anemia-iron deficiency		434.91	CVA		V03.81	HIB		V76.44	Screen, prosate
	281.0	Anemia-pernicious		266.2	Deficiency, folic acid B12		V65.44	HIV counseling		V76.47	Screen, vagina
	285.9	Anemia-unspecified		311	Depression		401.1	Hypertension, benign		216.5	Sebaceous cyst
	413.9	Angina, pectoris, oyher/unspecified		250.01	Diabetes, type I, juvenile type		401.9	Hypertension, unspecified		706.2	Sebaceous cyst
	300.00	Anxiety state, NOS		787.91	Diarrhea		401.0	Hypertension, malignant		786.05	Shortness of Breath
	300.4	Anxiety reaction		780.4	Dizziness		V04.81	Influenza		701.9	Skin tag
	716.90	Arthritis, NOS		V06.1	DTP		271.3	Lactose intolerance		845.00	Strain, ankle
	493.20	Asthma; chronic obstruction		V06.3	DTP + polio		573.9	Liver Disease		307.81	Tension headache
	493.00	Asthma; extrinic		536.8	Dyspepsia		724.5	Low Back Pain		V06.5	Tetanus - distheria (Td)
	493.10	Asthma; intrinsic		788.1	Dysuria		346.9	Migraine		305.1	Tobacco dependence
	493.90	Asthmas; unspecified		782.3	Edema		V06.4	MMR		788.41	Urinary frequency
	427.31	Atrial fibulation		530.81	Esophageal reflux		278.01	Obesity/Morbid		599.0	Unrinary tract infection, NOS
	724.5	Backache, unspecified		530.11	Esophagitis reflux		715.90	Osteoarthritis		V05.3	Viral hepatitis
	790.6	Blood chemistry		530.10	Esophagitis, unspecified		719.43	Pain in joint, forearm		368.40	Visual field defect, unspecified
	E906.3	Cat bite		780.6	Fever		625.4	PMS		V20.2	Well Child Exam
	786.50	Chest Pain		789.07	Generalized abdominal pain		486	Pneumonia			
	428.0	CHF		V72.3	Gynecological examiniation		V25.01	Prescription of oral contraceptivess			

DIAGNOSIS: (IF NOT CHECKED ABOVE)
372.00 Conjunctivitis

PROCEDURES: (IF NOT CHECKED ABOVE)

RETURN APPOINTMENT INFORMATION:
(DAYS) (WKS.) (MOS.) (PRN)

RECEIVED BY:
☐ CASH
☐ CREDIT CARD
☐ CHECK
____

TODAY'S FEE	*$48.00*
AMOUNT RECEIVED	*——*
BALANCE	*$48.00*

Figure C.26 Encounter form (Superbill) for Tonya McWilliams (Chapter 4).

Goode Medical Clinic
1234 Larsen Avenue
Saint Paul, Minnesota 55316

Phone: (555) 555-1234
Fax: (555) 555-5678

PATIENT NAME	CHART #	DATE		
Jerry Silversmith		*3/1/2010*	☐ MEDI-MEDI ☐ SELF PAY ☐ MEDICARE	☐ MEDICAL ☐ PRIVATE ☐ HMO___

☐	CPT/Md	DESCRIPTION	FEE
OFFICE VISIT - NEW PATIENT			
	99202	Focused Ex.	
	99203	Detailed Ex.	
	99204	Comprehensive Ex.	
	99205	Complex Ex.	
OFFICE VISIT - ESTABLISHED PATIENT			
	99212	Focused Ex.	
✓	99213	Expanded Ex.	*$48.00*
	99214	Detailed Ex.	
	99215	Complex Ex.	
PREVENTATIVE MEDICINE - NEW PATIENT			
	99381	< 1 year old	
	99382	1-4 year old	
	99383	5-11 year old	
	99384	12-17 year old	
	99385	18-39 year old	
	99386	40-64 year old	
	99387	65 + year old	
PREVENTATIVE MEDICINE - ESTABLISHED PATIENT			
	99391	< 1 year old	
	99392	1-4 year old	
	99393	5-11 year old	
	99394	12-17 year old	
	99395	18-39 year old	
	99396	40-64 year old	
	99397	65 + year old	

☐	CPT/Md	DESCRIPTION	FEE
LAB STUDIES			
	36415	Venipucture	
	81000	Urinalysis	
	81003	- w/o Micro	
	84703	HCG (Urine, Pregnancy)	
	82948	Glucose	
	82270	Hemoccult	
	85025	CBC -diff.	
	85018	Hemoglobin	
	88174	Pap Smear	
	87210	KOH/ Saline Wet Mount	
	87430	Strep Antigen	
	87070	Throat Culture	
	80053	Chem profile	
	80061	Lipid profile	
	82465	Cholesterol	
	99000	Handling fee	
X-RAY			
	70210	Sinuses	
	70360	Neck Soft Tissue	
	71010	CXR (PA only)	
	71020	Chest 2V	
	72040	C-Spine 2V	
	72100	Lumbrosacral	
	73030	Shoulder 2V	
	73070	Elbow 2V	
	73120	Hand 2V	
	73560	Knee 2V	
	73620	Foot 2V	
	74000	KUB	

☐	CPT/Md	DESCRIPTION	FEE
PROCEDURES			
	92551	Audiometry	
	29705	Cast Removal Full Arm/Leg	
	2900__	Casting (by location)	
	92567	Ear Check	
	69210	Ear Wax Rem. 1 2	
	93000	EKG	
	93005	EKG tracing only	
	93010	EKG Int. and Rep	
	11750	Excision Nail	
	94375	Respiratory Flow Volume	
	93224	Holter up to 48 hours	
	10060	I & D Abscess Simple	
	10061	I & D Abscess Comp.	
	94761	Oximetry w/Exercise	
	94726	Plethysmography	
	94760	Pulse Oximetry	
	11100	Skin Bx	
	94010	Spirometry	
	99173	Visual Acuity	
	17110	Wart destruction up to 14	
	17111	Wart destruction 15 lesions +	
	11042	Wound Debrid.	

☐	CPT/Md	DESCRIPTION	FEE
INJECTIONS			
	90655	Influenza 6-35 months	
	90656	Influenza 3 years +	
	90732	Pneumoccal	
	J0295	Ampicillin, 1.5 gr	
	J2001	Liocaine for IV infusion 10mg	
	J1885	Toradol 15mg	
	90720	DTP - HIB	
	90746	HEP B - HIB	
	90707	MMR	
	86580	PPD	
	90732	Pneumovax	
	90716	Varicella	
	82607	Vitamin B12 Inj.	
	90712	Polio oral use (OPV)	
	90713	Polio injection (IPV)	
	90714	Td preservative free 7 yrs +	
	90718	Td 7 years +	
	95115	Allergy inj., single	
	95117	Allergy inj., multiple	
OTHER			

DIAGNOSTIC CODES (ICD-9-CM)

Code	Description	Code	Description	Code	Description	Code	Description
789.0__	Abdominal Pain	564.0	Constipation	784.0	Headache	782.1	Rash or ezanthem
682.__	Abscess/Cellulitis	692.6	Contact dermatitis due to plants	414.9	Heart Dis., Coronary	714.0	Rheumatoid Arthritis
995.3	Allergic Reaction	692.9	Contact dermatitis, NOS	599.70	Hematuria	V70.0	Routine general exam
331	Alzheimer's	V25.09	Contraceptive management	455.6	Hemorrhoids	V76.10	Screen, breast
285.__	Anemia, other & unspec	923.10	Contusion, forearm	573.3	Hepatitus, NOS	V76.2	Screen, cervix
280.9	Anemia-iron deficiency	434.91	CVA	V03.81	HIB	V76.44	Screen, prosate
281.0	Anemia-pernicious	266.2	Deficiency, folic acid B12	V65.44	HIV counseling	V76.47	Screen, vagina
285.9	Anemia-unspecified	311	Depression	401.1	Hypertension, benign	216.5	Sebaceous cyst
413.9	Angina, pectoris, oyher/unspecified	250.01	Diabetes, type I, juvenile type	401.9	Hypertension, unspecified	706.2	Sebaceous cyst
300.00	Anxiety state, NOS	787.91	Diarrhea	401.0	Hypertension, malignant	786.05	Shortness of Breath
300.4	Anxiety reaction	780.4	Dizziness	V04.81	Influenza	701.9	Skin tag
716.90	Arthritis, NOS	V06.1	DTP	271.3	Lactose intolerance	845.00	Strain, ankle
493.20	Asthma; chronic obstruction	V06.3	DTP + polio	573.9	Liver Disease	307.81	Tension headache
493.00	Asthma; extrinic	536.8	Dyspepsia	724.5	Low Back Pain	V06.5	Tetanus - distheria (Td)
493.10	Asthma; intrinsic	788.1	Dysuria	346.9	Migraine	305.1	Tobacco dependence
493.90	Asthmas; unspecified	782.3	Edema	V06.4	MMR	788.41	Urinary frequency
427.31	Atrial fibulation	530.81	Esophageal reflux	278.01	Obesity/Morbid	599.0	Unrinary tract infection, NOS
724.5	Backache, unspecified	530.11	Esophagitis reflux	715.90	Osteoarthritis	V05.3	Viral hepatitis
790.6	Blood chemistry	530.10	Esophagitis, unspecified	719.43	Pain in joint, forearm	368.40	Visual field defect, unspecified
E906.3	Cat bite	780.6	Fever	625.4	PMS	V20.2	Well Child Exam
786.50	Chest Pain	789.07	Generalized abdominal pain	486	Pneumonia		
428.0	CHF	V72.3	Gynecological examiniation	V25.01	Prescription of oral contraceptivess		

DIAGNOSIS: (IF NOT CHECKED ABOVE)		RECEIVED BY:	TODAY'S FEE	*$48.00*
250.00 Diabetes mellitus without mention of complication		☐ CASH ☐ CREDIT CARD ☐ CHECK # ______	AMOUNT RECEIVED	———
PROCEDURES: (IF NOT CHECKED ABOVE)	RETURN APPOINTMENT INFORMATION: (DAYS) (WKS.) (MOS.) (PRN)		BALANCE	*$48.00*

Figure C.27 Encounter form (Superbill) for Jerry Silversmith (Chapter 4).

Goode Medical Clinic
1234 Larsen Avenue
Saint Paul, Minnesota 55316

Phone: (555) 555-1234
Fax: (555) 555-5678

PATIENT NAME	CHART #	DATE		
Tim Butler		*3/2/2010*	☐ MEDI-MEDI ☐ SELF PAY ☐ MEDICARE	☐ MEDICAL ☐ PRIVATE ☐ HMO_______

☐	CPT/Md	DESCRIPTION	FEE	☐	CPT/Md	DESCRIPTION	FEE	☐	CPT/Md	DESCRIPTION	FEE	☐	CPT/Md	DESCRIPTION	FEE
OFFICE VISIT - NEW PATIENT				**LAB STUDIES**				**PROCEDURES**				**INJECTIONS**			
	99202	Focused Ex.			36415	Venipucture			92551	Audiometry			90655	Influenza 6-35 months	
	99203	Detailed Ex.			81000	Urinalysis			29705	Cast Removal Full Arm/Leg			90656	Influenza 3 years +	
	99204	Comprehensive Ex.			81003	- w/o Micro			2900__	Casting (by location)			90732	Pneumoccal	
	99205	Complex Ex.			84703	HCG (Urine, Pregnancy)			92567	Ear Check			J0295	Ampicillin, 1.5 gr	
OFFICE VISIT - ESTABLISHED PATIENT					82948	Glucose			69210	Ear Wax Rem. 1 2			J2001	Liocaine for IV infusion 10mg	
	99212	Focused Ex.			82270	Hemoccult			93000	EKG			J1885	Toradol 15mg	
✓	99213	Expanded Ex.	*$48.00*		85025	CBC -diff.			93005	EKG tracing only			90720	DTP - HIB	
	99214	Detailed Ex.			85018	Hemoglobin			93010	EKG Int. and Rep			90746	HEP B - HIB	
	99215	Complex Ex.			88174	Pap Smear			11750	Excision Nail			90707	MMR	
PREVENTATIVE MEDICINE - NEW PATIENT					87210	KOH/ Saline Wet Mount			94375	Respiratory Flow Volume			86580	PPD	
	99381	< 1 year old			87430	Strep Antigen			93224	Holter up to 48 hours			90732	Pneumovax	
	99382	1-4 year old			87070	Throat Culture			10060	I & D Abscess Simple			90716	Varicella	
	99383	5-11 year old			80053	Chem profile			10061	I & D Abscess Comp.			82607	Vitamin B12 Inj.	
	99384	12-17 year old			80061	Lipid profile			94761	Oximetry w/Exercise			90712	Polio oral use (OPV)	
	99385	18-39 year old			82465	Cholesterol			94726	Plethysmography			90713	Polio injection (IPV)	
	99386	40-64 year old			99000	Handling fee			94760	Pulse Oximetry			90714	Td preservative free 7 yrs +	
	99387	65 + year old		**X-RAY**					11100	Skin Bx			90718	Td 7 years +	
PREVENTATIVE MEDICINE - ESTABLISHED PATIENT					70210	Sinuses			94010	Spirometry			95115	Allergy inj., single	
	99391	< 1 year old			70360	Neck Soft Tissue			99173	Visual Acuity			95117	Allergy inj., multiple	
	99392	1-4 year old			71010	CXR (PA only)			17110	Wart destruction up to 14					
	99393	5-11 year old			71020	Chest 2V			17111	Wart destruction 15 lesions +					
	99394	12-17 year old			72040	C-Spine 2V			11042	Wound Debrid.		**OTHER**			
	99395	18-39 year old			72100	Lumbrosacral									
	99396	40-64 year old			73030	Shoulder 2V									
	99397	65 + year old			73070	Elbow 2V									
✓	*87880*	*Detection Strep A*	*$20.00*		73120	Hand 2V									
					73560	Knee 2V									
					73620	Foot 2V									
					74000	KUB									

DIAGNOSTIC CODES (ICD-9-CM)

☐	Code	Description	☐	Code	Description	☐	Code	Description	☐	Code	Description
	789.0__	Abdominal Pain		564.0	Constipation		784.0	Headache		782.1	Rash or ezanthem
	682.__	Abscess/Cellulitis		692.6	Contact dermatitis due to plants		414.9	Heart Dis., Coronary		714.0	Rheumatoid Arthritis
	995.3	Allergic Reaction		692.9	Contact dermatitis, NOS		599.70	Hematuria		V70.0	Routine general exam
	331	Alzheimer's		V25.09	Contraceptive management		455.6	Hemorrhoids		V76.10	Screen, breast
	285.__	Anemia, other & unspec		923.10	Contusion, forearm		573.3	Hepatitus, NOS		V76.2	Screen, cervix
	280.9	Anemia-iron deficiency		434.91	CVA		V03.81	HIB		V76.44	Screen, prosate
	281.0	Anemia-pernicious		266.2	Deficiency, folic acid B12		V65.44	HIV counseling		V76.47	Screen, vagina
	285.9	Anemia-unspecified		311	Depression		401.1	Hypertension, benign		216.5	Sebaceous cyst
	413.9	Angina, pectoris, oyher/unspecified		250.01	Diabetes, type I, juvenile type		401.9	Hypertension, unspecified		706.2	Sebaceous cyst
	300.00	Anxiety state, NOS		787.91	Diarrhea		401.0	Hypertension, malignant		786.05	Shortness of Breath
	300.4	Anxiety reaction		780.4	Dizziness		V04.81	Influenza		701.9	Skin tag
	716.90	Arthritis, NOS		V06.1	DTP		271.3	Lactose intolerance		845.00	Strain, ankle
	493.20	Asthma; chronic obstruction		V06.3	DTP + polio		573.9	Liver Disease		307.81	Tension headache
	493.00	Asthma; extrinic		536.8	Dyspepsia		724.5	Low Back Pain		V06.5	Tetanus - distheria (Td)
	493.10	Asthma; intrinsic		788.1	Dysuria		346.9	Migraine		305.1	Tobacco dependence
	493.90	Asthmas; unspecified		782.3	Edema		V06.4	MMR		788.41	Urinary frequency
	427.31	Atrial fibulation		530.81	Esophageal reflux		278.01	Obesity/Morbid		599.0	Unrinary tract infection, NOS
	724.5	Backache, unspecified		530.11	Esophagitis reflux		715.90	Osteoarthritis		V05.3	Viral hepatitis
	790.6	Blood chemistry		530.10	Esophagitis, unspecified		719.43	Pain in joint, forearm		368.40	Visual field defect, unspecified
	E906.3	Cat bite		780.6	Fever		625.4	PMS		V20.2	Well Child Exam
	786.50	Chest Pain		789.07	Generalized abdominal pain		486	Pneumonia			
	428.0	CHF		V72.3	Gynecological examiniation		V25.01	Prescription of oral contraceptivess			

DIAGNOSIS: (IF NOT CHECKED ABOVE)		RECEIVED BY:	TODAY'S FEE	*$68.00*
034.0 Strep Throat		☐ CASH ☐ CREDIT CARD ☐ CHECK # :__________	AMOUNT RECEIVED	*———*
PROCEDURES: (IF NOT CHECKED ABOVE)	RETURN APPOINTMENT INFORMATION: (DAYS) (WKS.) (MOS.) (PRN)		BALANCE	*$68.00*

Figure C.28 Encounter form (Superbill) for Tim Butler (Chapter 4).

BCBS of MN
1355 Insurance Carrier Loop
Minneapolis, MN 55111
(763)555-0426

Remittance advice

Elsevier Clinic
1234 College Avenue
St. Paul, MN 55316

Page: 1 of 1
Date: XX/XX/XX
Group Practice ID#: 593XX
Check number: 45678

Patient name	DOS	Procedure code	Units	Total charge	Allowable	Provider responsibility	Co-pay	Amount paid
Portman, Peter	03/01/2010	99213	1	48.00	38.40	9.60		38.40
Ashuri, Lee	03/02/2010	99213	1	48.00	38.40	9.60		38.40
McWilliams, Tonya	03/02/2010	99213	1	48.00	38.40	9.60		38.40

Total charges $144.00 Total provider responsibility $28.80 Total co-pay 0 Total paid $115.20

Figure C.29 Remittance Advice — Blue Cross and Blue Shield for patients Portman, Ashuri, and McWilliams

First Med
7 Medical Blvd.
Detroit, MI 48266
(555)555-2220

Remittance advice

Elsevier Clinic
1234 College Avenue
St. Paul, MN 55316

Page: 1 of 1
Date: XX/XX/XX
Group Practice ID#: 593XX
Check number: 901234

Patient name	DOS	Procedure code	Units	Total charge	Allowable	Provider responsibility	Co-pay	Amount paid
Silversmith, Jerry	03/01/2010	99213	1	48.00	38.40	9.60		38.40
Butler, Tim	03/02/2010	99213	1	48.00	38.40	9.60		38.40
	03/02/2010	87880	1	20.00	16.00	4.00		16.00

Total charges $116.00 Total provider responsibility $23.20 Total co-pay 0 Total paid $92.80

Figure C.30 Remittance Advice—First Med for patients Silversmith and Butler (Chapter 4).

Patient Registration Information

Account # :
Insurance # :
Co-Payment: $

Please PRINT AND complete ALL sections below!

PATIENT'S PERSONAL INFORMATION Marital Status ☒ Single ☐ Married ☐ Divorced ☐ Widowed Sex: ☒ Male ☐ Female

Name: Simpson (last name) David (first name) (initial)

Street address: 2300 Highland Avenue (Apt #) City: St. Paul State: MN Zip: 55100

Home phone: (555) 555-8765 Work phone: (555) 213-6789 Social Security # 234-XX-5678

Date of Birth: 12 (month) / 12 (day) / 68 (year)

Employer / Name of School Cola Coke Corporation ☒ Full Time ☐ Part Time

PATIENT'S / RESPONSIBLE PARTY INFORMATION

Responsible party: Self Date of Birth:

Relationship to Patient: ☒ Self ☐ Spouse ☐ Other Social Security # - -

Responsible party's home phone: ( )

Address: (Apt #) City: State: Zip:

Employer's name: Cola Coke Corporation Phone number: (555) 638-3245

Address: 97 Walnut Avenue City: St. Paul State: MN Zip: 55100

Name of Parent/Guardian:

PATIENT'S INSURANCE INFORMATION Please present insurance cards to receptionist.

PRIMARY insurance company's name: Blue Cross/Blue Shield

Insurance address: XXX Blue Cross Blvd. City: Eagan State: MN Zip: 55122

Name of insured: David Simpson Date of Birth: 12/12/68 Relationship to insured: ☒ Self ☐ Spouse ☐ Other ☐ Child

Insurance ID number: 234XX5678 Group number: DS-3456-CC

Does your insurance cover medication? Yes

EMERGENCY CONTACT

Name of person not living with you: Lisa Simpson Relationship: sister

Address: 83 Lesser Union Circle City: North St. Paul State: MN Zip: 55136

Phone number: (555) 434-2222

Assignment of Benefits • Financial Agreement

I hereby give lifetime authorization for payment of insurance benefits to be made directly to Your Name Clinic ,and any assisting physicians, for services rendered. I understand that I am financially responsible for all charges whether or not they are covered by insurance. In the event of default, I agree to pay all costs of collection, and reasonable attorney's fees. I hereby authorize this healthcare provider to release all information necessary to secure the payment of benefits.

I further agree that a photocopy of this agreement shall be as valid as the original.

Date: XX/XX/XXXX Your Signature: David Simpson

FORM # 58-8423 • BIBBERO SYSTEMS, INC.• PETALUMA, CA.• TO ORDER CALL TOLL FREE :800-BIBBERO (800-242-2376) • FAX (800) 242-9330 (REV.7/94)

Figure C.31 Registration form for David Simpson (Chapter 4).

Patient Registration Information

Account # :
Insurance # :
Co-Payment: $

Please PRINT AND complete ALL sections below!

PATIENT'S PERSONAL INFORMATION Marital Status ☒ Single ❑ Married ❑ Divorced ❑ Widowed Sex: ❑ Male ☒ Female

Name: Jones (last name) Melissa (first name) (initial)

Street address: 2300 Porch Street (Apt #) City: St. Paul State: MN Zip: 55100

Home phone: (555) 453-6789 Work phone: (555) 753-0123 Social Security # 456 - XX - 7891

Date of Birth: 8 (month) / 12 (day) / 1972 (year)

Employer / Name of School Everyday Consultants ☒ Full Time ❑ Part Time

PATIENT'S / RESPONSIBLE PARTY INFORMATION

Responsible party: Self Date of Birth:

Relationship to Patient: ☒ Self ❑ Spouse ❑ Other See above Social Security # - -

Responsible party's home phone: ( )

Address: See above (Apt #) City: State: Zip:

Employer's name: Everyday Consultants Phone number: (555) 631-4567

Address: 10 Red Street City: St. Paul State: MN Zip: 55100

Name of Parent/Guardian:

PATIENT'S INSURANCE INFORMATION Please present insurance cards to receptionist.

PRIMARY insurance company's name: Blue Cross/Blue Shield

Insurance address: XXX Blue Cross Blvd. City: Eagan State: MN Zip: 55122

Name of insured: Melissa Jones Date of Birth: 8/12/72 Relationship to insured: ☒ Self ☐ Spouse ☐ Other ☐ Child

Insurance ID number: 456XX7891 Group number: EC-9876-MJ

Does your insurance cover medication? Yes

EMERGENCY CONTACT

Name of person not living with you: Amy Jones Relationship: Cousin

Address: 7 Cedar Circle City: Minneapolis State: MN Zip: 55111

Phone number: (555) 838-1234

Assignment of Benefits • Financial Agreement

I hereby give lifetime authorization for payment of insurance benefits to be made directly to Your Name Clinic ,and any assisting physicians, for services rendered. I understand that I am financially responsible for all charges whether or not they are covered by insurance. In the event of default, I agree to pay all costs of collection, and reasonable attorney's fees. I hereby authorize this healthcare provider to release all information necessary to secure the payment of benefits.
I further agree that a photocopy of this agreement shall be as valid as the original.

Date: XX/XX/XXXX Your Signature: Melissa Jones

FORM # 58-8423 • BIBBERO SYSTEMS, INC.• PETALUMA, CA.• TO ORDER CALL TOLL FREE :800-BIBBERO (800-242-2376) • FAX (800) 242-9330 (REV.7/94)

Figure C.32 Registration form for Melissa Jones (Chapter 4).

Account # :
Insurance # :
Co-Payment: $

Patient Registration Information

Please PRINT AND complete ALL sections below!

PATIENT'S PERSONAL INFORMATION Marital Status ❑ Single ☒ Married ❑ Divorced ❑ Widowed Sex: ❑ Male ☒ Female

Name: Potter (last name) Anne (first name) ___ (initial)

Street address: 2340 Lucas Avenue (Apt # ___) City: St. Paul State: MN Zip: 55100

Home phone: (555) 532-0987 Work phone: (___) ___ Social Security # 789 - XX - 0123

Date of Birth: 03 (month) / 04 (day) / 1946 (year)

Employer / Name of School Self-employed ☒ Full Time ❑ Part Time

PATIENT'S / RESPONSIBLE PARTY INFORMATION

Responsible party: Richard Potter Date of Birth: 7/14/46

Relationship to Patient: ❑ Self ☒ Spouse ❑ Other ___ Social Security # 538 - XX - 7890

Responsible party's home phone: (___) See above

Address: See above (Apt # ___) City: ___ State: ___ Zip: ___

Employer's name: Richard Potter Industries Phone number: (555) 238-8901

Address: 2300 Skywalker Lane City: Edina State: MN Zip: 55280

Name of Parent/Guardian: ___

PATIENT'S INSURANCE INFORMATION Please present insurance cards to receptionist.

PRIMARY insurance company's name: First Med

Insurance address: One Medical Blvd. City: Detroit State: MI Zip: 48226

Name of insured: Richard Potter Date of Birth: 7/14/46 Relationship to insured: ☐ Self ☒ Spouse ☐ Other ☐ Child

Insurance ID number: 538XX7890 Group number: RP 234556

Does your insurance cover medication? Yes

EMERGENCY CONTACT

Name of person not living with you: Richard Potter Relationship: spouse

Address: See above City: ___ State: ___ Zip: ___

Phone number: (555) 238-8901 (work)

Assignment of Benefits • Financial Agreement

I hereby give lifetime authorization for payment of insurance benefits to be made directly to Your Name Clinic ,and any assisting physicians, for services rendered. I understand that I am financially responsible for all charges whether or not they are covered by insurance. In the event of default, I agree to pay all costs of collection, and reasonable attorney's fees. I hereby authorize this healthcare provider to release all information necessary to secure the payment of benefits.
I further agree that a photocopy of this agreement shall be as valid as the original.

Date: XX/XX/XXXX Your Signature: Anne Potter

FORM # 58-8423 • BIBBERO SYSTEMS, INC.• PETALUMA, CA.• TO ORDER CALL TOLL FREE :800-BIBBERO (800-242-2376) • FAX (800) 242-9330 (REV.7/94)

Figure C.33 Registration form for Anne Potter (Chapter 4).

Patient Registration Information

Account # : ____________
Insurance # : ____________
Co-Payment: $ ____________

Please PRINT AND complete ALL sections below!

PATIENT'S PERSONAL INFORMATION Marital Status ❑ Single ☒ Married ❑ Divorced ❑ Widowed Sex: ☒ Male ❑ Female

Name: *Potter* (last name) *Richard* (first name) ____ (initial)

Street address: *2340 Lucas Avenue* (Apt # ____) City: *St. Paul* State: *MN* Zip: *55100*

Home phone: (*555*) *532-0987* Work phone: (____) ____________ Social Security # *538* - *XX* - *7890*

Date of Birth: *7* (month) / *14* (day) / *46* (year)

Employer / Name of School *Richard Potter Industries* ☒ Full Time ❑ Part Time

PATIENT'S / RESPONSIBLE PARTY INFORMATION

Responsible party: *Self* Date of Birth: ____________

Relationship to Patient: ☒ Self ❑ Spouse ❑ Other ____________ Social Security # ____-____-____

Responsible party's home phone: (____) *See above*

Address: *See above* (Apt # ____) City: ____________ State: ____ Zip: ____

Employer's name: *Richard Potter Industries* Phone number: (*555*) *238-8901*

Address: *2300 Skywalker Lane* City: *Edina* State: *MN* Zip: *55280*

Name of Parent/Guardian: ____________

PATIENT'S INSURANCE INFORMATION Please present insurance cards to receptionist.

PRIMARY insurance company's name: *First Med*

Insurance address: *One Medical Blvd.* City: *Detroit* State: *MI* Zip: *48226*

Name of insured: *Richard Potter* Date of Birth: *7/14/46* Relationship to insured: ☒ Self ☐ Spouse ☐ Other ☐ Child

Insurance ID number: *538XX7890* Group number: *RP 234556*

Does your insurance cover medication? *Yes*

EMERGENCY CONTACT

Name of person not living with you: *Anne Potter* Relationship: *spouse*

Address: *See above* City: ____________ State: ____ Zip: ____

Phone number: (*555*) *532-0987*

Assignment of Benefits • Financial Agreement

I hereby give lifetime authorization for payment of insurance benefits to be made directly to *Your Name Clinic* ,and any assisting physicians, for services rendered. I understand that I am financially responsible for all charges whether or not they are covered by insurance. In the event of default, I agree to pay all costs of collection, and reasonable attorney's fees. I hereby authorize this healthcare provider to release all information necessary to secure the payment of benefits.

I further agree that a photocopy of this agreement shall be as valid as the original.

Date: *XX/XX/XXXX* Your Signature: *Richard Potter*

FORM # 58-8423 • BIBBERO SYSTEMS, INC.• PETALUMA, CA.• TO ORDER CALL TOLL FREE :800-BIBBERO (800-242-2376) • FAX (800) 242-9330 (REV.7/94)

Figure C.34 Registration form for Richard Potter (Chapter 4).

Patient Registration Information

Account # : ______
Insurance # : ______
Co-Payment: $ ______

Please PRINT AND complete ALL sections below!

PATIENT'S PERSONAL INFORMATION Marital Status ☒ Single ❑ Married ❑ Divorced ❑ Widowed Sex: ☒ Male ❑ Female

Name: Ruha (last name) Michael (first name) ____ (initial)

Street address: 1234 Cardinal Street (Apt # ____) City: St. Paul State: MN Zip: 55100

Home phone: (555) 555-0011 Work phone: (____) ______ Social Security # 456 - XX - 2334

Date of Birth: 2 (month) / 12 (day) / 2010 (year)

Employer / Name of School ______ ❑ Full Time ❑ Part Time

PATIENT'S / RESPONSIBLE PARTY INFORMATION

Responsible party: Daniel Ruha Date of Birth: 7/21/67

Relationship to Patient: ❑ Self ❑ Spouse ☒ Other father Social Security # 890 - XX - 7654

Responsible party's home phone: (____) See above

Address: ______ (Apt # ____) City: ______ State: ______ Zip: ______

Employer's name: Enigma Products Phone number: (555) 555-1209

Address: 4567 Birch Avenue City: Edina State: MN Zip: 55280

Name of Parent/Guardian: ______

PATIENT'S INSURANCE INFORMATION Please present insurance cards to receptionist.

PRIMARY insurance company's name: Blue Cross/ Blue Shield

Insurance address: XXX Blue Cross Blvd. City: Eagan State: MN Zip: 55122

Name of insured: Daniel Ruha Date of Birth: 7/21/67 Relationship to insured: ☐ Self ☐ Spouse ☐ Other ☒ Child

Insurance ID number: 890XX7654 Group number: DR-2334-AP

Does your insurance cover medication? Yes

EMERGENCY CONTACT

Name of person not living with you: Daniel Ruha Relationship: father

Address: See above City: ______ State: ______ Zip: ______

Phone number: (555) 555-4325 (work)

Assignment of Benefits • Financial Agreement

I hereby give lifetime authorization for payment of insurance benefits to be made directly to Your Name Clinic ,and any assisting physicians, for services rendered. I understand that I am financially responsible for all charges whether or not they are covered by insurance. In the event of default, I agree to pay all costs of collection, and reasonable attorney's fees. I hereby authorize this healthcare provider to release all information necessary to secure the payment of benefits.
I further agree that a photocopy of this agreement shall be as valid as the original.

Date: XX/XX/XXXX Your Signature: Daniel Ruha

FORM # 58-8423 • BIBBERO SYSTEMS, INC.• PETALUMA, CA.• TO ORDER CALL TOLL FREE :800-BIBBERO (800-242-2376) • FAX (800) 242-9330 (REV.7/94)

Figure C.35 Registration form for Michael Ruha (Chapter 4).

Goode Medical Clinic
1234 Larsen Avenue
Saint Paul, Minnesota 55316

Phone: (555) 555-1234
Fax: (555) 555-5678

PATIENT NAME	CHART #	DATE		
David Simpson		*3/9/2010*	☐ MEDI-MEDI ☐ SELF PAY ☐ MEDICARE	☐ MEDICAL ☐ PRIVATE ☐ HMO____

✓	CPT/Md	DESCRIPTION	FEE	✓	CPT/Md	DESCRIPTION	FEE	✓	CPT/Md	DESCRIPTION	FEE	✓	CPT/Md	DESCRIPTION	FEE
OFFICE VISIT - NEW PATIENT				**LAB STUDIES**				**PROCEDURES**				**INJECTIONS**			
	99202	Focused Ex.			36415	Venipucture			92551	Audiometry			90655	Influenza 6-35 months	
	99203	Detailed Ex.			81000	Urinalysis			29705	Cast Removal Full Arm/Leg			90656	Influenza 3 years +	
	99204	Comprehensive Ex.			81003	- w/o Micro			2900__	Casting (by location)			90732	Pneumoccal	
	99205	Complex Ex.			84703	HCG (Urine, Pregnancy)			92567	Ear Check			J0295	Ampicillin, 1.5 gr	
OFFICE VISIT - ESTABLISHED PATIENT					82948	Glucose			69210	Ear Wax Rem. 1 2			J2001	Licocaine for IV infusion 10mg	
	99212	Focused Ex.			82270	Hemoccult			93000	EKG			J1885	Toradol 15mg	
✓	99213	Expanded Ex.	*$48.00*		85025	CBC -diff.			93005	EKG tracing only			90720	DTP - HIB	
	99214	Detailed Ex.			85018	Hemoglobin			93010	EKG Int. and Rep			90746	HEP B - HIB	
	99215	Complex Ex.			88174	Pap Smear			11750	Excision Nail			90707	MMR	
PREVENTATIVE MEDICINE - NEW PATIENT					87210	KOH/ Saline Wet Mount			94375	Respiratory Flow Volume			86580	PPD	
	99381	< 1 year old			87430	Strep Antigen			93224	Holter up to 48 hours			90732	Pneumovax	
	99382	1-4 year old			87070	Throat Culture			10060	I & D Abscess Simple			90716	Varicella	
	99383	5-11 year old			80053	Chem profile			10061	I & D Abscess Comp.			82607	Vitamin B12 Inj.	
	99384	12-17 year old			80061	Lipid profile			94761	Oximetry w/Exercise			90712	Polio oral use (OPV)	
	99385	18-39 year old			82465	Cholesterol			94726	Plethysmography			90713	Polio injection (IPV)	
	99386	40-64 year old			99000	Handling fee			94760	Pulse Oximetry			90714	Td preservative free 7 yrs +	
	99387	65 + year old		**X-RAY**					11100	Skin Bx			90718	Td 7 years +	
PREVENTATIVE MEDICINE - ESTABLISHED PATIENT					70210	Sinuses			94010	Spirometry			95115	Allergy inj., single	
	99391	< 1 year old			70360	Neck Soft Tissue			99173	Visual Acuity			95117	Allergy inj., multiple	
	99392	1-4 year old			71010	CXR (PA only)			17110	Wart destruction up to 14					
	99393	5-11 year old			71020	Chest 2V			17111	Wart destruction 15 lesions +					
	99394	12-17 year old			72040	C-Spine 2V			11042	Wound Debrid.			**OTHER**		
	99395	18-39 year old			72100	Lumbrosacral									
	99396	40-64 year old			73030	Shoulder 2V									
	99397	65 + year old			73070	Elbow 2V									
					73120	Hand 2V									
					73560	Knee 2V									
					73620	Foot 2V									
					74000	KUB									

DIAGNOSTIC CODES (ICD-9-CM)

✓	Code	Description	✓	Code	Description	✓	Code	Description	✓	Code	Description
	789.0__	Abdominal Pain		564.0	Constipation		784.0	Headache		782.1	Rash or ezanthem
	682.__	Abscess/Cellulitis		692.6	Contact dermatitis due to plants		414.9	Heart Dis., Coronary		714.0	Rheumatoid Arthritis
	995.3	Allergic Reaction		692.9	Contact dermatitis, NOS		599.70	Hematuria		V70.0	Routine general exam
	331	Alzheimer's		V25.09	Contraceptive management		455.6	Hemorrhoids		V76.10	Screen, breast
	285.__	Anemia, other & unspec	✓	923.10	Contusion, forearm		573.3	Hepatitus, NOS		V76.2	Screen, cervix
	280.9	Anemia-iron deficiency		434.91	CVA		V03.81	HIB		V76.44	Screen, prosate
	281.0	Anemia-pernicious		266.2	Deficiency, folic acid B12		V65.44	HIV counseling		V76.47	Screen, vagina
	285.9	Anemia-unspecified		311	Depression		401.1	Hypertension, benign		216.5	Sebaceous cyst
	413.9	Angina, pectoris, oyher/unspecified		250.01	Diabetes, type I, juvenile type		401.9	Hypertension, unspecified		706.2	Sebaceous cyst
	300.00	Anxiety state, NOS		787.91	Diarrhea		401.0	Hypertension, malignant		786.05	Shortness of Breath
	300.4	Anxiety reaction		780.4	Dizziness		V04.81	Influenza		701.9	Skin tag
	716.90	Arthritis, NOS		V06.1	DTP		271.3	Lactose intolerance		845.00	Strain, ankle
	493.20	Asthma; chronic obstruction		V06.3	DTP + polio		573.9	Liver Disease		307.81	Tension headache
	493.00	Asthma; extrinic		536.8	Dyspepsia		724.5	Low Back Pain		V06.5	Tetanus - distheria (Td)
	493.10	Asthma; intrinsic		788.1	Dysuria		346.9	Migraine		305.1	Tobacco dependence
	493.90	Asthmas; unspecified		782.3	Edema		V06.4	MMR		788.41	Urinary frequency
	427.31	Atrial fibulation		530.81	Esophageal reflux		278.01	Obesity/Morbid		599.0	Unrinary tract infection, NOS
	724.5	Backache, unspecified		530.11	Esophagitis reflux		715.90	Osteoarthritis		V05.3	Viral hepatitis
	790.6	Blood chemistry		530.10	Esophagitis, unspecified		719.43	Pain in joint, forearm		368.40	Visual field defect, unspecified
	E906.3	Cat bite		780.6	Fever		625.4	PMS		V20.2	Well Child Exam
	786.50	Chest Pain		789.07	Generalized abdominal pain		486	Pneumonia			
	428.0	CHF		V72.3	Gynecological examiniation		V25.01	Prescription of oral contraceptivess			

DIAGNOSIS: (IF NOT CHECKED ABOVE)		RECEIVED BY:	TODAY'S FEE	*$48.00*
		☐ CASH	AMOUNT RECEIVED	———
PROCEDURES: (IF NOT CHECKED ABOVE)	RETURN APPOINTMENT INFORMATION: (DAYS) (WKS.) (MOS.) (PRN)	☐ CREDIT CARD ☐ CHECK # ________	BALANCE	*$48.00*

Figure C.36 Encounter form (Superbill) for David Simpson (Chapter 4).

Phone: (555) 555-1234
Fax: (555) 555-5678

Goode Medical Clinic

1234 Larsen Avenue
Saint Paul, Minnesota 55316

PATIENT NAME	CHART #	DATE		
Melissa Jones		*3/9/2010*	☐ MEDI-MEDI ☐ SELF PAY ☐ MEDICARE	☐ MEDICAL ☐ PRIVATE ☐ HMO_______

☐	CPT/Md	DESCRIPTION	FEE	☐	CPT/Md	DESCRIPTION	FEE	☐	CPT/Md	DESCRIPTION	FEE	☐	CPT/Md	DESCRIPTION	FEE
OFFICE VISIT - NEW PATIENT				**LAB STUDIES**				**PROCEDURES**				**INJECTIONS**			
	99202	Focused Ex.			36415	Venipucture			92551	Audiometry			90655	Influenza 6-35 months	
	99203	Detailed Ex.			81000	Urinalysis			29705	Cast Removal Full Arm/Leg			90656	Influenza 3 years +	
	99204	Comprehensive Ex.			81003	- w/o Micro			2900__	Casting (by location)			90732	Pneumoccal	
	99205	Complex Ex.			84703	HCG (Urine, Pregnancy)			92567	Ear Check			J0295	Ampicillin, 1.5 gr	
OFFICE VISIT - ESTABLISHED PATIENT					82948	Glucose			69210	Ear Wax Rem. 1 2			J2001	Liocaine for IV infusion 10mg	
	99212	Focused Ex.			82270	Hemoccult			93000	EKG			J1885	Toradol 15mg	
✓	99213	Expanded Ex.	*$48.00*		85025	CBC -diff.			93005	EKG tracing only			90720	DTP - HIB	
	99214	Detailed Ex.			85018	Hemoglobin			93010	EKG Int. and Rep			90746	HEP B - HIB	
	99215	Complex Ex.			88174	Pap Smear			11750	Excision Nail			90707	MMR	
PREVENTATIVE MEDICINE - NEW PATIENT					87210	KOH/ Saline Wet Mount			94375	Respiratory Flow Volume			86580	PPD	
	99381	< 1 year old			87430	Strep Antigen			93224	Holter up to 48 hours			90732	Pneumovax	
	99382	1-4 year old			87070	Throat Culture			10060	I & D Abscess Simple			90716	Varicella	
	99383	5-11 year old			80053	Chem profile			10061	I & D Abscess Comp.			82607	Vitamin B12 Inj.	
	99384	12-17 year old			80061	Lipid profile			94761	Oximetry w/Exercise			90712	Polio oral use (OPV)	
	99385	18-39 year old			82465	Cholesterol			94726	Plethysmography			90713	Polio injection (IPV)	
	99386	40-64 year old			99000	Handling fee			94760	Pulse Oximetry			90714	Td preservative free 7 yrs +	
	99387	65 + year old		**X-RAY**					11100	Skin Bx			90718	Td 7 years +	
PREVENTATIVE MEDICINE - ESTABLISHED PATIENT					70210	Sinuses			94010	Spirometry			95115	Allergy inj., single	
	99391	< 1 year old			70360	Neck Soft Tissue			99173	Visual Acuity			95117	Allergy inj., multiple	
	99392	1-4 year old			71010	CXR (PA only)			17110	Wart destruction up to 14					
	99393	5-11 year old			71020	Chest 2V			17111	Wart destruction 15 lesions +					
	99394	12-17 year old			72040	C-Spine 2V			11042	Wound Debrid.		**OTHER**			
	99395	18-39 year old			72100	Lumbrosacral									
	99396	40-64 year old			73030	Shoulder 2V									
	99397	65 + year old			73070	Elbow 2V									
					73120	Hand 2V									
					73560	Knee 2V									
					73620	Foot 2V									
					74000	KUB									

DIAGNOSTIC CODES (ICD-9-CM)

	Code	Description		Code	Description		Code	Description		Code	Description
	789.0__	Abdominal Pain		564.0	Constipation		784.0	Headache		782.1	Rash or ezanthem
	682.__	Abscess/Cellulitis		692.6	Contact dermatitis due to plants		414.9	Heart Dis., Coronary		714.0	Rheumatoid Arthritis
	995.3	Allergic Reaction	✓	692.9	Contact dermatitis, NOS		599.70	Hematuria		V70.0	Routine general exam
	331	Alzheimer's		V25.09	Contraceptive management		455.6	Hemorrhoids		V76.10	Screen, breast
	285.__	Anemia, other & unspec		923.10	Contusion, forearm		573.3	Hepatitus, NOS		V76.2	Screen, cervix
	280.9	Anemia-iron deficiency		434.91	CVA		V03.81	HIB		V76.44	Screen, prosate
	281.0	Anemia-pernicious		266.2	Deficiency, folic acid B12		V65.44	HIV counseling		V76.47	Screen, vagina
	285.9	Anemia-unspecified		311	Depression		401.1	Hypertension, benign		216.5	Sebaceous cyst
	413.9	Angina, pectoris, oyher/unspecified		250.01	Diabetes, type I, juvenile type		401.9	Hypertension, unspecified		706.2	Sebaceous cyst
	300.00	Anxiety state, NOS		787.91	Diarrhea		401.0	Hypertension, malignant		786.05	Shortness of Breath
	300.4	Anxiety reaction		780.4	Dizziness		V04.81	Influenza		701.9	Skin tag
	716.90	Arthritis, NOS		V06.1	DTP		271.3	Lactose intolerance		845.00	Strain, ankle
	493.20	Asthma; chronic obstruction		V06.3	DTP + polio		573.9	Liver Disease		307.81	Tension headache
	493.00	Asthma; extrinic		536.8	Dyspepsia		724.5	Low Back Pain		V06.5	Tetanus - distheria (Td)
	493.10	Asthma; intrinsic		788.1	Dysuria		346.9	Migraine		305.1	Tobacco dependence
	493.90	Asthmas; unspecified		782.3	Edema		V06.4	MMR		788.41	Urinary frequency
	427.31	Atrial fibulation		530.81	Esophageal reflux		278.01	Obesity/Morbid		599.0	Unrinary tract infection, NOS
	724.5	Backache, unspecified		530.11	Esophagitis reflux		715.90	Osteoarthritis		V05.3	Viral hepatitis
	790.6	Blood chemistry		530.10	Esophagitis, unspecified		719.43	Pain in joint, forearm		368.40	Visual field defect, unspecified
	E906.3	Cat bite		780.6	Fever		625.4	PMS		V20.2	Well Child Exam
	786.50	Chest Pain		789.07	Generalized abdominal pain		486	Pneumonia			
	428.0	CHF		V72.3	Gynecological examiniation		V25.01	Prescription of oral contraceptivess			

DIAGNOSIS: (IF NOT CHECKED ABOVE)		RECEIVED BY: ☐ CASH ☐ CREDIT CARD ☐ CHECK # ________	TODAY'S FEE	*$48.00*
PROCEDURES: (IF NOT CHECKED ABOVE)	RETURN APPOINTMENT INFORMATION: (DAYS) (WKS.) (MOS.) (PRN)		AMOUNT RECEIVED	———
			BALANCE	*$48.00*

Figure C.37 Encounter form (Superbill) for Melissa Jones (Chapter 4).

Goode Medical Clinic

1234 Larsen Avenue
Saint Paul, Minnesota 55316

Phone: (555) 555-1234
Fax: (555) 555-5678

PATIENT NAME	CHART #	DATE		
Anne Potter		*3/9/2010*	☐ MEDI-MEDI ☐ SELF PAY ☐ MEDICARE	☐ MEDICAL ☐ PRIVATE ☐ HMO____

✓	CPT/Md	DESCRIPTION	FEE	✓	CPT/Md	DESCRIPTION	FEE	✓	CPT/Md	DESCRIPTION	FEE	✓	CPT/Md	DESCRIPTION	FEE
OFFICE VISIT - NEW PATIENT				LAB STUDIES				PROCEDURES				INJECTIONS			
	99202	Focused Ex.			36415	Venipucture			92551	Audiometry			90655	Influenza 6-35 months	
	99203	Detailed Ex.			81000	Urinalysis			29705	Cast Removal Full Arm/Leg			90656	Influenza 3 years +	
	99204	Comprehensive Ex.			81003	- w/o Micro			2900__	Casting (by location)			90732	Pneumoccal	
	99205	Complex Ex.			84703	HCG (Urine, Pregnancy)			92567	Ear Check			J0295	Ampicillin, 1.5 gr	
OFFICE VISIT - ESTABLISHED PATIENT					82948	Glucose			69210	Ear Wax Rem. 1 2			J2001	Liocaine for IV infusion 10mg	
	99212	Focused Ex.			82270	Hemoccult			93000	EKG			J1885	Toradol 15mg	
	99213	Expanded Ex.			85025	CBC -diff.			93005	EKG tracing only			90720	DTP - HIB	
	99214	Detailed Ex.			85018	Hemoglobin			93010	EKG Int. and Rep			90746	HEP B - HIB	
	99215	Complex Ex.		✓	88174	Pap Smear	*$35.00*		11750	Excision Nail			90707	MMR	
PREVENTATIVE MEDICINE - NEW PATIENT					87210	KOH/ Saline Wet Mount			94375	Respiratory Flow Volume			86580	PPD	
	99381	< 1 year old			87430	Strep Antigen			93224	Holter up to 48 hours			90732	Pneumovax	
	99382	1-4 year old			87070	Throat Culture			10060	I & D Abscess Simple			90716	Varicella	
	99383	5-11 year old			80053	Chem profile			10061	I & D Abscess Comp.			82607	Vitamin B12 Inj.	
	99384	12-17 year old			80061	Lipid profile			94761	Oximetry w/Exercise			90712	Polio oral use (OPV)	
	99385	18-39 year old			82465	Cholesterol			94726	Plethysmography			90713	Polio injection (IPV)	
✓	99386	40-64 year old	*$85.00*	✓	99000	Handling fee	*$10.00*		94760	Pulse Oximetry			90714	Td preservative free 7 yrs +	
	99387	65 + year old		X-RAY					11100	Skin Bx			90718	Td 7 years +	
PREVENTATIVE MEDICINE - ESTABLISHED PATIENT					70210	Sinuses			94010	Spirometry			95115	Allergy inj., single	
	99391	< 1 year old			70360	Neck Soft Tissue			99173	Visual Acuity			95117	Allergy inj., multiple	
	99392	1-4 year old			71010	CXR (PA only)			17110	Wart destruction up to 14					
	99393	5-11 year old			71020	Chest 2V			17111	Wart destruction 15 lesions +					
	99394	12-17 year old			72040	C-Spine 2V			11042	Wound Debrid.			OTHER		
	99395	18-39 year old			72100	Lumbrosacral									
	99396	40-64 year old			73030	Shoulder 2V									
	99397	65 + year old			73070	Elbow 2V									
✓	*80050*	*Gen Health Screen*	*$45.00*		73120	Hand 2V									
					73560	Knee 2V									
					73620	Foot 2V									
					74000	KUB									

DIAGNOSTIC CODES (ICD-9-CM)

✓	Code	Description	✓	Code	Description	✓	Code	Description	✓	Code	Description
	789.0__	Abdominal Pain		564.0	Constipation		784.0	Headache		782.1	Rash or ezanthem
	682.__	Abscess/Cellulitis		692.6	Contact dermatitis due to plants		414.9	Heart Dis., Coronary		714.0	Rheumatoid Arthritis
	995.3	Allergic Reaction		692.9	Contact dermatitis, NOS		599.70	Hematuria		V70.0	Routine general exam
	331	Alzheimer's		V25.09	Contraceptive management		455.6	Hemorrhoids		V76.10	Screen, breast
	285.__	Anemia, other & unspec		923.10	Contusion, forearm		573.3	Hepatitus, NOS		V76.2	Screen, cervix
	280.9	Anemia-iron deficiency		434.91	CVA		V03.81	HIB		V76.44	Screen, prosate
	281.0	Anemia-pernicious		266.2	Deficiency, folic acid B12		V65.44	HIV counseling		V76.47	Screen, vagina
	285.9	Anemia-unspecified		311	Depression		401.1	Hypertension, benign		216.5	Sebaceous cyst
	413.9	Angina, pectoris, oyher/unspecified		250.01	Diabetes, type I, juvenile type		401.9	Hypertension, unspecified		706.2	Sebaceous cyst
	300.00	Anxiety state, NOS		787.91	Diarrhea		401.0	Hypertension, malignant		786.05	Shortness of Breath
	300.4	Anxiety reaction		780.4	Dizziness		V04.81	Influenza		701.9	Skin tag
	716.90	Arthritis, NOS		V06.1	DTP		271.3	Lactose intolerance		845.00	Strain, ankle
	493.20	Asthma; chronic obstruction		V06.3	DTP + polio		573.9	Liver Disease		307.81	Tension headache
	493.00	Asthma; extrinic		536.8	Dyspepsia		724.5	Low Back Pain		V06.5	Tetanus - distheria (Td)
	493.10	Asthma; intrinsic		788.1	Dysuria		346.9	Migraine		305.1	Tobacco dependence
	493.90	Asthmas; unspecified		782.3	Edema		V06.4	MMR		788.41	Urinary frequency
	427.31	Atrial fibulation		530.81	Esophageal reflux		278.01	Obesity/Morbid		599.0	Unrinary tract infection, NOS
	724.5	Backache, unspecified		530.11	Esophagitis reflux		715.90	Osteoarthritis		V05.3	Viral hepatitis
	790.6	Blood chemistry		530.10	Esophagitis, unspecified		719.43	Pain in joint, forearm		368.40	Visual field defect, unspecified
	E906.3	Cat bite		780.6	Fever		625.4	PMS		V20.2	Well Child Exam
	786.50	Chest Pain		789.07	Generalized abdominal pain		486	Pneumonia			
	428.0	CHF	✓	V72.3	Gynecological examiniation		V25.01	Prescription of oral contraceptivess			

DIAGNOSIS: (IF NOT CHECKED ABOVE)

PROCEDURES: (IF NOT CHECKED ABOVE)

RETURN APPOINTMENT INFORMATION:

(DAYS) (WKS.) (MOS.) (PRN)

RECEIVED BY:

☐ CASH
☐ CREDIT CARD
☐ CHECK
#________

TODAY'S FEE	*$175.00*
AMOUNT RECEIVED	*——*
BALANCE	*$175.00*

Figure C.38 Encounter form (Superbill) for Anne Potter (Chapter 4).

Goode Medical Clinic
1234 Larsen Avenue
Saint Paul, Minnesota 55316

Phone: (555) 555-1234
Fax: (555) 555-5678

PATIENT NAME	CHART #	DATE		
Richard Potter		*3/9/2010*	☐ MEDI-MEDI ☐ SELF PAY ☐ MEDICARE	☐ MEDICAL ☐ PRIVATE ☐ HMO_______

✓	CPT/Md	DESCRIPTION	FEE	✓	CPT/Md	DESCRIPTION	FEE	✓	CPT/Md	DESCRIPTION	FEE	✓	CPT/Md	DESCRIPTION	FEE
OFFICE VISIT - NEW PATIENT				**LAB STUDIES**				**PROCEDURES**				**INJECTIONS**			
	99202	Focused Ex.			36415	Venipuncture			92551	Audiometry			90655	Influenza 6-35 months	
	99203	Detailed Ex.			81000	Urinalysis			29705	Cast Removal Full Arm/Leg			90656	Influenza 3 years +	
	99204	Comprehensive Ex.			81003	- w/o Micro			2900__	Casting (by location)			90732	Pneumoccal	
	99205	Complex Ex.			84703	HCG (Urine, Pregnancy)			92567	Ear Check			J0295	Ampicillin, 1.5 gr	
OFFICE VISIT - ESTABLISHED PATIENT					82948	Glucose			69210	Ear Wax Rem. 1 2			J2001	Liocaine for IV infusion 10mg	
	99212	Focused Ex.			82270	Hemoccult			93000	EKG			J1885	Toradol 15mg	
	99213	Expanded Ex.			85025	CBC -diff.			93005	EKG tracing only			90720	DTP - HIB	
	99214	Detailed Ex.			85018	Hemoglobin			93010	EKG Int. and Rep			90746	HEP B - HIB	
	99215	Complex Ex.			88174	Pap Smear			11750	Excision Nail			90707	MMR	
PREVENTATIVE MEDICINE - NEW PATIENT					87210	KOH/ Saline Wet Mount			94375	Respiratory Flow Volume			86580	PPD	
	99381	< 1 year old			87430	Strep Antigen			93224	Holter up to 48 hours			90732	Pneumovax	
	99382	1-4 year old			87070	Throat Culture			10060	I & D Abscess Simple			90716	Varicella	
	99383	5-11 year old			80053	Chem profile			10061	I & D Abscess Comp.			82607	Vitamin B12 Inj.	
	99384	12-17 year old			80061	Lipid profile			94761	Oximetry w/Exercise			90712	Polio oral use (OPV)	
	99385	18-39 year old			82465	Cholesterol			94726	Plethysmography			90713	Polio injection (IPV)	
✓	99386	40-64 year old	*$85.00*		99000	Handling fee			94760	Pulse Oximetry			90714	Td preservative free 7 yrs +	
	99387	65 + year old		**X-RAY**					11100	Skin Bx			90718	Td 7 years +	
PREVENTATIVE MEDICINE - ESTABLISHED PATIENT					70210	Sinuses			94010	Spirometry			95115	Allergy inj., single	
	99391	< 1 year old			70360	Neck Soft Tissue			99173	Visual Acuity			95117	Allergy inj., multiple	
	99392	1-4 year old			71010	CXR (PA only)			17110	Wart destruction up to 14					
	99393	5-11 year old			71020	Chest 2V			17111	Wart destruction 15 lesions +					
	99394	12-17 year old			72040	C-Spine 2V			11042	Wound Debrid.		**OTHER**			
	99395	18-39 year old			72100	Lumbrosacral									
	99396	40-64 year old			73030	Shoulder 2V									
	99397	65 + year old			73070	Elbow 2V									
✓	*80050*	*Gen Health Panel*	*$45.00*		73120	Hand 2V									
					73560	Knee 2V									
					73620	Foot 2V									
					74000	KUB									

DIAGNOSTIC CODES (ICD-9-CM)

✓	Code	Description	✓	Code	Description	✓	Code	Description	✓	Code	Description
	789.0__	Abdominal Pain		564.0	Constipation		784.0	Headache		782.1	Rash or ezanthem
	682.__	Abscess/Cellulitis		692.6	Contact dermatitis due to plants		414.9	Heart Dis., Coronary		714.0	Rheumatoid Arthritis
	995.3	Allergic Reaction		692.9	Contact dermatitis, NOS		599.70	Hematuria	✓	V70.0	Routine general exam
	331	Alzheimer's		V25.09	Contraceptive management		455.6	Hemorrhoids		V76.10	Screen, breast
	285.__	Anemia, other & unspec		923.10	Contusion, forearm		573.3	Hepatitus, NOS		V76.2	Screen, cervix
	280.9	Anemia-iron deficiency		434.91	CVA		V03.81	HIB		V76.44	Screen, prosate
	281.0	Anemia-pernicious		266.2	Deficiency, folic acid B12		V65.44	HIV counseling		V76.47	Screen, vagina
	285.9	Anemia-unspecified		311	Depression		401.1	Hypertension, benign		216.5	Sebaceous cyst
	413.9	Angina, pectoris, oyher/unspecified		250.01	Diabetes, type I, juvenile type		401.9	Hypertension, unspecified		706.2	Sebaceous cyst
	300.00	Anxiety state, NOS		787.91	Diarrhea		401.0	Hypertension, malignant		786.05	Shortness of Breath
	300.4	Anxiety reaction		780.4	Dizziness		V04.81	Influenza		701.9	Skin tag
	716.90	Arthritis, NOS		V06.1	DTP		271.3	Lactose intolerance		845.00	Strain, ankle
	493.20	Asthma; chronic obstruction		V06.3	DTP + polio		573.9	Liver Disease		307.81	Tension headache
	493.00	Asthma; extrinic		536.8	Dyspepsia		724.5	Low Back Pain		V06.5	Tetanus - distheria (Td)
	493.10	Asthma; intrinsic		788.1	Dysuria		346.9	Migraine		305.1	Tobacco dependence
	493.90	Asthmas; unspecified		782.3	Edema		V06.4	MMR		788.41	Urinary frequency
	427.31	Atrial fibulation		530.81	Esophageal reflux		278.01	Obesity/Morbid		599.0	Unrinary tract infection, NOS
	724.5	Backache, unspecified		530.11	Esophagitis reflux		715.90	Osteoarthritis		V05.3	Viral hepatitis
	790.6	Blood chemistry		530.10	Esophagitis, unspecified		719.43	Pain in joint, forearm		368.40	Visual field defect, unspecified
	E906.3	Cat bite		780.6	Fever		625.4	PMS		V20.2	Well Child Exam
	786.50	Chest Pain		789.07	Generalized abdominal pain		486	Pneumonia			
	428.0	CHF		V72.3	Gynecological examiniation		V25.01	Prescription of oral contraceptivess			

DIAGNOSIS: (IF NOT CHECKED ABOVE)		RECEIVED BY:	TODAY'S FEE	*$130.00*
PROCEDURES: (IF NOT CHECKED ABOVE)	RETURN APPOINTMENT INFORMATION: (DAYS) (WKS.) (MOS.) (PRN)	☐ CASH ☐ CREDIT CARD ☐ CHECK # _________	AMOUNT RECEIVED	———
			BALANCE	*$130.00*

Figure C.39 Encounter form (Superbill) for Richard Potter (Chapter 4).

Goode Medical Clinic
1234 Larsen Avenue
Saint Paul, Minnesota 55316

Phone: (555) 555-1234
Fax: (555) 555-5678

PATIENT NAME	CHART #	DATE		
Michael Ruha		*3/9/2010*	☐ MEDI-MEDI ☐ SELF PAY ☐ MEDICARE	☐ MEDICAL ☐ PRIVATE ☐ HMO______

☐	CPT/Md	DESCRIPTION	FEE	☐	CPT/Md	DESCRIPTION	FEE	☐	CPT/Md	DESCRIPTION	FEE	☐	CPT/Md	DESCRIPTION	FEE
OFFICE VISIT - NEW PATIENT				**LAB STUDIES**				**PROCEDURES**				**INJECTIONS**			
	99202	Focused Ex.			36415	Venipucture			92551	Audiometry			90655	Influenza 6-35 months	
	99203	Detailed Ex.			81000	Urinalysis			29705	Cast Removal Full Arm/Leg			90656	Influenza 3 years +	
	99204	Comprehensive Ex.			81003	- w/o Micro			2900__	Casting (by location)			90732	Pneumoccal	
	99205	Complex Ex.			84703	HCG (Urine, Pregnancy)			92567	Ear Check			J0295	Ampicillin, 1.5 gr	
OFFICE VISIT - ESTABLISHED PATIENT					82948	Glucose			69210	Ear Wax Rem. 1 2			J2001	Liocaine for IV infusion 10mg	
	99212	Focused Ex.			82270	Hemoccult			93000	EKG			J1885	Toradol 15mg	
	99213	Expanded Ex.			85025	CBC -diff.			93005	EKG tracing only			90720	DTP - HIB	
	99214	Detailed Ex.			85018	Hemoglobin			93010	EKG Int. and Rep			90746	HEP B - HIB	
	99215	Complex Ex.			88174	Pap Smear			11750	Excision Nail			90707	MMR	
PREVENTATIVE MEDICINE - NEW PATIENT					87210	KOH/ Saline Wet Mount			94375	Respiratory Flow Volume			86580	PPD	
✓	99381	< 1 year old	*$50.00*		87430	Strep Antigen			93224	Holter up to 48 hours			90732	Pneumovax	
	99382	1-4 year old			87070	Throat Culture			10060	I & D Abscess Simple			90716	Varicella	
	99383	5-11 year old			80053	Chem profile			10061	I & D Abscess Comp.			82607	Vitamin B12 Inj.	
	99384	12-17 year old			80061	Lipid profile			94761	Oximetry w/Exercise			90712	Polio oral use (OPV)	
	99385	18-39 year old			82465	Cholesterol			94726	Plethysmography			90713	Polio injection (IPV)	
	99386	40-64 year old			99000	Handling fee			94760	Pulse Oximetry			90714	Td preservative free 7 yrs +	
	99387	65 + year old		**X-RAY**					11100	Skin Bx			90718	Td 7 years +	
PREVENTATIVE MEDICINE - ESTABLISHED PATIENT					70210	Sinuses			94010	Spirometry			95115	Allergy inj., single	
	99391	< 1 year old			70360	Neck Soft Tissue			99173	Visual Acuity			95117	Allergy inj., multiple	
	99392	1-4 year old			71010	CXR (PA only)			17110	Wart destruction up to 14					
	99393	5-11 year old			71020	Chest 2V			17111	Wart destruction 15 lesions +					
	99394	12-17 year old			72040	C-Spine 2V			11042	Wound Debrid.		**OTHER**			
	99395	18-39 year old			72100	Lumbrosacral									
	99396	40-64 year old			73030	Shoulder 2V									
	99397	65 + year old			73070	Elbow 2V									
					73120	Hand 2V									
					73560	Knee 2V									
					73620	Foot 2V									
					74000	KUB									

DIAGNOSTIC CODES (ICD-9-CM)

☐	Code	Description	☐	Code	Description	☐	Code	Description	☐	Code	Description
	789.0__	Abdominal Pain		564.0	Constipation		784.0	Headache		782.1	Rash or ezanthem
	682.__	Abscess/Cellulitis		692.6	Contact dermatitis due to plants		414.9	Heart Dis., Coronary		714.0	Rheumatoid Arthritis
	995.3	Allergic Reaction		692.9	Contact dermatitis, NOS		599.70	Hematuria		V70.0	Routine general exam
	331	Alzheimer's		V25.09	Contraceptive management		455.6	Hemorrhoids		V76.10	Screen, breast
	285.__	Anemia, other & unspec		923.10	Contusion, forearm		573.3	Hepatitus, NOS		V76.2	Screen, cervix
	280.9	Anemia-iron deficiency		434.91	CVA		V03.81	HIB		V76.44	Screen, prosate
	281.0	Anemia-pernicious		266.2	Deficiency, folic acid B12		V65.44	HIV counseling		V76.47	Screen, vagina
	285.9	Anemia-unspecified		311	Depression		401.1	Hypertension, benign		216.5	Sebaceous cyst
	413.9	Angina, pectoris, oyher/unspecified		250.01	Diabetes, type I, juvenile type		401.9	Hypertension, unspecified		706.2	Sebaceous cyst
	300.00	Anxiety state, NOS		787.91	Diarrhea		401.0	Hypertension, malignant		786.05	Shortness of Breath
	300.4	Anxiety reaction		780.4	Dizziness		V04.81	Influenza		701.9	Skin tag
	716.90	Arthritis, NOS		V06.1	DTP		271.3	Lactose intolerance		845.00	Strain, ankle
	493.20	Asthma; chronic obstruction		V06.3	DTP + polio		573.9	Liver Disease		307.81	Tension headache
	493.00	Asthma; extrinic		536.8	Dyspepsia		724.5	Low Back Pain		V06.5	Tetanus - distheria (Td)
	493.10	Asthma; intrinsic		788.1	Dysuria		346.9	Migraine		305.1	Tobacco dependence
	493.90	Asthmas; unspecified		782.3	Edema		V06.4	MMR		788.41	Urinary frequency
	427.31	Atrial fibulation		530.81	Esophageal reflux		278.01	Obesity/Morbid		599.0	Unrinary tract infection, NOS
	724.5	Backache, unspecified		530.11	Esophagitis reflux		715.90	Osteoarthritis		V05.3	Viral hepatitis
	790.6	Blood chemistry		530.10	Esophagitis, unspecified		719.43	Pain in joint, forearm		368.40	Visual field defect, unspecified
	E906.3	Cat bite		780.6	Fever		625.4	PMS	✓	V20.2	Well Child Exam
	786.50	Chest Pain		789.07	Generalized abdominal pain		486	Pneumonia			
	428.0	CHF		V72.3	Gynecological examiniation		V25.01	Prescription of oral contraceptivess			

DIAGNOSIS: (IF NOT CHECKED ABOVE)		RECEIVED BY:	TODAY'S FEE	*$50.00*
		☐ CASH	AMOUNT RECEIVED	——
PROCEDURES: (IF NOT CHECKED ABOVE)	RETURN APPOINTMENT INFORMATION:	☐ CREDIT CARD		
	(DAYS) (WKS.) (MOS.) (PRN)	☐ CHECK # __________	BALANCE	*$50.00*

Figure C.40 Encounter form (Superbill) for Michael Ruha (Chapter 4).

BCBS of MN
1355 Insurance Carrier Loop
Minneapolis, MN 55111
(763)555-0426

Remittance advice

Elsevier Clinic
1234 College Avenue
St. Paul, MN 55316

Page: 1 of 1
Date: XX/XX/XX
Group Practice ID#: 567XX
Check number: 45678

Patient name	DOS	Procedure code	Units	Total charge	Allowable	Provider responsibility	Co-pay	Amount paid
Simpson, David	03/09/2010	99213	1	48.00	39.00	9.00		39.00
Jones, Melissa	03/09/2010	99213	1	48.00	39.00	9.00		39.00
Ruha, Michael	03/09/2010	99381	1	50.00	48.00	2.00		48.00

Total charges $146.00 Total provider responsibility $20.00 Total co-pay 0 Total paid $126.00

Figure C.41 Remittance Advice — Blue Cross and Blue Shield for patients Simpson, Jones, and Ruha (Chapter 4).

First Med
7 Medical Blvd.
Detroit, MI 48266
(555)555-2220

Remittance advice

Elsevier Clinic
1234 College Avenue
St. Paul, MN 55316

Page: 1 of 1
Date: XX/XX/XX
Group Practice ID#: 567XX
Check number: 90123

Patient name	DOS	Procedure code	Units	Total charge	Allowable	Provider responsibility	Co-pay	Amount paid
Potter, Anne	03/09/2010	99386	1	85.00	80.00	5.00	0	80.00
	03/09/2010	80050	1	45.00	20.00	25.00	0	20.00
	03/09/2010	99000	1	10.00	4.00	6.00	0	4.00
	03/09/2010	88155	1	35.00	30.00	5.00	0	30.00
Potter, Richard	03/09/2010	99386	1	85.00	80.00	5.00	0	80.00
	03/09/2010	80050	1	45.00	20.00	25.00	0	20.00

Total charges $305.00 Total provider responsibility $71.00 Total co-pay 0 Total paid $234.00

Figure C.42 Remittance Advice—First Med for patients Anne Potter and Richard Potter (Chapter 4).

Patient Registration Information

Account # : ______
Insurance # : ______
Co-Payment: $ ______

Please PRINT AND complete ALL sections below!

PATIENT'S PERSONAL INFORMATION Marital Status ❑ Single ❑ Married ❑ Divorced ☒ Widowed Sex: ☒ Male ❑ Female

Name: Kenner (last name) Ben (first name) ____ (initial)

Street address: 100 Cottage Land (Apt # ____) City: St. Paul State: MN Zip: 55100

Home phone: (555) 555-3823 Work phone: (____) ______ Social Security # 883 - XX - 9023

Date of Birth: 7 (month) / 23 (day) / 1946 (year)

Employer / Name of School ______ ❑ Full Time ❑ Part Time

PATIENT'S / RESPONSIBLE PARTY INFORMATION

Responsible party: Ben Kenner Date of Birth: ______

Relationship to Patient: ☒ Self ❑ Spouse ❑ Other ______ Social Security # ____-____-____

Responsible party's home phone: (____) ______

Address: ______ (Apt # ____) City: ______ State: ______ Zip: ______

Employer's name: Retired Phone number: (____) ______

Address: ______ City: ______ State: ______ Zip: ______

Name of Parent/Guardian: ______

PATIENT'S INSURANCE INFORMATION Please present insurance cards to receptionist.

PRIMARY insurance company's name: Medicare

Insurance address: 233 North Michigan Ave City: Chicago State: IL Zip: 60601

Name of insured: Ben Kenner Date of Birth: ______ Relationship to insured: ☒ Self ☐ Spouse ☐ Other ☐ Child

Insurance ID number: 883XX9023A Group number: ______

Does your insurance cover medication? Yes

EMERGENCY CONTACT

Name of person not living with you: ______ Relationship: ______

Address: ______ City: ______ State: ______ Zip: ______

Phone number: (____) ______

Assignment of Benefits • Financial Agreement

I hereby give lifetime authorization for payment of insurance benefits to be made directly to Your Name Clinic ,and any assisting physicians, for services rendered. I understand that I am financially responsible for all charges whether or not they are covered by insurance. In the event of default, I agree to pay all costs of collection, and reasonable attorney's fees. I hereby authorize this healthcare provider to release all information necessary to secure the payment of benefits.

I further agree that a photocopy of this agreement shall be as valid as the original.

Date: XX/XX/XXXX Your Signature: Ben Kenner

FORM # 58-8423 • BIBBERO SYSTEMS, INC.• PETALUMA, CA.• TO ORDER CALL TOLL FREE :800-BIBBERO (800-242-2376) • FAX (800) 242-9330 (REV.7/94)

Figure C.43 Registration form for Ben Kenner (Chapter 5).

Patient Registration Information

Account # : ______
Insurance # : ______
Co-Payment: $ ______

Please PRINT AND complete ALL sections below!

PATIENT'S PERSONAL INFORMATION Marital Status ☒ Single ☐ Married ☐ Divorced ☐ Widowed Sex: ☒ Male ☐ Female

Name: Daniels (last name) Ewan (first name) ____ (initial)

Street address: 4232 Peach Avenue (Apt # ____) City: Cottageville State: MN Zip: 55111

Home phone: (555) 555-9382 Work phone: (555) 555-1283 Social Security # 092 - XX - 3822

Date of Birth: 10 (month) / 09 (day) / 1982 (year)

Employer / Name of School ______ ☐ Full Time ☐ Part Time

PATIENT'S / RESPONSIBLE PARTY INFORMATION

Responsible party: Ewan Daniels Date of Birth: 10/09/1982

Relationship to Patient: ☒ Self ☐ Spouse ☐ Other ______ Social Security # ____-____-____

Responsible party's home phone: (____) See above

Address: ______ (Apt # ____) City: ______ State: ______ Zip: ______

Employer's name: Country Star Inn Phone number: (555) 555-3542

Address: Country Road 23 City: Eagan State: MN Zip: 55122

Name of Parent/Guardian: ______

PATIENT'S INSURANCE INFORMATION Please present insurance cards to receptionist.

PRIMARY insurance company's name: Star Insurance

Insurance address: 55 Steeple Street City: St. Paul State: MN Zip: 55100

Name of insured: Ewan Daniels Date of Birth: ______ Relationship to insured: ☒ Self ☐ Spouse ☐ Other ☐ Child

Insurance ID number: SI-823209 Group number: ______

Does your insurance cover medication? No

EMERGENCY CONTACT

Name of person not living with you: Warren Danials Relationship: Brother

Address: ______ City: ______ State: ______ Zip: ______

Phone number: (555) 555-4324

Assignment of Benefits • Financial Agreement

I hereby give lifetime authorization for payment of insurance benefits to be made directly to Your Name Clinic ,and any assisting physicians, for services rendered. I understand that I am financially responsible for all charges whether or not they are covered by insurance. In the event of default, I agree to pay all costs of collection, and reasonable attorney's fees. I hereby authorize this healthcare provider to release all information necessary to secure the payment of benefits.
I further agree that a photocopy of this agreement shall be as valid as the original.

Date: XX/XX/XXXX Your Signature: Ewan Daniels

FORM # 58-8423 • BIBBERO SYSTEMS, INC.• PETALUMA, CA.• TO ORDER CALL TOLL FREE :800-BIBBERO (800-242-2376) • FAX (800) 242-9330 (REV.7/94)

Figure C.44 Registration form for Ewan Daniels (Chapter 5).

Patient Registration Information

Account # : ______
Insurance # : ______
Co-Payment: $ ______

Please PRINT AND complete ALL sections below!

PATIENT'S PERSONAL INFORMATION Marital Status ☒ Single ☐ Married ☐ Divorced ☐ Widowed Sex: ☐ Male ☒ Female

Name: Franks (last name) Jean (first name) ____ (initial)

Street address: P.O. BOX-532 (Apt # ____) City: St. Paul State: MN Zip: 55100

Home phone: (555) 555-0101 Work phone: (____) ______ Social Security # 111 - XX - 0002

Date of Birth: 4 (month) / 23 (day) / 43 (year)

Employer / Name of School Retired ☐ Full Time ☐ Part Time

PATIENT'S / RESPONSIBLE PARTY INFORMATION

Responsible party: Self Date of Birth: ______

Relationship to Patient: ☒ Self ☐ Spouse ☐ Other ______ Social Security # ____-____-____

Responsible party's home phone: (____) See above

Address: ______ (Apt # ____) City: ______ State: ______ Zip: ______

Employer's name: n/a Phone number: (____) ______

Address: ______ City: ______ State: ______ Zip: ______

Name of Parent/Guardian: ______

PATIENT'S INSURANCE INFORMATION Please present insurance cards to receptionist.

PRIMARY insurance company's name: Medicare

Insurance address: 233 North Michigan Avenue City: Chicago State: IL Zip: 60601

Name of insured: Jean Franks Date of Birth: 4/23/43 Relationship to insured: ☒ Self ☐ Spouse ☐ Other ☐ Child

Insurance ID number: 111XX0002A Group number: ______

Does your insurance cover medication? Yes

EMERGENCY CONTACT

Name of person not living with you: Cindy Savannah Relationship: daughter

Address: 47 South Spruce Street City: Minneapolis State: MN Zip: 55111

Phone number: (555) 555-8328

Assignment of Benefits • Financial Agreement

I hereby give lifetime authorization for payment of insurance benefits to be made directly to Your Name Clinic, and any assisting physicians, for services rendered. I understand that I am financially responsible for all charges whether or not they are covered by insurance. In the event of default, I agree to pay all costs of collection, and reasonable attorney's fees. I hereby authorize this healthcare provider to release all information necessary to secure the payment of benefits.

I further agree that a photocopy of this agreement shall be as valid as the original.

Date: XX/XX/XXXX Your Signature: Jean Franks

FORM # 58-8423 • BIBBERO SYSTEMS, INC.• PETALUMA, CA.• TO ORDER CALL TOLL FREE :800-BIBBERO (800-242-2376) • FAX (800) 242-9330 (REV.7/94)

Figure C.45 Registration form for Jean Franks (Chapter 5).

Goode Medical Clinic

1234 Larsen Avenue
Saint Paul, Minnesota 55316

Phone: (555) 555-1234
Fax: (555) 555-5678

PATIENT NAME	CHART #	DATE		
Ben Kenner		*3/10/2010*	☐ MEDI-MEDI ☐ SELF PAY ☐ MEDICARE	☐ MEDICAL ☐ PRIVATE ☐ HMO____

√	CPT/Md	DESCRIPTION	FEE	√	CPT/Md	DESCRIPTION	FEE	√	CPT/Md	DESCRIPTION	FEE	√	CPT/Md	DESCRIPTION	FEE
OFFICE VISIT - NEW PATIENT				**LAB STUDIES**				**PROCEDURES**				**INJECTIONS**			
	99202	Focused Ex.			36415	Venipucture			92551	Audiometry			90655	Influenza 6-35 months	
	99203	Detailed Ex.			81000	Urinalysis			29705	Cast Removal Full Arm/Leg			90656	Influenza 3 years +	
	99204	Comprehensive Ex.			81003	- w/o Micro			2900__	Casting (by location)			90732	Pneumoccal	
	99205	Complex Ex.			84703	HCG (Urine, Pregnancy)			92567	Ear Check			J0295	Ampicillin, 1.5 gr	
OFFICE VISIT - ESTABLISHED PATIENT					82948	Glucose			69210	Ear Wax Rem. 1 2			J2001	Liocaine for IV infusion 10mg	
	99212	Focused Ex.			82270	Hemoccult		√	93000	EKG	*$55.00*		J1885	Toradol 15mg	
	99213	Expanded Ex.			85025	CBC -diff.			93005	EKG tracing only			90720	DTP - HIB	
	99214	Detailed Ex.			85018	Hemoglobin			93010	EKG Int. and Rep			90746	HEP B - HIB	
	99215	Complex Ex.			88174	Pap Smear			11750	Excision Nail			90707	MMR	
PREVENTATIVE MEDICINE - NEW PATIENT					87210	KOH/ Saline Wet Mount			94375	Respiratory Flow Volume			86580	PPD	
	99381	< 1 year old			87430	Strep Antigen			93224	Holter up to 48 hours			90732	Pneumovax	
	99382	1-4 year old			87070	Throat Culture			10060	I & D Abscess Simple			90716	Varicella	
	99383	5-11 year old			80053	Chem profile			10061	I & D Abscess Comp.			82607	Vitamin B12 Inj.	
	99384	12-17 year old			80061	Lipid profile			94761	Oximetry w/Exercise			90712	Polio oral use (OPV)	
	99385	18-39 year old			82465	Cholesterol			94726	Plethysmography			90713	Polio injection (IPV)	
	99386	40-64 year old		√	99000	Handling fee	*$10.00*		94760	Pulse Oximetry			90714	Td preservative free 7 yrs +	
	99387	65 + year old		**X-RAY**					11100	Skin Bx			90718	Td 7 years +	
PREVENTATIVE MEDICINE - ESTABLISHED PATIENT					70210	Sinuses			94010	Spirometry			95115	Allergy inj., single	
	99391	< 1 year old			70360	Neck Soft Tissue			99173	Visual Acuity			95117	Allergy inj., multiple	
	99392	1-4 year old			71010	CXR (PA only)			17110	Wart destruction up to 14					
	99393	5-11 year old			71020	Chest 2V			17111	Wart destruction 15 lesions +					
	99394	12-17 year old			72040	C-Spine 2V			11042	Wound Debrid.		**OTHER**			
	99395	18-39 year old			72100	Lumbrosacral									
	99396	40-64 year old			73030	Shoulder 2V									
√	99397	65 + year old	*$90.00*		73070	Elbow 2V									
					73120	Hand 2V									
					73560	Knee 2V									
					73620	Foot 2V									
√	*80050*	*Gen Health Panel*	*$45.00*		74000	KUB									

DIAGNOSTIC CODES (ICD-9-CM)

√	Code	Description	√	Code	Description	√	Code	Description	√	Code	Description
	789.0__	Abdominal Pain		564.0	Constipation		784.0	Headache		782.1	Rash or ezanthem
	682.__	Abscess/Cellulitis		692.6	Contact dermatitis due to plants		414.9	Heart Dis., Coronary		714.0	Rheumatoid Arthritis
	995.3	Allergic Reaction		692.9	Contact dermatitis, NOS		599.70	Hematuria	√	V70.0	Routine general exam
	331	Alzheimer's		V25.09	Contraceptive management		455.6	Hemorrhoids		V76.10	Screen, breast
	285.__	Anemia, other & unspec		923.10	Contusion, forearm		573.3	Hepatitus, NOS		V76.2	Screen, cervix
	280.9	Anemia-iron deficiency		434.91	CVA		V03.81	HIB		V76.44	Screen, prosate
	281.0	Anemia-pernicious		266.2	Deficiency, folic acid B12		V65.44	HIV counseling		V76.47	Screen, vagina
	285.9	Anemia-unspecified		311	Depression		401.1	Hypertension, benign		216.5	Sebaceous cyst
	413.9	Angina, pectoris, oyher/unspecified		250.01	Diabetes, type I, juvenile type		401.9	Hypertension, unspecified		706.2	Sebaceous cyst
	300.00	Anxiety state, NOS		787.91	Diarrhea		401.0	Hypertension, malignant		786.05	Shortness of Breath
	300.4	Anxiety reaction		780.4	Dizziness		V04.81	Influenza		701.9	Skin tag
	716.90	Arthritis, NOS		V06.1	DTP		271.3	Lactose intolerance		845.00	Strain, ankle
	493.20	Asthma; chronic obstruction		V06.3	DTP + polio		573.9	Liver Disease		307.81	Tension headache
	493.00	Asthma; extrinic		536.8	Dyspepsia		724.5	Low Back Pain		V06.5	Tetanus - distheria (Td)
	493.10	Asthma; intrinsic		788.1	Dysuria		346.9	Migraine		305.1	Tobacco dependence
	493.90	Asthmas; unspecified		782.3	Edema		V06.4	MMR		788.41	Urinary frequency
	427.31	Atrial fibulation		530.81	Esophageal reflux		278.01	Obesity/Morbid		599.0	Unrinary tract infection, NOS
	724.5	Backache, unspecified		530.11	Esophagitis reflux		715.90	Osteoarthritis		V05.3	Viral hepatitis
	790.6	Blood chemistry		530.10	Esophagitis, unspecified		719.43	Pain in joint, forearm		368.40	Visual field defect, unspecified
	E906.3	Cat bite		780.6	Fever		625.4	PMS		V20.2	Well Child Exam
	786.50	Chest Pain		789.07	Generalized abdominal pain		486	Pneumonia			
	428.0	CHF		V72.3	Gynecological examiniation		V25.01	Prescription of oral contraceptivess			

DIAGNOSIS: (IF NOT CHECKED ABOVE)		RECEIVED BY:	TODAY'S FEE	*$200.00*
PROCEDURES: (IF NOT CHECKED ABOVE)	RETURN APPOINTMENT INFORMATION:	☐ CASH ☐ CREDIT CARD	AMOUNT RECEIVED	——
	(DAYS) (WKS.) (MOS.) (PRN)	☐ CHECK # ________	BALANCE	*$200.00*

Figure C.46 Encounter form (Superbill) for Ben Kenner (Chapter 5).

Goode Medical Clinic

1234 Larsen Avenue
Saint Paul, Minnesota 55316

Phone: (555) 555-1234
Fax: (555) 555-5678

PATIENT NAME	CHART #	DATE		
Ewan Daniels		3/10/2010	☐ MEDI-MEDI ☐ SELF PAY ☐ MEDICARE	☐ MEDICAL ☐ PRIVATE ☐ HMO____

✓	CPT/Md	DESCRIPTION	FEE
	OFFICE VISIT - NEW PATIENT		
	99202	Focused Ex.	
✓	99203	Detailed Ex.	$80.00
	99204	Comprehensive Ex.	
	99205	Complex Ex.	
	OFFICE VISIT - ESTABLISHED PATIENT		
	99212	Focused Ex.	
	99213	Expanded Ex.	
	99214	Detailed Ex.	
	99215	Complex Ex.	
	PREVENTATIVE MEDICINE - NEW PATIENT		
	99381	< 1 year old	
	99382	1-4 year old	
	99383	5-11 year old	
	99384	12-17 year old	
	99385	18-39 year old	
	99386	40-64 year old	
	99387	65 + year old	
	PREVENTATIVE MEDICINE - ESTABLISHED PATIENT		
	99391	< 1 year old	
	99392	1-4 year old	
	99393	5-11 year old	
	99394	12-17 year old	
	99395	18-39 year old	
	99396	40-64 year old	
	99397	65 + year old	

✓	CPT/Md	DESCRIPTION	FEE
	LAB STUDIES		
	36415	Venipucture	
	81000	Urinalysis	
	81003	- w/o Micro	
	84703	HCG (Urine, Pregnancy)	
	82948	Glucose	
	82270	Hemoccult	
	85025	CBC -diff.	
	85018	Hemoglobin	
	88174	Pap Smear	
	87210	KOH/ Saline Wet Mount	
	87430	Strep Antigen	
	87070	Throat Culture	
	80053	Chem profile	
	80061	Lipid profile	
	82465	Cholesterol	
	99000	Handling fee	
	X-RAY		
	70210	Sinuses	
	70360	Neck Soft Tissue	
	71010	CXR (PA only)	
	71020	Chest 2V	
	72040	C-Spine 2V	
	72100	Lumbrosacral	
	73030	Shoulder 2V	
	73070	Elbow 2V	
	73120	Hand 2V	
	73560	Knee 2V	
	73620	Foot 2V	
	74000	KUB	

✓	CPT/Md	DESCRIPTION	FEE
	PROCEDURES		
	92551	Audiometry	
	29705	Cast Removal Full Arm/Leg	
	2900__	Casting (by location)	
	92567	Ear Check	
	69210	Ear Wax Rem. 1 2	
	93000	EKG	
	93005	EKG tracing only	
	93010	EKG Int. and Rep	
	11750	Excision Nail	
	94375	Respiratory Flow Volume	
	93224	Holter up to 48 hours	
	10060	I & D Abscess Simple	
	10061	I & D Abscess Comp.	
	94761	Oximetry w/Exercise	
	94726	Plethysmography	
	94760	Pulse Oximetry	
	11100	Skin Bx	
	94010	Spirometry	
	99173	Visual Acuity	
	17110	Wart destruction up to 14	
	17111	Wart destruction 15 lesions +	
	11042	Wound Debrid.	

✓	CPT/Md	DESCRIPTION	FEE
	INJECTIONS		
	90655	Influenza 6-35 months	
	90656	Influenza 3 years +	
	90732	Pneumoccal	
	J0295	Ampicillin, 1.5 gr	
	J2001	Liocaine for IV infusion 10mg	
	J1885	Toradol 15mg	
	90720	DTP - HIB	
	90746	HEP B - HIB	
	90707	MMR	
	86580	PPD	
	90732	Pneumovax	
	90716	Varicella	
	82607	Vitamin B12 Inj.	
	90712	Polio oral use (OPV)	
	90713	Polio injection (IPV)	
	90714	Td preservative free 7 yrs +	
	90718	Td 7 years +	
	95115	Allergy inj., single	
	95117	Allergy inj., multiple	
	OTHER		

DIAGNOSTIC CODES (ICD-9-CM)

Code	Description	Code	Description	Code	Description	Code	Description
789.0__	Abdominal Pain	564.0	Constipation	784.0	Headache	782.1	Rash or ezanthem
682.__	Abscess/Cellulitis	692.6	Contact dermatitis due to plants	414.9	Heart Dis., Coronary	714.0	Rheumatoid Arthritis
995.3	Allergic Reaction	692.9	Contact dermatitis, NOS	599.70	Hematuria	V70.0	Routine general exam
331	Alzheimer's	V25.09	Contraceptive management	455.6	Hemorrhoids	V76.10	Screen, breast
285.__	Anemia, other & unspec	923.10	Contusion, forearm	573.3	Hepatitus, NOS	V76.2	Screen, cervix
280.9	Anemia-iron deficiency	434.91	CVA	V03.81	HIB	V76.44	Screen, prosate
281.0	Anemia-pernicious	266.2	Deficiency, folic acid B12	V65.44	HIV counseling	V76.47	Screen, vagina
285.9	Anemia-unspecified	311	Depression	401.1	Hypertension, benign	216.5	Sebaceous cyst
413.9	Angina, pectoris, oyher/unspecified	250.01	Diabetes, type I, juvenile type	401.9	Hypertension, unspecified	706.2	Sebaceous cyst
300.00	Anxiety state, NOS	787.91	Diarrhea	401.0	Hypertension, malignant	786.05	Shortness of Breath
300.4	Anxiety reaction	780.4	Dizziness	V04.81	Influenza	701.9	Skin tag
716.90	Arthritis, NOS	V06.1	DTP	271.3	Lactose intolerance	845.00	Strain, ankle
493.20	Asthma; chronic obstruction	V06.3	DTP + polio	573.9	Liver Disease	307.81	Tension headache
493.00	Asthma; extrinic	536.8	Dyspepsia	724.5	Low Back Pain	V06.5	Tetanus - distheria (Td)
493.10	Asthma; intrinsic	788.1	Dysuria	346.9	Migraine	305.1	Tobacco dependence
493.90	Asthmas; unspecified	782.3	Edema	V06.4	MMR	788.41	Urinary frequency
427.31	Atrial fibulation	530.81	Esophageal reflux	278.01	Obesity/Morbid	599.0	Unrinary tract infection, NOS
724.5	Backache, unspecified	530.11	Esophagitis reflux	715.90	Osteoarthritis	V05.3	Viral hepatitis
790.6	Blood chemistry	530.10	Esophagitis, unspecified	719.43	Pain in joint, forearm	368.40	Visual field defect, unspecified
E906.3	Cat bite	780.6	Fever	625.4	PMS	V20.2	Well Child Exam
786.50	Chest Pain	789.07	Generalized abdominal pain	486	Pneumonia		
428.0	CHF	V72.3	Gynecological examiniation	V25.01	Prescription of oral contraceptivess		

DIAGNOSIS: (IF NOT CHECKED ABOVE)

465.9 Upper Respiratory Infection

PROCEDURES: (IF NOT CHECKED ABOVE)

RETURN APPOINTMENT INFORMATION:

(DAYS) (WKS.) (MOS.) (PRN)

RECEIVED BY:

☐ CASH
☐ CREDIT CARD
☐ CHECK
#________

TODAY'S FEE	$80.00
AMOUNT RECEIVED	——
BALANCE	$80.00

Figure C.47 Encounter form (Superbill) for Ewan Daniels (Chapter 5).

Goode Medical Clinic

1234 Larsen Avenue
Saint Paul, Minnesota 55316

Phone: (555) 555-1234
Fax: (555) 555-5678

PATIENT NAME	CHART #	DATE		
Jean Franks		*3/10/2010*	☐ MEDI-MEDI ☐ SELF PAY ☐ MEDICARE	☐ MEDICAL ☐ PRIVATE ☐ HMO___

✓	CPT/Md	DESCRIPTION	FEE
	OFFICE VISIT - NEW PATIENT		
	99202	Focused Ex.	
✓	99203	Detailed Ex.	*$80.00*
	99204	Comprehensive Ex.	
	99205	Complex Ex.	
	OFFICE VISIT - ESTABLISHED PATIENT		
	99212	Focused Ex.	
	99213	Expanded Ex.	
	99214	Detailed Ex.	
	99215	Complex Ex.	
	PREVENTATIVE MEDICINE - NEW PATIENT		
	99381	< 1 year old	
	99382	1-4 year old	
	99383	5-11 year old	
	99384	12-17 year old	
	99385	18-39 year old	
	99386	40-64 year old	
	99387	65 + year old	
	PREVENTATIVE MEDICINE - ESTABLISHED PATIENT		
	99391	< 1 year old	
	99392	1-4 year old	
	99393	5-11 year old	
	99394	12-17 year old	
	99395	18-39 year old	
	99396	40-64 year old	
	99397	65 + year old	

✓	CPT/Md	DESCRIPTION	FEE
	LAB STUDIES		
	36415	Venipucture	
	81000	Urinalysis	
	81003	- w/o Micro	
	84703	HCG (Urine, Pregnancy)	
	82948	Glucose	
	82270	Hemoccult	
	85025	CBC -diff.	
	85018	Hemoglobin	
	88174	Pap Smear	
	87210	KOH/ Saline Wet Mount	
	87430	Strep Antigen	
	87070	Throat Culture	
	80053	Chem profile	
	80061	Lipid profile	
	82465	Cholesterol	
	99000	Handling fee	
	X-RAY		
	70210	Sinuses	
	70360	Neck Soft Tissue	
	71010	CXR (PA only)	
	71020	Chest 2V	
	72040	C-Spine 2V	
	72100	Lumbrosacral	
	73030	Shoulder 2V	
	73070	Elbow 2V	
	73120	Hand 2V	
	73560	Knee 2V	
	73620	Foot 2V	
	74000	KUB	

✓	CPT/Md	DESCRIPTION	FEE
	PROCEDURES		
	92551	Audiometry	
	29705	Cast Removal Full Arm/Leg	
	2900__	Casting (by location)	
	92567	Ear Check	
	69210	Ear Wax Rem. 1 2	
	93000	EKG	
	93005	EKG tracing only	
	93010	EKG Int. and Rep	
	11750	Excision Nail	
	94375	Respiratory Flow Volume	
	93224	Holter up to 48 hours	
	10060	I & D Abscess Simple	
	10061	I & D Abscess Comp.	
	94761	Oximetry w/Exercise	
	94726	Plethysmography	
	94760	Pulse Oximetry	
	11100	Skin Bx	
	94010	Spirometry	
	99173	Visual Acuity	
	17110	Wart destruction up to 14	
	17111	Wart destruction 15 lesions +	
	11042	Wound Debrid.	

✓	CPT/Md	DESCRIPTION	FEE
	INJECTIONS		
	90655	Influenza 6-35 months	
	90656	Influenza 3 years +	
	90732	Pneumoccal	
	J0295	Ampicillin, 1.5 gr	
	J2001	Liocaine for IV infusion 10mg	
	J1885	Toradol 15mg	
	90720	DTP - HIB	
	90746	HEP B - HIB	
	90707	MMR	
	86580	PPD	
	90732	Pneumovax	
	90716	Varicella	
	82607	Vitamin B12 Inj.	
	90712	Polio oral use (OPV)	
	90713	Polio injection (IPV)	
	90714	Td preservative free 7 yrs +	
	90718	Td 7 years +	
	95115	Allergy inj., single	
	95117	Allergy inj., multiple	
	OTHER		

DIAGNOSTIC CODES (ICD-9-CM)

Code	Description	Code	Description	Code	Description	Code	Description
789.0__	Abdominal Pain	564.0	Constipation	784.0	Headache	782.1	Rash or ezanthem
682.__	Abscess/Cellulitis	692.6	Contact dermatitis due to plants	414.9	Heart Dis., Coronary	714.0	Rheumatoid Arthritis
995.3	Allergic Reaction	692.9	Contact dermatitis, NOS	599.70	Hematuria	V70.0	Routine general exam
331	Alzheimer's	V25.09	Contraceptive management	455.6	Hemorrhoids	V76.10	Screen, breast
285.__	Anemia, other & unspec	923.10	Contusion, forearm	573.3	Hepatitus, NOS	V76.2	Screen, cervix
280.9	Anemia-iron deficiency	434.91	CVA	V03.81	HIB	V76.44	Screen, prosate
281.0	Anemia-pernicious	266.2	Deficiency, folic acid B12	V65.44	HIV counseling	V76.47	Screen, vagina
285.9	Anemia-unspecified	311	Depression	401.1	Hypertension, benign	216.5	Sebaceous cyst
413.9	Angina, pectoris, oyher/unspecified	250.01	Diabetes, type I, juvenile type	401.9	Hypertension, unspecified	706.2	Sebaceous cyst
300.00	Anxiety state, NOS	787.91	Diarrhea	401.0	Hypertension, malignant	786.05	Shortness of Breath
300.4	Anxiety reaction	780.4	Dizziness	V04.81	Influenza	701.9	Skin tag
716.90	Arthritis, NOS	V06.1	DTP	271.3	Lactose intolerance	845.00	Strain, ankle
493.20	Asthma; chronic obstruction	V06.3	DTP + polio	573.9	Liver Disease	307.81	Tension headache
493.00	Asthma; extrinic	536.8	Dyspepsia	724.5	Low Back Pain	V06.5	Tetanus - distheria (Td)
493.10	Asthma; intrinsic	788.1	Dysuria	346.9	Migraine	305.1	Tobacco dependence
493.90	Asthmas; unspecified	782.3	Edema	V06.4	MMR	788.41	Urinary frequency
427.31	Atrial fibulation	530.81	Esophageal reflux	278.01	Obesity/Morbid	599.0	Unrinary tract infection, NOS
724.5	Backache, unspecified	530.11	Esophagitis reflux	715.90	Osteoarthritis	V05.3	Viral hepatitis
790.6	Blood chemistry	530.10	Esophagitis, unspecified	719.43	Pain in joint, forearm	368.40	Visual field defect, unspecified
E906.3	Cat bite	780.6	Fever	625.4	PMS	V20.2	Well Child Exam
786.50	Chest Pain	789.07	Generalized abdominal pain	486	Pneumonia		
428.0	CHF	V72.3	Gynecological examiniation	V25.01	Prescription of oral contraceptivess		

DIAGNOSIS: (IF NOT CHECKED ABOVE)

724.2 Low backpain

PROCEDURES: (IF NOT CHECKED ABOVE)

RETURN APPOINTMENT INFORMATION:

(DAYS) (WKS.) (MOS.) (PRN)

RECEIVED BY:

☐ CASH
☐ CREDIT CARD
☐ CHECK
#______

TODAY'S FEE	*$80.00*
AMOUNT RECEIVED	———
BALANCE	*$80.00*

Figure C.48 Encounter form (Superbill) for Jean Franks (Chapter 5).

Medicare Part B
233 N. Michigan Avenue
Chicago, IL 60601
(555)555-1000 Ext. 123

Remittance advice

Elsevier Clinic
1234 College Avenue
St. Paul, MN 55316

Page: 1 of 1
Date: XX/XX/XX
Group Practice ID#: 567XX
Check number: 45612

Patient name	DOS	Procedure code	Units	Total charge	Allowable	Provider responsibility	Co-pay	Amount paid
Kenner, Ben	03/10/2010	99397	1	90.00	72.00	18.00	0	72.00
	03/10/2010	80050	1	45.00	36.00	9.00	0	36.00
	03/10/2010	99000	1	10.00	8.00	2.00	0	8.00
	03/10/2010	93000	1	55.00	44.00	11.00	0	44.00

Total charges $200.00 Total provider responsibility $40.00 Total co-pay 0 Total paid $160.00

Figure C.49 Remittance Advice—Medicare for Ben Kenner (Chapter 5).

Star Insurance
45 Country Farm Lane
Woodsfield, MN 55432
(555)555-1212

Remittance advice

Elsevier Clinic
1234 College Avenue
St. Paul, MN 55316

Page: 1 of 1
Date: XX/XX/XX
Group Practice ID#: 567XX
Check number: 36985

Patient name	DOS	Procedure code	Units	Total charge	Allowable	Provider responsibility	Co-pay	Amount paid
Daniels, Ewan	03/10/2010	99203	1	80.00	72.00	8.00	20.00	52.00

Total charges $80.00 Total provider responsibility $8.00 Total co-pay $20.00 Total paid $52.00

Figure C.50 Remittance Advice—Star Insurance for Ewan Daniels (Chapter 5).

Goode Medical Clinic
William B. Goode, MD

Patient Registration Information

Account # : ______
Insurance # : ______
Co-Payment: $ ______

Please PRINT AND complete ALL sections below!

PATIENT'S PERSONAL INFORMATION Marital Status ☐ Single ☒ Married ☐ Divorced ☐ Widowed Sex: ☒ Male ☐ Female

Name: Cross (last name) Raymond (first name) ______ (initial)

Street address: 7534 76th Street (Apt # 4) City: St. Paul State: MN Zip: 55100

Home phone: (555) 555-1234 Work phone: (555) 555-5678 Social Security # 111-XX-1234

Date of Birth: 4 (month) / 12 (day) / 43 (year)

Employer / Name of School: Window Appliances ☒ Full Time ☐ Part Time

PATIENT'S / RESPONSIBLE PARTY INFORMATION

Responsible party: see above Date of Birth: ______

Relationship to Patient: ☒ Self ☐ Spouse ☐ Other ______ Social Security # ___-___-___

Responsible party's home phone: (____) see above

Address: ______ (Apt # ____) City: ______ State: ______ Zip: ______

Employer's name: Window Appliances Phone number: (555) 555-2345

Address: 987 West Carter Street City: St. Paul State: MN Zip: 55100

Name of Parent/Guardian: ______

PATIENT'S INSURANCE INFORMATION Please present insurance cards to receptionist.

PRIMARY insurance company's name: BC/BS

Insurance address: 1355 Insurance Carrier Loop City: Minneapolis State: MN Zip: 55401

Name of insured: Raymond Cross Date of Birth: 4/12/43 Relationship to insured: ☒ Self ☐ Spouse ☐ Other ☐ Child

Insurance ID number: RC-1234-WA Group number: 567890

Does your insurance cover medication? Yes

EMERGENCY CONTACT

Name of person not living with you: Selma Cross Relationship: Mother

Address: 1624 Westgate Drive City: St. Paul State: MN Zip: 55100

Phone number: (555) 555-0987

Assignment of Benefits • Financial Agreement

I hereby give lifetime authorization for payment of insurance benefits to be made directly to Goode Medical Clinic, and any assisting physicians, for services rendered. I understand that I am financially responsible for all charges whether or not they are covered by insurance. In the event of default, I agree to pay all costs of collection, and reasonable attorney's fees. I hereby authorize this healthcare provider to release all information necessary to secure the payment of benefits.

I further agree that a photocopy of this agreement shall be as valid as the original.

Date: XX/XX/XXXX Your Signature: Raymond Cross

FORM # 58-8423 • BIBBERO SYSTEMS, INC.• PETALUMA, CA.• TO ORDER CALL TOLL FREE :800-BIBBERO (800-242-2376) • FAX (800) 242-9330 (REV.7/94)

Figure C.51 Registration form for Raymond Cross (Appendix A: Day 1).

Goode Medical Clinic
William B. Goode, MD

Patient Registration Information

Account # :
Insurance # :
Co-Payment: $

Please PRINT AND complete ALL sections below!

PATIENT'S PERSONAL INFORMATION Marital Status ☒ Single ☐ Married ☐ Divorced ☐ Widowed Sex: ☐ Male ☒ Female

Name: Jackson (last name) Debra (first name) A (initial)

Street address: 1397 Bruce Street (Apt #) City: St. Paul State: MN Zip: 55100

Home phone: (555) 555-6789 Work phone: ( ) same Social Security # 999 - XX - 1098

Date of Birth: 10 (month) / 28 (day) / 72 (year)

Employer / Name of School Jackson Consultants ☒ Full Time ☐ Part Time

PATIENT'S / RESPONSIBLE PARTY INFORMATION

Responsible party: self Date of Birth:

Relationship to Patient: ☒ Self ☐ Spouse ☐ Other Social Security # - -

Responsible party's home phone: ( ) see above

Address: (Apt #) City: State: Zip:

Employer's name: Jackson Consultants Phone number: (555) 555-6789

Address: same as home City: State: Zip:

Name of Parent/Guardian:

PATIENT'S INSURANCE INFORMATION Please present insurance cards to receptionist.

PRIMARY insurance company's name: Blue Cross/Blue Shield

Insurance address: 1355 Insurance Carrier Loop City: Minneapolis State: MN Zip: 55401

Name of insured: Dabra Jackson Date of Birth: 10/28/72 Relationship to insured: ☒ Self ☐ Spouse ☐ Other ☐ Child

Insurance ID number: DJ-1098-JC Group number: 001234

Does your insurance cover medication? Yes

EMERGENCY CONTACT

Name of person not living with you: Bill Johanson Relationship: friend

Address: 1393 Bruce Street City: St. Paul State: MN Zip: 55100

Phone number: (555) 555-8201

Assignment of Benefits • Financial Agreement

I hereby give lifetime authorization for payment of insurance benefits to be made directly to Goode Medical Clinic, and any assisting physicians, for services rendered. I understand that I am financially responsible for all charges whether or not they are covered by insurance. In the event of default, I agree to pay all costs of collection, and reasonable attorney's fees. I hereby authorize this healthcare provider to release all information necessary to secure the payment of benefits.

I further agree that a photocopy of this agreement shall be as valid as the original.

Date: XX/XX/XXXX Your Signature: Debra Jackson

FORM # 58-8423 • BIBBERO SYSTEMS, INC.• PETALUMA, CA.• TO ORDER CALL TOLL FREE :800-BIBBERO (800-242-2376) • FAX (800) 242-9330 (REV.7/94)

Figure C.52 Registration form for Debra Jackson (Appendix A: Day 1).

Phone: (555) 555-1234
Fax: (555) 555-5678

Goode Medical Clinic
1234 Larsen Avenue
Saint Paul, Minnesota 55316

PATIENT NAME	CHART #	DATE		
Raymond Cross		*XX/XX/XXXX*	☐ MEDI-MEDI ☐ SELF PAY ☐ MEDICARE	☒ MEDICAL ☐ PRIVATE ☐ HMO___

✓	CPT/Md	DESCRIPTION	FEE
	OFFICE VISIT - NEW PATIENT		
	99202	Focused Ex.	
	99203	Detailed Ex.	
	99204	Comprehensive Ex.	
	99205	Complex Ex.	
	OFFICE VISIT - ESTABLISHED PATIENT		
	99212	Focused Ex.	
	99213	Expanded Ex.	
	99214	Detailed Ex.	
	99215	Complex Ex.	
	PREVENTATIVE MEDICINE - NEW PATIENT		
	99381	< 1 year old	
	99382	1-4 year old	
	99383	5-11 year old	
	99384	12-17 year old	
	99385	18-39 year old	
✓	99386	40-64 year old	*$85.*
	99387	65 + year old	
	PREVENTATIVE MEDICINE - ESTABLISHED PATIENT		
	99391	< 1 year old	
	99392	1-4 year old	
	99393	5-11 year old	
	99394	12-17 year old	
	99395	18-39 year old	
	99396	40-64 year old	
	99397	65 + year old	

✓	CPT/Md	DESCRIPTION	FEE
	LAB STUDIES		
	36415	Venipucture	
✓	81000	Urinalysis *—01*	*$78.*
	81003	- w/o Micro	
	84703	HCG (Urine, Pregnancy)	
	82948	Glucose	
	82270	Hemoccult	
✓	85025	CBC -diff.	*$120.*
	85018	Hemoglobin	
	88174	Pap Smear	
	87210	KOH/ Saline Wet Mount	
	87430	Strep Antigen	
	87070	Throat Culture	
	80053	Chem profile	
	80061	Lipid profile	
	82465	Cholesterol	
	99000	Handling fee	
	X-RAY		
	70210	Sinuses	
	70360	Neck Soft Tissue	
	71010	CXR (PA only)	
	71020	Chest 2V	
	72040	C-Spine 2V	
	72100	Lumbrosacral	
	73030	Shoulder 2V	
	73070	Elbow 2V	
	73120	Hand 2V	
	73560	Knee 2V	
	73620	Foot 2V	
	74000	KUB	

✓	CPT/Md	DESCRIPTION	FEE
	PROCEDURES		
	92551	Audiometry	
	29705	Cast Removal Full Arm/Leg	
	2900__	Casting (by location)	
	92567	Ear Check	
	69210	Ear Wax Rem. 1 2	
✓	93000	EKG	*$50.*
	93005	EKG tracing only	
	93010	EKG Int. and Rep	
	11750	Excision Nail	
	94375	Respiratory Flow Volume	
	93224	Holter up to 48 hours	
	10060	I & D Abscess Simple	
	10061	I & D Abscess Comp.	
	94761	Oximetry w/Exercise	
	94726	Plethysmography	
	94760	Pulse Oximetry	
	11100	Skin Bx	
	94010	Spirometry	
	99173	Visual Acuity	
	17110	Wart destruction up to 14	
	17111	Wart destruction 15 lesions +	
	11042	Wound Debrid.	

✓	CPT/Md	DESCRIPTION	FEE
	INJECTIONS		
	90655	Influenza 6-35 months	
	90656	Influenza 3 years +	
	90732	Pneumoccal	
	J0295	Ampicillin, 1.5 gr	
	J2001	Liocaine for IV infusion 10mg	
	J1885	Toradol 15mg	
	90720	DTP - HIB	
	90746	HEP B - HIB	
	90707	MMR	
	86580	PPD	
	90732	Pneumovax	
	90716	Varicella	
	82607	Vitamin B12 Inj.	
	90712	Polio oral use (OPV)	
	90713	Polio injection (IPV)	
	90714	Td preservative free 7 yrs +	
	90718	Td 7 years +	
	95115	Allergy inj., single	
	95117	Allergy inj., multiple	
	OTHER		

DIAGNOSTIC CODES (ICD-9-CM)

✓	Code	Description	✓	Code	Description	✓	Code	Description	✓	Code	Description
	789.0__	Abdominal Pain		564.0	Constipation		784.0	Headache		782.1	Rash or ezanthem
	682.__	Abscess/Cellulitis		692.6	Contact dermatitis due to plants		414.9	Heart Dis., Coronary		714.0	Rheumatoid Arthritis
	995.3	Allergic Reaction		692.9	Contact dermatitis, NOS		599.70	Hematuria	✓	V70.0	Routine general exam
	331	Alzheimer's		V25.09	Contraceptive management		455.6	Hemorrhoids		V76.10	Screen, breast
	285.__	Anemia, other & unspec		923.10	Contusion, forearm		573.3	Hepatitus, NOS		V76.2	Screen, cervix
	280.9	Anemia-iron deficiency		434.91	CVA		V03.81	HIB		V76.44	Screen, prosate
	281.0	Anemia-pernicious		266.2	Deficiency, folic acid B12		V65.44	HIV counseling		V76.47	Screen, vagina
	285.9	Anemia-unspecified		311	Depression		401.1	Hypertension, benign		216.5	Sebaceous cyst
	413.9	Angina, pectoris, oyher/unspecified		250.01	Diabetes, type I, juvenile type		401.9	Hypertension, unspecified		706.2	Sebaceous cyst
	300.00	Anxiety state, NOS		787.91	Diarrhea		401.0	Hypertension, malignant		786.05	Shortness of Breath
	300.4	Anxiety reaction		780.4	Dizziness		V04.81	Influenza		701.9	Skin tag
	716.90	Arthritis, NOS		V06.1	DTP		271.3	Lactose intolerance		845.00	Strain, ankle
	493.20	Asthma; chronic obstruction		V06.3	DTP + polio		573.9	Liver Disease		307.81	Tension headache
	493.00	Asthma; extrinic		536.8	Dyspepsia		724.5	Low Back Pain		V06.5	Tetanus - distheria (Td)
	493.10	Asthma; intrinsic		788.1	Dysuria		346.9	Migraine		305.1	Tobacco dependence
	493.90	Asthmas; unspecified		782.3	Edema		V06.4	MMR		788.41	Urinary frequency
	427.31	Atrial fibulation		530.81	Esophageal reflux		278.01	Obesity/Morbid		599.0	Unrinary tract infection, NOS
	724.5	Backache, unspecified		530.11	Esophagitis reflux		715.90	Osteoarthritis		V05.3	Viral hepatitis
	790.6	Blood chemistry		530.10	Esophagitis, unspecified		719.43	Pain in joint, forearm		368.40	Visual field defect, unspecified
	E906.3	Cat bite		780.6	Fever		625.4	PMS		V20.2	Well Child Exam
	786.50	Chest Pain		789.07	Generalized abdominal pain		486	Pneumonia			
	428.0	CHF		V72.3	Gynecological examiniation		V25.01	Prescription of oral contraceptivess			

DIAGNOSIS: (IF NOT CHECKED ABOVE)

PROCEDURES: (IF NOT CHECKED ABOVE)

RETURN APPOINTMENT INFORMATION:
follow-up as needed
(DAYS) (WKS.) (MOS.) (PRN)

RECEIVED BY:
☐ CASH
☐ CREDIT CARD
☐ CHECK
____

TODAY'S FEE	*$333.—*
AMOUNT RECEIVED	*——*
BALANCE	*$333.—*

Figure C.53 Encounter form (Superbill) for Raymond Cross (Appendix A: Day 1).

Goode Medical Clinic
William B. Goode, MD

Patient Registration Information

Account # :
Insurance # :
Co-Payment: $

Please PRINT AND complete ALL sections below!

PATIENT'S PERSONAL INFORMATION Marital Status ☒ Single ☐ Married ☐ Divorced ☐ Widowed Sex: ☐ Male ☒ Female

Name: Carter (last name) Tiffany (first name) (initial)

Street address: 123 Dexter Street (Apt # 9) City: Minneapolis State: MN Zip: 55100

Home phone: (555) 555-4795 Work phone: (555) 555-9324 Social Security # 999 - XX - 1234

Date of Birth: 10 (month) / 28 (day) / 72 (year)

Employer / Name of School Uptown Clothes ☒ Full Time ☐ Part Time

PATIENT'S / RESPONSIBLE PARTY INFORMATION

Responsible party: Tiffany Carter Date of Birth: 3/12/76

Relationship to Patient: ☒ Self ☐ Spouse ☐ Other Social Security # - -

Responsible party's home phone: ( ) see above

Address: (Apt #) City: State: Zip:

Employer's name: Uptown Clothes Phone number: (555) 555-9324

Address: 453 Uptown Clothes City: Minneapolis State: MN Zip: 55100

Name of Parent/Guardian:

PATIENT'S INSURANCE INFORMATION Please present insurance cards to receptionist.

PRIMARY insurance company's name: Blue Cross/Blue Shield

Insurance address: 1355 Insurance Carrier Loop City: Minneapolis State: MN Zip: 55401

Name of insured: Tiffany Carter Date of Birth: 4/12/43 Relationship to insured: ☒ Self ☐ Spouse ☐ Other ☐ Child

Insurance ID number: TC-5432-UC Group number: 21098

Does your insurance cover medication? Yes

EMERGENCY CONTACT

Name of person not living with you: Mike Carter Relationship: brother

Address: 834 Fairview Road, #4B City: St. Paul State: MN Zip: 55100

Phone number: (555) 555-1765

Assignment of Benefits • Financial Agreement

I hereby give lifetime authorization for payment of insurance benefits to be made directly to Goode Medical Clinic ,and any assisting physicians, for services rendered. I understand that I am financially responsible for all charges whether or not they are covered by insurance. In the event of default, I agree to pay all costs of collection, and reasonable attorney's fees. I hereby authorize this healthcare provider to release all information necessary to secure the payment of benefits.
I further agree that a photocopy of this agreement shall be as valid as the original.

Date: XX/XX/XXXX Your Signature: Tiffany Carter

FORM # 58-8423 • BIBBERO SYSTEMS, INC.• PETALUMA, CA.• TO ORDER CALL TOLL FREE :800-BIBBERO (800-242-2376) • FAX (800) 242-9330 (REV.7/94)

Figure C.54 Registration form for Tiffany Carter (Appendix A: Day 1).

Goode Medical Clinic
1234 Larsen Avenue
Saint Paul, Minnesota 55316

Phone: (555) 555-1234
Fax: (555) 555-5678

PATIENT NAME	CHART #	DATE		
Debra Jackson		*XX/XX/XXXX*	☐ MEDI-MEDI ☐ SELF PAY ☐ MEDICARE	☒ MEDICAL ☐ PRIVATE ☐ HMO______

☐	CPT/Md	DESCRIPTION	FEE	☐	CPT/Md	DESCRIPTION	FEE	☐	CPT/Md	DESCRIPTION	FEE	☐	CPT/Md	DESCRIPTION	FEE
OFFICE VISIT - NEW PATIENT				**LAB STUDIES**				**PROCEDURES**				**INJECTIONS**			
	99202	Focused Ex.			36415	Venipucture			92551	Audiometry			90655	Influenza 6-35 months	
	99203	Detailed Ex.		✓	81000	Urinalysis *—01*	*$78.*		29705	Cast Removal Full Arm/Leg			90656	Influenza 3 years +	
	99204	Comprehensive Ex.			81003	- w/o Micro			2900__	Casting (by location)			90732	Pneumoccal	
	99205	Complex Ex.			84703	HCG (Urine, Pregnancy)			92567	Ear Check			J0295	Ampicillin, 1.5 gr	
OFFICE VISIT - ESTABLISHED PATIENT					82948	Glucose			69210	Ear Wax Rem. 1 2			J2001	Liocaine for IV infusion 10mg	
	99212	Focused Ex.			82270	Hemoccult		✓	93000	EKG	*$50.*		J1885	Toradol 15mg	
	99213	Expanded Ex.		✓	85025	CBC -diff.	*$120.*		93005	EKG tracing only			90720	DTP - HIB	
	99214	Detailed Ex.			85018	Hemoglobin			93010	EKG Int. and Rep			90746	HEP B - HIB	
	99215	Complex Ex.			88174	Pap Smear			11750	Excision Nail			90707	MMR	
PREVENTATIVE MEDICINE - NEW PATIENT					87210	KOH/ Saline Wet Mount			94375	Respiratory Flow Volume			86580	PPD	
	99381	< 1 year old			87430	Strep Antigen			93224	Holter up to 48 hours			90732	Pneumovax	
	99382	1-4 year old			87070	Throat Culture			10060	I & D Abscess Simple			90716	Varicella	
	99383	5-11 year old			80053	Chem profile			10061	I & D Abscess Comp.			82607	Vitamin B12 Inj.	
	99384	12-17 year old			80061	Lipid profile			94761	Oximetry w/Exercise			90712	Polio oral use (OPV)	
✓	99385	18-39 year old	*$85.*		82465	Cholesterol			94726	Plethysmography			90713	Polio injection (IPV)	
	99386	40-64 year old			99000	Handling fee			94760	Pulse Oximetry			90714	Td preservative free 7 yrs +	
	99387	65 + year old		**X-RAY**					11100	Skin Bx			90718	Td 7 years +	
PREVENTATIVE MEDICINE - ESTABLISHED PATIENT					70210	Sinuses			94010	Spirometry			95115	Allergy inj., single	
	99391	< 1 year old			70360	Neck Soft Tissue			99173	Visual Acuity			95117	Allergy inj., multiple	
	99392	1-4 year old			71010	CXR (PA only)			17110	Wart destruction up to 14					
	99393	5-11 year old			71020	Chest 2V			17111	Wart destruction 15 lesions +					
	99394	12-17 year old			72040	C-Spine 2V			11042	Wound Debrid.			**OTHER**		
	99395	18-39 year old			72100	Lumbrosacral									
	99396	40-64 year old			73030	Shoulder 2V									
	99397	65 + year old			73070	Elbow 2V									
					73120	Hand 2V									
					73560	Knee 2V									
					73620	Foot 2V									
					74000	KUB									

DIAGNOSTIC CODES (ICD-9-CM)

☐	Code	Description	☐	Code	Description	☐	Code	Description	☐	Code	Description
	789.0__	Abdominal Pain		564.0	Constipation		784.0	Headache		782.1	Rash or ezanthem
	682.__	Abscess/Cellulitis		692.6	Contact dermatitis due to plants		414.9	Heart Dis., Coronary		714.0	Rheumatoid Arthritis
	995.3	Allergic Reaction		692.9	Contact dermatitis, NOS		599.70	Hematuria	✓	V70.0	Routine general exam
	331	Alzheimer's		V25.09	Contraceptive management		455.6	Hemorrhoids		V76.10	Screen, breast
	285.__	Anemia, other & unspec		923.10	Contusion, forearm		573.3	Hepatitus, NOS		V76.2	Screen, cervix
	280.9	Anemia-iron deficiency		434.91	CVA		V03.81	HIB		V76.44	Screen, prosate
	281.0	Anemia-pernicious		266.2	Deficiency, folic acid B12		V65.44	HIV counseling		V76.47	Screen, vagina
	285.9	Anemia-unspecified		311	Depression		401.1	Hypertension, benign		216.5	Sebaceous cyst
	413.9	Angina, pectoris, oyher/unspecified		250.01	Diabetes, type I, juvenile type		401.9	Hypertension, unspecified		706.2	Sebaceous cyst
	300.00	Anxiety state, NOS		787.91	Diarrhea		401.0	Hypertension, malignant		786.05	Shortness of Breath
	300.4	Anxiety reaction		780.4	Dizziness		V04.81	Influenza		701.9	Skin tag
	716.90	Arthritis, NOS		V06.1	DTP		271.3	Lactose intolerance		845.00	Strain, ankle
	493.20	Asthma; chronic obstruction		V06.3	DTP + polio		573.9	Liver Disease		307.81	Tension headache
	493.00	Asthma; extrinic		536.8	Dyspepsia		724.5	Low Back Pain		V06.5	Tetanus - distheria (Td)
	493.10	Asthma; intrinsic		788.1	Dysuria		346.9	Migraine		305.1	Tobacco dependence
	493.90	Asthmas; unspecified		782.3	Edema		V06.4	MMR		788.41	Urinary frequency
	427.31	Atrial fibulation		530.81	Esophageal reflux		278.01	Obesity/Morbid		599.0	Unrinary tract infection, NOS
	724.5	Backache, unspecified		530.11	Esophagitis reflux		715.90	Osteoarthritis		V05.3	Viral hepatitis
	790.6	Blood chemistry		530.10	Esophagitis, unspecified		719.43	Pain in joint, forearm		368.40	Visual field defect, unspecified
	E906.3	Cat bite		780.6	Fever		625.4	PMS		V20.2	Well Child Exam
	786.50	Chest Pain		789.07	Generalized abdominal pain		486	Pneumonia			
	428.0	CHF		V72.3	Gynecological examiniation		V25.01	Prescription of oral contraceptivess			

DIAGNOSIS: (IF NOT CHECKED ABOVE)		RECEIVED BY:	TODAY'S FEE	*$333.—*
		☒ CASH	AMOUNT RECEIVED	*$10. co-pay*
PROCEDURES: (IF NOT CHECKED ABOVE)	RETURN APPOINTMENT INFORMATION: (DAYS) (WKS.) (MOS.) (PRN)	☐ CREDIT CARD ☐ CHECK # ____________	BALANCE	*$323.—*

Figure C.55 Encounter form (Superbill) for Debra Jackson (Appendix A: Day 1).

Goode Medical Clinic
1234 Larsen Avenue
Saint Paul, Minnesota 55316

Phone: (555) 555-1234
Fax: (555) 555-5678

PATIENT NAME	CHART #	DATE		
Tiffany Carter		*XX/XX/XXXX*	☐ MEDI-MEDI ☐ SELF PAY ☐ MEDICARE	☒ MEDICAL ☐ PRIVATE ☐ HMO____

☐	CPT/Md	DESCRIPTION	FEE
	OFFICE VISIT - NEW PATIENT		
	99202	Focused Ex.	
✓	99203	Detailed Ex. *Lev.3*	*$80.*
	99204	Comprehensive Ex.	
	99205	Complex Ex.	
	OFFICE VISIT - ESTABLISHED PATIENT		
	99212	Focused Ex.	
	99213	Expanded Ex.	
	99214	Detailed Ex.	
	99215	Complex Ex.	
	PREVENTATIVE MEDICINE - NEW PATIENT		
	99381	< 1 year old	
	99382	1-4 year old	
	99383	5-11 year old	
	99384	12-17 year old	
	99385	18-39 year old	
	99386	40-64 year old	
	99387	65 + year old	
	PREVENTATIVE MEDICINE - ESTABLISHED PATIENT		
	99391	< 1 year old	
	99392	1-4 year old	
	99393	5-11 year old	
	99394	12-17 year old	
	99395	18-39 year old	
	99396	40-64 year old	
	99397	65 + year old	

☐	CPT/Md	DESCRIPTION	FEE
	LAB STUDIES		
	36415	Venipucture	
	81000	Urinalysis	
	81003	- w/o Micro	
	84703	HCG (Urine, Pregnancy)	
	82948	Glucose	
	82270	Hemoccult	
	85025	CBC -diff.	
	85018	Hemoglobin	
	88174	Pap Smear	
	87210	KOH/ Saline Wet Mount	
	87430	Strep Antigen	
	87070	Throat Culture	
	80053	Chem profile	
	80061	Lipid profile	
	82465	Cholesterol	
	99000	Handling fee	
	X-RAY		
	70210	Sinuses	
	70360	Neck Soft Tissue	
	71010	CXR (PA only)	
	71020	Chest 2V	
	72040	C-Spine 2V	
	72100	Lumbrosacral	
	73030	Shoulder 2V	
	73070	Elbow 2V	
	73120	Hand 2V	
	73560	Knee 2V	
	73620	Foot 2V	
	74000	KUB	

☐	CPT/Md	DESCRIPTION	FEE
	PROCEDURES		
	92551	Audiometry	
	29705	Cast Removal Full Arm/Leg	
	2900__	Casting (by location)	
	92567	Ear Check	
	69210	Ear Wax Rem. 1 2	
	93000	EKG	
	93005	EKG tracing only	
	93010	EKG Int. and Rep	
	11750	Excision Nail	
	94375	Respiratory Flow Volume	
	93224	Holter up to 48 hours	
	10060	I & D Abscess Simple	
	10061	I & D Abscess Comp.	
	94761	Oximetry w/Exercise	
	94726	Plethysmography	
	94760	Pulse Oximetry	
	11100	Skin Bx	
	94010	Spirometry	
	99173	Visual Acuity	
	17110	Wart destruction up to 14	
	17111	Wart destruction 15 lesions +	
	11042	Wound Debrid.	

☐	CPT/Md	DESCRIPTION	FEE
	INJECTIONS		
	90655	Influenza 6-35 months	
	90656	Influenza 3 years +	
	90732	Pneumoccal	
	J0295	Ampicillin, 1.5 gr	
	J2001	Liocaine for IV infusion 10mg	
	J1885	Toradol 15mg	
	90720	DTP - HIB	
	90746	HEP B - HIB	
	90707	MMR	
	86580	PPD	
	90732	Pneumovax	
	90716	Varicella	
	82607	Vitamin B12 Inj.	
	90712	Polio oral use (OPV)	
	90713	Polio injection (IPV)	
	90714	Td preservative free 7 yrs +	
	90718	Td 7 years +	
	95115	Allergy inj., single	
	95117	Allergy inj., multiple	
	OTHER		

DIAGNOSTIC CODES (ICD-9-CM)

☐	Code	Description	☐	Code	Description	☐	Code	Description	☐	Code	Description
	789.0__	Abdominal Pain		564.0	Constipation		784.0	Headache		782.1	Rash or ezanthem
	682.__	Abscess/Cellulitis		692.6	Contact dermatitis due to plants		414.9	Heart Dis., Coronary		714.0	Rheumatoid Arthritis
	995.3	Allergic Reaction	✓	692.9	Contact dermatitis, NOS		599.70	Hematuria		V70.0	Routine general exam
	331	Alzheimer's		V25.09	Contraceptive management		455.6	Hemorrhoids		V76.10	Screen, breast
	285.__	Anemia, other & unspec		923.10	Contusion, forearm		573.3	Hepatitus, NOS		V76.2	Screen, cervix
	280.9	Anemia-iron deficiency		434.91	CVA		V03.81	HIB		V76.44	Screen, prosate
	281.0	Anemia-pernicious		266.2	Deficiency, folic acid B12		V65.44	HIV counseling		V76.47	Screen, vagina
	285.9	Anemia-unspecified		311	Depression		401.1	Hypertension, benign		216.5	Sebaceous cyst
	413.9	Angina, pectoris, oyher/unspecified		250.01	Diabetes, type I, juvenile type		401.9	Hypertension, unspecified		706.2	Sebaceous cyst
	300.00	Anxiety state, NOS		787.91	Diarrhea		401.0	Hypertension, malignant		786.05	Shortness of Breath
	300.4	Anxiety reaction		780.4	Dizziness		V04.81	Influenza		701.9	Skin tag
	716.90	Arthritis, NOS		V06.1	DTP		271.3	Lactose intolerance		845.00	Strain, ankle
	493.20	Asthma; chronic obstruction		V06.3	DTP + polio		573.9	Liver Disease		307.81	Tension headache
	493.00	Asthma; extrinic		536.8	Dyspepsia		724.5	Low Back Pain		V06.5	Tetanus - distheria (Td)
	493.10	Asthma; intrinsic		788.1	Dysuria		346.9	Migraine		305.1	Tobacco dependence
	493.90	Asthmas; unspecified		782.3	Edema		V06.4	MMR		788.41	Urinary frequency
	427.31	Atrial fibulation		530.81	Esophageal reflux		278.01	Obesity/Morbid		599.0	Unrinary tract infection, NOS
	724.5	Backache, unspecified		530.11	Esophagitis reflux		715.90	Osteoarthritis		V05.3	Viral hepatitis
	790.6	Blood chemistry		530.10	Esophagitis, unspecified		719.43	Pain in joint, forearm		368.40	Visual field defect, unspecified
	E906.3	Cat bite		780.6	Fever		625.4	PMS		V20.2	Well Child Exam
	786.50	Chest Pain		789.07	Generalized abdominal pain		486	Pneumonia			
	428.0	CHF		V72.3	Gynecological examiniation		V25.01	Prescription of oral contraceptivess			

DIAGNOSIS: (IF NOT CHECKED ABOVE)

PROCEDURES: (IF NOT CHECKED ABOVE)

RETURN APPOINTMENT INFORMATION: *follow-up*
(DAYS) (*1* WKS.) (MOS.) (PRN)

RECEIVED BY:		
	TODAY'S FEE	*$80.—*
☐ CASH ☐ CREDIT CARD	AMOUNT RECEIVED	*$10. copay*
☒ CHECK # *1045*	BALANCE	*$70.—*

Figure C.56 Encounter form (Superbill) for Tiffany Carter (Appendix A: Day 1).

Goode Medical Clinic
William B. Goode, MD

Patient Registration Information

Account # :
Insurance # :
Co-Payment: $

Please PRINT AND complete ALL sections below!

PATIENT'S PERSONAL INFORMATION Marital Status ❑ Single ❑ Married ☒ Divorced ❑ Widowed Sex: ❑ Male ☒ Female

Name: Mann (last name) Cindy (first name) (initial)

Street address: P.O.BOX 876 (Apt # 9) City: St. Paul State: MN Zip: 55100

Home phone: (555) 555-2945 Work phone: (555) 555-1245 Social Security # 111 - XX - 8603

Date of Birth: 09 (month) / 12 (day) / 1962 (year)

Employer / Name of School Mall of Minnesota ☒ Full Time ❑ Part Time

PATIENT'S / RESPONSIBLE PARTY INFORMATION

Responsible party: Self Date of Birth:

Relationship to Patient: ☒ Self ❑ Spouse ❑ Other Social Security # - -

Responsible party's home phone: ( ) See above

Address: (Apt #) City: State: Zip:

Employer's name: Mall of MN Phone number: (555) 555-5678

Address: 12 American Drive City: St. Paul State: MN Zip: 55401

Name of Parent/Guardian:

PATIENT'S INSURANCE INFORMATION Please present insurance cards to receptionist.

PRIMARY insurance company's name: First Med

Insurance address: 1324 Insurance Carrier Loop City: Minneapolis State: MN Zip: 55401

Name of insured: Cindy Mann Date of Birth: 9/12/62 Relationship to insured: ☒ Self ☐ Spouse ☐ Other ☐ Child

Insurance ID number: 111XX8603 Group number: C8603 M

Does your insurance cover medication? No

EMERGENCY CONTACT

Name of person not living with you: Anna Simpson Relationship: friend

Address: 27A South 1st Street City: St. Paul State: MN Zip: 55100

Phone number: (555) 555-4763

Assignment of Benefits • Financial Agreement

I hereby give lifetime authorization for payment of insurance benefits to be made directly to Goode Medical Clinic ,and any assisting physicians, for services rendered. I understand that I am financially responsible for all charges whether or not they are covered by insurance. In the event of default, I agree to pay all costs of collection, and reasonable attorney's fees. I hereby authorize this healthcare provider to release all information necessary to secure the payment of benefits.

I further agree that a photocopy of this agreement shall be as valid as the original.

Date: XX/XX/XXXX Your Signature: Cindy Mann

FORM # 58-8423 • BIBBERO SYSTEMS, INC.• PETALUMA, CA.• TO ORDER CALL TOLL FREE :800-BIBBERO (800-242-2376) • FAX (800) 242-9330 (REV.7/94)

Figure C.57 Registration form for Cindy Mann (Appendix A: Day 2).

Goode Medical Clinic
1234 Larsen Avenue
Saint Paul, Minnesota 55316

Phone: (555) 555-1234
Fax: (555) 555-5678

PATIENT NAME	CHART #	DATE		
Cindy Mann		*XX/XX/XXXX*	☐ MEDI-MEDI ☐ SELF PAY ☐ MEDICARE	☒ MEDICAL ☐ PRIVATE ☐ HMO___

✓	CPT/Md	DESCRIPTION	FEE	✓	CPT/Md	DESCRIPTION	FEE	✓	CPT/Md	DESCRIPTION	FEE	✓	CPT/Md	DESCRIPTION	FEE
OFFICE VISIT - NEW PATIENT				**LAB STUDIES**				**PROCEDURES**				**INJECTIONS**			
	99202	Focused Ex.			36415	Venipuncture			92551	Audiometry			90655	Influenza 6-35 months	
✓	99203	Detailed Ex.	*$80.*		81000	Urinalysis			29705	Cast Removal Full Arm/Leg			90656	Influenza 3 years +	
	99204	Comprehensive Ex.			81003	- w/o Micro			2900__	Casting (by location)			90732	Pneumoccal	
	99205	Complex Ex.			84703	HCG (Urine, Pregnancy)			92567	Ear Check			J0295	Ampicillin, 1.5 gr	
OFFICE VISIT - ESTABLISHED PATIENT					82948	Glucose			69210	Ear Wax Rem. 1 2			J2001	Licocaine for IV infusion 10mg	
	99212	Focused Ex.			82270	Hemoccult			93000	EKG			J1885	Toradol 15mg	
	99213	Expanded Ex.			85025	CBC -diff.			93005	EKG tracing only			90720	DTP - HIB	
	99214	Detailed Ex.			85018	Hemoglobin			93010	EKG Int. and Rep			90746	HEP B - HIB	
	99215	Complex Ex.			88174	Pap Smear			11750	Excision Nail			90707	MMR	
PREVENTATIVE MEDICINE - NEW PATIENT					87210	KOH/ Saline Wet Mount			94375	Respiratory Flow Volume			86580	PPD	
	99381	< 1 year old			87430	Strep Antigen			93224	Holter up to 48 hours			90732	Pneumovax	
	99382	1-4 year old			87070	Throat Culture			10060	I & D Abscess Simple			90716	Varicella	
	99383	5-11 year old			80053	Chem profile			10061	I & D Abscess Comp.			82607	Vitamin B12 Inj.	
	99384	12-17 year old			80061	Lipid profile			94761	Oximetry w/Exercise			90712	Polio oral use (OPV)	
	99385	18-39 year old			82465	Cholesterol			94726	Plethysmography			90713	Polio injection (IPV)	
	99386	40-64 year old			99000	Handling fee			94760	Pulse Oximetry			90714	Td preservative free 7 yrs +	
	99387	65 + year old		**X-RAY**					11100	Skin Bx			90718	Td 7 years +	
PREVENTATIVE MEDICINE - ESTABLISHED PATIENT					70210	Sinuses			94010	Spirometry			95115	Allergy inj., single	
	99391	< 1 year old			70360	Neck Soft Tissue			99173	Visual Acuity			95117	Allergy inj., multiple	
	99392	1-4 year old			71010	CXR (PA only)			17110	Wart destruction up to 14					
	99393	5-11 year old			71020	Chest 2V			17111	Wart destruction 15 lesions +					
	99394	12-17 year old			72040	C-Spine 2V			11042	Wound Debrid.		**OTHER**			
	99395	18-39 year old			72100	Lumbrosacral									
	99396	40-64 year old			73030	Shoulder 2V									
	99397	65 + year old			73070	Elbow 2V									
					73120	Hand 2V									
					73560	Knee 2V									
					73620	Foot 2V									
					74000	KUB									

DIAGNOSTIC CODES (ICD-9-CM)

✓	Code	Description	✓	Code	Description	✓	Code	Description	✓	Code	Description
	789.0__	Abdominal Pain		564.0	Constipation		784.0	Headache		782.1	Rash or ezanthem
	682.__	Abscess/Cellulitis		692.6	Contact dermatitis due to plants		414.9	Heart Dis., Coronary		714.0	Rheumatoid Arthritis
	995.3	Allergic Reaction		692.9	Contact dermatitis, NOS		599.70	Hematuria		V70.0	Routine general exam
	331	Alzheimer's		V25.09	Contraceptive management		455.6	Hemorrhoids		V76.10	Screen, breast
	285.__	Anemia, other & unspec		923.10	Contusion, forearm		573.3	Hepatitus, NOS		V76.2	Screen, cervix
	280.9	Anemia-iron deficiency		434.91	CVA		V03.81	HIB		V76.44	Screen, prosate
	281.0	Anemia-pernicious		266.2	Deficiency, folic acid B12		V65.44	HIV counseling		V76.47	Screen, vagina
	285.9	Anemia-unspecified		311	Depression		401.1	Hypertension, benign		216.5	Sebaceous cyst
	413.9	Angina, pectoris, oyher/unspecified		250.01	Diabetes, type I, juvenile type		401.9	Hypertension, unspecified		706.2	Sebaceous cyst
	300.00	Anxiety state, NOS		787.91	Diarrhea		401.0	Hypertension, malignant		786.05	Shortness of Breath
	300.4	Anxiety reaction		780.4	Dizziness		V04.81	Influenza		701.9	Skin tag
	716.90	Arthritis, NOS		V06.1	DTP		271.3	Lactose intolerance		845.00	Strain, ankle
	493.20	Asthma; chronic obstruction		V06.3	DTP + polio		573.9	Liver Disease		307.81	Tension headache
	493.00	Asthma; extrinic		536.8	Dyspepsia		724.5	Low Back Pain		V06.5	Tetanus - distheria (Td)
	493.10	Asthma; intrinsic		788.1	Dysuria		346.9	Migraine		305.1	Tobacco dependence
	493.90	Asthmas; unspecified		782.3	Edema		V06.4	MMR		788.41	Urinary frequency
	427.31	Atrial fibulation		530.81	Esophageal reflux		278.01	Obesity/Morbid		599.0	Unrinary tract infection, NOS
	724.5	Backache, unspecified		530.11	Esophagitis reflux		715.90	Osteoarthritis		V05.3	Viral hepatitis
	790.6	Blood chemistry		530.10	Esophagitis, unspecified		719.43	Pain in joint, forearm		368.40	Visual field defect, unspecified
	E906.3	Cat bite	✓	780.6	Fever		625.4	PMS		V20.2	Well Child Exam
	786.50	Chest Pain		789.07	Generalized abdominal pain		486	Pneumonia			
	428.0	CHF		V72.3	Gynecological examiniation		V25.01	Prescription of oral contraceptivess			

DIAGNOSIS: (IF NOT CHECKED ABOVE)

PROCEDURES: (IF NOT CHECKED ABOVE)

RETURN APPOINTMENT INFORMATION:

(DAYS) (WKS.) (MOS.) (PRN)

RECEIVED BY:	TODAY'S FEE	*$80.—*
☐ CASH ☐ CREDIT CARD ☐ CHECK # ________	AMOUNT RECEIVED	———
	BALANCE	*$80.—*

Figure C.58 Encounter form (Superbill) for Cindy Mann (Appendix A: Day 2).

Goode Medical Clinic
William B. Goode, MD

Patient Registration Information

Account # :
Insurance # :
Co-Payment: $

Please PRINT AND complete ALL sections below!

PATIENT'S PERSONAL INFORMATION Marital Status ❑ Single ☒ Married ❑ Divorced ❑ Widowed Sex: ☒ Male ❑ Female

Name: Gorge (last name) Curtis (first name) (initial)

Street address: 123 University St. (Apt #) City: St. Paul State: MN Zip: 55100

Home phone: (555) 555-2716 Work phone: ( ) Social Security # 888 - XX - 1234

Date of Birth: 4 (month) / 23 (day) / 39 (year)

Employer / Name of School n/a ❑ Full Time ❑ Part Time

PATIENT'S / RESPONSIBLE PARTY INFORMATION

Responsible party: Self Date of Birth:

Relationship to Patient: ☒ Self ❑ Spouse ❑ Other Social Security # - -

Responsible party's home phone: ( ) Same as above

Address: (Apt #) City: State: Zip:

Employer's name: n/a Phone number:( )

Address: City: State: Zip:

Name of Parent/Guardian:

PATIENT'S INSURANCE INFORMATION Please present insurance cards to receptionist.

PRIMARY insurance company's name:

Insurance address: City: State: Zip:

Name of insured: Date of Birth: Relationship to insured: ☐ Self ☐ Spouse ☐ Other ☐ Child

Insurance ID number: Group number:

Does your insurance cover medication?

EMERGENCY CONTACT

Name of person ~~not~~ living with you: Sandy Gorge Relationship: Spouse

Address: Same as above City: State: Zip:

Phone number: ( ) Same as above

Assignment of Benefits • Financial Agreement

I hereby give lifetime authorization for payment of insurance benefits to be made directly to Goode Medical Clinic ,and any assisting physicians, for services rendered. I understand that I am financially responsible for all charges whether or not they are covered by insurance. In the event of default, I agree to pay all costs of collection, and reasonable attorney's fees. I hereby authorize this healthcare provider to release all information necessary to secure the payment of benefits.

I further agree that a photocopy of this agreement shall be as valid as the original.

Date: XX/XX/XXXX Your Signature: Curtis Gorge

FORM # 58-8423 • BIBBERO SYSTEMS, INC.• PETALUMA, CA.• TO ORDER CALL TOLL FREE :800-BIBBERO (800-242-2376) • FAX (800) 242-9330 (REV.7/94)

Figure C.59 Registration form for Curtis Gorge (Appendix A: Day 2).

Goode Medical Clinic
1234 Larsen Avenue
Saint Paul, Minnesota 55316

Phone: (555) 555-1234
Fax: (555) 555-5678

PATIENT NAME	CHART #	DATE		
Curtis Gorge		*XX/XX/XXXX*	☐ MEDI-MEDI ■ SELF PAY ☒ MEDICARE	☐ MEDICAL ☐ PRIVATE ☐ HMO____

☐	CPT/Md	DESCRIPTION	FEE	☐	CPT/Md	DESCRIPTION	FEE	☐	CPT/Md	DESCRIPTION	FEE	☐	CPT/Md	DESCRIPTION	FEE
OFFICE VISIT - NEW PATIENT				**LAB STUDIES**				**PROCEDURES**				**INJECTIONS**			
	99202	Focused Ex.			36415	Venipuncture			92551	Audiometry			90655	Influenza 6-35 months	
✓	99203	Detailed Ex.	*$80.*		81000	Urinalysis			29705	Cast Removal Full Arm/Leg			90656	Influenza 3 years +	
	99204	Comprehensive Ex.			81003	- w/o Micro			2900__	Casting (by location)			90732	Pneumoccal	
	99205	Complex Ex.			84703	HCG (Urine, Pregnancy)			92567	Ear Check			J0295	Ampicillin, 1.5 gr	
OFFICE VISIT - ESTABLISHED PATIENT					82948	Glucose			69210	Ear Wax Rem. 1 2			J2001	Liocaine for IV infusion 10mg	
	99212	Focused Ex.			82270	Hemoccult			93000	EKG			J1885	Toradol 15mg	
	99213	Expanded Ex.			85025	CBC -diff.			93005	EKG tracing only			90720	DTP - HIB	
	99214	Detailed Ex.			85018	Hemoglobin			93010	EKG Int. and Rep			90746	HEP B - HIB	
	99215	Complex Ex.			88174	Pap Smear			11750	Excision Nail			90707	MMR	
PREVENTATIVE MEDICINE - NEW PATIENT					87210	KOH/ Saline Wet Mount			94375	Respiratory Flow Volume			86580	PPD	
	99381	< 1 year old			87430	Strep Antigen			93224	Holter up to 48 hours			90732	Pneumovax	
	99382	1-4 year old			87070	Throat Culture			10060	I & D Abscess Simple			90716	Varicella	
	99383	5-11 year old			80053	Chem profile			10061	I & D Abscess Comp.			82607	Vitamin B12 Inj.	
	99384	12-17 year old			80061	Lipid profile			94761	Oximetry w/Exercise			90712	Polio oral use (OPV)	
	99385	18-39 year old			82465	Cholesterol			94726	Plethysmography			90713	Polio injection (IPV)	
	99386	40-64 year old			99000	Handling fee			94760	Pulse Oximetry			90714	Td preservative free 7 yrs +	
	99387	65 + year old		**X-RAY**					11100	Skin Bx			90718	Td 7 years +	
PREVENTATIVE MEDICINE - ESTABLISHED PATIENT					70210	Sinuses			94010	Spirometry			95115	Allergy inj., single	
	99391	< 1 year old			70360	Neck Soft Tissue			99173	Visual Acuity			95117	Allergy inj., multiple	
	99392	1-4 year old			71010	CXR (PA only)			17110	Wart destruction up to 14					
	99393	5-11 year old			71020	Chest 2V			17111	Wart destruction 15 lesions +					
	99394	12-17 year old			72040	C-Spine 2V			11042	Wound Debrid.		**OTHER**			
	99395	18-39 year old			72100	Lumbrosacral									
	99396	40-64 year old			73030	Shoulder 2V									
	99397	65 + year old			73070	Elbow 2V									
					73120	Hand 2V									
					73560	Knee 2V									
					73620	Foot 2V									
					74000	KUB									

DIAGNOSTIC CODES (ICD-9-CM)

☐	Code	Description	☐	Code	Description	☐	Code	Description	☐	Code	Description
	789.0__	Abdominal Pain		564.0	Constipation		784.0	Headache		782.1	Rash or ezanthem
	682.__	Abscess/Cellulitis		692.6	Contact dermatitis due to plants		414.9	Heart Dis., Coronary		714.0	Rheumatoid Arthritis
	995.3	Allergic Reaction		692.9	Contact dermatitis, NOS		599.70	Hematuria		V70.0	Routine general exam
	331	Alzheimer's		V25.09	Contraceptive management		455.6	Hemorrhoids		V76.10	Screen, breast
	285.__	Anemia, other & unspec		923.10	Contusion, forearm		573.3	Hepatitus, NOS		V76.2	Screen, cervix
	280.9	Anemia-iron deficiency		434.91	CVA		V03.81	HIB		V76.44	Screen, prosate
	281.0	Anemia-pernicious		266.2	Deficiency, folic acid B12		V65.44	HIV counseling		V76.47	Screen, vagina
	285.9	Anemia-unspecified		311	Depression		401.1	Hypertension, benign		216.5	Sebaceous cyst
	413.9	Angina, pectoris, oyher/unspecified		250.01	Diabetes, type I, juvenile type		401.9	Hypertension, unspecified		706.2	Sebaceous cyst
	300.00	Anxiety state, NOS		787.91	Diarrhea		401.0	Hypertension, malignant		786.05	Shortness of Breath
	300.4	Anxiety reaction		780.4	Dizziness		V04.81	Influenza		701.9	Skin tag
	716.90	Arthritis, NOS		V06.1	DTP		271.3	Lactose intolerance		845.00	Strain, ankle
	493.20	Asthma; chronic obstruction		V06.3	DTP + polio		573.9	Liver Disease		307.81	Tension headache
	493.00	Asthma; extrinic		536.8	Dyspepsia		724.5	Low Back Pain		V06.5	Tetanus - distheria (Td)
	493.10	Asthma; intrinsic		788.1	Dysuria		346.9	Migraine		305.1	Tobacco dependence
	493.90	Asthmas; unspecified		782.3	Edema		V06.4	MMR		788.41	Urinary frequency
	427.31	Atrial fibulation		530.81	Esophageal reflux		278.01	Obesity/Morbid		599.0	Unrinary tract infection, NOS
	724.5	Backache, unspecified		530.11	Esophagitis reflux		715.90	Osteoarthritis		V05.3	Viral hepatitis
	790.6	Blood chemistry		530.10	Esophagitis, unspecified		719.43	Pain in joint, forearm		368.40	Visual field defect, unspecified
	E906.3	Cat bite		780.6	Fever		625.4	PMS		V20.2	Well Child Exam
	786.50	Chest Pain		789.07	Generalized abdominal pain		486	Pneumonia			
	428.0	CHF		V72.3	Gynecological examiniation		V25.01	Prescription of oral contraceptivess			

DIAGNOSIS: (IF NOT CHECKED ABOVE)

Cough — 786.2

PROCEDURES: (IF NOT CHECKED ABOVE)

RETURN APPOINTMENT INFORMATION:

(DAYS) (WKS.) (MOS.) (PRN)

RECEIVED BY:

☐ CASH
☐ CREDIT CARD
☒ CHECK
2903

TODAY'S FEE	*$80.—*
AMOUNT RECEIVED	*$50.—*
BALANCE	*$30.—*

Figure C.60 Encounter form (Superbill) for Curtis Gorge (Appendix A: Day 2).

Goode Medical Clinic
William B. Goode, MD

Patient Registration Information

Account # :
Insurance # :
Co-Payment: $

Please PRINT AND complete ALL sections below!

PATIENT'S PERSONAL INFORMATION Marital Status ☐ Single ☒ Married ☐ Divorced ☐ Widowed Sex: ☐ Male ☒ Female

Name: Stone (last name) Lynn (first name) J (initial)
Street address: 10 France Avenue (Apt # ___) City: St. Paul State: MN Zip: 55100
Home phone: (555) 555-6419 Work phone: (___) 555-1118 Social Security # 901 - XX - 2345
Date of Birth: 12 (month) / 9 (day) / 67 (year)
Employer / Name of School MN Interior Designs ☒ Full Time ☐ Part Time

PATIENT'S / RESPONSIBLE PARTY INFORMATION

Responsible party: Donald Stone Date of Birth: 3/15/66
Relationship to Patient: ☒ Self ☐ Spouse ☐ Other Social Security # 178 - XX - 4653
Responsible party's home phone: (___) see as above
Address: (Apt # ___) City: State: Zip:
Employer's name: Stone Architects Phone number: (555) 555-9012
Address: 678 80th Street City: Minneapolis State: MN Zip: 55401
Name of Parent/Guardian:

PATIENT'S INSURANCE INFORMATION Please present insurance cards to receptionist.

PRIMARY insurance company's name: Blue Cross/Blue Shield
Insurance address: 1355 Insurance Carrier Loop City: Minneapolis State: MN Zip: 55401
Name of insured: Donald Stone Date of Birth: 3/15/66 Relationship to insured: ☐ Self ☐ Spouse ☐ Other ☐ Child
Insurance ID number: DS-0123-SA Group number: 45678
Does your insurance cover medication? Yes

EMERGENCY CONTACT

Name of person not living with you: Donald Stone (at work) Relationship: Spouse
Address: 678 80th Street City: Minneapolis State: MN Zip: 55401
Phone number: (555) 555-4332

Assignment of Benefits • Financial Agreement

I hereby give lifetime authorization for payment of insurance benefits to be made directly to Goode Medical Clinic ,and any assisting physicians, for services rendered. I understand that I am financially responsible for all charges whether or not they are covered by insurance. In the event of default, I agree to pay all costs of collection, and reasonable attorney's fees. I hereby authorize this healthcare provider to release all information necessary to secure the payment of benefits.
I further agree that a photocopy of this agreement shall be as valid as the original.

Date: XX/XX/XXXX Your Signature: Lynn Stone

FORM # 58-8423 • BIBBERO SYSTEMS, INC.• PETALUMA, CA.• TO ORDER CALL TOLL FREE :800-BIBBERO (800-242-2376) • FAX (800) 242-9330 (REV.7/94)

Figure C.61 Registration form for Lynn Stone (Appendix A: Day 2).

Goode Medical Clinic

1234 Larsen Avenue
Saint Paul, Minnesota 55316

Phone: (555) 555-1234
Fax: (555) 555-5678

PATIENT NAME	CHART #	DATE		
Lynn Stone		*XX/XX/XXXX*	☐ MEDI-MEDI ☐ SELF PAY ☐ MEDICARE	☒ MEDICAL ☐ PRIVATE ☐ HMO________

☐	CPT/Md	DESCRIPTION	FEE
	OFFICE VISIT - NEW PATIENT		
	99202	Focused Ex.	
✓	99203	Detailed Ex.	*$80.*
	99204	Comprehensive Ex.	
	99205	Complex Ex.	
	OFFICE VISIT - ESTABLISHED PATIENT		
	99212	Focused Ex.	
	99213	Expanded Ex.	
	99214	Detailed Ex.	
	99215	Complex Ex.	
	PREVENTATIVE MEDICINE - NEW PATIENT		
	99381	< 1 year old	
	99382	1-4 year old	
	99383	5-11 year old	
	99384	12-17 year old	
	99385	18-39 year old	
	99386	40-64 year old	
	99387	65 + year old	
	PREVENTATIVE MEDICINE - ESTABLISHED PATIENT		
	99391	< 1 year old	
	99392	1-4 year old	
	99393	5-11 year old	
	99394	12-17 year old	
	99395	18-39 year old	
	99396	40-64 year old	
	99397	65 + year old	

☐	CPT/Md	DESCRIPTION	FEE
	LAB STUDIES		
	36415	Venipuncture	
	81000	Urinalysis	
	81003	- w/o Micro	
	84703	HCG (Urine, Pregnancy)	
	82948	Glucose	
	82270	Hemoccult	
	85025	CBC -diff.	
	85018	Hemoglobin	
	88174	Pap Smear	
	87210	KOH/ Saline Wet Mount	
	87430	Strep Antigen	
	87070	Throat Culture	
	80053	Chem profile	
	80061	Lipid profile	
	82465	Cholesterol	
	99000	Handling fee	
	X-RAY		
	70210	Sinuses	
	70360	Neck Soft Tissue	
	71010	CXR (PA only)	
	71020	Chest 2V	
	72040	C-Spine 2V	
	72100	Lumbrosacral	
	73030	Shoulder 2V	
	73070	Elbow 2V	
	73120	Hand 2V	
	73560	Knee 2V	
	73620	Foot 2V	
	74000	KUB	

☐	CPT/Md	DESCRIPTION	FEE
	PROCEDURES		
	92551	Audiometry	
	29705	Cast Removal Full Arm/Leg	
	2900__	Casting (by location)	
	92567	Ear Check	
	69210	Ear Wax Rem. 1 2	
	93000	EKG	
	93005	EKG tracing only	
	93010	EKG Int. and Rep	
	11750	Excision Nail	
	94375	Respiratory Flow Volume	
	93224	Holter up to 48 hours	
	10060	I & D Abscess Simple	
	10061	I & D Abscess Comp.	
	94761	Oximetry w/Exercise	
	94726	Plethysmography	
	94760	Pulse Oximetry	
	11100	Skin Bx	
	94010	Spirometry	
	99173	Visual Acuity	
	17110	Wart destruction up to 14	
	17111	Wart destruction 15 lesions +	
	11042	Wound Debrid.	

☐	CPT/Md	DESCRIPTION	FEE
	INJECTIONS		
	90655	Influenza 6-35 months	
	90656	Influenza 3 years +	
	90732	Pneumoccal	
	J0295	Ampicillin, 1.5 gr	
	J2001	Liocaine for IV infusion 10mg	
	J1885	Toradol 15mg	
	90720	DTP - HIB	
	90746	HEP B - HIB	
	90707	MMR	
	86580	PPD	
	90732	Pneumovax	
	90716	Varicella	
	82607	Vitamin B12 Inj.	
	90712	Polio oral use (OPV)	
	90713	Polio injection (IPV)	
	90714	Td preservative free 7 yrs +	
	90718	Td 7 years +	
	95115	Allergy inj., single	
	95117	Allergy inj., multiple	
	OTHER		

DIAGNOSTIC CODES (ICD-9-CM)

☐	Code	Description	☐	Code	Description	☐	Code	Description	☐	Code	Description
	789.0__	Abdominal Pain		564.0	Constipation		784.0	Headache		782.1	Rash or ezanthem
	682.__	Abscess/Cellulitis		692.6	Contact dermatitis due to plants		414.9	Heart Dis., Coronary		714.0	Rheumatoid Arthritis
	995.3	Allergic Reaction		692.9	Contact dermatitis, NOS		599.70	Hematuria		V70.0	Routine general exam
	331	Alzheimer's		V25.09	Contraceptive management		455.6	Hemorrhoids		V76.10	Screen, breast
	285.__	Anemia, other & unspec		923.10	Contusion, forearm		573.3	Hepatitus, NOS		V76.2	Screen, cervix
	280.9	Anemia-iron deficiency		434.91	CVA		V03.81	HIB		V76.44	Screen, prosate
	281.0	Anemia-pernicious		266.2	Deficiency, folic acid B12		V65.44	HIV counseling		V76.47	Screen, vagina
	285.9	Anemia-unspecified		311	Depression		401.1	Hypertension, benign		216.5	Sebaceous cyst
	413.9	Angina, pectoris, oyher/unspecified		250.01	Diabetes, type I, juvenile type		401.9	Hypertension, unspecified		706.2	Sebaceous cyst
	300.00	Anxiety state, NOS		787.91	Diarrhea		401.0	Hypertension, malignant		786.05	Shortness of Breath
	300.4	Anxiety reaction		780.4	Dizziness		V04.81	Influenza		701.9	Skin tag
	716.90	Arthritis, NOS		V06.1	DTP		271.3	Lactose intolerance		845.00	Strain, ankle
	493.20	Asthma; chronic obstruction		V06.3	DTP + polio		573.9	Liver Disease		307.81	Tension headache
	493.00	Asthma; extrinic		536.8	Dyspepsia		724.5	Low Back Pain		V06.5	Tetanus - distheria (Td)
	493.10	Asthma; intrinsic		788.1	Dysuria		346.9	Migraine		305.1	Tobacco dependence
	493.90	Asthmas; unspecified		782.3	Edema		V06.4	MMR		788.41	Urinary frequency
	427.31	Atrial fibulation		530.81	Esophageal reflux		278.01	Obesity/Morbid		599.0	Unrinary tract infection, NOS
	724.5	Backache, unspecified		530.11	Esophagitis reflux		715.90	Osteoarthritis		V05.3	Viral hepatitis
	790.6	Blood chemistry		530.10	Esophagitis, unspecified		719.43	Pain in joint, forearm		368.40	Visual field defect, unspecified
	E906.3	Cat bite		780.6	Fever		625.4	PMS		V20.2	Well Child Exam
	786.50	Chest Pain		789.07	Generalized abdominal pain		486	Pneumonia			
	428.0	CHF		V72.3	Gynecological examiniation		V25.01	Prescription of oral contraceptivess			

DIAGNOSIS: (IF NOT CHECKED ABOVE)
Fatigue — 780.79

PROCEDURES: (IF NOT CHECKED ABOVE)

RETURN APPOINTMENT INFORMATION:
follow-up
(*3* DAYS) (WKS.) (MOS.) (PRN)

RECEIVED BY:
☐ CASH
☐ CREDIT CARD
☐ CHECK
#________

TODAY'S FEE	*$80.00*
AMOUNT RECEIVED	——
BALANCE	*$80.00*

Figure C.62 Encounter form (Superbill) for Lynn Stone (Appendix A: Day 2).

Goode Medical Clinic
William B. Goode, MD

Patient Registration Information

Account # :
Insurance # :
Co-Payment: $

Please PRINT AND complete ALL sections below!

PATIENT'S PERSONAL INFORMATION Marital Status ☒ Single ❑ Married ❑ Divorced ❑ Widowed Sex: ☒ Male ❑ Female

Name: Hill (last name) Dylan (first name) (initial)

Street address: 123 Edina Avenue (Apt #) City: St. Paul State: MN Zip: 55100

Home phone: (555) 555-5678 Work phone: (555) 555-6275 Social Security # 345 - XX - 5538

Date of Birth: 01 (month) / 20 (day) / 1952 (year)

Employer / Name of School Brick and Concrete, Inc. ☒ Full Time ❑ Part Time

PATIENT'S / RESPONSIBLE PARTY INFORMATION

Responsible party: self Date of Birth:

Relationship to Patient: ☒ Self ❑ Spouse ❑ Other Social Security # - -

Responsible party's home phone: ( ) see as above

Address: (Apt #) City: State: Zip:

Employer's name: Brick and Concrete, Inc. Phone number: (555) 555-6275

Address: Cty. Road C City: Shorenem State: MN Zip: 55000

Name of Parent/Guardian:

PATIENT'S INSURANCE INFORMATION Please present insurance cards to receptionist.

PRIMARY insurance company's name: First Med

Insurance address: 1324 Insurance Carrier Loop City: Minneapolis State: MN Zip: 55401

Name of insured: Dylan Hill Date of Birth: 01/20/52 Relationship to insured: ☐ Self ☐ Spouse ☐ Other ☐ Child

Insurance ID number: 345XX5538 Group number:

Does your insurance cover medication? Yes

EMERGENCY CONTACT

Name of person not living with you: Marcy Hill Relationship: sister

Address: 145 Lakeshore Drive City: Edina State: MN Zip: 55436

Phone number: (555) 555-3339

Assignment of Benefits • Financial Agreement

I hereby give lifetime authorization for payment of insurance benefits to be made directly to Goode Medical Clinic ,and any assisting physicians, for services rendered. I understand that I am financially responsible for all charges whether or not they are covered by insurance. In the event of default, I agree to pay all costs of collection, and reasonable attorney's fees. I hereby authorize this healthcare provider to release all information necessary to secure the payment of benefits.

I further agree that a photocopy of this agreement shall be as valid as the original.

Date: XX/XX/XXXX Your Signature: Dylan Hill

FORM # 58-8423 • BIBBERO SYSTEMS, INC.• PETALUMA, CA.• TO ORDER CALL TOLL FREE :800-BIBBERO (800-242-2376) • FAX (800) 242-9330 (REV.7/94)

Figure C.63 Registration form for Dylan Hill (Appendix A: Day 2).

Phone: (555) 555-1234
Fax: (555) 555-5678

Goode Medical Clinic

1234 Larsen Avenue
Saint Paul, Minnesota 55316

PATIENT NAME	CHART #	DATE		
Dylan Hill		*XX/XX/XXXX*	☐ MEDI-MEDI ☐ SELF PAY ☐ MEDICARE	☐ MEDICAL ☒ PRIVATE ☐ HMO____

☐	CPT/Md	DESCRIPTION	FEE	☐	CPT/Md	DESCRIPTION	FEE	☐	CPT/Md	DESCRIPTION	FEE	☐	CPT/Md	DESCRIPTION	FEE
OFFICE VISIT - NEW PATIENT				**LAB STUDIES**				**PROCEDURES**				**INJECTIONS**			
	99202	Focused Ex.			36415	Venipucture			92551	Audiometry			90655	Influenza 6-35 months	
	99203	Detailed Ex.		✓	81000	Urinalysis *—01*	*$78.*		29705	Cast Removal Full Arm/Leg			90656	Influenza 3 years +	
	99204	Comprehensive Ex.			81003	- w/o Micro			2900__	Casting (by location)			90732	Pneumoccal	
	99205	Complex Ex.			84703	HCG (Urine, Pregnancy)			92567	Ear Check			J0295	Ampicillin, 1.5 gr	
OFFICE VISIT - ESTABLISHED PATIENT					82948	Glucose			69210	Ear Wax Rem. 1 2			J2001	Liocaine for IV infusion 10mg	
	99212	Focused Ex.			82270	Hemoccult		✓	93000	EKG */ECG*	*$50.*		J1885	Toradol 15mg	
	99213	Expanded Ex.		✓	85025	CBC -diff.	*$120.*		93005	EKG tracing only			90720	DTP - HIB	
	99214	Detailed Ex.			85018	Hemoglobin			93010	EKG Int. and Rep			90746	HEP B - HIB	
	99215	Complex Ex.			88174	Pap Smear			11750	Excision Nail			90707	MMR	
PREVENTATIVE MEDICINE - NEW PATIENT					87210	KOH/ Saline Wet Mount			94375	Respiratory Flow Volume			86580	PPD	
	99381	< 1 year old			87430	Strep Antigen			93224	Holter up to 48 hours			90732	Pneumovax	
	99382	1-4 year old			87070	Throat Culture			10060	I & D Abscess Simple			90716	Varicella	
	99383	5-11 year old			80053	Chem profile			10061	I & D Abscess Comp.			82607	Vitamin B12 Inj.	
	99384	12-17 year old			80061	Lipid profile			94761	Oximetry w/Exercise			90712	Polio oral use (OPV)	
	99385	18-39 year old			82465	Cholesterol			94726	Plethysmography			90713	Polio injection (IPV)	
✓	99386	40-64 year old	*$85.*		99000	Handling fee			94760	Pulse Oximetry			90714	Td preservative free 7 yrs +	
	99387	65 + year old		**X-RAY**					11100	Skin Bx			90718	Td 7 years +	
PREVENTATIVE MEDICINE - ESTABLISHED PATIENT					70210	Sinuses			94010	Spirometry			95115	Allergy inj., single	
	99391	< 1 year old			70360	Neck Soft Tissue			99173	Visual Acuity			95117	Allergy inj., multiple	
	99392	1-4 year old			71010	CXR (PA only)			17110	Wart destruction up to 14					
	99393	5-11 year old			71020	Chest 2V			17111	Wart destruction 15 lesions +					
	99394	12-17 year old			72040	C-Spine 2V			11042	Wound Debrid.		**OTHER**			
	99395	18-39 year old			72100	Lumbrosacral									
	99396	40-64 year old			73030	Shoulder 2V									
	99397	65 + year old			73070	Elbow 2V									
					73120	Hand 2V									
					73560	Knee 2V									
					73620	Foot 2V									
					74000	KUB									

DIAGNOSTIC CODES (ICD-9-CM)

☐	Code	Description	☐	Code	Description	☐	Code	Description	☐	Code	Description
	789.0__	Abdominal Pain		564.0	Constipation		784.0	Headache		782.1	Rash or ezanthem
	682.__	Abscess/Cellulitis		692.6	Contact dermatitis due to plants		414.9	Heart Dis., Coronary		714.0	Rheumatoid Arthritis
	995.3	Allergic Reaction		692.9	Contact dermatitis, NOS		599.70	Hematuria	✓	V70.0	Routine general exam
	331	Alzheimer's		V25.09	Contraceptive management		455.6	Hemorrhoids		V76.10	Screen, breast
	285.__	Anemia, other & unspec		923.10	Contusion, forearm		573.3	Hepatitus, NOS		V76.2	Screen, cervix
	280.9	Anemia-iron deficiency		434.91	CVA		V03.81	HIB		V76.44	Screen, prosate
	281.0	Anemia-pernicious		266.2	Deficiency, folic acid B12		V65.44	HIV counseling		V76.47	Screen, vagina
	285.9	Anemia-unspecified		311	Depression		401.1	Hypertension, benign		216.5	Sebaceous cyst
	413.9	Angina, pectoris, oyher/unspecified		250.01	Diabetes, type I, juvenile type		401.9	Hypertension, unspecified		706.2	Sebaceous cyst
	300.00	Anxiety state, NOS		787.91	Diarrhea		401.0	Hypertension, malignant		786.05	Shortness of Breath
	300.4	Anxiety reaction		780.4	Dizziness		V04.81	Influenza		701.9	Skin tag
	716.90	Arthritis, NOS		V06.1	DTP		271.3	Lactose intolerance		845.00	Strain, ankle
	493.20	Asthma; chronic obstruction		V06.3	DTP + polio		573.9	Liver Disease		307.81	Tension headache
	493.00	Asthma; extrinic		536.8	Dyspepsia		724.5	Low Back Pain		V06.5	Tetanus - distheria (Td)
	493.10	Asthma; intrinsic		788.1	Dysuria		346.9	Migraine		305.1	Tobacco dependence
	493.90	Asthmas; unspecified		782.3	Edema		V06.4	MMR		788.41	Urinary frequency
	427.31	Atrial fibulation		530.81	Esophageal reflux		278.01	Obesity/Morbid		599.0	Unrinary tract infection, NOS
	724.5	Backache, unspecified		530.11	Esophagitis reflux		715.90	Osteoarthritis		V05.3	Viral hepatitis
	790.6	Blood chemistry		530.10	Esophagitis, unspecified		719.43	Pain in joint, forearm		368.40	Visual field defect, unspecified
	E906.3	Cat bite		780.6	Fever		625.4	PMS		V20.2	Well Child Exam
	786.50	Chest Pain		789.07	Generalized abdominal pain		486	Pneumonia			
	428.0	CHF		V72.3	Gynecological examiniation		V25.01	Prescription of oral contraceptivess			

DIAGNOSIS: (IF NOT CHECKED ABOVE)		RECEIVED BY:	TODAY'S FEE	*$333.—*
		☐ CASH	AMOUNT RECEIVED	
PROCEDURES: (IF NOT CHECKED ABOVE)	RETURN APPOINTMENT INFORMATION: *appt. 3rd wk of every* (DAYS) (WKS.) ((MOS.)) (PRN)	☐ CREDIT CARD ☐ CHECK # ________	BALANCE	*$333.—*

Figure C.64 Encounter form (Superbill) for Dylan Hill (Appendix A: Day 2).

Goode Medical Clinic
William B. Goode, MD

Patient Registration Information

Account # :
Insurance # :
Co-Payment: $

Please PRINT AND complete ALL sections below!

PATIENT'S PERSONAL INFORMATION Marital Status ☒ Single ❑ Married ❑ Divorced ❑ Widowed Sex: ❑ Male ❑ Female

Name: Hutton (last name) Nancy (first name) (initial)

Street address: 7654 Randelph Ave. (Apt # ____) City: St. Paul State: MN Zip: 55100

Home phone: (555) 555-8826 Work phone: (555) 555-4732 Social Security # 123 - XX - 9046

Date of Birth: 4 (month) / 30 (day) / 60 (year)

Employer / Name of School WITC Community College ☒ Full Time ❑ Part Time

PATIENT'S / RESPONSIBLE PARTY INFORMATION

Responsible party: self Date of Birth:

Relationship to Patient: ☒ Self ❑ Spouse ❑ Other ____ Social Security # ____ - ____ - ____

Responsible party's home phone: (____) see above

Address: see above (Apt # ____) City: ____ State: ____ Zip: ____

Employer's name: WITC Comm. Coll Phone number: (555) 555-4732

Address: 100 Community Lane City: St. Paul State: MN Zip: 55100

Name of Parent/Guardian:

PATIENT'S INSURANCE INFORMATION Please present insurance cards to receptionist.

PRIMARY insurance company's name: First Med

Insurance address: 1324 Insurance Carrier Loop City: Minneapolis State: MN Zip: 55401

Name of insured: self Date of Birth: ____ Relationship to insured: ☒ Self ☐ Spouse ☐ Other ☐ Child

Insurance ID number: 123XX9046 Group number: 89012

Does your insurance cover medication? Yes

EMERGENCY CONTACT

Name of person not living with you: Carrie Hutton Relationship: parent

Address: 4003 Lighthouse Way City: Minneapolis State: MN Zip: 55401

Phone number: (555) 555-1379

Assignment of Benefits • Financial Agreement

I hereby give lifetime authorization for payment of insurance benefits to be made directly to Goode Medical Clinic ,and any assisting physicians, for services rendered. I understand that I am financially responsible for all charges whether or not they are covered by insurance. In the event of default, I agree to pay all costs of collection, and reasonable attorney's fees. I hereby authorize this healthcare provider to release all information necessary to secure the payment of benefits.
I further agree that a photocopy of this agreement shall be as valid as the original.

Date: XX/XX/XXXX Your Signature: Nancy Hutton

FORM # 58-8423 • BIBBERO SYSTEMS, INC.• PETALUMA, CA.• TO ORDER CALL TOLL FREE :800-BIBBERO (800-242-2376) • FAX (800) 242-9330 (REV.7/94)

Figure C.65 Registration form for Nancy Hutton (Appendix A: Day 2).

Goode Medical Clinic

Phone: (555) 555-1234
Fax: (555) 555-5678

1234 Larsen Avenue
Saint Paul, Minnesota 55316

PATIENT NAME	CHART #	DATE		
Nancy Hutton		XX/XX/XXXX	☐ MEDI-MEDI ☐ SELF PAY ☐ MEDICARE	☐ MEDICAL ☒ PRIVATE ☐ HMO___

✓	CPT/Md	DESCRIPTION	FEE
OFFICE VISIT - NEW PATIENT			
	99202	Focused Ex.	
	99203	Detailed Ex.	
	99204	Comprehensive Ex.	
	99205	Complex Ex.	
OFFICE VISIT - ESTABLISHED PATIENT			
	99212	Focused Ex.	
	99213	Expanded Ex.	
	99214	Detailed Ex.	
	99215	Complex Ex.	
PREVENTATIVE MEDICINE - NEW PATIENT			
	99381	< 1 year old	
	99382	1-4 year old	
	99383	5-11 year old	
	99384	12-17 year old	
	99385	18-39 year old	
✓	99386	40-64 year old	$85.
	99387	65 + year old	
PREVENTATIVE MEDICINE - ESTABLISHED PATIENT			
	99391	< 1 year old	
	99392	1-4 year old	
	99393	5-11 year old	
	99394	12-17 year old	
	99395	18-39 year old	
	99396	40-64 year old	
	99397	65 + year old	

✓	CPT/Md	DESCRIPTION	FEE
LAB STUDIES			
	36415	Venipucture	
✓	81000	Urinalysis —1	$78.
	81003	- w/o Micro	
	84703	HCG (Urine, Pregnancy)	
	82948	Glucose	
	82270	Hemoccult	
✓	85025	CBC -diff.	$120.
	85018	Hemoglobin	
	88174	Pap Smear	
	87210	KOH/ Saline Wet Mount	
	87430	Strep Antigen	
	87070	Throat Culture	
	80053	Chem profile	
	80061	Lipid profile	
	82465	Cholesterol	
	99000	Handling fee	
X-RAY			
	70210	Sinuses	
	70360	Neck Soft Tissue	
	71010	CXR (PA only)	
	71020	Chest 2V	
	72040	C-Spine 2V	
	72100	Lumbrosacral	
	73030	Shoulder 2V	
	73070	Elbow 2V	
	73120	Hand 2V	
	73560	Knee 2V	
	73620	Foot 2V	
	74000	KUB	

✓	CPT/Md	DESCRIPTION	FEE
PROCEDURES			
	92551	Audiometry	
	29705	Cast Removal Full Arm/Leg	
	2900_	Casting (by location)	
	92567	Ear Check	
	69210	Ear Wax Rem. 1 2	
✓	93000	EKG ECG	$50.
	93005	EKG tracing only	
	93010	EKG Int. and Rep	
	11750	Excision Nail	
	94375	Respiratory Flow Volume	
	93224	Holter up to 48 hours	
	10060	I & D Abscess Simple	
	10061	I & D Abscess Comp.	
	94761	Oximetry w/Exercise	
	94726	Plethysmography	
	94760	Pulse Oximetry	
	11100	Skin Bx	
	94010	Spirometry	
	99173	Visual Acuity	
	17110	Wart destruction up to 14	
	17111	Wart destruction 15 lesions +	
	11042	Wound Debrid.	

✓	CPT/Md	DESCRIPTION	FEE
INJECTIONS			
	90655	Influenza 6-35 months	
	90656	Influenza 3 years +	
	90732	Pneumoccal	
	J0295	Ampicillin, 1.5 gr	
	J2001	Liocaine for IV infusion 10mg	
	J1885	Toradol 15mg	
	90720	DTP - HIB	
	90746	HEP B - HIB	
	90707	MMR	
	86580	PPD	
	90732	Pneumovax	
	90716	Varicella	
	82607	Vitamin B12 Inj.	
	90712	Polio oral use (OPV)	
	90713	Polio injection (IPV)	
	90714	Td preservative free 7 yrs +	
	90718	Td 7 years +	
	95115	Allergy inj., single	
	95117	Allergy inj., multiple	
OTHER			

DIAGNOSTIC CODES (ICD-9-CM)

✓	Code	Description	✓	Code	Description	✓	Code	Description	✓	Code	Description
	789.0__	Abdominal Pain		564.0	Constipation		784.0	Headache		782.1	Rash or ezanthem
	682.__	Abscess/Cellulitis		692.6	Contact dermatitis due to plants		414.9	Heart Dis., Coronary		714.0	Rheumatoid Arthritis
	995.3	Allergic Reaction		692.9	Contact dermatitis, NOS		599.70	Hematuria	✓	V70.0	Routine general exam
	331	Alzheimer's		V25.09	Contraceptive management		455.6	Hemorrhoids		V76.10	Screen, breast
	285.__	Anemia, other & unspec		923.10	Contusion, forearm		573.3	Hepatitus, NOS		V76.2	Screen, cervix
	280.9	Anemia-iron deficiency		434.91	CVA		V03.81	HIB		V76.44	Screen, prosate
	281.0	Anemia-pernicious		266.2	Deficiency, folic acid B12		V65.44	HIV counseling		V76.47	Screen, vagina
	285.9	Anemia-unspecified		311	Depression		401.1	Hypertension, benign		216.5	Sebaceous cyst
	413.9	Angina, pectoris, oyher/unspecified		250.01	Diabetes, type I, juvenile type		401.9	Hypertension, unspecified		706.2	Sebaceous cyst
	300.00	Anxiety state, NOS		787.91	Diarrhea		401.0	Hypertension, malignant		786.05	Shortness of Breath
	300.4	Anxiety reaction		780.4	Dizziness		V04.81	Influenza		701.9	Skin tag
	716.90	Arthritis, NOS		V06.1	DTP		271.3	Lactose intolerance		845.00	Strain, ankle
	493.20	Asthma; chronic obstruction		V06.3	DTP + polio		573.9	Liver Disease		307.81	Tension headache
	493.00	Asthma; extrinic		536.8	Dyspepsia		724.5	Low Back Pain		V06.5	Tetanus - distheria (Td)
	493.10	Asthma; intrinsic		788.1	Dysuria		346.9	Migraine		305.1	Tobacco dependence
	493.90	Asthmas; unspecified		782.3	Edema		V06.4	MMR		788.41	Urinary frequency
	427.31	Atrial fibulation		530.81	Esophageal reflux		278.01	Obesity/Morbid		599.0	Unrinary tract infection, NOS
	724.5	Backache, unspecified		530.11	Esophagitis reflux		715.90	Osteoarthritis		V05.3	Viral hepatitis
	790.6	Blood chemistry		530.10	Esophagitis, unspecified		719.43	Pain in joint, forearm		368.40	Visual field defect, unspecified
	E906.3	Cat bite		780.6	Fever		625.4	PMS		V20.2	Well Child Exam
	786.50	Chest Pain		789.07	Generalized abdominal pain		486	Pneumonia			
	428.0	CHF		V72.3	Gynecological examiniation		V25.01	Prescription of oral contraceptivess			

DIAGNOSIS: (IF NOT CHECKED ABOVE)		RECEIVED BY:	TODAY'S FEE	$333.—
		☒ CASH	AMOUNT RECEIVED	$20. —
PROCEDURES: (IF NOT CHECKED ABOVE)	RETURN APPOINTMENT INFORMATION: (DAYS) (WKS.) (MOS.) (PRN)	☐ CREDIT CARD ☐ CHECK # ________	BALANCE	$313.—

Figure C.66 Encounter form (Superbill) for Nancy Hutton (Appendix A: Day 2).

Goode Medical Clinic
William B. Goode, MD

Patient Registration Information

Account # : ____
Insurance # : ____
Co-Payment: $ ____

Please PRINT AND complete ALL sections below!

PATIENT'S PERSONAL INFORMATION Marital Status ☐ Single ☐ Married ☒ Divorced ☐ Widowed Sex: ☒ Male ☐ Female

Name: Jones (last name) Robert (first name) ____ (initial)

Street address: 543 Marketplace Rd. (Apt # ____) City: St. Paul State: MN Zip: 55100

Home phone: (555) 555-4567 Work phone: (____) ____ Social Security # 890 - XX - 1234

Date of Birth: 7 (month) / 9 (day) / 43 (year)

Employer / Name of School n/a ☐ Full Time ☐ Part Time

PATIENT'S / RESPONSIBLE PARTY INFORMATION

Responsible party: Self Date of Birth: ____

Relationship to Patient: ☒ Self ☐ Spouse ☐ Other ____ Social Security # ____ - ____ - ____

Responsible party's home phone: (____) see above info.

Address: see above info. (Apt # ____) City: ____ State: ____ Zip: ____

Employer's name: n/a Phone number: (____) ____

Address: ____ City: ____ State: ____ Zip: ____

Name of Parent/Guardian: ____

PATIENT'S INSURANCE INFORMATION Please present insurance cards to receptionist.

PRIMARY insurance company's name: Medicare-Part B

Insurance address: 4502 Wisconsin Ave City: Milwaskee State: MN Zip: 53201

Name of insured: Robert Jones Date of Birth: ____ Relationship to insured: ☒ Self ☐ Spouse ☐ Other ☐ Child

Insurance ID number: 890XX1234 Group number: ____

Does your insurance cover medication? yes

EMERGENCY CONTACT

Name of person not living with you: ____ Relationship: ____

Address: ____ City: ____ State: ____ Zip: ____

Phone number: (____) ____

Assignment of Benefits • Financial Agreement

I hereby give lifetime authorization for payment of insurance benefits to be made directly to Goode Medical Clinic ,and any assisting physicians, for services rendered. I understand that I am financially responsible for all charges whether or not they are covered by insurance. In the event of default, I agree to pay all costs of collection, and reasonable attorney's fees. I hereby authorize this healthcare provider to release all information necessary to secure the payment of benefits.

I further agree that a photocopy of this agreement shall be as valid as the original.

Date: XX/XX/XXXX Your Signature: Robert Jones

FORM # 58-8423 • BIBBERO SYSTEMS, INC.• PETALUMA, CA.• TO ORDER CALL TOLL FREE :800-BIBBERO (800-242-2376) • FAX (800) 242-9330 (REV.7/94)

Figure C.67 Registration form for Robert Jones (Appendix A: Day 2).

Phone: (555) 555-1234
Fax: (555) 555-5678

Goode Medical Clinic
1234 Larsen Avenue
Saint Paul, Minnesota 55316

PATIENT NAME	CHART #	DATE		
Robert Jones		XX/XX/XXXX	☐ MEDI-MEDI ☐ SELF PAY ☒ MEDICARE	☐ MEDICAL ☐ PRIVATE ☐ HMO____

✓	CPT/Md	DESCRIPTION	FEE	✓	CPT/Md	DESCRIPTION	FEE	✓	CPT/Md	DESCRIPTION	FEE	✓	CPT/Md	DESCRIPTION	FEE
OFFICE VISIT - NEW PATIENT				**LAB STUDIES**				**PROCEDURES**				**INJECTIONS**			
	99202	Focused Ex.			36415	Venipuncture			92551	Audiometry			90655	Influenza 6-35 months	
	99203	Detailed Ex.			81000	Urinalysis			29705	Cast Removal Full Arm/Leg			90656	Influenza 3 years +	
✓	99204	Comprehensive Ex.	$100.		81003	- w/o Micro			2900__	Casting (by location)			90732	Pneumoccal	
	99205	Complex Ex.			84703	HCG (Urine, Pregnancy)			92567	Ear Check			J0295	Ampicillin, 1.5 gr	
OFFICE VISIT - ESTABLISHED PATIENT					82948	Glucose			69210	Ear Wax Rem. 1 2			J2001	Liocaine for IV infusion 10mg	
	99212	Focused Ex.			82270	Hemoccult		✓	93000	EKG /ECG	$50.		J1885	Toradol 15mg	
	99213	Expanded Ex.			85025	CBC -diff.			93005	EKG tracing only			90720	DTP - HIB	
	99214	Detailed Ex.			85018	Hemoglobin			93010	EKG Int. and Rep			90746	HEP B - HIB	
	99215	Complex Ex.			88174	Pap Smear			11750	Excision Nail			90707	MMR	
PREVENTATIVE MEDICINE - NEW PATIENT					87210	KOH/ Saline Wet Mount			94375	Respiratory Flow Volume			86580	PPD	
	99381	< 1 year old			87430	Strep Antigen			93224	Holter up to 48 hours			90732	Pneumovax	
	99382	1-4 year old			87070	Throat Culture			10060	I & D Abscess Simple			90716	Varicella	
	99383	5-11 year old			80053	Chem profile			10061	I & D Abscess Comp.			82607	Vitamin B12 Inj.	
	99384	12-17 year old			80061	Lipid profile			94761	Oximetry w/Exercise			90712	Polio oral use (OPV)	
	99385	18-39 year old			82465	Cholesterol			94726	Plethysmography			90713	Polio injection (IPV)	
	99386	40-64 year old			99000	Handling fee			94760	Pulse Oximetry			90714	Td preservative free 7 yrs +	
	99387	65 + year old		**X-RAY**					11100	Skin Bx			90718	Td 7 years +	
PREVENTATIVE MEDICINE - ESTABLISHED PATIENT					70210	Sinuses			94010	Spirometry			95115	Allergy inj., single	
	99391	< 1 year old			70360	Neck Soft Tissue			99173	Visual Acuity			95117	Allergy inj., multiple	
	99392	1-4 year old			71010	CXR (PA only)			17110	Wart destruction up to 14					
	99393	5-11 year old			71020	Chest 2V			17111	Wart destruction 15 lesions +					
	99394	12-17 year old			72040	C-Spine 2V			11042	Wound Debrid.		**OTHER**			
	99395	18-39 year old			72100	Lumbrosacral									
	99396	40-64 year old			73030	Shoulder 2V									
	99397	65 + year old			73070	Elbow 2V									
					73120	Hand 2V									
					73560	Knee 2V									
					73620	Foot 2V									
					74000	KUB									

DIAGNOSTIC CODES (ICD-9-CM)

✓	Code	Description	✓	Code	Description	✓	Code	Description	✓	Code	Description
	789.0__	Abdominal Pain		564.0	Constipation		784.0	Headache		782.1	Rash or ezanthem
	682.__	Abscess/Cellulitis		692.6	Contact dermatitis due to plants		414.9	Heart Dis., Coronary		714.0	Rheumatoid Arthritis
	995.3	Allergic Reaction		692.9	Contact dermatitis, NOS		599.70	Hematuria		V70.0	Routine general exam
	331	Alzheimer's		V25.09	Contraceptive management		455.6	Hemorrhoids		V76.10	Screen, breast
	285.__	Anemia, other & unspec		923.10	Contusion, forearm		573.3	Hepatitus, NOS		V76.2	Screen, cervix
	280.9	Anemia-iron deficiency		434.91	CVA		V03.81	HIB		V76.44	Screen, prosate
	281.0	Anemia-pernicious		266.2	Deficiency, folic acid B12		V65.44	HIV counseling		V76.47	Screen, vagina
	285.9	Anemia-unspecified		311	Depression		401.1	Hypertension, benign		216.5	Sebaceous cyst
	413.9	Angina, pectoris, oyher/unspecified		250.01	Diabetes, type I, juvenile type		401.9	Hypertension, unspecified		706.2	Sebaceous cyst
	300.00	Anxiety state, NOS		787.91	Diarrhea		401.0	Hypertension, malignant		786.05	Shortness of Breath
	300.4	Anxiety reaction		780.4	Dizziness		V04.81	Influenza		701.9	Skin tag
	716.90	Arthritis, NOS		V06.1	DTP		271.3	Lactose intolerance		845.00	Strain, ankle
	493.20	Asthma; chronic obstruction		V06.3	DTP + polio		573.9	Liver Disease		307.81	Tension headache
	493.00	Asthma; extrinic		536.8	Dyspepsia		724.5	Low Back Pain		V06.5	Tetanus - distheria (Td)
	493.10	Asthma; intrinsic		788.1	Dysuria		346.9	Migraine		305.1	Tobacco dependence
	493.90	Asthmas; unspecified		782.3	Edema		V06.4	MMR		788.41	Urinary frequency
	427.31	Atrial fibulation		530.81	Esophageal reflux		278.01	Obesity/Morbid		599.0	Unrinary tract infection, NOS
	724.5	Backache, unspecified		530.11	Esophagitis reflux		715.90	Osteoarthritis		V05.3	Viral hepatitis
	790.6	Blood chemistry		530.10	Esophagitis, unspecified		719.43	Pain in joint, forearm		368.40	Visual field defect, unspecified
	E906.3	Cat bite		780.6	Fever		625.4	PMS		V20.2	Well Child Exam
✓	786.50	Chest Pain		789.07	Generalized abdominal pain		486	Pneumonia			
	428.0	CHF		V72.3	Gynecological examiniation		V25.01	Prescription of oral contraceptivess			

DIAGNOSIS: (IF NOT CHECKED ABOVE)		RECEIVED BY:	TODAY'S FEE	$150.—
786.59 Chest pain pressure, tightness ↗ use this code		☐ CASH ☐ CREDIT CARD ☐ CHECK # ________	AMOUNT RECEIVED	——
PROCEDURES: (IF NOT CHECKED ABOVE)	RETURN APPOINTMENT INFORMATION: (DAYS) (WKS.) (MOS.) (PRN)		BALANCE	$150.00

Figure C.68 Encounter form (Superbill) for Robert Jones (Appendix A: Day 2).

Goode Medical Clinic
William B. Goode, MD

Patient Registration Information

Account # :
Insurance # :
Co-Payment: $

Please PRINT AND complete ALL sections below!

PATIENT'S PERSONAL INFORMATION Marital Status ☒ Single ☐ Married ☐ Divorced ☐ Widowed Sex: ☒ Male ☐ Female

Name: Paul (last name) Sammy (first name) ___ (initial)

Street address: 234 Hardy Drive (Apt # ___) City: St. Paul State: MN Zip: 55100

Home phone: (555) 555-2203 Work phone: (___) ___ Social Security # 789 - XX - 0123

Date of Birth: 5 (month) / 13 (day) / 1997 (year)

Employer / Name of School ___ ☐ Full Time ☐ Part Time

PATIENT'S / RESPONSIBLE PARTY INFORMATION

Responsible party: John Paul Date of Birth: 8/29/72

Relationship to Patient: ☐ Self ☐ Spouse ☒ Other Parent Social Security # 150 - XX - 6674

Responsible party's home phone: (___) same as above

Address: ___ (Apt # ___) City: ___ State: ___ Zip: ___

Employer's name: Music Records, Inc. Phone number: (555) 555-6000

Address: 901 80th Street City: St. Paul State: MN Zip: 55100

Name of Parent/Guardian: John and Debbie Paul

PATIENT'S INSURANCE INFORMATION Please present insurance cards to receptionist.

PRIMARY insurance company's name: Blue Cross/Blue Shield

Insurance address: 1355 Insurance Carrier Loop City: Minneapolis State: MN Zip: 55401

Name of insured: John Paul Date of Birth: 8/29/72 Relationship to insured: ☐ Self ☐ Spouse ☐ Other ☒ Child

Insurance ID number: SP-4567-MR Group number: 90123

Does your insurance cover medication? Yes

EMERGENCY CONTACT

Name of person ~~not~~ living with you: Debbie Paul Relationship: mother

Address: see above City: ___ State: ___ Zip: ___

Phone number: (555) 555-2203 or (555) 555-1316 (wk)

Assignment of Benefits • Financial Agreement

I hereby give lifetime authorization for payment of insurance benefits to be made directly to Goode Medical Clinic ,and any assisting physicians, for services rendered. I understand that I am financially responsible for all charges whether or not they are covered by insurance. In the event of default, I agree to pay all costs of collection, and reasonable attorney's fees. I hereby authorize this healthcare provider to release all information necessary to secure the payment of benefits.
I further agree that a photocopy of this agreement shall be as valid as the original.

Date: XX/XX/XXXX Your Signature: Debbie Paul

FORM # 58-8423 • BIBBERO SYSTEMS, INC.• PETALUMA, CA.• TO ORDER CALL TOLL FREE :800-BIBBERO (800-242-2376) • FAX (800) 242-9330 (REV.7/94)

Figure C.69 Registration form for Sammy Paul (Appendix A: Day 2).

Goode Medical Clinic
1234 Larsen Avenue
Saint Paul, Minnesota 55316

Phone: (555) 555-1234
Fax: (555) 555-5678

PATIENT NAME	CHART #	DATE		
Sammy Paul		XX/XX/XXXX	☐ MEDI-MEDI ☐ SELF PAY ☐ MEDICARE	☒ MEDICAL ☐ PRIVATE ☐ HMO___

✓	CPT/Md	DESCRIPTION	FEE	✓	CPT/Md	DESCRIPTION	FEE	✓	CPT/Md	DESCRIPTION	FEE	✓	CPT/Md	DESCRIPTION	FEE
OFFICE VISIT - NEW PATIENT				**LAB STUDIES**				**PROCEDURES**				**INJECTIONS**			
√	99202	Focused Ex.	$60.		36415	Venipucture			92551	Audiometry			90655	Influenza 6-35 months	
	99203	Detailed Ex.			81000	Urinalysis			29705	Cast Removal Full Arm/Leg			90656	Influenza 3 years +	
	99204	Comprehensive Ex.			81003	- w/o Micro			2900__	Casting (by location)			90732	Pneumoccal	
	99205	Complex Ex.			84703	HCG (Urine, Pregnancy)			92567	Ear Check			J0295	Ampicillin, 1.5 gr	
OFFICE VISIT - ESTABLISHED PATIENT					82948	Glucose			69210	Ear Wax Rem. 1 2			J2001	Liocaine for IV infusion 10mg	
	99212	Focused Ex.			82270	Hemoccult			93000	EKG			J1885	Toradol 15mg	
	99213	Expanded Ex.			85025	CBC -diff.			93005	EKG tracing only			90720	DTP - HIB	
	99214	Detailed Ex.			85018	Hemoglobin			93010	EKG Int. and Rep			90746	HEP B - HIB	
	99215	Complex Ex.			88174	Pap Smear			11750	Excision Nail			90707	MMR	
PREVENTATIVE MEDICINE - NEW PATIENT					87210	KOH/ Saline Wet Mount			94375	Respiratory Flow Volume			86580	PPD	
	99381	< 1 year old			87430	Strep Antigen			93224	Holter up to 48 hours			90732	Pneumovax	
	99382	1-4 year old			87070	Throat Culture			10060	I & D Abscess Simple			90716	Varicella	
	99383	5-11 year old			80053	Chem profile			10061	I & D Abscess Comp.			82607	Vitamin B12 Inj.	
	99384	12-17 year old			80061	Lipid profile			94761	Oximetry w/Exercise			90712	Polio oral use (OPV)	
	99385	18-39 year old			82465	Cholesterol			94726	Plethysmography			90713	Polio injection (IPV)	
	99386	40-64 year old			99000	Handling fee			94760	Pulse Oximetry			90714	Td preservative free 7 yrs +	
	99387	65 + year old		**X-RAY**					11100	Skin Bx			90718	Td 7 years +	
PREVENTATIVE MEDICINE - ESTABLISHED PATIENT					70210	Sinuses			94010	Spirometry			95115	Allergy inj., single	
	99391	< 1 year old			70360	Neck Soft Tissue			99173	Visual Acuity			95117	Allergy inj., multiple	
	99392	1-4 year old			71010	CXR (PA only)			17110	Wart destruction up to 14					
	99393	5-11 year old			71020	Chest 2V			17111	Wart destruction 15 lesions +					
	99394	12-17 year old			72040	C-Spine 2V			11042	Wound Debrid.		**OTHER**			
	99395	18-39 year old			72100	Lumbrosacral									
	99396	40-64 year old			73030	Shoulder 2V									
	99397	65 + year old			73070	Elbow 2V									
					73120	Hand 2V									
					73560	Knee 2V									
					73620	Foot 2V									
					74000	KUB									

DIAGNOSTIC CODES (ICD-9-CM)

	Code	Description		Code	Description		Code	Description		Code	Description
	789.0__	Abdominal Pain		564.0	Constipation		784.0	Headache		782.1	Rash or ezanthem
	682.__	Abscess/Cellulitis		692.6	Contact dermatitis due to plants		414.9	Heart Dis., Coronary		714.0	Rheumatoid Arthritis
	995.3	Allergic Reaction		692.9	Contact dermatitis, NOS		599.70	Hematuria		V70.0	Routine general exam
	331	Alzheimer's		V25.09	Contraceptive management		455.6	Hemorrhoids		V76.10	Screen, breast
	285.__	Anemia, other & unspec		923.10	Contusion, forearm		573.3	Hepatitus, NOS		V76.2	Screen, cervix
	280.9	Anemia-iron deficiency		434.91	CVA		V03.81	HIB		V76.44	Screen, prosate
	281.0	Anemia-pernicious		266.2	Deficiency, folic acid B12		V65.44	HIV counseling		V76.47	Screen, vagina
	285.9	Anemia-unspecified		311	Depression		401.1	Hypertension, benign		216.5	Sebaceous cyst
	413.9	Angina, pectoris, oyher/unspecified		250.01	Diabetes, type I, juvenile type		401.9	Hypertension, unspecified		706.2	Sebaceous cyst
	300.00	Anxiety state, NOS		787.91	Diarrhea		401.0	Hypertension, malignant		786.05	Shortness of Breath
	300.4	Anxiety reaction		780.4	Dizziness		V04.81	Influenza		701.9	Skin tag
	716.90	Arthritis, NOS		V06.1	DTP		271.3	Lactose intolerance		845.00	Strain, ankle
	493.20	Asthma; chronic obstruction		V06.3	DTP + polio		573.9	Liver Disease		307.81	Tension headache
	493.00	Asthma; extrinic		536.8	Dyspepsia		724.5	Low Back Pain		V06.5	Tetanus - distheria (Td)
	493.10	Asthma; intrinsic		788.1	Dysuria		346.9	Migraine		305.1	Tobacco dependence
	493.90	Asthmas; unspecified		782.3	Edema		V06.4	MMR		788.41	Urinary frequency
	427.31	Atrial fibulation		530.81	Esophageal reflux		278.01	Obesity/Morbid		599.0	Unrinary tract infection, NOS
	724.5	Backache, unspecified		530.11	Esophagitis reflux		715.90	Osteoarthritis		V05.3	Viral hepatitis
	790.6	Blood chemistry		530.10	Esophagitis, unspecified		719.43	Pain in joint, forearm		368.40	Visual field defect, unspecified
	E906.3	Cat bite		780.6	Fever		625.4	PMS		V20.2	Well Child Exam
	786.50	Chest Pain		789.07	Generalized abdominal pain		486	Pneumonia			
	428.0	CHF		V72.3	Gynecological examiniation		V25.01	Prescription of oral contraceptivess			

DIAGNOSIS: (IF NOT CHECKED ABOVE)		RECEIVED BY:	TODAY'S FEE	$60.—
Otitis externa, infective (380.10)		☐ CASH	AMOUNT RECEIVED	——
PROCEDURES: (IF NOT CHECKED ABOVE)	RETURN APPOINTMENT INFORMATION:	☐ CREDIT CARD ☐ CHECK		
	(DAYS) (WKS.) (MOS.) (PRN)	# ________	BALANCE	$60.—

Figure C.70 Encounter form (Superbill) for Sammy Paul (Appendix A: Day 2).

Goode Medical Clinic
William B. Goode, MD

Patient Registration Information

Account # :
Insurance # :
Co-Payment: $

Please PRINT AND complete ALL sections below!

PATIENT'S PERSONAL INFORMATION Marital Status ☒ Single ☐ Married ☐ Divorced ☐ Widowed Sex: ☒ Male ☐ Female

Name: Smith (last name) Danny (first name) (initial)
Street address: 4567 Hamline Ave. (Apt #) City: St. Paul State: MN Zip: 55100
Home phone: (555) 555-8901 Work phone: ( ) Social Security # 185-XX-8996
Date of Birth: 07 (month) / 12 (day) / 1999 (year)
Employer / Name of School ☐ Full Time ☐ Part Time

PATIENT'S / RESPONSIBLE PARTY INFORMATION

Responsible party: Doug Smith Date of Birth: 12/04/1969
Relationship to Patient: ☐ Self ☐ Spouse ☒ Other parent Social Security # 201-XX-6653
Responsible party's home phone: ( ) see above
Address: (Apt #) City: State: Zip:
Employer's name: Movie Producers Phone number: (555) 555-1908
Address: 500 Warehouse Street City: Minneapolis State: MN Zip: 55111
Name of Parent/Guardian: Doug and Ann Smith

PATIENT'S INSURANCE INFORMATION Please present insurance cards to receptionist.

PRIMARY insurance company's name: Blue Cross and Blue Shield
Insurance address: 1355 Insurance Carrier Loop City: Minneapolis State: MN Zip: 55401
Name of insured: Doug Smith Date of Birth: 12/4/69 Relationship to insured: ☐ Self ☐ Spouse ☐ Other ☒ Child
Insurance ID number: DS-0123-MP Group number: 67890
Does your insurance cover medication? Yes

EMERGENCY CONTACT

Name of person not living with you: Doug Smith Relationship: father
Address: see above City: State: Zip:
Phone number: (555) 555-1119 (cell phone)

Assignment of Benefits • Financial Agreement

I hereby give lifetime authorization for payment of insurance benefits to be made directly to Goode Medical Clinic, and any assisting physicians, for services rendered. I understand that I am financially responsible for all charges whether or not they are covered by insurance. In the event of default, I agree to pay all costs of collection, and reasonable attorney's fees. I hereby authorize this healthcare provider to release all information necessary to secure the payment of benefits.
I further agree that a photocopy of this agreement shall be as valid as the original.

Date: XX/XX/XXXX Your Signature: Doug Smith

FORM # 58-8423 • BIBBERO SYSTEMS, INC.• PETALUMA, CA.• TO ORDER CALL TOLL FREE :800-BIBBERO (800-242-2376) • FAX (800) 242-9330 (REV.7/94)

Figure C.71 Registration form for Danny Smith (Appendix A: Day 3).

Goode Medical Clinic

1234 Larsen Avenue
Saint Paul, Minnesota 55316

Phone: (555) 555-1234
Fax: (555) 555-5678

PATIENT NAME	CHART #	DATE		
Danny Smith		*XX/XX/XXXX*	☐ MEDI-MEDI ☐ SELF PAY ☐ MEDICARE	☒ MEDICAL ☐ PRIVATE ☐ HMO____

✓	CPT/Md	DESCRIPTION	FEE	✓	CPT/Md	DESCRIPTION	FEE	✓	CPT/Md	DESCRIPTION	FEE	✓	CPT/Md	DESCRIPTION	FEE
OFFICE VISIT - NEW PATIENT				**LAB STUDIES**				**PROCEDURES**				**INJECTIONS**			
	99202	Focused Ex.			36415	Venipucture			92551	Audiometry			90655	Influenza 6-35 months	
√	99203	Detailed Ex.	*$80.00*		81000	Urinalysis			29705	Cast Removal Full Arm/Leg			90656	Influenza 3 years +	
	99204	Comprehensive Ex.			81003	- w/o Micro			2900__	Casting (by location)			90732	Pneumoccal	
	99205	Complex Ex.			84703	HCG (Urine, Pregnancy)			92567	Ear Check			J0295	Ampicillin, 1.5 gr	
OFFICE VISIT - ESTABLISHED PATIENT					82948	Glucose			69210	Ear Wax Rem. 1 2			J2001	Liocaine for IV infusion 10mg	
	99212	Focused Ex.			82270	Hemoccult			93000	EKG			J1885	Toradol 15mg	
	99213	Expanded Ex.			85025	CBC -diff.			93005	EKG tracing only			90720	DTP - HIB	
	99214	Detailed Ex.			85018	Hemoglobin			93010	EKG Int. and Rep			90746	HEP B - HIB	
	99215	Complex Ex.			88174	Pap Smear			11750	Excision Nail			90707	MMR	
PREVENTATIVE MEDICINE - NEW PATIENT					87210	KOH/ Saline Wet Mount			94375	Respiratory Flow Volume			86580	PPD	
	99381	< 1 year old			87430	Strep Antigen			93224	Holter up to 48 hours			90732	Pneumovax	
	99382	1-4 year old			87070	Throat Culture			10060	I & D Abscess Simple			90716	Varicella	
	99383	5-11 year old			80053	Chem profile			10061	I & D Abscess Comp.			82607	Vitamin B12 Inj.	
	99384	12-17 year old			80061	Lipid profile			94761	Oximetry w/Exercise			90712	Polio oral use (OPV)	
	99385	18-39 year old			82465	Cholesterol			94726	Plethysmography			90713	Polio injection (IPV)	
	99386	40-64 year old			99000	Handling fee			94760	Pulse Oximetry			90714	Td preservative free 7 yrs +	
	99387	65 + year old		**X-RAY**					11100	Skin Bx			90718	Td 7 years +	
PREVENTATIVE MEDICINE - ESTABLISHED PATIENT					70210	Sinuses			94010	Spirometry			95115	Allergy inj., single	
	99391	< 1 year old			70360	Neck Soft Tissue			99173	Visual Acuity			95117	Allergy inj., multiple	
	99392	1-4 year old			71010	CXR (PA only)			17110	Wart destruction up to 14					
	99393	5-11 year old			71020	Chest 2V			17111	Wart destruction 15 lesions +					
	99394	12-17 year old			72040	C-Spine 2V			11042	Wound Debrid.			**OTHER**		
	99395	18-39 year old			72100	Lumbrosacral									
	99396	40-64 year old			73030	Shoulder 2V									
	99397	65 + year old			73070	Elbow 2V									
					73120	Hand 2V									
					73560	Knee 2V									
					73620	Foot 2V									
					74000	KUB									

DIAGNOSTIC CODES (ICD-9-CM)

✓	Code	Description	✓	Code	Description	✓	Code	Description	✓	Code	Description
	789.0__	Abdominal Pain		564.0	Constipation		784.0	Headache		782.1	Rash or ezanthem
	682.__	Abscess/Cellulitis		692.6	Contact dermatitis due to plants		414.9	Heart Dis., Coronary		714.0	Rheumatoid Arthritis
	995.3	Allergic Reaction		692.9	Contact dermatitis, NOS		599.70	Hematuria		V70.0	Routine general exam
	331	Alzheimer's		V25.09	Contraceptive management		455.6	Hemorrhoids		V76.10	Screen, breast
	285.__	Anemia, other & unspec		923.10	Contusion, forearm		573.3	Hepatitus, NOS		V76.2	Screen, cervix
	280.9	Anemia-iron deficiency		434.91	CVA		V03.81	HIB		V76.44	Screen, prosate
	281.0	Anemia-pernicious		266.2	Deficiency, folic acid B12		V65.44	HIV counseling		V76.47	Screen, vagina
	285.9	Anemia-unspecified		311	Depression		401.1	Hypertension, benign		216.5	Sebaceous cyst
	413.9	Angina, pectoris, oyher/unspecified		250.01	Diabetes, type I, juvenile type		401.9	Hypertension, unspecified		706.2	Sebaceous cyst
	300.00	Anxiety state, NOS		787.91	Diarrhea		401.0	Hypertension, malignant		786.05	Shortness of Breath
	300.4	Anxiety reaction		780.4	Dizziness		V04.81	Influenza		701.9	Skin tag
	716.90	Arthritis, NOS		V06.1	DTP		271.3	Lactose intolerance		845.00	Strain, ankle
	493.20	Asthma; chronic obstruction		V06.3	DTP + polio		573.9	Liver Disease		307.81	Tension headache
	493.00	Asthma; extrinic		536.8	Dyspepsia		724.5	Low Back Pain		V06.5	Tetanus - distheria (Td)
	493.10	Asthma; intrinsic		788.1	Dysuria		346.9	Migraine		305.1	Tobacco dependence
	493.90	Asthmas; unspecified		782.3	Edema		V06.4	MMR		788.41	Urinary frequency
	427.31	Atrial fibulation		530.81	Esophageal reflux		278.01	Obesity/Morbid		599.0	Unrinary tract infection, NOS
	724.5	Backache, unspecified		530.11	Esophagitis reflux		715.90	Osteoarthritis		V05.3	Viral hepatitis
	790.6	Blood chemistry		530.10	Esophagitis, unspecified		719.43	Pain in joint, forearm		368.40	Visual field defect, unspecified
	E906.3	Cat bite		780.6	Fever		625.4	PMS		V20.2	Well Child Exam
	786.50	Chest Pain		789.07	Generalized abdominal pain		486	Pneumonia			
	428.0	CHF		V72.3	Gynecological examiniation		V25.01	Prescription of oral contraceptivess			

DIAGNOSIS: (IF NOT CHECKED ABOVE)
932 Penny up nostril (right)

PROCEDURES: (IF NOT CHECKED ABOVE)

RETURN APPOINTMENT INFORMATION:
follow-up in
(*2* DAYS) (WKS.) (MOS.) (PRN)

RECEIVED BY:
☐ CASH
☐ CREDIT CARD
☐ CHECK
\# __________

TODAY'S FEE	*$80.—*
AMOUNT RECEIVED	*——*
BALANCE	*$80.—*

Figure C.72 Encounter form (Superbill) for Danny Smith (Appendix A: Day 3).

BCBS of MN
1355 Insurance Carrier Loop
Minneapolis, MN 55111
(763)555-0426

Remittance advice

Goode Medical Clinic
1612 Southwest Blvd.
St. Paul, MN 55100

Page: 1 of 1
Date: XX/XX/XX
Group Practice ID#: 567XX
Check number: 345678

Patient name	DOS	Procedure code	Units	Total charge	Allowable	Provider responsibility	Co-pay	Amount paid
Cross, Raymond	02/04/2013	99386	1	85.00	31.50	53.50	0	31.50
	02/04/2013	93000	1	50.00	27.00	23.00	0	27.00
	02/04/2013	81001	1	78.00	43.00	35.00	0	43.00
	02/04/2013	85023	1	120.00	50.00	70.00	0	50.00
Jackson, Debra	02/04/2013	99385	1	85.00	36.00	49.00	10.00	26.00
	02/04/2013	93000	1	50.00	27.00	23.00	0	27.00
	02/04/2013	81001	1	78.00	43.00	35.00	0	43.00
	02/04/2013	85023	1	120.00	50.00	70.00	0	50.00
Carter, Tiffany	02/04/2013	99203	1	80.00	76.00	4.00	10.00	66.00
Stone, Lynn	02/05/2013	99203	1	80.00	76.00	4.00	0	76.00
Paul, Sammy	02/05/2013	99202	1	60.00	56.00	4.00	0	56.00

Total charges $886.00 Total provider responsibility $370.50 Total co-pay $20.00 Total paid $495.50

Figure C.73 Remittance Advice—Blue Cross and Blue Shield (Appendix A: Day 4).

First Med EGHP Claims
1324 Insurance Carrier Loop
Minneapolis, MN 55111
(763) 345-9124

Remittance advice

Page: 1 of 1
Date: XX/XX/XX
Group Practice ID#: 567XX
Check number: 890123

Goode Medical Clinic
1612 Southwest Blvd.
St. Paul, MN 55100

Patient name	DOS	Procedure code	Units	Total charge	Allowable	Provider responsibility	Co-pay	Amount paid
Mann, Cindy	02/05/2013	99203	1	80.00	76.00	4.00	0	76.00
Hill, Dylan	02/05/2013	99386	1	85.00	31.50	53.50	0	31.50
	02/05/2013	93000	1	50.00	27.00	23.00	0	27.00
	02/05/2013	81001	1	78.00	43.00	35.00	0	43.00
	02/05/2013	85023	1	120.00	50.00	70.00	0	50.00
Hutton, Nancy	02/05/2013	99386	1	85.00	31.50	53.50	20.00	11.50
	02/05/2013	93000	1	50.00	27.00	23.00	0	27.00
	02/05/2013	81001	1	78.00	43.00	35.00	0	43.00
	02/05/2013	85023	1	120.00	50.00	70.00	0	50.00

Total charges $746.00 Total provider responsibility $367.00 Total co-pay 0 Total paid $359.00

Figure C.74 Remittance Advice—First Med Insurance (Appendix A: Day 4).

Goode Medical Clinic
William B. Goode, MD

Patient Registration Information

Account # : ________
Insurance # : ________
Co-Payment: $ ________

Please PRINT AND complete ALL sections below!

PATIENT'S PERSONAL INFORMATION Marital Status ☒ Single ☐ Married ☐ Divorced ☐ Widowed Sex: ☒ Male ☐ Female

Name: Johnson (last name) Mike (first name) ____ (initial)

Street address: 200 Penny Lane (Apt # ____) City: Grove State: MN Zip: 55102

Home phone: (555) 555-1297 Work phone: (555) 555-3344 Social Security # 901 - XX - 2354

Date of Birth: 7 (month) / 23 (day) / 56 (year)

Employer / Name of School Dept. of Transportation, MN. ☒ Full Time ☐ Part Time

PATIENT'S / RESPONSIBLE PARTY INFORMATION

Responsible party: me Date of Birth: ________

Relationship to Patient: ☒ Self ☐ Spouse ☐ Other ________ Social Security # ____-____-____

Responsible party's home phone: (____) see above info.

Address: ________ (Apt # ____) City: ________ State: ____ Zip: ____

Employer's name: State of Minnesota, DOT Phone number: (555) XXX-7168

Address: ________ City: ________ State: ____ Zip: ____

Name of Parent/Guardian: ________

PATIENT'S INSURANCE INFORMATION Please present insurance cards to receptionist.

PRIMARY insurance company's name: Blue Cross/Blue Shield

Insurance address: 1355 Insurance Carrier Loop City: Minneapolis State: MN Zip: 55401

Name of insured: me Date of Birth: ________ Relationship to insured: ☒ Self ☐ Spouse ☐ Other ☐ Child

Insurance ID number: MJ-0123-MN Group number: 63251

Does your insurance cover medication? yes

EMERGENCY CONTACT

Name of person not living with you: James Carter Relationship: friend

Address: 603 State Road, #3A City: St. Paul State: MN Zip: 55100

Phone number: (555) 555-7713

Assignment of Benefits • Financial Agreement

I hereby give lifetime authorization for payment of insurance benefits to be made directly to Goode Medical Clinic ,and any assisting physicians, for services rendered. I understand that I am financially responsible for all charges whether or not they are covered by insurance. In the event of default, I agree to pay all costs of collection, and reasonable attorney's fees. I hereby authorize this healthcare provider to release all information necessary to secure the payment of benefits.

I further agree that a photocopy of this agreement shall be as valid as the original.

Date: XX/XX/XXXX Your Signature: Mike Johnson

FORM # 58-8423 • BIBBERO SYSTEMS, INC.• PETALUMA, CA.• TO ORDER CALL TOLL FREE :800-BIBBERO (800-242-2376) • FAX (800) 242-9330 (REV.7/94)

Figure C.75 Registration form for Mike Johnson (Appendix A: Day 4).

Goode Medical Clinic
William B. Goode, MD

Patient Registration Information

Account # :
Insurance # :
Co-Payment: $

Please PRINT AND complete ALL sections below!

PATIENT'S PERSONAL INFORMATION Marital Status ❑ Single ❑ Married ❑ Divorced ☒ Widowed Sex: ❑ Male ☒ Female

Name: Taylor (last name) Lynn (first name) (initial)

Street address: 900 Craft Street (Apt #) City: St. Paul State: MN Zip: 55100

Home phone: (555) 555-5562 Work phone: ( ) Social Security # 165 - XX - 6369

Date of Birth: 11 (month) / 7 (day) / 36 (year)

Employer / Name of School ❑ Full Time ❑ Part Time

PATIENT'S / RESPONSIBLE PARTY INFORMATION

Responsible party: self Date of Birth:

Relationship to Patient: ☒ Self ❑ Spouse ❑ Other Social Security # - -

Responsible party's home phone: ( ) see above

Address: (Apt #) City: State: Zip:

Employer's name: n/a Phone number:( )

Address: City: State: Zip:

Name of Parent/Guardian:

PATIENT'S INSURANCE INFORMATION Please present insurance cards to receptionist.

PRIMARY insurance company's name: Medicare-Part B

Insurance address: 4502 Wisconsin Ave City: Milwaukee State: MN Zip: 53201

Name of insured: Lynn Taylor Date of Birth: Relationship to insured: ☒ Self ☐ Spouse ☐ Other ☐ Child

Insurance ID number: 165XX6369 CA Group number:

Does your insurance cover medication? Yes

EMERGENCY CONTACT

Name of person not living with you: Mary Smith Relationship: friend

Address: 902 Craft Street City: St. Paul State: MN Zip: 55100

Phone number: (555) 555-0842

Assignment of Benefits • Financial Agreement

I hereby give lifetime authorization for payment of insurance benefits to be made directly to Goode Medical Clinic ,and any assisting physicians, for services rendered. I understand that I am financially responsible for all charges whether or not they are covered by insurance. In the event of default, I agree to pay all costs of collection, and reasonable attorney's fees. I hereby authorize this healthcare provider to release all information necessary to secure the payment of benefits.
I further agree that a photocopy of this agreement shall be as valid as the original.

Date: XX/XX/XXXX Your Signature: Lynn Taylor

FORM # 58-8423 • BIBBERO SYSTEMS, INC.• PETALUMA, CA.• TO ORDER CALL TOLL FREE :800-BIBBERO (800-242-2376) • FAX (800) 242-9330 (REV.7/94)

Figure C.76 Registration form for Lynn Taylor (Appendix A: Day 4).

Goode Medical Clinic

1234 Larsen Avenue
Saint Paul, Minnesota 55316

Phone: (555) 555-1234
Fax: (555) 555-5678

PATIENT NAME	CHART #	DATE		
Lynn Taylor		*XX/XX/XXXX*	☐ MEDI-MEDI ☒ SELF PAY ☒ MEDICARE	☐ MEDICAL ☐ PRIVATE ☐ HMO____

✓	CPT/Md	DESCRIPTION	FEE	✓	CPT/Md	DESCRIPTION	FEE	✓	CPT/Md	DESCRIPTION	FEE	✓	CPT/Md	DESCRIPTION	FEE
OFFICE VISIT - NEW PATIENT				**LAB STUDIES**				**PROCEDURES**				**INJECTIONS**			
	99202	Focused Ex.			36415	Venipucture			92551	Audiometry			90655	Influenza 6-35 months	
✓	99203	Detailed Ex.	*$80.*		81000	Urinalysis			29705	Cast Removal Full Arm/Leg			90656	Influenza 3 years +	
	99204	Comprehensive Ex.			81003	- w/o Micro			2900__	Casting (by location)			90732	Pneumoccal	
	99205	Complex Ex.			84703	HCG (Urine, Pregnancy)			92567	Ear Check			J0295	Ampicillin, 1.5 gr	
OFFICE VISIT - ESTABLISHED PATIENT					82948	Glucose			69210	Ear Wax Rem. 1 2			J2001	Liocaine for IV infusion 10mg	
	99212	Focused Ex.			82270	Hemoccult			93000	EKG			J1885	Toradol 15mg	
	99213	Expanded Ex.			85025	CBC -diff.			93005	EKG tracing only			90720	DTP - HIB	
	99214	Detailed Ex.			85018	Hemoglobin			93010	EKG Int. and Rep			90746	HEP B - HIB	
	99215	Complex Ex.			88174	Pap Smear			11750	Excision Nail			90707	MMR	
PREVENTATIVE MEDICINE - NEW PATIENT					87210	KOH/ Saline Wet Mount			94375	Respiratory Flow Volume			86580	PPD	
	99381	< 1 year old			87430	Strep Antigen			93224	Holter up to 48 hours			90732	Pneumovax	
	99382	1-4 year old			87070	Throat Culture			10060	I & D Abscess Simple			90716	Varicella	
	99383	5-11 year old			80053	Chem profile			10061	I & D Abscess Comp.			82607	Vitamin B12 Inj.	
	99384	12-17 year old			80061	Lipid profile			94761	Oximetry w/Exercise			90712	Polio oral use (OPV)	
	99385	18-39 year old			82465	Cholesterol			94726	Plethysmography			90713	Polio injection (IPV)	
	99386	40-64 year old			99000	Handling fee			94760	Pulse Oximetry			90714	Td preservative free 7 yrs +	
	99387	65 + year old		**X-RAY**					11100	Skin Bx			90718	Td 7 years +	
PREVENTATIVE MEDICINE - ESTABLISHED PATIENT					70210	Sinuses			94010	Spirometry			95115	Allergy inj., single	
	99391	< 1 year old			70360	Neck Soft Tissue			99173	Visual Acuity			95117	Allergy inj., multiple	
	99392	1-4 year old			71010	CXR (PA only)			17110	Wart destruction up to 14					
	99393	5-11 year old			71020	Chest 2V			17111	Wart destruction 15 lesions +					
	99394	12-17 year old			72040	C-Spine 2V			11042	Wound Debrid.		**OTHER**			
	99395	18-39 year old			72100	Lumbrosacral									
	99396	40-64 year old			73030	Shoulder 2V									
	99397	65 + year old			73070	Elbow 2V									
					73120	Hand 2V									
					73560	Knee 2V									
					73620	Foot 2V									
					74000	KUB									

DIAGNOSTIC CODES (ICD-9-CM)

✓	Code	Description	✓	Code	Description	✓	Code	Description	✓	Code	Description
	789.0__	Abdominal Pain		564.0	Constipation		784.0	Headache		782.1	Rash or ezanthem
	682.__	Abscess/Cellulitis		692.6	Contact dermatitis due to plants		414.9	Heart Dis., Coronary		714.0	Rheumatoid Arthritis
	995.3	Allergic Reaction		692.9	Contact dermatitis, NOS		599.70	Hematuria		V70.0	Routine general exam
	331	Alzheimer's		V25.09	Contraceptive management		455.6	Hemorrhoids		V76.10	Screen, breast
	285.__	Anemia, other & unspec		923.10	Contusion, forearm		573.3	Hepatitus, NOS		V76.2	Screen, cervix
	280.9	Anemia-iron deficiency		434.91	CVA		V03.81	HIB		V76.44	Screen, prosate
	281.0	Anemia-pernicious		266.2	Deficiency, folic acid B12		V65.44	HIV counseling		V76.47	Screen, vagina
	285.9	Anemia-unspecified		311	Depression		401.1	Hypertension, benign		216.5	Sebaceous cyst
	413.9	Angina, pectoris, oyher/unspecified		250.01	Diabetes, type I, juvenile type		401.9	Hypertension, unspecified		706.2	Sebaceous cyst
	300.00	Anxiety state, NOS		787.91	Diarrhea		401.0	Hypertension, malignant		786.05	Shortness of Breath
	300.4	Anxiety reaction		780.4	Dizziness		V04.81	Influenza		701.9	Skin tag
✓	716.90	Arthritis, NOS		V06.1	DTP		271.3	Lactose intolerance		845.00	Strain, ankle
	493.20	Asthma; chronic obstruction		V06.3	DTP + polio		573.9	Liver Disease		307.81	Tension headache
	493.00	Asthma; extrinic		536.8	Dyspepsia		724.5	Low Back Pain		V06.5	Tetanus - distheria (Td)
	493.10	Asthma; intrinsic		788.1	Dysuria		346.9	Migraine		305.1	Tobacco dependence
	493.90	Asthmas; unspecified		782.3	Edema		V06.4	MMR		788.41	Urinary frequency
	427.31	Atrial fibulation		530.81	Esophageal reflux		278.01	Obesity/Morbid		599.0	Unrinary tract infection, NOS
	724.5	Backache, unspecified		530.11	Esophagitis reflux		715.90	Osteoarthritis		V05.3	Viral hepatitis
	790.6	Blood chemistry		530.10	Esophagitis, unspecified		719.43	Pain in joint, forearm		368.40	Visual field defect, unspecified
	E906.3	Cat bite		780.6	Fever		625.4	PMS		V20.2	Well Child Exam
	786.50	Chest Pain		789.07	Generalized abdominal pain		486	Pneumonia			
	428.0	CHF		V72.3	Gynecological examiniation		V25.01	Prescription of oral contraceptivess			

DIAGNOSIS: (IF NOT CHECKED ABOVE)		RECEIVED BY:	TODAY'S FEE	*$80.—*
PROCEDURES: (IF NOT CHECKED ABOVE)	RETURN APPOINTMENT INFORMATION: (DAYS) (WKS.) (MOS.) (PRN)	☐ CASH ☐ CREDIT CARD ☐ CHECK # ________	AMOUNT RECEIVED	*$0.00*
			BALANCE	*$80.00*

Figure C.77 Encounter form (Superbill) for Lynn Taylor (Appendix A: Day 4).

Goode Medical Clinic
1234 Larsen Avenue
Saint Paul, Minnesota 55316

Phone: (555) 555-1234
Fax: (555) 555-5678

PATIENT NAME	CHART #	DATE		
Tiffany Carter		*XX/XX/XXXX*	☐ MEDI-MEDI ☐ SELF PAY ☐ MEDICARE	☒ MEDICAL ☐ PRIVATE ☐ HMO_______

✓	CPT/Md	DESCRIPTION	FEE	✓	CPT/Md	DESCRIPTION	FEE	✓	CPT/Md	DESCRIPTION	FEE	✓	CPT/Md	DESCRIPTION	FEE
OFFICE VISIT - NEW PATIENT				**LAB STUDIES**				**PROCEDURES**				**INJECTIONS**			
	99202	Focused Ex.			36415	Venipucture			92551	Audiometry			90655	Influenza 6-35 months	
	99203	Detailed Ex.			81000	Urinalysis			29705	Cast Removal Full Arm/Leg			90656	Influenza 3 years +	
	99204	Comprehensive Ex.			81003	- w/o Micro			2900__	Casting (by location)			90732	Pneumoccal	
	99205	Complex Ex.			84703	HCG (Urine, Pregnancy)			92567	Ear Check			J0295	Ampicillin, 1.5 gr	
OFFICE VISIT - ESTABLISHED PATIENT					82948	Glucose			69210	Ear Wax Rem. 1 2			J2001	Liocaine for IV infusion 10mg	
	99212	Focused Ex.			82270	Hemoccult			93000	EKG			J1885	Toradol 15mg	
✓	99213	Expanded Ex.	*$48.*		85025	CBC -diff.			93005	EKG tracing only			90720	DTP - HIB	
	99214	Detailed Ex.			85018	Hemoglobin			93010	EKG Int. and Rep			90746	HEP B - HIB	
	99215	Complex Ex.			88174	Pap Smear			11750	Excision Nail			90707	MMR	
PREVENTATIVE MEDICINE - NEW PATIENT					87210	KOH/ Saline Wet Mount			94375	Respiratory Flow Volume			86580	PPD	
	99381	< 1 year old			87430	Strep Antigen			93224	Holter up to 48 hours			90732	Pneumovax	
	99382	1-4 year old			87070	Throat Culture			10060	I & D Abscess Simple			90716	Varicella	
	99383	5-11 year old			80053	Chem profile			10061	I & D Abscess Comp.			82607	Vitamin B12 Inj.	
	99384	12-17 year old			80061	Lipid profile			94761	Oximetry w/Exercise			90712	Polio oral use (OPV)	
	99385	18-39 year old			82465	Cholesterol			94726	Plethysmography			90713	Polio injection (IPV)	
	99386	40-64 year old			99000	Handling fee			94760	Pulse Oximetry			90714	Td preservative free 7 yrs +	
	99387	65 + year old		**X-RAY**					11100	Skin Bx			90718	Td 7 years +	
PREVENTATIVE MEDICINE - ESTABLISHED PATIENT					70210	Sinuses			94010	Spirometry			95115	Allergy inj., single	
	99391	< 1 year old			70360	Neck Soft Tissue			99173	Visual Acuity			95117	Allergy inj., multiple	
	99392	1-4 year old			71010	CXR (PA only)			17110	Wart destruction up to 14					
	99393	5-11 year old			71020	Chest 2V			17111	Wart destruction 15 lesions +					
	99394	12-17 year old			72040	C-Spine 2V			11042	Wound Debrid.		**OTHER**			
	99395	18-39 year old			72100	Lumbrosacral									
	99396	40-64 year old			73030	Shoulder 2V									
	99397	65 + year old			73070	Elbow 2V									
					73120	Hand 2V									
					73560	Knee 2V									
					73620	Foot 2V									
					74000	KUB									

DIAGNOSTIC CODES (ICD-9-CM)

✓	Code	Description	✓	Code	Description	✓	Code	Description	✓	Code	Description
	789.0__	Abdominal Pain		564.0	Constipation		784.0	Headache		782.1	Rash or ezanthem
	682.__	Abscess/Cellulitis		692.6	Contact dermatitis due to plants		414.9	Heart Dis., Coronary		714.0	Rheumatoid Arthritis
	995.3	Allergic Reaction	✓	692.9	Contact dermatitis, NOS		599.70	Hematuria		V70.0	Routine general exam
	331	Alzheimer's		V25.09	Contraceptive management		455.6	Hemorrhoids		V76.10	Screen, breast
	285.__	Anemia, other & unspec		923.10	Contusion, forearm		573.3	Hepatitus, NOS		V76.2	Screen, cervix
	280.9	Anemia-iron deficiency		434.91	CVA		V03.81	HIB		V76.44	Screen, prosate
	281.0	Anemia-pernicious		266.2	Deficiency, folic acid B12		V65.44	HIV counseling		V76.47	Screen, vagina
	285.9	Anemia-unspecified		311	Depression		401.1	Hypertension, benign		216.5	Sebaceous cyst
	413.9	Angina, pectoris, oyher/unspecified		250.01	Diabetes, type I, juvenile type		401.9	Hypertension, unspecified		706.2	Sebaceous cyst
	300.00	Anxiety state, NOS		787.91	Diarrhea		401.0	Hypertension, malignant		786.05	Shortness of Breath
	300.4	Anxiety reaction		780.4	Dizziness		V04.81	Influenza		701.9	Skin tag
	716.90	Arthritis, NOS		V06.1	DTP		271.3	Lactose intolerance		845.00	Strain, ankle
	493.20	Asthma; chronic obstruction		V06.3	DTP + polio		573.9	Liver Disease		307.81	Tension headache
	493.00	Asthma; extrinic		536.8	Dyspepsia		724.5	Low Back Pain		V06.5	Tetanus - distheria (Td)
	493.10	Asthma; intrinsic		788.1	Dysuria		346.9	Migraine		305.1	Tobacco dependence
	493.90	Asthmas; unspecified		782.3	Edema		V06.4	MMR		788.41	Urinary frequency
	427.31	Atrial fibulation		530.81	Esophageal reflux		278.01	Obesity/Morbid		599.0	Unrinary tract infection, NOS
	724.5	Backache, unspecified		530.11	Esophagitis reflux		715.90	Osteoarthritis		V05.3	Viral hepatitis
	790.6	Blood chemistry		530.10	Esophagitis, unspecified		719.43	Pain in joint, forearm		368.40	Visual field defect, unspecified
	E906.3	Cat bite		780.6	Fever		625.4	PMS		V20.2	Well Child Exam
	786.50	Chest Pain		789.07	Generalized abdominal pain		486	Pneumonia			
	428.0	CHF		V72.3	Gynecological examiniation		V25.01	Prescription of oral contraceptivess			

DIAGNOSIS: (IF NOT CHECKED ABOVE)
Detergents — E861.0

PROCEDURES: (IF NOT CHECKED ABOVE)

RETURN APPOINTMENT INFORMATION:
follow-up 1 week
(*12* DAYS) (WKS.) (MOS.) (PRN)

RECEIVED BY:
☐ CASH
☐ CREDIT CARD
☐ CHECK
#________

TODAY'S FEE	*$48.—*
AMOUNT RECEIVED	*———*
BALANCE	*$48.—*

Figure C.78 Encounter form (Superbill) for Tiffany Carter (Appendix A: Day 4).

Goode Medical Clinic

1234 Larsen Avenue
Saint Paul, Minnesota 55316

Phone: (555) 555-1234
Fax: (555) 555-5678

PATIENT NAME	CHART #	DATE		
Mike Johnson		*XX/XX/XXXX*	☐ MEDI-MEDI ☐ SELF PAY ☐ MEDICARE	☒ MEDICAL ☐ PRIVATE ☐ HMO___

☐	CPT/Md	DESCRIPTION	FEE	☐	CPT/Md	DESCRIPTION	FEE	☐	CPT/Md	DESCRIPTION	FEE	☐	CPT/Md	DESCRIPTION	FEE
OFFICE VISIT - NEW PATIENT				**LAB STUDIES**				**PROCEDURES**				**INJECTIONS**			
	99202	Focused Ex.			36415	Venipucture			92551	Audiometry			90655	Influenza 6-35 months	
	99203	Detailed Ex.			81000	Urinalysis			29705	Cast Removal Full Arm/Leg			90656	Influenza 3 years +	
√	99204	Comprehensive Ex.	*$100.*		81003	- w/o Micro			2900__	Casting (by location)			90732	Pneumoccal	
	99205	Complex Ex.			84703	HCG (Urine, Pregnancy)			92567	Ear Check			J0295	Ampicillin, 1.5 gr	
OFFICE VISIT - ESTABLISHED PATIENT				√	82948	Glucose	*$25.*		69210	Ear Wax Rem. 1 2			J2001	Liocaine for IV infusion 10mg	
	99212	Focused Ex.			82270	Hemoccult			93000	EKG			J1885	Toradol 15mg	
	99213	Expanded Ex.			85025	CBC -diff.			93005	EKG tracing only			90720	DTP - HIB	
	99214	Detailed Ex.			85018	Hemoglobin			93010	EKG Int. and Rep			90746	HEP B - HIB	
	99215	Complex Ex.			88174	Pap Smear			11750	Excision Nail			90707	MMR	
PREVENTATIVE MEDICINE - NEW PATIENT					87210	KOH/ Saline Wet Mount			94375	Respiratory Flow Volume			86580	PPD	
	99381	< 1 year old			87430	Strep Antigen			93224	Holter up to 48 hours			90732	Pneumovax	
	99382	1-4 year old			87070	Throat Culture			10060	I & D Abscess Simple			90716	Varicella	
	99383	5-11 year old			80053	Chem profile			10061	I & D Abscess Comp.			82607	Vitamin B12 Inj.	
	99384	12-17 year old			80061	Lipid profile			94761	Oximetry w/Exercise			90712	Polio oral use (OPV)	
	99385	18-39 year old			82465	Cholesterol			94726	Plethysmography			90713	Polio injection (IPV)	
	99386	40-64 year old			99000	Handling fee			94760	Pulse Oximetry			90714	Td preservative free 7 yrs +	
	99387	65 + year old		**X-RAY**					11100	Skin Bx			90718	Td 7 years +	
PREVENTATIVE MEDICINE - ESTABLISHED PATIENT					70210	Sinuses			94010	Spirometry			95115	Allergy inj., single	
	99391	< 1 year old			70360	Neck Soft Tissue			99173	Visual Acuity			95117	Allergy inj., multiple	
	99392	1-4 year old			71010	CXR (PA only)			17110	Wart destruction up to 14					
	99393	5-11 year old			71020	Chest 2V			17111	Wart destruction 15 lesions +					
	99394	12-17 year old			72040	C-Spine 2V			11042	Wound Debrid.		**OTHER**			
	99395	18-39 year old			72100	Lumbrosacral									
	99396	40-64 year old			73030	Shoulder 2V									
	99397	65 + year old			73070	Elbow 2V									
					73120	Hand 2V									
					73560	Knee 2V									
					73620	Foot 2V									
					74000	KUB									

DIAGNOSTIC CODES (ICD-9-CM)

☐	Code	Description	☐	Code	Description	☐	Code	Description	☐	Code	Description
	789.0__	Abdominal Pain		564.0	Constipation		784.0	Headache		782.1	Rash or ezanthem
	682.__	Abscess/Cellulitis		692.6	Contact dermatitis due to plants		414.9	Heart Dis., Coronary		714.0	Rheumatoid Arthritis
	995.3	Allergic Reaction		692.9	Contact dermatitis, NOS		599.70	Hematuria		V70.0	Routine general exam
	331	Alzheimer's		V25.09	Contraceptive management		455.6	Hemorrhoids		V76.10	Screen, breast
	285.__	Anemia, other & unspec		923.10	Contusion, forearm		573.3	Hepatitus, NOS		V76.2	Screen, cervix
	280.9	Anemia-iron deficiency		434.91	CVA		V03.81	HIB		V76.44	Screen, prosate
	281.0	Anemia-pernicious		266.2	Deficiency, folic acid B12		V65.44	HIV counseling		V76.47	Screen, vagina
	285.9	Anemia-unspecified		311	Depression		401.1	Hypertension, benign		216.5	Sebaceous cyst
	413.9	Angina, pectoris, oyher/unspecified		250.01	Diabetes, type I, juvenile type	√	401.9	Hypertension, unspecified		706.2	Sebaceous cyst
	300.00	Anxiety state, NOS		787.91	Diarrhea		401.0	Hypertension, malignant		786.05	Shortness of Breath
	300.4	Anxiety reaction		780.4	Dizziness		V04.81	Influenza		701.9	Skin tag
	716.90	Arthritis, NOS		V06.1	DTP		271.3	Lactose intolerance		845.00	Strain, ankle
	493.20	Asthma; chronic obstruction		V06.3	DTP + polio		573.9	Liver Disease		307.81	Tension headache
	493.00	Asthma; extrinic		536.8	Dyspepsia		724.5	Low Back Pain		V06.5	Tetanus - distheria (Td)
	493.10	Asthma; intrinsic		788.1	Dysuria		346.9	Migraine		305.1	Tobacco dependence
	493.90	Asthmas; unspecified		782.3	Edema		V06.4	MMR		788.41	Urinary frequency
	427.31	Atrial fibulation		530.81	Esophageal reflux		278.01	Obesity/Morbid		599.0	Unrinary tract infection, NOS
	724.5	Backache, unspecified		530.11	Esophagitis reflux		715.90	Osteoarthritis		V05.3	Viral hepatitis
	790.6	Blood chemistry		530.10	Esophagitis, unspecified		719.43	Pain in joint, forearm		368.40	Visual field defect, unspecified
	E906.3	Cat bite		780.6	Fever		625.4	PMS		V20.2	Well Child Exam
	786.50	Chest Pain		789.07	Generalized abdominal pain		486	Pneumonia			
	428.0	CHF		V72.3	Gynecological examiniation		V25.01	Prescription of oral contraceptivess			

DIAGNOSIS: (IF NOT CHECKED ABOVE)		RECEIVED BY:	TODAY'S FEE	*$125.—*
Diabetes — 250.03		☐ CASH	AMOUNT RECEIVED	*——*
PROCEDURES: (IF NOT CHECKED ABOVE)	RETURN APPOINTMENT INFORMATION:	☐ CREDIT CARD		
	(DAYS) (*1* WKS.) (MOS.) (PRN)	☐ CHECK # ________	BALANCE	*$125.—*

Figure C.79 Encounter form (Superbill) for Mike Johnson (Appendix A: Day 4).

Goode Medical Clinic
William B. Goode, MD

Patient Registration Information

Account # :
Insurance # :
Co-Payment: $

Please PRINT AND complete ALL sections below!

PATIENT'S PERSONAL INFORMATION Marital Status ☒ Single ☐ Married ☐ Divorced ☐ Widowed Sex: ☐ Male ☒ Female

Name: Tschida (last name) Sara (first name) (initial)

Street address: 100 Carter Street (Apt #) City: Grove State: MN Zip: 55102

Home phone: (555) 555-3636 Work phone: ( ) Social Security # 890 - XX - 8115

Date of Birth: 8 (month) / 8 (day) / 1977 (year)

Employer / Name of School Self-employed ☐ Full Time ☐ Part Time

PATIENT'S / RESPONSIBLE PARTY INFORMATION

Responsible party: Self Date of Birth:

Relationship to Patient: ☒ Self ☐ Spouse ☐ Other Social Security # - -

Responsible party's home phone: ( ) see above

Address: (Apt #) City: State: Zip:

Employer's name: n/a Phone number:( )

Address: City: State: Zip:

Name of Parent/Guardian:

PATIENT'S INSURANCE INFORMATION Please present insurance cards to receptionist.

PRIMARY insurance company's name: None

Insurance address: City: State: Zip:

Name of insured: Date of Birth: Relationship to insured: ☐ Self ☐ Spouse ☐ Other ☐ Child

Insurance ID number: Group number:

Does your insurance cover medication?

EMERGENCY CONTACT

Name of person not living with you: Becky Tschida Relationship: Sister

Address: 4 Steeplechase Lane City: Bayview State: MN Zip: 55362

Phone number: (555) 555-6663

Assignment of Benefits • Financial Agreement

I hereby give lifetime authorization for payment of insurance benefits to be made directly to Goode Medical Clinic ,and any assisting physicians, for services rendered. I understand that I am financially responsible for all charges whether or not they are covered by insurance. In the event of default, I agree to pay all costs of collection, and reasonable attorney's fees. I hereby authorize this healthcare provider to release all information necessary to secure the payment of benefits.

I further agree that a photocopy of this agreement shall be as valid as the original.

Date: XX/XX/XXXX Your Signature: Sara Tschida

FORM # 58-8423 • BIBBERO SYSTEMS, INC.• PETALUMA, CA.• TO ORDER CALL TOLL FREE :800-BIBBERO (800-242-2376) • FAX (800) 242-9330 (REV.7/94)

Figure C.80 Registration form for Sara Tschida (Appendix A: Day 4).

Goode Medical Clinic
1234 Larsen Avenue
Saint Paul, Minnesota 55316

Phone: (555) 555-1234
Fax: (555) 555-5678

PATIENT NAME	CHART #	DATE		
Sara Tschida		XX/XX/XXXX	☐ MEDI-MEDI ☒ SELF PAY ☐ MEDICARE	☐ MEDICAL ☐ PRIVATE ☐ HMO___

☐	CPT/Md	DESCRIPTION	FEE	☐	CPT/Md	DESCRIPTION	FEE	☐	CPT/Md	DESCRIPTION	FEE	☐	CPT/Md	DESCRIPTION	FEE
OFFICE VISIT - NEW PATIENT				LAB STUDIES				PROCEDURES				INJECTIONS			
	99202	Focused Ex.			36415	Venipucture			92551	Audiometry			90655	Influenza 6-35 months	
	99203	Detailed Ex.		✓	81000	Urinalysis —1	$78.		29705	Cast Removal Full Arm/Leg			90656	Influenza 3 years +	
	99204	Comprehensive Ex.			81003	- w/o Micro			2900__	Casting (by location)			90732	Pneumoccal	
	99205	Complex Ex.			84703	HCG (Urine, Pregnancy)			92567	Ear Check			J0295	Ampicillin, 1.5 gr	
OFFICE VISIT - ESTABLISHED PATIENT					82948	Glucose			69210	Ear Wax Rem. 1 2			J2001	Liocaine for IV infusion 10mg	
	99212	Focused Ex.			82270	Hemoccult		✓	93000	EKG / ECG	$50.		J1885	Toradol 15mg	
	99213	Expanded Ex.			85025	CBC -diff.			93005	EKG tracing only			90720	DTP - HIB	
	99214	Detailed Ex.			85018	Hemoglobin			93010	EKG Int. and Rep			90746	HEP B - HIB	
	99215	Complex Ex.		✓	88174	Pap Smear	$45.		11750	Excision Nail			90707	MMR	
PREVENTATIVE MEDICINE - NEW PATIENT					87210	KOH/ Saline Wet Mount			94375	Respiratory Flow Volume			86580	PPD	
	99381	< 1 year old			87430	Strep Antigen			93224	Holter up to 48 hours			90732	Pneumovax	
	99382	1-4 year old			87070	Throat Culture			10060	I & D Abscess Simple			90716	Varicella	
	99383	5-11 year old			80053	Chem profile			10061	I & D Abscess Comp.			82607	Vitamin B12 Inj.	
	99384	12-17 year old			80061	Lipid profile			94761	Oximetry w/Exercise			90712	Polio oral use (OPV)	
✓	99385	18-39 year old	$85.		82465	Cholesterol			94726	Plethysmography			90713	Polio injection (IPV)	
	99386	40-64 year old			99000	Handling fee			94760	Pulse Oximetry			90714	Td preservative free 7 yrs +	
	99387	65 + year old		X-RAY					11100	Skin Bx			90718	Td 7 years +	
PREVENTATIVE MEDICINE - ESTABLISHED PATIENT					70210	Sinuses			94010	Spirometry			95115	Allergy inj., single	
	99391	< 1 year old			70360	Neck Soft Tissue			99173	Visual Acuity			95117	Allergy inj., multiple	
	99392	1-4 year old			71010	CXR (PA only)			17110	Wart destruction up to 14					
	99393	5-11 year old			71020	Chest 2V			17111	Wart destruction 15 lesions +					
	99394	12-17 year old			72040	C-Spine 2V			11042	Wound Debrid.		OTHER			
	99395	18-39 year old			72100	Lumbrosacral									
	99396	40-64 year old			73030	Shoulder 2V									
	99397	65 + year old			73070	Elbow 2V									
					73120	Hand 2V									
					73560	Knee 2V									
					73620	Foot 2V									
					74000	KUB									

DIAGNOSTIC CODES (ICD-9-CM)

☐	Code	Description	☐	Code	Description	☐	Code	Description	☐	Code	Description
	789.0__	Abdominal Pain		564.0	Constipation		784.0	Headache		782.1	Rash or ezanthem
	682.__	Abscess/Cellulitis		692.6	Contact dermatitis due to plants		414.9	Heart Dis., Coronary		714.0	Rheumatoid Arthritis
	995.3	Allergic Reaction		692.9	Contact dermatitis, NOS		599.70	Hematuria	✓	V70.0	Routine general exam
	331	Alzheimer's		V25.09	Contraceptive management		455.6	Hemorrhoids		V76.10	Screen, breast
	285.__	Anemia, other & unspec		923.10	Contusion, forearm		573.3	Hepatitus, NOS		V76.2	Screen, cervix
	280.9	Anemia-iron deficiency		434.91	CVA		V03.81	HIB		V76.44	Screen, prosate
	281.0	Anemia-pernicious		266.2	Deficiency, folic acid B12		V65.44	HIV counseling		V76.47	Screen, vagina
	285.9	Anemia-unspecified		311	Depression		401.1	Hypertension, benign		216.5	Sebaceous cyst
	413.9	Angina, pectoris, oyher/unspecified		250.01	Diabetes, type I, juvenile type		401.9	Hypertension, unspecified		706.2	Sebaceous cyst
	300.00	Anxiety state, NOS		787.91	Diarrhea		401.0	Hypertension, malignant		786.05	Shortness of Breath
	300.4	Anxiety reaction		780.4	Dizziness		V04.81	Influenza		701.9	Skin tag
	716.90	Arthritis, NOS		V06.1	DTP		271.3	Lactose intolerance		845.00	Strain, ankle
	493.20	Asthma; chronic obstruction		V06.3	DTP + polio		573.9	Liver Disease		307.81	Tension headache
	493.00	Asthma; extrinic		536.8	Dyspepsia		724.5	Low Back Pain		V06.5	Tetanus - distheria (Td)
	493.10	Asthma; intrinsic		788.1	Dysuria		346.9	Migraine		305.1	Tobacco dependence
	493.90	Asthmas; unspecified		782.3	Edema		V06.4	MMR		788.41	Urinary frequency
	427.31	Atrial fibulation		530.81	Esophageal reflux		278.01	Obesity/Morbid		599.0	Unrinary tract infection, NOS
	724.5	Backache, unspecified		530.11	Esophagitis reflux		715.90	Osteoarthritis		V05.3	Viral hepatitis
	790.6	Blood chemistry		530.10	Esophagitis, unspecified		719.43	Pain in joint, forearm		368.40	Visual field defect, unspecified
	E906.3	Cat bite		780.6	Fever		625.4	PMS		V20.2	Well Child Exam
	786.50	Chest Pain		789.07	Generalized abdominal pain		486	Pneumonia			
	428.0	CHF		V72.3	Gynecological examiniation		V25.01	Prescription of oral contraceptivess			

DIAGNOSIS: (IF NOT CHECKED ABOVE)		RECEIVED BY:	TODAY'S FEE	$258.00
PROCEDURES: (IF NOT CHECKED ABOVE)	RETURN APPOINTMENT INFORMATION: (DAYS) (WKS.) (MOS.) (PRN)	☐ CASH ☐ CREDIT CARD ☒ CHECK # 4324	AMOUNT RECEIVED	$258.00
			BALANCE	$0.00

Figure C.81 Encounter form (Superbill) for Sara Tschida (Appendix A: Day 4).

Goode Medical Clinic
William B. Goode, MD

Patient Registration Information

Account # :
Insurance # :
Co-Payment: $

Please PRINT AND complete ALL sections below!

PATIENT'S PERSONAL INFORMATION Marital Status ❑ Single ☒ Married ❑ Divorced ❑ Widowed Sex: ☒ Male ❑ Female

Name: Burns (last name) Adam (first name) G. (initial)
Street address: 2300 Mayo Drive (Apt #) City: St. Paul State: MN Zip: 55100
Home phone: (555) 555-8323 Work phone: (555) 555-6507 Social Security # 116 - XX - 8124
Date of Birth: 2 (month) / 2 (day) / 1953 (year)
Employer / Name of School Regions Clinic ☒ Full Time ❑ Part Time

PATIENT'S / RESPONSIBLE PARTY INFORMATION

Responsible party: self Date of Birth: 2/2/53
Relationship to Patient: ☒ Self ❑ Spouse ❑ Other Social Security # - -
Responsible party's home phone: (555) 555-8323
Address: 2300 Mayo Drive (Apt #) City: St. Paul State: MN Zip: 55100
Employer's name: Regions Clinic Phone number: (555) 555-7879
Address: 100 Regions Road City: St. Paul State: MN Zip: 55100
Name of Parent/Guardian:

PATIENT'S INSURANCE INFORMATION Please present insurance cards to receptionist.

PRIMARY insurance company's name: Blue Cross/Blue Shield
Insurance address: 1355 Insurance Carrier Loop City: Minneapolis State: MN Zip: 55401
Name of insured: Adam Burns Date of Birth: Relationship to insured: ☒ Self ☐ Spouse ☐ Other ☐ Child
Insurance ID number: AB-4567-RC Group number: 87654
Does your insurance cover medication? Yes

EMERGENCY CONTACT

Name of person not living with you: Marlo Burns Relationship: Spouse
Address: 2300 Mayo Drive City: St. Paul State: MN Zip: 55100
Phone number: (555) 555-8323

Assignment of Benefits • Financial Agreement

I hereby give lifetime authorization for payment of insurance benefits to be made directly to Goode Medical Clinic, and any assisting physicians, for services rendered. I understand that I am financially responsible for all charges whether or not they are covered by insurance. In the event of default, I agree to pay all costs of collection, and reasonable attorney's fees. I hereby authorize this healthcare provider to release all information necessary to secure the payment of benefits.
I further agree that a photocopy of this agreement shall be as valid as the original.

Date: xx/xx/xxxx Your Signature: Adam Burns

FORM # 58-8423 • BIBBERO SYSTEMS, INC.• PETALUMA, CA.• TO ORDER CALL TOLL FREE :800-BIBBERO (800-242-2376) • FAX (800) 242-9330 (REV.7/94)

Figure C.82 Registration form for Adam Burns (Appendix A: Day 4).

Goode Medical Clinic
1234 Larsen Avenue
Saint Paul, Minnesota 55316

Phone: (555) 555-1234
Fax: (555) 555-5678

PATIENT NAME	CHART #	DATE		
Adam Burns		*XX/XX/XXXX*	☐ MEDI-MEDI ☐ SELF PAY ☐ MEDICARE	☒ MEDICAL ☐ PRIVATE ☐ HMO_____

☐	CPT/Md	DESCRIPTION	FEE	☐	CPT/Md	DESCRIPTION	FEE	☐	CPT/Md	DESCRIPTION	FEE	☐	CPT/Md	DESCRIPTION	FEE
OFFICE VISIT - NEW PATIENT				**LAB STUDIES**				**PROCEDURES**				**INJECTIONS**			
	99202	Focused Ex.			36415	Venipucture			92551	Audiometry			90655	Influenza 6-35 months	
	99203	Detailed Ex.			81000	Urinalysis			29705	Cast Removal Full Arm/Leg			90656	Influenza 3 years +	
✓	99204	Comprehensive Ex.	*$100.*		81003	- w/o Micro			2900__	Casting (by location)			90732	Pneumoccal	
	99205	Complex Ex.			84703	HCG (Urine, Pregnancy)			92567	Ear Check			J0295	Ampicillin, 1.5 gr	
OFFICE VISIT - ESTABLISHED PATIENT					82948	Glucose			69210	Ear Wax Rem. 1 2			J2001	Liocaine for IV infusion 10mg	
	99212	Focused Ex.			82270	Hemoccult			93000	EKG			J1885	Toradol 15mg	
	99213	Expanded Ex.			85025	CBC -diff.			93005	EKG tracing only			90720	DTP - HIB	
	99214	Detailed Ex.			85018	Hemoglobin			93010	EKG Int. and Rep			90746	HEP B - HIB	
	99215	Complex Ex.			88174	Pap Smear			11750	Excision Nail			90707	MMR	
PREVENTATIVE MEDICINE - NEW PATIENT					87210	KOH/ Saline Wet Mount			94375	Respiratory Flow Volume			86580	PPD	
	99381	< 1 year old			87430	Strep Antigen			93224	Holter up to 48 hours			90732	Pneumovax	
	99382	1-4 year old			87070	Throat Culture			10060	I & D Abscess Simple			90716	Varicella	
	99383	5-11 year old			80053	Chem profile			10061	I & D Abscess Comp.			82607	Vitamin B12 Inj.	
	99384	12-17 year old			80061	Lipid profile			94761	Oximetry w/Exercise			90712	Polio oral use (OPV)	
	99385	18-39 year old			82465	Cholesterol			94726	Plethysmography			90713	Polio injection (IPV)	
	99386	40-64 year old			99000	Handling fee			94760	Pulse Oximetry			90714	Td preservative free 7 yrs +	
	99387	65 + year old		**X-RAY**					11100	Skin Bx			90718	Td 7 years +	
PREVENTATIVE MEDICINE - ESTABLISHED PATIENT					70210	Sinuses			94010	Spirometry			95115	Allergy inj., single	
	99391	< 1 year old			70360	Neck Soft Tissue			99173	Visual Acuity			95117	Allergy inj., multiple	
	99392	1-4 year old			71010	CXR (PA only)			17110	Wart destruction up to 14					
	99393	5-11 year old			71020	Chest 2V			17111	Wart destruction 15 lesions +					
	99394	12-17 year old			72040	C-Spine 2V			11042	Wound Debrid.		**OTHER**			
	99395	18-39 year old			72100	Lumbrosacral									
	99396	40-64 year old			73030	Shoulder 2V									
	99397	65 + year old			73070	Elbow 2V									
					73120	Hand 2V									
					73560	Knee 2V									
					73620	Foot 2V									
					74000	KUB									

DIAGNOSTIC CODES (ICD-9-CM)

☐	Code	Description	☐	Code	Description	☐	Code	Description	☐	Code	Description
	789.0__	Abdominal Pain		564.0	Constipation		784.0	Headache		782.1	Rash or ezanthem
	682.__	Abscess/Cellulitis		692.6	Contact dermatitis due to plants		414.9	Heart Dis., Coronary		714.0	Rheumatoid Arthritis
	995.3	Allergic Reaction		692.9	Contact dermatitis, NOS		599.70	Hematuria		V70.0	Routine general exam
	331	Alzheimer's		V25.09	Contraceptive management		455.6	Hemorrhoids		V76.10	Screen, breast
	285.__	Anemia, other & unspec		923.10	Contusion, forearm		573.3	Hepatitus, NOS		V76.2	Screen, cervix
	280.9	Anemia-iron deficiency		434.91	CVA		V03.81	HIB		V76.44	Screen, prosate
	281.0	Anemia-pernicious		266.2	Deficiency, folic acid B12		V65.44	HIV counseling		V76.47	Screen, vagina
	285.9	Anemia-unspecified		311	Depression		401.1	Hypertension, benign		216.5	Sebaceous cyst
	413.9	Angina, pectoris, oyher/unspecified		250.01	Diabetes, type I, juvenile type	✓	401.9	Hypertension, unspecified		706.2	Sebaceous cyst
	300.00	Anxiety state, NOS		787.91	Diarrhea		401.0	Hypertension, malignant		786.05	Shortness of Breath
	300.4	Anxiety reaction		780.4	Dizziness		V04.81	Influenza		701.9	Skin tag
	716.90	Arthritis, NOS		V06.1	DTP		271.3	Lactose intolerance		845.00	Strain, ankle
	493.20	Asthma; chronic obstruction		V06.3	DTP + polio		573.9	Liver Disease		307.81	Tension headache
	493.00	Asthma; extrinic		536.8	Dyspepsia		724.5	Low Back Pain		V06.5	Tetanus - distheria (Td)
	493.10	Asthma; intrinsic		788.1	Dysuria		346.9	Migraine		305.1	Tobacco dependence
	493.90	Asthmas; unspecified		782.3	Edema		V06.4	MMR		788.41	Urinary frequency
	427.31	Atrial fibulation		530.81	Esophageal reflux		278.01	Obesity/Morbid		599.0	Unrinary tract infection, NOS
	724.5	Backache, unspecified		530.11	Esophagitis reflux		715.90	Osteoarthritis		V05.3	Viral hepatitis
	790.6	Blood chemistry		530.10	Esophagitis, unspecified		719.43	Pain in joint, forearm		368.40	Visual field defect, unspecified
	E906.3	Cat bite		780.6	Fever		625.4	PMS		V20.2	Well Child Exam
	786.50	Chest Pain		789.07	Generalized abdominal pain		486	Pneumonia			
	428.0	CHF		V72.3	Gynecological examiniation		V25.01	Prescription of oral contraceptivess			

DIAGNOSIS: (IF NOT CHECKED ABOVE)		RECEIVED BY:	TODAY'S FEE	*$100.00*
		☐ CASH	AMOUNT RECEIVED	———
PROCEDURES: (IF NOT CHECKED ABOVE)	RETURN APPOINTMENT INFORMATION: *follow-up tomorrow* (*1* DAYS) (WKS.) (MOS.) (PRN)	☐ CREDIT CARD ☐ CHECK # ________	BALANCE	*$100.00*

Figure C.83 Encounter form (Superbill) for Adam Burns (Appendix A: Day 4).

Goode Medical Clinic
1234 Larsen Avenue
Saint Paul, Minnesota 55316

Phone: (555) 555-1234
Fax: (555) 555-5678

PATIENT NAME	CHART #	DATE		
Robert Jones		*XX/XX/XXXX*	☐ MEDI-MEDI ☐ SELF PAY ☒ MEDICARE	☐ MEDICAL ☐ PRIVATE ☐ HMO______

☐	CPT/Md	DESCRIPTION	FEE	☐	CPT/Md	DESCRIPTION	FEE	☐	CPT/Md	DESCRIPTION	FEE	☐	CPT/Md	DESCRIPTION	FEE
OFFICE VISIT - NEW PATIENT				**LAB STUDIES**				**PROCEDURES**				**INJECTIONS**			
	99202	Focused Ex.			36415	Venipucture			92551	Audiometry			90655	Influenza 6-35 months	
	99203	Detailed Ex.			81000	Urinalysis			29705	Cast Removal Full Arm/Leg			90656	Influenza 3 years +	
	99204	Comprehensive Ex.			81003	- w/o Micro			2900__	Casting (by location)			90732	Pneumoccal	
	99205	Complex Ex.			84703	HCG (Urine, Pregnancy)			92567	Ear Check			J0295	Ampicillin, 1.5 gr	
OFFICE VISIT - ESTABLISHED PATIENT					82948	Glucose			69210	Ear Wax Rem. 1 2			J2001	Liocaine for IV infusion 10mg	
	99212	Focused Ex.			82270	Hemoccult		✓	93000	EKG / *ECG*	*$50.*		J1885	Toradol 15mg	
✓	99213	Expanded Ex.	*$48.*		85025	CBC -diff.			93005	EKG tracing only			90720	DTP - HIB	
	99214	Detailed Ex.			85018	Hemoglobin			93010	EKG Int. and Rep			90746	HEP B - HIB	
	99215	Complex Ex.			88174	Pap Smear			11750	Excision Nail			90707	MMR	
PREVENTATIVE MEDICINE - NEW PATIENT					87210	KOH/ Saline Wet Mount			94375	Respiratory Flow Volume			86580	PPD	
	99381	< 1 year old			87430	Strep Antigen			93224	Holter up to 48 hours			90732	Pneumovax	
	99382	1-4 year old			87070	Throat Culture			10060	I & D Abscess Simple			90716	Varicella	
	99383	5-11 year old			80053	Chem profile			10061	I & D Abscess Comp.			82607	Vitamin B12 Inj.	
	99384	12-17 year old			80061	Lipid profile			94761	Oximetry w/Exercise			90712	Polio oral use (OPV)	
	99385	18-39 year old			82465	Cholesterol			94726	Plethysmography			90713	Polio injection (IPV)	
	99386	40-64 year old			99000	Handling fee			94760	Pulse Oximetry			90714	Td preservative free 7 yrs +	
	99387	65 + year old		**X-RAY**					11100	Skin Bx			90718	Td 7 years +	
PREVENTATIVE MEDICINE - ESTABLISHED PATIENT					70210	Sinuses			94010	Spirometry			95115	Allergy inj., single	
	99391	< 1 year old			70360	Neck Soft Tissue			99173	Visual Acuity			95117	Allergy inj., multiple	
	99392	1-4 year old			71010	CXR (PA only)			17110	Wart destruction up to 14					
	99393	5-11 year old			71020	Chest 2V			17111	Wart destruction 15 lesions +					
	99394	12-17 year old			72040	C-Spine 2V			11042	Wound Debrid.		**OTHER**			
	99395	18-39 year old			72100	Lumbrosacral									
	99396	40-64 year old			73030	Shoulder 2V									
	99397	65 + year old			73070	Elbow 2V									
					73120	Hand 2V									
					73560	Knee 2V									
					73620	Foot 2V									
					74000	KUB									

DIAGNOSTIC CODES (ICD-9-CM)

Code	Description	Code	Description	Code	Description	Code	Description
789.0__	Abdominal Pain	564.0	Constipation	784.0	Headache	782.1	Rash or ezanthem
682.__	Abscess/Cellulitis	692.6	Contact dermatitis due to plants	414.9	Heart Dis., Coronary	714.0	Rheumatoid Arthritis
995.3	Allergic Reaction	692.9	Contact dermatitis, NOS	599.70	Hematuria	V70.0	Routine general exam
331	Alzheimer's	V25.09	Contraceptive management	455.6	Hemorrhoids	V76.10	Screen, breast
285.__	Anemia, other & unspec	923.10	Contusion, forearm	573.3	Hepatitus, NOS	V76.2	Screen, cervix
280.9	Anemia-iron deficiency	434.91	CVA	V03.81	HIB	V76.44	Screen, prosate
281.0	Anemia-pernicious	266.2	Deficiency, folic acid B12	V65.44	HIV counseling	V76.47	Screen, vagina
285.9	Anemia-unspecified	311	Depression	401.1	Hypertension, benign	216.5	Sebaceous cyst
413.9	Angina, pectoris, oyher/unspecified	250.01	Diabetes, type I, juvenile type	401.9	Hypertension, unspecified	706.2	Sebaceous cyst
300.00	Anxiety state, NOS	787.91	Diarrhea	401.0	Hypertension, malignant	786.05	Shortness of Breath
300.4	Anxiety reaction	780.4	Dizziness	V04.81	Influenza	701.9	Skin tag
716.90	Arthritis, NOS	V06.1	DTP	271.3	Lactose intolerance	845.00	Strain, ankle
493.20	Asthma; chronic obstruction	V06.3	DTP + polio	573.9	Liver Disease	307.81	Tension headache
493.00	Asthma; extrinic	536.8	Dyspepsia	724.5	Low Back Pain	V06.5	Tetanus - distheria (Td)
493.10	Asthma; intrinsic	788.1	Dysuria	346.9	Migraine	305.1	Tobacco dependence
493.90	Asthmas; unspecified	782.3	Edema	V06.4	MMR	788.41	Urinary frequency
427.31	Atrial fibulation	530.81	Esophageal reflux	278.01	Obesity/Morbid	599.0	Unrinary tract infection, NOS
724.5	Backache, unspecified	530.11	Esophagitis reflux	715.90	Osteoarthritis	V05.3	Viral hepatitis
790.6	Blood chemistry	530.10	Esophagitis, unspecified	719.43	Pain in joint, forearm	368.40	Visual field defect, unspecified
E906.3	Cat bite	780.6	Fever	625.4	PMS	V20.2	Well Child Exam
786.50	Chest Pain	789.07	Generalized abdominal pain	486	Pneumonia		
428.0	CHF	V72.3	Gynecological examiniation	V25.01	Prescription of oral contraceptivess		

DIAGNOSIS: (IF NOT CHECKED ABOVE)

Old myocardial infarction (412)

PROCEDURES: (IF NOT CHECKED ABOVE)

RETURN APPOINTMENT INFORMATION:

(DAYS) (WKS.) (MOS.) (PRN)

RECEIVED BY:
☐ CASH
☐ CREDIT CARD
☐ CHECK
#________

TODAY'S FEE	*$98.00*
AMOUNT RECEIVED	——
BALANCE	*$98.00*

Figure C.84 Encounter form (Superbill) for Robert Jones (Appendix A: Day 4).

Medicare Part B
4502 Wisconsin Ave
Milwaukee WI 53201
(414)555-0943

Remittance advice

Goode Medical Clinic
1612 Southwest Blvd.
St. Paul, MN 55100

Page: 1 of 1
Date: XX/XX/XX
Group Practice ID#: 567XX
Check number: 23456

Patient name	DOS	Procedure code	Units	Total charge	Allowable	Provider responsibility	Co-pay	Amount paid
Jones, Robert	02/05/2013	99204	1	100.00	86.20	13.80	0	86.20
	02/05/2013	93000	1	50.00	18.00	32.00	0	18.00

Total charges $150.00 Total provider responsibility $45.80 Total co-pay 0 Total paid $104.20

Figure C.85 Remittance Advice—Medicare for Robert Jones (Appendix A: Day 4).

Medicare Part B
4502 Wisconsin Ave
Milwaukee WI 53201
(414)555-0943

Remittance advice

Goode Medical Clinic
1612 Southwest Blvd.
St. Paul, MN 55100

Page: 1 of 1
Date: XX/XX/XX
Group Practice ID#: 567XX
Check number: 7682342

Patient name	DOS	Procedure code	Units	Total charge	Allowable	Provider responsibility	Co-pay	Amount paid
Taylor, Lynn	02/07/2013	99203	1	80.00	68.60	11.40	0	68.60
Jones, Robert	02/07/2013	99213	1	48.00	28.60	19.40	0	28.60
	02/07/2013	93000	1	50.00	18.00	32.00	0	18.00

Total charges $178.00 Total provider responsibility $62.80 Total co-pay 0 Total paid $115.20

Figure C.86 Remittance Advice—Medicare for patients Taylor and Jones (Appendix A: Day 4).

BCBS of MN
1355 Insurance Carrier Loop
Minneapolis, MN 55111
(763)555-0426

Remittance advice

Goode Medical Clinic
1612 Southwest Blvd.
St. Paul, MN 55100

Page: 1 of 1
Date: XX/XX/XX
Group Practice ID#: 567XX
Check number: 345678

Patient name	DOS	Procedure code	Units	Total charge	Allowable	Provider responsibility	Co-pay	Amount paid
Smith, Danny	02/06/2013	99203	1	80.00	76.00	4.00		76.00
Johnson, Mike	02/07/2013	99204	1	100.00	96.00	4.00		96.00
	02/07/2013	82948	1	25.00	15.00	10.00		15.00
Carter, Tiffany	02/07/2013	99213	1	48.00	46.00	2.00		46.00
Burns, Adam	02/07/2013	99204	1	100.00	96.00	4.00		96.00

Total charges $353.00 Total provider responsibility $24.00 Total co-pay 0 Total paid $329.00

Figure C.87 Remittance Advice—Blue Cross and Blue Shield (Appendix A: Day 4).

Goode Medical Clinic
1234 Larsen Avenue
Saint Paul, Minnesota 55316

Phone: (555) 555-1234
Fax: (555) 555-5678

PATIENT NAME	CHART #	DATE		
Lynn Stone		*XX/XX/XXXX*	☐ MEDI-MEDI ☐ SELF PAY ☐ MEDICARE	☒ MEDICAL ☐ PRIVATE ☐ HMO____

☐	CPT/Md	DESCRIPTION	FEE	☐	CPT/Md	DESCRIPTION	FEE	☐	CPT/Md	DESCRIPTION	FEE	☐	CPT/Md	DESCRIPTION	FEE
OFFICE VISIT - NEW PATIENT				**LAB STUDIES**				**PROCEDURES**				**INJECTIONS**			
	99202	Focused Ex.			36415	Venipucture			92551	Audiometry			90655	Influenza 6-35 months	
	99203	Detailed Ex.			81000	Urinalysis			29705	Cast Removal Full Arm/Leg			90656	Influenza 3 years +	
	99204	Comprehensive Ex.			81003	- w/o Micro			2900__	Casting (by location)			90732	Pneumoccal	
	99205	Complex Ex.			84703	HCG (Urine, Pregnancy)			92567	Ear Check			J0295	Ampicillin, 1.5 gr	
OFFICE VISIT - ESTABLISHED PATIENT					82948	Glucose			69210	Ear Wax Rem. 1 2			J2001	Liocaine for IV infusion 10mg	
	99212	Focused Ex.			82270	Hemoccult			93000	EKG			J1885	Toradol 15mg	
✓	99213	Expanded Ex.	*$48.*		85025	CBC -diff.			93005	EKG tracing only			90720	DTP - HIB	
	99214	Detailed Ex.			85018	Hemoglobin			93010	EKG Int. and Rep			90746	HEP B - HIB	
	99215	Complex Ex.			88174	Pap Smear			11750	Excision Nail			90707	MMR	
PREVENTATIVE MEDICINE - NEW PATIENT					87210	KOH/ Saline Wet Mount			94375	Respiratory Flow Volume			86580	PPD	
	99381	< 1 year old			87430	Strep Antigen			93224	Holter up to 48 hours			90732	Pneumovax	
	99382	1-4 year old			87070	Throat Culture			10060	I & D Abscess Simple			90716	Varicella	
	99383	5-11 year old			80053	Chem profile			10061	I & D Abscess Comp.		✓	~~82607~~	Vitamin B12 Inj.	*$30.*
	99384	12-17 year old			80061	Lipid profile			94761	Oximetry w/Exercise			90712	Polio oral use (OPV)	
	99385	18-39 year old			82465	Cholesterol			94726	Plethysmography			90713	Polio injection (IPV)	
	99386	40-64 year old			99000	Handling fee			94760	Pulse Oximetry			90714	Td preservative free 7 yrs +	
	99387	65 + year old		**X-RAY**					11100	Skin Bx			90718	Td 7 years +	
PREVENTATIVE MEDICINE - ESTABLISHED PATIENT					70210	Sinuses			94010	Spirometry			95115	Allergy inj., single	
	99391	< 1 year old			70360	Neck Soft Tissue			99173	Visual Acuity			95117	Allergy inj., multiple	
	99392	1-4 year old			71010	CXR (PA only)			17110	Wart destruction up to 14					
	99393	5-11 year old			71020	Chest 2V			17111	Wart destruction 15 lesions +					
	99394	12-17 year old			72040	C-Spine 2V			11042	Wound Debrid.		**OTHER**			
	99395	18-39 year old			72100	Lumbrosacral									
	99396	40-64 year old			73030	Shoulder 2V									
	99397	65 + year old			73070	Elbow 2V									
					73120	Hand 2V									
					73560	Knee 2V									
					73620	Foot 2V									
					74000	KUB									

DIAGNOSTIC CODES (ICD-9-CM)

☐	Code	Description	☐	Code	Description	☐	Code	Description	☐	Code	Description
	789.0__	Abdominal Pain		564.0	Constipation		784.0	Headache		782.1	Rash or ezanthem
	682.__	Abscess/Cellulitis		692.6	Contact dermatitis due to plants		414.9	Heart Dis., Coronary		714.0	Rheumatoid Arthritis
	995.3	Allergic Reaction		692.9	Contact dermatitis, NOS		599.70	Hematuria		V70.0	Routine general exam
	331	Alzheimer's		V25.09	Contraceptive management		455.6	Hemorrhoids		V76.10	Screen, breast
✓	285. *9*	Anemia, other & unspec		923.10	Contusion, forearm		573.3	Hepatitus, NOS		V76.2	Screen, cervix
	280.9	Anemia-iron deficiency		434.91	CVA		V03.81	HIB		V76.44	Screen, prosate
	281.0	Anemia-pernicious		266.2	Deficiency, folic acid B12		V65.44	HIV counseling		V76.47	Screen, vagina
	285.9	Anemia-unspecified		311	Depression		401.1	Hypertension, benign		216.5	Sebaceous cyst
	413.9	Angina, pectoris, oyher/unspecified		250.01	Diabetes, type I, juvenile type		401.9	Hypertension, unspecified		706.2	Sebaceous cyst
	300.00	Anxiety state, NOS		787.91	Diarrhea		401.0	Hypertension, malignant		786.05	Shortness of Breath
	300.4	Anxiety reaction		780.4	Dizziness		V04.81	Influenza		701.9	Skin tag
	716.90	Arthritis, NOS		V06.1	DTP		271.3	Lactose intolerance		845.00	Strain, ankle
	493.20	Asthma; chronic obstruction		V06.3	DTP + polio		573.9	Liver Disease		307.81	Tension headache
	493.00	Asthma; extrinic		536.8	Dyspepsia		724.5	Low Back Pain		V06.5	Tetanus - distheria (Td)
	493.10	Asthma; intrinsic		788.1	Dysuria		346.9	Migraine		305.1	Tobacco dependence
	493.90	Asthmas; unspecified		782.3	Edema		V06.4	MMR		788.41	Urinary frequency
	427.31	Atrial fibulation		530.81	Esophageal reflux		278.01	Obesity/Morbid		599.0	Unrinary tract infection, NOS
	724.5	Backache, unspecified		530.11	Esophagitis reflux		715.90	Osteoarthritis		V05.3	Viral hepatitis
	790.6	Blood chemistry		530.10	Esophagitis, unspecified		719.43	Pain in joint, forearm		368.40	Visual field defect, unspecified
	E906.3	Cat bite		780.6	Fever		625.4	PMS		V20.2	Well Child Exam
	786.50	Chest Pain		789.07	Generalized abdominal pain		486	Pneumonia			
	428.0	CHF		V72.3	Gynecological examiniation		V25.01	Prescription of oral contraceptivess			

DIAGNOSIS: (IF NOT CHECKED ABOVE)		RECEIVED BY:	TODAY'S FEE	*$78.00*
PROCEDURES: (IF NOT CHECKED ABOVE)	RETURN APPOINTMENT INFORMATION:	☐ CASH ☐ CREDIT CARD ☐ CHECK #________	AMOUNT RECEIVED	———
use J3420 for B12 inj.	(DAYS) (WKS.) (MOS.) (PRN)		BALANCE	*$78.00*

Figure C.88 Encounter form (Superbill) for Lynn Stone (Appendix A: Day 5).

Goode Medical Clinic
William B. Goode, MD

Patient Registration Information

Account # :
Insurance # :
Co-Payment: $

Please PRINT AND complete ALL sections below!

PATIENT'S PERSONAL INFORMATION Marital Status ☒ Single ☐ Married ☐ Divorced ☐ Widowed Sex: ☒ Male ☐ Female

Name: Nelson (last name) Steve (first name) (initial)

Street address: 123 Ramsey Hill (Apt #) City: St. Paul State: MN Zip: 55100

Home phone: (555) 555-4545 Work phone: (555) 555-6756 Social Security # 456 - XX - 4382

Date of Birth: 11 (month) / 30 (day) / 76 (year)

Employer / Name of School Governs Bar ☒ Full Time ☐ Part Time

PATIENT'S / RESPONSIBLE PARTY INFORMATION

Responsible party: self (Steve Nelson) Date of Birth:

Relationship to Patient: ☒ Self ☐ Spouse ☐ Other Social Security # - -

Responsible party's home phone: ( )

Address: (Apt #) City: State: Zip:

Employer's name: Governs Bar Phone number: (555) 555-6756

Address: 900 8th Street City: St. Paul State: MN Zip: 55100

Name of Parent/Guardian:

PATIENT'S INSURANCE INFORMATION Please present insurance cards to receptionist.

PRIMARY insurance company's name: Blue Cross and Blue Shield

Insurance address: 1355 Insurance Carrier Loop City: Minneapolis State: MN Zip: 55401

Name of insured: Steve Nelson Date of Birth: Relationship to insured: ☒ Self ☐ Spouse ☐ Other ☐ Child

Insurance ID number: SN-4567-GB Group number: 56789

Does your insurance cover medication? yes

EMERGENCY CONTACT

Name of person not living with you: Peter Nelson Relationship: Father

Address: 29 Highgate Court City: Minneapolis State: MN Zip: 55100

Phone number: (555) 555-9999 (cell)

Assignment of Benefits • Financial Agreement

I hereby give lifetime authorization for payment of insurance benefits to be made directly to Goode Medical Clinic ,and any assisting physicians, for services rendered. I understand that I am financially responsible for all charges whether or not they are covered by insurance. In the event of default, I agree to pay all costs of collection, and reasonable attorney's fees. I hereby authorize this healthcare provider to release all information necessary to secure the payment of benefits.
I further agree that a photocopy of this agreement shall be as valid as the original.

Date: XX/XX/XXXX Your Signature: Steve Nelson

FORM # 58-8423 • BIBBERO SYSTEMS, INC.• PETALUMA, CA.• TO ORDER CALL TOLL FREE :800-BIBBERO (800-242-2376) • FAX (800) 242-9330 (REV.7/94)

Figure C.89 Registration form for Steve Nelson (Appendix A: Day 5).

Goode Medical Clinic
1234 Larsen Avenue
Saint Paul, Minnesota 55316

Phone: (555) 555-1234
Fax: (555) 555-5678

PATIENT NAME	CHART #	DATE		
Steve Nelson		*XX/XX/XXXX*	☐ MEDI-MEDI ☐ SELF PAY ☐ MEDICARE	☐ MEDICAL ☒ PRIVATE ☐ HMO___

✓	CPT/Md	DESCRIPTION	FEE	✓	CPT/Md	DESCRIPTION	FEE	✓	CPT/Md	DESCRIPTION	FEE	✓	CPT/Md	DESCRIPTION	FEE
OFFICE VISIT - NEW PATIENT				LAB STUDIES				PROCEDURES				INJECTIONS			
	99202	Focused Ex.			36415	Venipucture			92551	Audiometry			90655	Influenza 6-35 months	
✓	99203	Detailed Ex.	*$80.*		81000	Urinalysis			29705	Cast Removal Full Arm/Leg			90656	Influenza 3 years +	
	99204	Comprehensive Ex.			81003	- w/o Micro			2900__	Casting (by location)			90732	Pneumoccal	
	99205	Complex Ex.			84703	HCG (Urine, Pregnancy)			92567	Ear Check			J0295	Ampicillin, 1.5 gr	
OFFICE VISIT - ESTABLISHED PATIENT					82948	Glucose			69210	Ear Wax Rem. 1 2			J2001	Liocaine for IV infusion 10mg	
	99212	Focused Ex.			82270	Hemoccult			93000	EKG			J1885	Toradol 15mg	
	99213	Expanded Ex.			85025	CBC -diff.			93005	EKG tracing only			90720	DTP - HIB	
	99214	Detailed Ex.			85018	Hemoglobin			93010	EKG Int. and Rep			90746	HEP B - HIB	
	99215	Complex Ex.			88174	Pap Smear			11750	Excision Nail			90707	MMR	
PREVENTATIVE MEDICINE - NEW PATIENT					87210	KOH/ Saline Wet Mount			94375	Respiratory Flow Volume			86580	PPD	
	99381	< 1 year old			87430	Strep Antigen			93224	Holter up to 48 hours			90732	Pneumovax	
	99382	1-4 year old			87070	Throat Culture			10060	I & D Abscess Simple			90716	Varicella	
	99383	5-11 year old			80053	Chem profile			10061	I & D Abscess Comp.			82607	Vitamin B12 Inj.	
	99384	12-17 year old			80061	Lipid profile			94761	Oximetry w/Exercise			90712	Polio oral use (OPV)	
	99385	18-39 year old			82465	Cholesterol			94726	Plethysmography			90713	Polio injection (IPV)	
	99386	40-64 year old			99000	Handling fee			94760	Pulse Oximetry			90714	Td preservative free 7 yrs +	
	99387	65 + year old		X-RAY					11100	Skin Bx			90718	Td 7 years +	
PREVENTATIVE MEDICINE - ESTABLISHED PATIENT					70210	Sinuses			94010	Spirometry			95115	Allergy inj., single	
	99391	< 1 year old			70360	Neck Soft Tissue			99173	Visual Acuity			95117	Allergy inj., multiple	
	99392	1-4 year old			71010	CXR (PA only)			17110	Wart destruction up to 14					
	99393	5-11 year old			71020	Chest 2V			17111	Wart destruction 15 lesions +					
	99394	12-17 year old			72040	C-Spine 2V			11042	Wound Debrid.		OTHER			
	99395	18-39 year old			72100	Lumbrosacral									
	99396	40-64 year old			73030	Shoulder 2V									
	99397	65 + year old			73070	Elbow 2V									
					73120	Hand 2V									
					73560	Knee 2V									
					73620	Foot 2V									
					74000	KUB									

DIAGNOSTIC CODES (ICD-9-CM)

✓	Code	Description	✓	Code	Description	✓	Code	Description	✓	Code	Description
	789.0__	Abdominal Pain		564.0	Constipation		784.0	Headache		782.1	Rash or ezanthem
	682.__	Abscess/Cellulitis		692.6	Contact dermatitis due to plants		414.9	Heart Dis., Coronary		714.0	Rheumatoid Arthritis
	995.3	Allergic Reaction		692.9	Contact dermatitis, NOS		599.70	Hematuria		V70.0	Routine general exam
	331	Alzheimer's		V25.09	Contraceptive management		455.6	Hemorrhoids		V76.10	Screen, breast
	285.__	Anemia, other & unspec		923.10	Contusion, forearm		573.3	Hepatitus, NOS		V76.2	Screen, cervix
	280.9	Anemia-iron deficiency		434.91	CVA		V03.81	HIB		V76.44	Screen, prosate
	281.0	Anemia-pernicious		266.2	Deficiency, folic acid B12		V65.44	HIV counseling		V76.47	Screen, vagina
	285.9	Anemia-unspecified		311	Depression		401.1	Hypertension, benign		216.5	Sebaceous cyst
	413.9	Angina, pectoris, oyher/unspecified		250.01	Diabetes, type I, juvenile type		401.9	Hypertension, unspecified		706.2	Sebaceous cyst
	300.00	Anxiety state, NOS		787.91	Diarrhea		401.0	Hypertension, malignant		786.05	Shortness of Breath
	300.4	Anxiety reaction		780.4	Dizziness		V04.81	Influenza		701.9	Skin tag
	716.90	Arthritis, NOS		V06.1	DTP		271.3	Lactose intolerance		845.00	Strain, ankle
	493.20	Asthma; chronic obstruction		V06.3	DTP + polio		573.9	Liver Disease		307.81	Tension headache
	493.00	Asthma; extrinic		536.8	Dyspepsia	✓	724.5	Low Back Pain		V06.5	Tetanus - distheria (Td)
	493.10	Asthma; intrinsic		788.1	Dysuria		346.9	Migraine		305.1	Tobacco dependence
	493.90	Asthmas; unspecified		782.3	Edema		V06.4	MMR		788.41	Urinary frequency
	427.31	Atrial fibulation		530.81	Esophageal reflux		278.01	Obesity/Morbid		599.0	Unrinary tract infection, NOS
	724.5	Backache, unspecified		530.11	Esophagitis reflux		715.90	Osteoarthritis		V05.3	Viral hepatitis
	790.6	Blood chemistry		530.10	Esophagitis, unspecified		719.43	Pain in joint, forearm		368.40	Visual field defect, unspecified
	E906.3	Cat bite		780.6	Fever		625.4	PMS		V20.2	Well Child Exam
	786.50	Chest Pain		789.07	Generalized abdominal pain		486	Pneumonia			
	428.0	CHF		V72.3	Gynecological examiniation		V25.01	Prescription of oral contraceptivess			

DIAGNOSIS: (IF NOT CHECKED ABOVE)

Motor vehicle accident — E812.0

PROCEDURES: (IF NOT CHECKED ABOVE)

RETURN APPOINTMENT INFORMATION:

(DAYS) (WKS.) (MOS.) (PRN)

RECEIVED BY:

☐ CASH
☐ CREDIT CARD
☐ CHECK
\# __________

TODAY'S FEE	*$80.—*
AMOUNT RECEIVED	*—*
BALANCE	*$80.—*

Figure C.90 Encounter form (Superbill) for Steve Nelson (Appendix A: Day 5).

Goode Medical Clinic

1234 Larsen Avenue
Saint Paul, Minnesota 55316

Phone: (555) 555-1234
Fax: (555) 555-5678

PATIENT NAME	CHART #	DATE		
Danny Smith		XX/XX/XXXX	☐ MEDI-MEDI ☐ SELF PAY ☐ MEDICARE	☒ MEDICAL ☐ PRIVATE ☐ HMO______

✓	CPT/Md	DESCRIPTION	FEE	✓	CPT/Md	DESCRIPTION	FEE	✓	CPT/Md	DESCRIPTION	FEE	✓	CPT/Md	DESCRIPTION	FEE
OFFICE VISIT - NEW PATIENT				**LAB STUDIES**				**PROCEDURES**				**INJECTIONS**			
	99202	Focused Ex.			36415	Venipucture			92551	Audiometry			90655	Influenza 6-35 months	
	99203	Detailed Ex.			81000	Urinalysis			29705	Cast Removal Full Arm/Leg			90656	Influenza 3 years +	
	99204	Comprehensive Ex.			81003	- w/o Micro			2900__	Casting (by location)			90732	Pneumoccal	
	99205	Complex Ex.			84703	HCG (Urine, Pregnancy)			92567	Ear Check			J0295	Ampicillin, 1.5 gr	
OFFICE VISIT - ESTABLISHED PATIENT					82948	Glucose			69210	Ear Wax Rem. 1 2			J2001	Liocaine for IV infusion 10mg	
	99212	Focused Ex.			82270	Hemoccult			93000	EKG			J1885	Toradol 15mg	
✓	99213	Expanded Ex.	$48.		85025	CBC -diff.			93005	EKG tracing only			90720	DTP - HIB	
	99214	Detailed Ex.			85018	Hemoglobin			93010	EKG Int. and Rep			90746	HEP B - HIB	
	99215	Complex Ex.			88174	Pap Smear			11750	Excision Nail			90707	MMR	
PREVENTATIVE MEDICINE - NEW PATIENT					87210	KOH/ Saline Wet Mount			94375	Respiratory Flow Volume			86580	PPD	
	99381	< 1 year old			87430	Strep Antigen			93224	Holter up to 48 hours			90732	Pneumovax	
	99382	1-4 year old			87070	Throat Culture			10060	I & D Abscess Simple			90716	Varicella	
	99383	5-11 year old			80053	Chem profile			10061	I & D Abscess Comp.			82607	Vitamin B12 Inj.	
	99384	12-17 year old			80061	Lipid profile			94761	Oximetry w/Exercise			90712	Polio oral use (OPV)	
	99385	18-39 year old			82465	Cholesterol			94726	Plethysmography			90713	Polio injection (IPV)	
	99386	40-64 year old			99000	Handling fee			94760	Pulse Oximetry			90714	Td preservative free 7 yrs +	
	99387	65 + year old		**X-RAY**					11100	Skin Bx			90718	Td 7 years +	
PREVENTATIVE MEDICINE - ESTABLISHED PATIENT					70210	Sinuses			94010	Spirometry			95115	Allergy inj., single	
	99391	< 1 year old			70360	Neck Soft Tissue			99173	Visual Acuity			95117	Allergy inj., multiple	
	99392	1-4 year old			71010	CXR (PA only)			17110	Wart destruction up to 14					
	99393	5-11 year old			71020	Chest 2V			17111	Wart destruction 15 lesions +					
	99394	12-17 year old			72040	C-Spine 2V			11042	Wound Debrid.		**OTHER**			
	99395	18-39 year old			72100	Lumbrosacral									
	99396	40-64 year old			73030	Shoulder 2V									
	99397	65 + year old			73070	Elbow 2V									
					73120	Hand 2V									
					73560	Knee 2V									
					73620	Foot 2V									
					74000	KUB									

DIAGNOSTIC CODES (ICD-9-CM)

✓	Code	Description	✓	Code	Description	✓	Code	Description	✓	Code	Description
	789.0__	Abdominal Pain		564.0	Constipation		784.0	Headache		782.1	Rash or ezanthem
	682.__	Abscess/Cellulitis		692.6	Contact dermatitis due to plants		414.9	Heart Dis., Coronary		714.0	Rheumatoid Arthritis
	995.3	Allergic Reaction		692.9	Contact dermatitis, NOS		599.70	Hematuria		V70.0	Routine general exam
	331	Alzheimer's		V25.09	Contraceptive management		455.6	Hemorrhoids		V76.10	Screen, breast
	285.__	Anemia, other & unspec		923.10	Contusion, forearm		573.3	Hepatitus, NOS		V76.2	Screen, cervix
	280.9	Anemia-iron deficiency		434.91	CVA		V03.81	HIB		V76.44	Screen, prosate
	281.0	Anemia-pernicious		266.2	Deficiency, folic acid B12		V65.44	HIV counseling		V76.47	Screen, vagina
	285.9	Anemia-unspecified		311	Depression		401.1	Hypertension, benign		216.5	Sebaceous cyst
	413.9	Angina, pectoris, oyher/unspecified		250.01	Diabetes, type I, juvenile type		401.9	Hypertension, unspecified		706.2	Sebaceous cyst
	300.00	Anxiety state, NOS		787.91	Diarrhea		401.0	Hypertension, malignant		786.05	Shortness of Breath
	300.4	Anxiety reaction		780.4	Dizziness		V04.81	Influenza		701.9	Skin tag
	716.90	Arthritis, NOS		V06.1	DTP		271.3	Lactose intolerance		845.00	Strain, ankle
	493.20	Asthma; chronic obstruction		V06.3	DTP + polio		573.9	Liver Disease		307.81	Tension headache
	493.00	Asthma; extrinic		536.8	Dyspepsia		724.5	Low Back Pain		V06.5	Tetanus - distheria (Td)
	493.10	Asthma; intrinsic		788.1	Dysuria		346.9	Migraine		305.1	Tobacco dependence
	493.90	Asthmas; unspecified		782.3	Edema		V06.4	MMR		788.41	Urinary frequency
	427.31	Atrial fibulation		530.81	Esophageal reflux		278.01	Obesity/Morbid		599.0	Unrinary tract infection, NOS
	724.5	Backache, unspecified		530.11	Esophagitis reflux		715.90	Osteoarthritis		V05.3	Viral hepatitis
	790.6	Blood chemistry		530.10	Esophagitis, unspecified		719.43	Pain in joint, forearm		368.40	Visual field defect, unspecified
	E906.3	Cat bite		780.6	Fever		625.4	PMS		V20.2	Well Child Exam
	786.50	Chest Pain		789.07	Generalized abdominal pain		486	Pneumonia			
	428.0	CHF		V72.3	Gynecological examiniation		V25.01	Prescription of oral contraceptivess			

DIAGNOSIS: (IF NOT CHECKED ABOVE)

932 Penny up nostril (right)

PROCEDURES: (IF NOT CHECKED ABOVE)

RETURN APPOINTMENT INFORMATION:

(DAYS) (WKS.) (MOS.) (PRN)

RECEIVED BY:

☐ CASH
☐ CREDIT CARD
☐ CHECK
#__________

TODAY'S FEE	$48.
AMOUNT RECEIVED	
BALANCE	$48.

Figure C.91 Encounter form (Superbill) for Danny Smith (Appendix A: Day 5).

Goode Medical Clinic
1234 Larsen Avenue
Saint Paul, Minnesota 55316

Phone: (555) 555-1234
Fax: (555) 555-5678

PATIENT NAME	CHART #	DATE		
Adam Burns		*XX/XX/XXXX*	☐ MEDI-MEDI ☐ SELF PAY ☐ MEDICARE	☒ MEDICAL ☐ PRIVATE ☐ HMO____

✓	CPT/Md	DESCRIPTION	FEE
	OFFICE VISIT - NEW PATIENT		
	99202	Focused Ex.	
	99203	Detailed Ex.	
	99204	Comprehensive Ex.	
	99205	Complex Ex.	
	OFFICE VISIT - ESTABLISHED PATIENT		
	99212	Focused Ex.	
✓	99213	Expanded Ex.	*$48.*
	99214	Detailed Ex.	
	99215	Complex Ex.	
	PREVENTATIVE MEDICINE - NEW PATIENT		
	99381	< 1 year old	
	99382	1-4 year old	
	99383	5-11 year old	
	99384	12-17 year old	
	99385	18-39 year old	
	99386	40-64 year old	
	99387	65 + year old	
	PREVENTATIVE MEDICINE - ESTABLISHED PATIENT		
	99391	< 1 year old	
	99392	1-4 year old	
	99393	5-11 year old	
	99394	12-17 year old	
	99395	18-39 year old	
	99396	40-64 year old	
	99397	65 + year old	

✓	CPT/Md	DESCRIPTION	FEE
	LAB STUDIES		
	36415	Venipucture	
	81000	Urinalysis	
	81003	- w/o Micro	
	84703	HCG (Urine, Pregnancy)	
	82948	Glucose	
	82270	Hemoccult	
	85025	CBC -diff.	
	85018	Hemoglobin	
	88174	Pap Smear	
	87210	KOH/ Saline Wet Mount	
	87430	Strep Antigen	
	87070	Throat Culture	
	80053	Chem profile	
	80061	Lipid profile	
	82465	Cholesterol	
	99000	Handling fee	
	X-RAY		
	70210	Sinuses	
	70360	Neck Soft Tissue	
	71010	CXR (PA only)	
	71020	Chest 2V	
	72040	C-Spine 2V	
	72100	Lumbrosacral	
	73030	Shoulder 2V	
	73070	Elbow 2V	
	73120	Hand 2V	
	73560	Knee 2V	
	73620	Foot 2V	
	74000	KUB	

✓	CPT/Md	DESCRIPTION	FEE
	PROCEDURES		
	92551	Audiometry	
	29705	Cast Removal Full Arm/Leg	
	2900__	Casting (by location)	
	92567	Ear Check	
	69210	Ear Wax Rem. 1 2	
	93000	EKG	
	93005	EKG tracing only	
	93010	EKG Int. and Rep	
	11750	Excision Nail	
	94375	Respiratory Flow Volume	
	93224	Holter up to 48 hours	
	10060	I & D Abscess Simple	
	10061	I & D Abscess Comp.	
	94761	Oximetry w/Exercise	
	94726	Plethysmography	
	94760	Pulse Oximetry	
	11100	Skin Bx	
	94010	Spirometry	
	99173	Visual Acuity	
	17110	Wart destruction up to 14	
	17111	Wart destruction 15 lesions +	
	11042	Wound Debrid.	

✓	CPT/Md	DESCRIPTION	FEE
	INJECTIONS		
	90655	Influenza 6-35 months	
	90656	Influenza 3 years +	
	90732	Pneumoccal	
	J0295	Ampicillin, 1.5 gr	
	J2001	Liocaine for IV infusion 10mg	
	J1885	Toradol 15mg	
	90720	DTP - HIB	
	90746	HEP B - HIB	
	90707	MMR	
	86580	PPD	
	90732	Pneumovax	
	90716	Varicella	
	82607	Vitamin B12 Inj.	
	90712	Polio oral use (OPV)	
	90713	Polio injection (IPV)	
	90714	Td preservative free 7 yrs +	
	90718	Td 7 years +	
	95115	Allergy inj., single	
	95117	Allergy inj., multiple	
	OTHER		

DIAGNOSTIC CODES (ICD-9-CM)

✓	Code	Description	✓	Code	Description	✓	Code	Description	✓	Code	Description
	789.0__	Abdominal Pain		564.0	Constipation		784.0	Headache		782.1	Rash or ezanthem
	682.__	Abscess/Cellulitis		692.6	Contact dermatitis due to plants		414.9	Heart Dis., Coronary		714.0	Rheumatoid Arthritis
	995.3	Allergic Reaction		692.9	Contact dermatitis, NOS		599.70	Hematuria		V70.0	Routine general exam
	331	Alzheimer's		V25.09	Contraceptive management		455.6	Hemorrhoids		V76.10	Screen, breast
	285.__	Anemia, other & unspec		923.10	Contusion, forearm		573.3	Hepatitus, NOS		V76.2	Screen, cervix
	280.9	Anemia-iron deficiency		434.91	CVA		V03.81	HIB		V76.44	Screen, prosate
	281.0	Anemia-pernicious		266.2	Deficiency, folic acid B12		V65.44	HIV counseling		V76.47	Screen, vagina
	285.9	Anemia-unspecified		311	Depression		401.1	Hypertension, benign		216.5	Sebaceous cyst
	413.9	Angina, pectoris, oyher/unspecified		250.01	Diabetes, type I, juvenile type	✓	401.9	Hypertension, unspecified		706.2	Sebaceous cyst
	300.00	Anxiety state, NOS		787.91	Diarrhea		401.0	Hypertension, malignant		786.05	Shortness of Breath
	300.4	Anxiety reaction		780.4	Dizziness		V04.81	Influenza		701.9	Skin tag
	716.90	Arthritis, NOS		V06.1	DTP		271.3	Lactose intolerance		845.00	Strain, ankle
	493.20	Asthma; chronic obstruction		V06.3	DTP + polio		573.9	Liver Disease		307.81	Tension headache
	493.00	Asthma; extrinic		536.8	Dyspepsia		724.5	Low Back Pain		V06.5	Tetanus - distheria (Td)
	493.10	Asthma; intrinsic		788.1	Dysuria		346.9	Migraine		305.1	Tobacco dependence
	493.90	Asthmas; unspecified		782.3	Edema		V06.4	MMR		788.41	Urinary frequency
	427.31	Atrial fibulation		530.81	Esophageal reflux		278.01	Obesity/Morbid		599.0	Unrinary tract infection, NOS
	724.5	Backache, unspecified		530.11	Esophagitis reflux		715.90	Osteoarthritis		V05.3	Viral hepatitis
	790.6	Blood chemistry		530.10	Esophagitis, unspecified		719.43	Pain in joint, forearm		368.40	Visual field defect, unspecified
	E906.3	Cat bite		780.6	Fever		625.4	PMS		V20.2	Well Child Exam
	786.50	Chest Pain		789.07	Generalized abdominal pain		486	Pneumonia			
	428.0	CHF		V72.3	Gynecological examiniation		V25.01	Prescription of oral contraceptivess			

DIAGNOSIS: (IF NOT CHECKED ABOVE)		RECEIVED BY:	TODAY'S FEE	*$48.*
PROCEDURES: (IF NOT CHECKED ABOVE)	RETURN APPOINTMENT INFORMATION: *follow-up tomorrow* (*1* DAYS) (WKS.) (MOS.) (PRN)	☐ CASH ☐ CREDIT CARD ☐ CHECK # ________	AMOUNT RECEIVED BALANCE	 *$48.*

Figure C.92 Encounter form (Superbill) for Adam Burns (Appendix A: Day 5).

BCBS of MN
1355 Insurance Carrier Loop
Minneapolis, MN 55111
(763)555-0426

Remittance advice

Goode Medical Clinic
1612 Southwest Blvd.
St. Paul, MN 55100

Page: 1 of 1
Date: XX/XX/XX
Group Practice ID#: 567XX
Check number: 234567

Patient name	DOS	Procedure code	Units	Total charge	Allowable	Provider responsibility	Co-pay	Amount paid
Stone, Lynn	02/08/2013	99213	1	48.00	46.00	2.00	0	46.00
	02/08/2013	J3420	1	30.00	15.00	15.00	0	15.00

Total charges $78.00 Total provider responsibility $17.00 Total co-pay 0 Total paid $61.00

Figure C.93.1 Remittance Advice—Blue Cross and Blue Shield (Appendix A: Day 6).

BCBS of MN
1355 Insurance Carrier Loop
Minneapolis, MN 55111
(763)555-0426

Remittance advice

Goode Medical Clinic
1612 Southwest Blvd.
St. Paul, MN 55100

Page: 1 of 1
Date: XX/XX/XX
Group Practice ID#: 567XX
Check number: 890123

Patient name	DOS	Procedure code	Units	Total charge	Allowable	Provider responsibility	Co-pay	Amount paid
Smith, Danny	02/08/2013	99213	1	48.00	46.00	2.00	0	46.00

Total charges $48.00 Total provider responsibility $2.00 Total co-pay 0 Total paid $46.00

Figure C.93.2 Remittance Advice—Blue Cross and Blue Shield (Appendix A: Day 6).

BCBS of MN
1355 Insurance Carrier Loop
Minneapolis, MN 55111
(763)555-0426

Remittance advice

Goode Medical Clinic
1612 Southwest Blvd.
St. Paul, MN 55100

Page: 1 of 1
Date: XX/XX/XX
Group Practice ID#: 567XX
Check number: 456789

Patient name	DOS	Procedure code	Units	Total charge	Allowable	Provider responsibility	Co-pay	Amount paid
Burns, Adam	02/08/2013	99213	0	48.00	46.00	2.00	0	46.00

Total charges $48.00 Total provider responsibility $2.00 Total co-pay 0 Total paid $46.00

Figure C.93.3 Remittance Advice—Blue Cross and Blue Shield (Appendix A: Day 6).

State Farm Insurance Company of MN
3489 Walkahead Rd.
St. Paul, MN 55100
(763)555-6026

Remittance advice

Goode Medical Clinic
1612 Southwest Blvd.
St. Paul, MN 55100

Page: 1 of 1
Date of accident: 02/03/2013
Federal Tax ID #: 23-XX-12345
Check number: 234568

Patient name	DOS	Procedure code	Units	Total charge	Allowable	Provider responsibility	Co-pay	Amount paid
Nelson, Steve	02/08/2013	99203	1	80.00	80.00	0.00	0	80.00

Total charges $80.00 Total provider responsibility $0.00 Total co-pay 0 Total paid $80.00

Figure C.94 Remittance Advice—State Farm Insurance (Appendix A: Day 6).

Goode Medical Clinic

1234 Larsen Avenue
Saint Paul, Minnesota 55316

Phone: (555) 555-1234
Fax: (555) 555-5678

PATIENT NAME	CHART #	DATE		
Adam Burns		*XX/XX/XXXX*	☐ MEDI-MEDI ☐ SELF PAY ☐ MEDICARE	☒ MEDICAL ☐ PRIVATE ☐ HMO____

✓	CPT/Md	DESCRIPTION	FEE	✓	CPT/Md	DESCRIPTION	FEE	✓	CPT/Md	DESCRIPTION	FEE	✓	CPT/Md	DESCRIPTION	FEE
OFFICE VISIT - NEW PATIENT				**LAB STUDIES**				**PROCEDURES**				**INJECTIONS**			
	99202	Focused Ex.			36415	Venipucture			92551	Audiometry			90655	Influenza 6-35 months	
	99203	Detailed Ex.			81000	Urinalysis			29705	Cast Removal Full Arm/Leg			90656	Influenza 3 years +	
	99204	Comprehensive Ex.			81003	- w/o Micro			2900__	Casting (by location)			90732	Pneumoccal	
	99205	Complex Ex.			84703	HCG (Urine, Pregnancy)			92567	Ear Check			J0295	Ampicillin, 1.5 gr	
OFFICE VISIT - ESTABLISHED PATIENT					82948	Glucose			69210	Ear Wax Rem. 1 2			J2001	Liocaine for IV infusion 10mg	
	99212	Focused Ex.			82270	Hemoccult			93000	EKG			J1885	Toradol 15mg	
✓	99213	Expanded Ex.	*$48.*		85025	CBC -diff.			93005	EKG tracing only			90720	DTP - HIB	
	99214	Detailed Ex.			85018	Hemoglobin			93010	EKG Int. and Rep			90746	HEP B - HIB	
	99215	Complex Ex.			88174	Pap Smear			11750	Excision Nail			90707	MMR	
PREVENTATIVE MEDICINE - NEW PATIENT					87210	KOH/ Saline Wet Mount			94375	Respiratory Flow Volume			86580	PPD	
	99381	< 1 year old			87430	Strep Antigen			93224	Holter up to 48 hours			90732	Pneumovax	
	99382	1-4 year old			87070	Throat Culture			10060	I & D Abscess Simple			90716	Varicella	
	99383	5-11 year old			80053	Chem profile			10061	I & D Abscess Comp.			82607	Vitamin B12 Inj.	
	99384	12-17 year old			80061	Lipid profile			94761	Oximetry w/Exercise			90712	Polio oral use (OPV)	
	99385	18-39 year old			82465	Cholesterol			94726	Plethysmography			90713	Polio injection (IPV)	
	99386	40-64 year old			99000	Handling fee			94760	Pulse Oximetry			90714	Td preservative free 7 yrs +	
	99387	65 + year old		**X-RAY**					11100	Skin Bx			90718	Td 7 years +	
PREVENTATIVE MEDICINE - ESTABLISHED PATIENT					70210	Sinuses			94010	Spirometry			95115	Allergy inj., single	
	99391	< 1 year old			70360	Neck Soft Tissue			99173	Visual Acuity			95117	Allergy inj., multiple	
	99392	1-4 year old			71010	CXR (PA only)			17110	Wart destruction up to 14					
	99393	5-11 year old			71020	Chest 2V			17111	Wart destruction 15 lesions +					
	99394	12-17 year old			72040	C-Spine 2V			11042	Wound Debrid.		**OTHER**			
	99395	18-39 year old			72100	Lumbrosacral									
	99396	40-64 year old			73030	Shoulder 2V									
	99397	65 + year old			73070	Elbow 2V									
					73120	Hand 2V									
					73560	Knee 2V									
					73620	Foot 2V									
					74000	KUB									

DIAGNOSTIC CODES (ICD-9-CM)

✓	Code	Description	✓	Code	Description	✓	Code	Description	✓	Code	Description
	789.0__	Abdominal Pain		564.0	Constipation		784.0	Headache		782.1	Rash or ezanthem
	682.__	Abscess/Cellulitis		692.6	Contact dermatitis due to plants		414.9	Heart Dis., Coronary		714.0	Rheumatoid Arthritis
	995.3	Allergic Reaction		692.9	Contact dermatitis, NOS		599.70	Hematuria		V70.0	Routine general exam
	331	Alzheimer's		V25.09	Contraceptive management		455.6	Hemorrhoids		V76.10	Screen, breast
	285.__	Anemia, other & unspec		923.10	Contusion, forearm		573.3	Hepatitus, NOS		V76.2	Screen, cervix
	280.9	Anemia-iron deficiency		434.91	CVA		V03.81	HIB		V76.44	Screen, prosate
	281.0	Anemia-pernicious		266.2	Deficiency, folic acid B12		V65.44	HIV counseling		V76.47	Screen, vagina
	285.9	Anemia-unspecified		311	Depression		401.1	Hypertension, benign		216.5	Sebaceous cyst
	413.9	Angina, pectoris, oyher/unspecified		250.01	Diabetes, type I, juvenile type	✓	401.9	Hypertension, unspecified		706.2	Sebaceous cyst
	300.00	Anxiety state, NOS		787.91	Diarrhea		401.0	Hypertension, malignant		786.05	Shortness of Breath
	300.4	Anxiety reaction		780.4	Dizziness		V04.81	Influenza		701.9	Skin tag
	716.90	Arthritis, NOS		V06.1	DTP		271.3	Lactose intolerance		845.00	Strain, ankle
	493.20	Asthma; chronic obstruction		V06.3	DTP + polio		573.9	Liver Disease		307.81	Tension headache
	493.00	Asthma; extrinic		536.8	Dyspepsia		724.5	Low Back Pain		V06.5	Tetanus - distheria (Td)
	493.10	Asthma; intrinsic		788.1	Dysuria		346.9	Migraine		305.1	Tobacco dependence
	493.90	Asthmas; unspecified		782.3	Edema		V06.4	MMR		788.41	Urinary frequency
	427.31	Atrial fibulation		530.81	Esophageal reflux		278.01	Obesity/Morbid		599.0	Unrinary tract infection, NOS
	724.5	Backache, unspecified		530.11	Esophagitis reflux		715.90	Osteoarthritis		V05.3	Viral hepatitis
	790.6	Blood chemistry		530.10	Esophagitis, unspecified		719.43	Pain in joint, forearm		368.40	Visual field defect, unspecified
	E906.3	Cat bite		780.6	Fever		625.4	PMS		V20.2	Well Child Exam
	786.50	Chest Pain		789.07	Generalized abdominal pain		486	Pneumonia			
	428.0	CHF		V72.3	Gynecological examiniation		V25.01	Prescription of oral contraceptivess			

DIAGNOSIS: (IF NOT CHECKED ABOVE)		RECEIVED BY:	TODAY'S FEE	*$48.—*
		☐ CASH	AMOUNT RECEIVED	*——*
PROCEDURES: (IF NOT CHECKED ABOVE)	RETURN APPOINTMENT INFORMATION:	☐ CREDIT CARD		
	(DAYS) (*1* WKS.) (MOS.) (PRN)	☐ CHECK # ________	BALANCE	*$48.—*

Figure C.95 Encounter form (Superbill) for Adam Burns (Appendix A: Day 6).

Goode Medical Clinic
1234 Larsen Avenue
Saint Paul, Minnesota 55316

Phone: (555) 555-1234
Fax: (555) 555-5678

PATIENT NAME	CHART #	DATE		
Tiffany Carter		*XX/XX/XXXX*	☐ MEDI-MEDI ☐ SELF PAY ☐ MEDICARE	☒ MEDICAL ☐ PRIVATE ☐ HMO___

✓	CPT/Md	DESCRIPTION	FEE	✓	CPT/Md	DESCRIPTION	FEE	✓	CPT/Md	DESCRIPTION	FEE	✓	CPT/Md	DESCRIPTION	FEE
OFFICE VISIT - NEW PATIENT				**LAB STUDIES**				**PROCEDURES**				**INJECTIONS**			
	99202	Focused Ex.			36415	Venipucture			92551	Audiometry			90655	Influenza 6-35 months	
	99203	Detailed Ex.			81000	Urinalysis			29705	Cast Removal Full Arm/Leg			90656	Influenza 3 years +	
	99204	Comprehensive Ex.			81003	- w/o Micro			2900__	Casting (by location)			90732	Pneumoccal	
	99205	Complex Ex.			84703	HCG (Urine, Pregnancy)			92567	Ear Check			J0295	Ampicillin, 1.5 gr	
OFFICE VISIT - ESTABLISHED PATIENT					82948	Glucose			69210	Ear Wax Rem. 1 2			J2001	Liocaine for IV infusion 10mg	
	99212	Focused Ex.			82270	Hemoccult			93000	EKG			J1885	Toradol 15mg	
√	99213	Expanded Ex.	*$48.*		85025	CBC -diff.			93005	EKG tracing only			90720	DTP - HIB	
	99214	Detailed Ex.			85018	Hemoglobin			93010	EKG Int. and Rep			90746	HEP B - HIB	
	99215	Complex Ex.			88174	Pap Smear			11750	Excision Nail			90707	MMR	
PREVENTATIVE MEDICINE - NEW PATIENT					87210	KOH/ Saline Wet Mount			94375	Respiratory Flow Volume			86580	PPD	
	99381	< 1 year old			87430	Strep Antigen			93224	Holter up to 48 hours			90732	Pneumovax	
	99382	1-4 year old			87070	Throat Culture			10060	I & D Abscess Simple			90716	Varicella	
	99383	5-11 year old			80053	Chem profile			10061	I & D Abscess Comp.			82607	Vitamin B12 Inj.	
	99384	12-17 year old			80061	Lipid profile			94761	Oximetry w/Exercise			90712	Polio oral use (OPV)	
	99385	18-39 year old			82465	Cholesterol			94726	Plethysmography			90713	Polio injection (IPV)	
	99386	40-64 year old			99000	Handling fee			94760	Pulse Oximetry			90714	Td preservative free 7 yrs +	
	99387	65 + year old		**X-RAY**					11100	Skin Bx			90718	Td 7 years +	
PREVENTATIVE MEDICINE - ESTABLISHED PATIENT					70210	Sinuses			94010	Spirometry			95115	Allergy inj., single	
	99391	< 1 year old			70360	Neck Soft Tissue			99173	Visual Acuity			95117	Allergy inj., multiple	
	99392	1-4 year old			71010	CXR (PA only)			17110	Wart destruction up to 14					
	99393	5-11 year old			71020	Chest 2V			17111	Wart destruction 15 lesions +					
	99394	12-17 year old			72040	C-Spine 2V			11042	Wound Debrid.		**OTHER**			
	99395	18-39 year old			72100	Lumbrosacral									
	99396	40-64 year old			73030	Shoulder 2V									
	99397	65 + year old			73070	Elbow 2V									
					73120	Hand 2V									
					73560	Knee 2V									
					73620	Foot 2V									
					74000	KUB									

DIAGNOSTIC CODES (ICD-9-CM)

✓	Code	Description	✓	Code	Description	✓	Code	Description	✓	Code	Description
	789.0__	Abdominal Pain		564.0	Constipation		784.0	Headache		782.1	Rash or ezanthem
	682.__	Abscess/Cellulitis		692.6	Contact dermatitis due to plants		414.9	Heart Dis., Coronary		714.0	Rheumatoid Arthritis
	995.3	Allergic Reaction	√	692.9	Contact dermatitis, NOS		599.70	Hematuria		V70.0	Routine general exam
	331	Alzheimer's		V25.09	Contraceptive management		455.6	Hemorrhoids		V76.10	Screen, breast
	285.__	Anemia, other & unspec		923.10	Contusion, forearm		573.3	Hepatitus, NOS		V76.2	Screen, cervix
	280.9	Anemia-iron deficiency		434.91	CVA		V03.81	HIB		V76.44	Screen, prosate
	281.0	Anemia-pernicious		266.2	Deficiency, folic acid B12		V65.44	HIV counseling		V76.47	Screen, vagina
	285.9	Anemia-unspecified		311	Depression		401.1	Hypertension, benign		216.5	Sebaceous cyst
	413.9	Angina, pectoris, oyher/unspecified		250.01	Diabetes, type I, juvenile type		401.9	Hypertension, unspecified		706.2	Sebaceous cyst
	300.00	Anxiety state, NOS		787.91	Diarrhea		401.0	Hypertension, malignant		786.05	Shortness of Breath
	300.4	Anxiety reaction		780.4	Dizziness		V04.81	Influenza		701.9	Skin tag
	716.90	Arthritis, NOS		V06.1	DTP		271.3	Lactose intolerance		845.00	Strain, ankle
	493.20	Asthma; chronic obstruction		V06.3	DTP + polio		573.9	Liver Disease		307.81	Tension headache
	493.00	Asthma; extrinic		536.8	Dyspepsia		724.5	Low Back Pain		V06.5	Tetanus - distheria (Td)
	493.10	Asthma; intrinsic		788.1	Dysuria		346.9	Migraine		305.1	Tobacco dependence
	493.90	Asthmas; unspecified		782.3	Edema		V06.4	MMR		788.41	Urinary frequency
	427.31	Atrial fibulation		530.81	Esophageal reflux		278.01	Obesity/Morbid		599.0	Unrinary tract infection, NOS
	724.5	Backache, unspecified		530.11	Esophagitis reflux		715.90	Osteoarthritis		V05.3	Viral hepatitis
	790.6	Blood chemistry		530.10	Esophagitis, unspecified		719.43	Pain in joint, forearm		368.40	Visual field defect, unspecified
	E906.3	Cat bite		780.6	Fever		625.4	PMS		V20.2	Well Child Exam
	786.50	Chest Pain		789.07	Generalized abdominal pain		486	Pneumonia			
	428.0	CHF		V72.3	Gynecological examiniation		V25.01	Prescription of oral contraceptivess			

DIAGNOSIS: (IF NOT CHECKED ABOVE)		RECEIVED BY:	TODAY'S FEE	*$48.—*
Detergents — E861.0		☐ CASH	AMOUNT RECEIVED	*—*
PROCEDURES: (IF NOT CHECKED ABOVE)	RETURN APPOINTMENT INFORMATION:	☐ CREDIT CARD		
	(DAYS) (WKS.) (MOS.) (PRN)	☐ CHECK # ______	BALANCE	*$48.—*

Figure C.96 Encounter form (Superbill) for Tiffany Carter (Appendix A: Day 7).

Goode Medical Clinic
William B. Goode, MD

Patient Registration Information

Account # :
Insurance # :
Co-Payment: $

Please PRINT AND complete ALL sections below!

PATIENT'S PERSONAL INFORMATION Marital Status ☑ Single ☐ Married ☐ Divorced ☐ Widowed Sex: ☐ Male ☑ Female

Name: Brown (last name) Addison (first name) (initial)

Street address: 4567 Dexter St. (Apt #) City: Minneapolis State: MN Zip: 55000

Home phone: (555) 555-1234 Work phone: (555) 555-5678 Social Security # 123 - XX - 4567

Date of Birth: 01 (month) / 02 (day) / 80 (year)

Employer / Name of School Pine Trees, Inc. ☑ Full Time ☐ Part Time

PATIENT'S / RESPONSIBLE PARTY INFORMATION

Responsible party: self Date of Birth:

Relationship to Patient: ☑ Self ☐ Spouse ☐ Other Social Security # - -

Responsible party's home phone: ( )

Address: (Apt #) City: State: Zip:

Employer's name: Phone number:( )

Address: City: State: Zip:

Name of Parent/Guardian:

PATIENT'S INSURANCE INFORMATION Please present insurance cards to receptionist.

PRIMARY insurance company's name:

Insurance address: City: State: Zip:

Name of insured: Date of Birth: Relationship to insured: ☐ Self ☐ Spouse ☐ Other ☐ Child

Insurance ID number: Group number:

Does your insurance cover medication?

EMERGENCY CONTACT

Name of person not living with you: Mike Brown Relationship: Father

Address: 9876 Carter Street City: Minneapolis State: MN Zip: 55000

Phone number: (555) 555-6183

Assignment of Benefits • Financial Agreement

I hereby give lifetime authorization for payment of insurance benefits to be made directly to Goode Medical Clinic ,and any assisting physicians, for services rendered. I understand that I am financially responsible for all charges whether or not they are covered by insurance. In the event of default, I agree to pay all costs of collection, and reasonable attorney's fees. I hereby authorize this healthcare provider to release all information necessary to secure the payment of benefits.
I further agree that a photocopy of this agreement shall be as valid as the original.

Date: XX/XX/XXXX Your Signature: Addison Brown

FORM # 58-8423 • BIBBERO SYSTEMS, INC.• PETALUMA, CA.• TO ORDER CALL TOLL FREE :800-BIBBERO (800-242-2376) • FAX (800) 242-9330 (REV.7/94)

Figure C.97 Registration form for Addison Brown (Appendix A: Day 7).

Goode Medical Clinic
1234 Larsen Avenue
Saint Paul, Minnesota 55316

Phone: (555) 555-1234
Fax: (555) 555-5678

PATIENT NAME	CHART #	DATE		
Addison Brown			☐ MEDI-MEDI ☐ SELF PAY ☐ MEDICARE	☐ MEDICAL ☐ PRIVATE ☐ HMO_____

✓	CPT/Md	DESCRIPTION	FEE	✓	CPT/Md	DESCRIPTION	FEE	✓	CPT/Md	DESCRIPTION	FEE	✓	CPT/Md	DESCRIPTION	FEE
OFFICE VISIT - NEW PATIENT				**LAB STUDIES**				**PROCEDURES**				**INJECTIONS**			
	99202	Focused Ex.			36415	Venipucture			92551	Audiometry			90655	Influenza 6-35 months	
	99203	Detailed Ex.			81000	Urinalysis			29705	Cast Removal Full Arm/Leg			90656	Influenza 3 years +	
✓	99204	Comprehensive Ex.	*$100.00*		81003	- w/o Micro			2900__	Casting (by location)			90732	Pneumoccal	
	99205	Complex Ex.			84703	HCG (Urine, Pregnancy)			92567	Ear Check			J0295	Ampicillin, 1.5 gr	
OFFICE VISIT - ESTABLISHED PATIENT					82948	Glucose			69210	Ear Wax Rem. 1 2			J2001	Liocaine for IV infusion 10mg	
	99212	Focused Ex.			82270	Hemoccult			93000	EKG			J1885	Toradol 15mg	
	99213	Expanded Ex.			85025	CBC -diff.			93005	EKG tracing only			90720	DTP - HIB	
	99214	Detailed Ex.			85018	Hemoglobin			93010	EKG Int. and Rep			90746	HEP B - HIB	
	99215	Complex Ex.			88174	Pap Smear			11750	Excision Nail			90707	MMR	
PREVENTATIVE MEDICINE - NEW PATIENT					87210	KOH/ Saline Wet Mount			94375	Respiratory Flow Volume			86580	PPD	
	99381	< 1 year old			87430	Strep Antigen			93224	Holter up to 48 hours			90732	Pneumovax	
	99382	1-4 year old			87070	Throat Culture			10060	I & D Abscess Simple			90716	Varicella	
	99383	5-11 year old			80053	Chem profile			10061	I & D Abscess Comp.			82607	Vitamin B12 Inj.	
	99384	12-17 year old			80061	Lipid profile			94761	Oximetry w/Exercise			90712	Polio oral use (OPV)	
	99385	18-39 year old			82465	Cholesterol			94726	Plethysmography			90713	Polio injection (IPV)	
	99386	40-64 year old			99000	Handling fee			94760	Pulse Oximetry			90714	Td preservative free 7 yrs +	
	99387	65 + year old		**X-RAY**					11100	Skin Bx			90718	Td 7 years +	
PREVENTATIVE MEDICINE - ESTABLISHED PATIENT					70210	Sinuses			94010	Spirometry			95115	Allergy inj., single	
	99391	< 1 year old			70360	Neck Soft Tissue			99173	Visual Acuity			95117	Allergy inj., multiple	
	99392	1-4 year old			71010	CXR (PA only)			17110	Wart destruction up to 14					
	99393	5-11 year old			71020	Chest 2V			17111	Wart destruction 15 lesions +					
	99394	12-17 year old			72040	C-Spine 2V			11042	Wound Debrid.			**OTHER**		
	99395	18-39 year old			72100	Lumbrosacral									
	99396	40-64 year old			73030	Shoulder 2V									
	99397	65 + year old			73070	Elbow 2V									
					73120	Hand 2V									
					73560	Knee 2V									
					73620	Foot 2V									
					74000	KUB									

DIAGNOSTIC CODES (ICD-9-CM)

Code	Description	Code	Description	Code	Description	Code	Description
789.0__	Abdominal Pain	564.0	Constipation	784.0	Headache	782.1	Rash or ezanthem
682.__	Abscess/Cellulitis	692.6	Contact dermatitis due to plants	414.9	Heart Dis., Coronary	714.0	Rheumatoid Arthritis
995.3	Allergic Reaction	692.9	Contact dermatitis, NOS	599.70	Hematuria	V70.0	Routine general exam
331	Alzheimer's	V25.09	Contraceptive management	455.6	Hemorrhoids	V76.10	Screen, breast
285.__	Anemia, other & unspec	923.10	Contusion, forearm	573.3	Hepatitus, NOS	V76.2	Screen, cervix
280.9	Anemia-iron deficiency	434.91	CVA	V03.81	HIB	V76.44	Screen, prosate
281.0	Anemia-pernicious	266.2	Deficiency, folic acid B12	V65.44	HIV counseling	V76.47	Screen, vagina
285.9	Anemia-unspecified	311	Depression	401.1	Hypertension, benign	216.5	Sebaceous cyst
413.9	Angina, pectoris, oyher/unspecified	250.01	Diabetes, type I, juvenile type	401.9	Hypertension, unspecified	706.2	Sebaceous cyst
300.00	Anxiety state, NOS	787.91	Diarrhea	401.0	Hypertension, malignant	786.05	Shortness of Breath
300.4	Anxiety reaction	780.4	Dizziness	V04.81	Influenza	701.9	Skin tag
716.90	Arthritis, NOS	V06.1	DTP	271.3	Lactose intolerance	845.00	Strain, ankle
493.20	Asthma; chronic obstruction	V06.3	DTP + polio	573.9	Liver Disease	307.81	Tension headache
493.00	Asthma; extrinic	536.8	Dyspepsia	724.5	Low Back Pain	V06.5	Tetanus - distheria (Td)
493.10	Asthma; intrinsic	788.1	Dysuria	346.9	Migraine	305.1	Tobacco dependence
493.90	Asthmas; unspecified	782.3	Edema	V06.4	MMR	788.41	Urinary frequency
427.31	Atrial fibulation	530.81	Esophageal reflux	278.01	Obesity/Morbid	599.0	Unrinary tract infection, NOS
724.5	Backache, unspecified	530.11	Esophagitis reflux	715.90	Osteoarthritis	V05.3	Viral hepatitis
790.6	Blood chemistry	530.10	Esophagitis, unspecified	719.43	Pain in joint, forearm	368.40	Visual field defect, unspecified
E906.3	Cat bite	780.6	Fever	625.4	PMS	V20.2	Well Child Exam
786.50	Chest Pain	789.07	Generalized abdominal pain	486	Pneumonia		
428.0	CHF	V72.3	Gynecological examiniation	V25.01	Prescription of oral contraceptivess		

DIAGNOSIS: (IF NOT CHECKED ABOVE)		RECEIVED BY:	TODAY'S FEE	*$100.00*
780.4 Vertigo		☐ CASH	AMOUNT RECEIVED	—
PROCEDURES: (IF NOT CHECKED ABOVE)	RETURN APPOINTMENT INFORMATION:	☐ CREDIT CARD		
	(DAYS) (WKS.) (MOS.) (PRN)	☐ CHECK # ______	BALANCE	*$100.00*

Figure C.98 Encounter form (Superbill) for Addison Brown (Appendix A: Day 7).

Goode Medical Clinic
William B. Goode, MD

Patient Registration Information

Account # :
Insurance # :
Co-Payment: $

Please PRINT AND complete ALL sections below!

PATIENT'S PERSONAL INFORMATION Marital Status ❑ Single ☒ Married ❑ Divorced ❑ Widowed Sex: ☒ Male ❑ Female

Name: Rose (last name) Cody (first name) (initial)

Street address: 2345 Rose Ave. (Apt #) City: Minneapolis State: MN Zip: 55000

Home phone: (555) 555-9354 Work phone: (555) 555-1614 Social Security # 987 - XX - 1243

Date of Birth: 09 / 25 / 71 (month / day / year)

Employer / Name of School Big Pictures, LLC ☒ Full Time ❑ Part Time

PATIENT'S / RESPONSIBLE PARTY INFORMATION

Responsible party: self Date of Birth:

Relationship to Patient: ☒ Self ❑ Spouse ❑ Other Social Security # - -

Responsible party's home phone: ( )

Address: (Apt #) City: State: Zip:

Employer's name: Phone number:( )

Address: City: State: Zip:

Name of Parent/Guardian:

PATIENT'S INSURANCE INFORMATION Please present insurance cards to receptionist.

PRIMARY insurance company's name: Blue Cross/ Blue Shield

Insurance address: 1355 Insurance Carrier Loop City: Minneapolis State: MN Zip: 55401

Name of insured: Cody Rose Date of Birth: 9-25-71 Relationship to insured: ☒ Self ☐ Spouse ☐ Other ☐ Child

Insurance ID number: CR-67890-BP Group number: 88945

Does your insurance cover medication? Yes

EMERGENCY CONTACT

Name of person ~~not~~ living with you: Brenda Rose Relationship: Wife

Address: 2345 Rose Ave. City: Minneapolis State: MN Zip: 55000

Phone number: (555) 555-9354 (home) 555-555-7530 (cell)

Assignment of Benefits • Financial Agreement

I hereby give lifetime authorization for payment of insurance benefits to be made directly to Goode Medical Clinic ,and any assisting physicians, for services rendered. I understand that I am financially responsible for all charges whether or not they are covered by insurance. In the event of default, I agree to pay all costs of collection, and reasonable attorney's fees. I hereby authorize this healthcare provider to release all information necessary to secure the payment of benefits.

I further agree that a photocopy of this agreement shall be as valid as the original.

Date: XX/XX/XXXX Your Signature: Cody Rose

FORM # 58-8423 • BIBBERO SYSTEMS, INC.• PETALUMA, CA.• TO ORDER CALL TOLL FREE :800-BIBBERO (800-242-2376) • FAX (800) 242-9330 (REV.7/94)

Figure C.99 Registration form for Cody Rose (Appendix A: Day 8).

Goode Medical Clinic
1234 Larsen Avenue
Saint Paul, Minnesota 55316

Phone: (555) 555-1234
Fax: (555) 555-5678

PATIENT NAME	CHART #	DATE		
Cody Rose			☐ MEDI-MEDI ☐ SELF PAY ☐ MEDICARE	☐ MEDICAL ☐ PRIVATE ☐ HMO____

☐	CPT/Md	DESCRIPTION	FEE
OFFICE VISIT - NEW PATIENT			
	99202	Focused Ex.	
✓	99203	Detailed Ex.	*$80.00*
	99204	Comprehensive Ex.	
	99205	Complex Ex.	
OFFICE VISIT - ESTABLISHED PATIENT			
	99212	Focused Ex.	
	99213	Expanded Ex.	
	99214	Detailed Ex.	
	99215	Complex Ex.	
PREVENTATIVE MEDICINE - NEW PATIENT			
	99381	< 1 year old	
	99382	1-4 year old	
	99383	5-11 year old	
	99384	12-17 year old	
	99385	18-39 year old	
	99386	40-64 year old	
	99387	65 + year old	
PREVENTATIVE MEDICINE - ESTABLISHED PATIENT			
	99391	< 1 year old	
	99392	1-4 year old	
	99393	5-11 year old	
	99394	12-17 year old	
	99395	18-39 year old	
	99396	40-64 year old	
	99397	65 + year old	

☐	CPT/Md	DESCRIPTION	FEE
LAB STUDIES			
	36415	Venipucture	
	81000	Urinalysis	
	81003	- w/o Micro	
	84703	HCG (Urine, Pregnancy)	
	82948	Glucose	
	82270	Hemoccult	
	85025	CBC -diff.	
	85018	Hemoglobin	
	88174	Pap Smear	
	87210	KOH/ Saline Wet Mount	
	87430	Strep Antigen	
	87070	Throat Culture	
	80053	Chem profile	
	80061	Lipid profile	
	82465	Cholesterol	
	99000	Handling fee	
X-RAY			
	70210	Sinuses	
	70360	Neck Soft Tissue	
	71010	CXR (PA only)	
	71020	Chest 2V	
	72040	C-Spine 2V	
	72100	Lumbrosacral	
	73030	Shoulder 2V	
	73070	Elbow 2V	
	73120	Hand 2V	
	73560	Knee 2V	
	73620	Foot 2V	
	74000	KUB	

☐	CPT/Md	DESCRIPTION	FEE
PROCEDURES			
	92551	Audiometry	
	29705	Cast Removal Full Arm/Leg	
	2900__	Casting (by location)	
	92567	Ear Check	
	69210	Ear Wax Rem. 1 2	
	93000	EKG	
	93005	EKG tracing only	
	93010	EKG Int. and Rep	
	11750	Excision Nail	
	94375	Respiratory Flow Volume	
	93224	Holter up to 48 hours	
	10060	I & D Abscess Simple	
	10061	I & D Abscess Comp.	
	94761	Oximetry w/Exercise	
	94726	Plethysmography	
	94760	Pulse Oximetry	
	11100	Skin Bx	
	94010	Spirometry	
	99173	Visual Acuity	
	17110	Wart destruction up to 14	
	17111	Wart destruction 15 lesions +	
	11042	Wound Debrid.	

☐	CPT/Md	DESCRIPTION	FEE
INJECTIONS			
	90655	Influenza 6-35 months	
	90656	Influenza 3 years +	
	90732	Pneumoccal	
	J0295	Ampicillin, 1.5 gr	
	J2001	Liocaine for IV infusion 10mg	
	J1885	Toradol 15mg	
	90720	DTP - HIB	
	90746	HEP B - HIB	
	90707	MMR	
	86580	PPD	
	90732	Pneumovax	
	90716	Varicella	
	82607	Vitamin B12 Inj.	
	90712	Polio oral use (OPV)	
	90713	Polio injection (IPV)	
	90714	Td preservative free 7 yrs +	
	90718	Td 7 years +	
	95115	Allergy inj., single	
	95117	Allergy inj., multiple	
OTHER			

DIAGNOSTIC CODES (ICD-9-CM)

Code	Description	Code	Description	Code	Description	Code	Description
789.0__	Abdominal Pain	564.0	Constipation	784.0	Headache	782.1	Rash or ezanthem
682.__	Abscess/Cellulitis	692.6	Contact dermatitis due to plants	414.9	Heart Dis., Coronary	714.0	Rheumatoid Arthritis
995.3	Allergic Reaction	692.9	Contact dermatitis, NOS	599.70	Hematuria	V70.0	Routine general exam
331	Alzheimer's	V25.09	Contraceptive management	455.6	Hemorrhoids	V76.10	Screen, breast
285.__	Anemia, other & unspec	923.10	Contusion, forearm	573.3	Hepatitus, NOS	V76.2	Screen, cervix
280.9	Anemia-iron deficiency	434.91	CVA	V03.81	HIB	V76.44	Screen, prosate
281.0	Anemia-pernicious	266.2	Deficiency, folic acid B12	V65.44	HIV counseling	V76.47	Screen, vagina
285.9	Anemia-unspecified	311	Depression	401.1	Hypertension, benign	216.5	Sebaceous cyst
413.9	Angina, pectoris, oyher/unspecified	250.01	Diabetes, type I, juvenile type	401.9	Hypertension, unspecified	706.2	Sebaceous cyst
300.00	Anxiety state, NOS	787.91	Diarrhea	401.0	Hypertension, malignant	786.05	Shortness of Breath
300.4	Anxiety reaction	780.4	Dizziness	V04.81	Influenza	701.9	Skin tag
716.90	Arthritis, NOS	V06.1	DTP	271.3	Lactose intolerance	845.00	Strain, ankle
493.20	Asthma; chronic obstruction	V06.3	DTP + polio	573.9	Liver Disease	307.81	Tension headache
493.00	Asthma; extrinic	536.8	Dyspepsia	724.5	Low Back Pain	V06.5	Tetanus - distheria (Td)
493.10	Asthma; intrinsic	788.1	Dysuria	346.9	Migraine	305.1	Tobacco dependence
493.90	Asthmas; unspecified	782.3	Edema	V06.4	MMR	788.41	Urinary frequency
427.31	Atrial fibulation	530.81	Esophageal reflux	278.01	Obesity/Morbid	599.0	Unrinary tract infection, NOS
724.5	Backache, unspecified	530.11	Esophagitis reflux	715.90	Osteoarthritis	V05.3	Viral hepatitis
790.6	Blood chemistry	530.10	Esophagitis, unspecified	719.43	Pain in joint, forearm	368.40	Visual field defect, unspecified
E906.3	Cat bite	780.6	Fever	625.4	PMS	V20.2	Well Child Exam
786.50	Chest Pain	789.07	Generalized abdominal pain	486	Pneumonia		
428.0	CHF	V72.3	Gynecological examiniation	V25.01	Prescription of oral contraceptivess		

DIAGNOSIS: (IF NOT CHECKED ABOVE)

354.0 Carpal Tunnel Syndrome

PROCEDURES: (IF NOT CHECKED ABOVE)

RETURN APPOINTMENT INFORMATION:

(DAYS) (WKS.) (MOS.) (PRN)

RECEIVED BY:

☐ CASH
☐ CREDIT CARD
☐ CHECK
#________

TODAY'S FEE	*$80.00*
AMOUNT RECEIVED	—
BALANCE	*$80.00*

Figure C.100 Encounter form (Superbill) for Cody Rose (Appendix A: Day 8).

Goode Medical Clinic
William B. Goode, MD

Patient Registration Information

Account # : ______
Insurance # : ______
Co-Payment: $ ______

Please PRINT AND complete ALL sections below!

PATIENT'S PERSONAL INFORMATION Marital Status ❑ Single ☒ Married ❑ Divorced ❑ Widowed Sex: ❑ Male ☒ Female

Name: Brooks (last name) Louise (first name) E. (initial)

Street address: 3333 Winter Lane (Apt # ____) City: Minneapolis State: MN Zip: 55000

Home phone: (555) 555-3216 Work phone: (555) 555-0011 Social Security # 243 - XX - 8109

Date of Birth: 07 (month) / 05 (day) / 1975 (year)

Employer / Name of School: Dreamy Cheese ☒ Full Time ❑ Part Time

PATIENT'S / RESPONSIBLE PARTY INFORMATION

Responsible party: self Date of Birth: ______

Relationship to Patient: ☒ Self ❑ Spouse ❑ Other ______ Social Security # ____-____-____

Responsible party's home phone: (____) ______

Address: ______ (Apt # ____) City: ______ State: ______ Zip: ______

Employer's name: ______ Phone number: (____) ______

Address: ______ City: ______ State: ______ Zip: ______

Name of Parent/Guardian: ______

PATIENT'S INSURANCE INFORMATION Please present insurance cards to receptionist.

PRIMARY insurance company's name: First Med

Insurance address: 1324 Insurance Carrier Loop City: Minneapolis State: MN Zip: 55401

Name of insured: Louise Brooks Date of Birth: 7-5-75 Relationship to insured: ☒ Self ☐ Spouse ☐ Other ☐ Child

Insurance ID number: LB02314 Group number: 654

Does your insurance cover medication? No

EMERGENCY CONTACT

Name of person ~~not~~ living with you: Robert Brooks Relationship: husband

Address: 3333 Winter Lane City: Minneapolis State: MN Zip: 55000

Phone number: (555) 555-6849 (cell)

Assignment of Benefits • Financial Agreement

I hereby give lifetime authorization for payment of insurance benefits to be made directly to Goode Medical Clinic, and any assisting physicians, for services rendered. I understand that I am financially responsible for all charges whether or not they are covered by insurance. In the event of default, I agree to pay all costs of collection, and reasonable attorney's fees. I hereby authorize this healthcare provider to release all information necessary to secure the payment of benefits.
I further agree that a photocopy of this agreement shall be as valid as the original.

Date: XX/XX/XXXX Your Signature: Louise Brooks

FORM # 58-8423 • BIBBERO SYSTEMS, INC.• PETALUMA, CA.• TO ORDER CALL TOLL FREE :800-BIBBERO (800-242-2376) • FAX (800) 242-9330 (REV.7/94)

Figure C.101 Registration form for Louise Brooks (Appendix A: Day 8).

Goode Medical Clinic
1234 Larsen Avenue
Saint Paul, Minnesota 55316

Phone: (555) 555-1234
Fax: (555) 555-5678

PATIENT NAME	CHART #	DATE	☐ MEDI-MEDI ☐ SELF PAY ☐ MEDICARE	☐ MEDICAL ☐ PRIVATE ☐ HMO______
Louise Brooks				

✓	CPT/Md	DESCRIPTION	FEE	✓	CPT/Md	DESCRIPTION	FEE	✓	CPT/Md	DESCRIPTION	FEE	✓	CPT/Md	DESCRIPTION	FEE
OFFICE VISIT - NEW PATIENT				**LAB STUDIES**				**PROCEDURES**				**INJECTIONS**			
	99202	Focused Ex.			36415	Venipucture			92551	Audiometry			90655	Influenza 6-35 months	
✓	99203	Detailed Ex.	*$80.00*		81000	Urinalysis			29705	Cast Removal Full Arm/Leg			90656	Influenza 3 years +	
	99204	Comprehensive Ex.			81003	- w/o Micro			2900__	Casting (by location)			90732	Pneumoccal	
	99205	Complex Ex.			84703	HCG (Urine, Pregnancy)			92567	Ear Check			J0295	Ampicillin, 1.5 gr	
OFFICE VISIT - ESTABLISHED PATIENT					82948	Glucose			69210	Ear Wax Rem. 1 2			J2001	Liocaine for IV infusion 10mg	
	99212	Focused Ex.			82270	Hemoccult			93000	EKG			J1885	Toradol 15mg	
	99213	Expanded Ex.			85025	CBC -diff.			93005	EKG tracing only			90720	DTP - HIB	
	99214	Detailed Ex.			85018	Hemoglobin			93010	EKG Int. and Rep			90746	HEP B - HIB	
	99215	Complex Ex.			88174	Pap Smear			11750	Excision Nail			90707	MMR	
PREVENTATIVE MEDICINE - NEW PATIENT					87210	KOH/ Saline Wet Mount			94375	Respiratory Flow Volume			86580	PPD	
	99381	< 1 year old			87430	Strep Antigen			93224	Holter up to 48 hours			90732	Pneumovax	
	99382	1-4 year old			87070	Throat Culture			10060	I & D Abscess Simple			90716	Varicella	
	99383	5-11 year old			80053	Chem profile			10061	I & D Abscess Comp.			82607	Vitamin B12 Inj.	
	99384	12-17 year old			80061	Lipid profile			94761	Oximetry w/Exercise			90712	Polio oral use (OPV)	
	99385	18-39 year old			82465	Cholesterol			94726	Plethysmography			90713	Polio injection (IPV)	
	99386	40-64 year old			99000	Handling fee			94760	Pulse Oximetry			90714	Td preservative free 7 yrs +	
	99387	65 + year old		**X-RAY**					11100	Skin Bx			90718	Td 7 years +	
PREVENTATIVE MEDICINE - ESTABLISHED PATIENT					70210	Sinuses			94010	Spirometry			95115	Allergy inj., single	
	99391	< 1 year old			70360	Neck Soft Tissue			99173	Visual Acuity			95117	Allergy inj., multiple	
	99392	1-4 year old			71010	CXR (PA only)			17110	Wart destruction up to 14					
	99393	5-11 year old			71020	Chest 2V			17111	Wart destruction 15 lesions +					
	99394	12-17 year old			72040	C-Spine 2V			11042	Wound Debrid.		**OTHER**			
	99395	18-39 year old			72100	Lumbrosacral									
	99396	40-64 year old			73030	Shoulder 2V									
	99397	65 + year old			73070	Elbow 2V									
					73120	Hand 2V									
					73560	Knee 2V									
					73620	Foot 2V									
					74000	KUB									

DIAGNOSTIC CODES (ICD-9-CM)

✓	Code	Description	✓	Code	Description	✓	Code	Description	✓	Code	Description
	789.0__	Abdominal Pain		564.0	Constipation		784.0	Headache		782.1	Rash or ezanthem
	682.__	Abscess/Cellulitis		692.6	Contact dermatitis due to plants		414.9	Heart Dis., Coronary		714.0	Rheumatoid Arthritis
	995.3	Allergic Reaction		692.9	Contact dermatitis, NOS		599.70	Hematuria		V70.0	Routine general exam
	331	Alzheimer's		V25.09	Contraceptive management		455.6	Hemorrhoids		V76.10	Screen, breast
	285.__	Anemia, other & unspec		923.10	Contusion, forearm		573.3	Hepatitus, NOS		V76.2	Screen, cervix
	280.9	Anemia-iron deficiency		434.91	CVA		V03.81	HIB		V76.44	Screen, prosate
	281.0	Anemia-pernicious		266.2	Deficiency, folic acid B12		V65.44	HIV counseling		V76.47	Screen, vagina
	285.9	Anemia-unspecified		311	Depression		401.1	Hypertension, benign		216.5	Sebaceous cyst
	413.9	Angina, pectoris, oyher/unspecified		250.01	Diabetes, type I, juvenile type		401.9	Hypertension, unspecified		706.2	Sebaceous cyst
	300.00	Anxiety state, NOS		787.91	Diarrhea		401.0	Hypertension, malignant		786.05	Shortness of Breath
	300.4	Anxiety reaction		780.4	Dizziness		V04.81	Influenza		701.9	Skin tag
	716.90	Arthritis, NOS		V06.1	DTP		271.3	Lactose intolerance		845.00	Strain, ankle
	493.20	Asthma; chronic obstruction		V06.3	DTP + polio		573.9	Liver Disease		307.81	Tension headache
	493.00	Asthma; extrinic		536.8	Dyspepsia		724.5	Low Back Pain		V06.5	Tetanus - distheria (Td)
	493.10	Asthma; intrinsic		788.1	Dysuria		346.9	Migraine		305.1	Tobacco dependence
	493.90	Asthmas; unspecified		782.3	Edema		V06.4	MMR		788.41	Urinary frequency
	427.31	Atrial fibulation		530.81	Esophageal reflux		278.01	Obesity/Morbid		599.0	Unrinary tract infection, NOS
	724.5	Backache, unspecified		530.11	Esophagitis reflux		715.90	Osteoarthritis		V05.3	Viral hepatitis
	790.6	Blood chemistry		530.10	Esophagitis, unspecified		719.43	Pain in joint, forearm		368.40	Visual field defect, unspecified
	E906.3	Cat bite		780.6	Fever		625.4	PMS		V20.2	Well Child Exam
	786.50	Chest Pain		789.07	Generalized abdominal pain		486	Pneumonia			
	428.0	CHF		V72.3	Gynecological examiniation		V25.01	Prescription of oral contraceptivess			

DIAGNOSIS: (IF NOT CHECKED ABOVE)		RECEIVED BY:	TODAY'S FEE	*$80.00*
716.90 Arthritis, NOS		☐ CASH	AMOUNT RECEIVED	*—*
PROCEDURES: (IF NOT CHECKED ABOVE)	RETURN APPOINTMENT INFORMATION:	☐ CREDIT CARD		
	(DAYS) (WKS.) (MOS.) (PRN)	☐ CHECK # ________	BALANCE	*$80.00*

Figure C.102 Encounter form (Superbill) for Louise Brooks (Appendix A: Day 8).

Goode Medical Clinic
William B. Goode, MD

Patient Registration Information

Account # :
Insurance # :
Co-Payment: $

Please PRINT AND complete ALL sections below!

PATIENT'S PERSONAL INFORMATION Marital Status ❑ Single ☒ Married ❑ Divorced ❑ Widowed Sex: ☒ Male ❑ Female

Name: Camon (last name) Tim (first name) (initial)

Street address: 2007 Packer St. (Apt #) City: Minneapolis State: MN Zip: 55000

Home phone: (555) 555-8143 Work phone: (555) 555-1226 Social Security # 701 - XX - 8338

Date of Birth: 11 (month) / 18 (day) / 1969 (year)

Employer / Name of School Paper Mill ☒ Full Time ❑ Part Time

PATIENT'S / RESPONSIBLE PARTY INFORMATION

Responsible party: self Date of Birth:

Relationship to Patient: ☒ Self ❑ Spouse ❑ Other Social Security # - -

Responsible party's home phone: ( )

Address: (Apt #) City: State: Zip:

Employer's name: Phone number:( )

Address: City: State: Zip:

Name of Parent/Guardian:

PATIENT'S INSURANCE INFORMATION Please present insurance cards to receptionist.

PRIMARY insurance company's name: First Med

Insurance address: 1324 Insurance Carrier Loop City: Minneapolis State: MN Zip: 55401

Name of insured: Timothy Camon Date of Birth: 11-18-69 Relationship to insured: ☒ Self ☐ Spouse ☐ Other ☐ Child

Insurance ID number: TC 77598 Group number: 567

Does your insurance cover medication? No

EMERGENCY CONTACT

Name of person not living with you: Nikki Camon Relationship: wife

Address: 2007 Packer Street City: Minneapolis State: MN Zip: 55000

Phone number: (555) 555-8143 (home) 555-555-7160 (work)

Assignment of Benefits • Financial Agreement

I hereby give lifetime authorization for payment of insurance benefits to be made directly to Goode Medical Clinic ,and any assisting physicians, for services rendered. I understand that I am financially responsible for all charges whether or not they are covered by insurance. In the event of default, I agree to pay all costs of collection, and reasonable attorney's fees. I hereby authorize this healthcare provider to release all information necessary to secure the payment of benefits.
I further agree that a photocopy of this agreement shall be as valid as the original.

Date: XX/XX/XXXX Your Signature: Tim Camon

FORM # 58-8423 • BIBBERO SYSTEMS, INC.• PETALUMA, CA.• TO ORDER CALL TOLL FREE :800-BIBBERO (800-242-2376) • FAX (800) 242-9330 (REV.7/94)

Figure C.103 Registration form for Tim Camon (Appendix A: Day 8).

Goode Medical Clinic
1234 Larsen Avenue
Saint Paul, Minnesota 55316

Phone: (555) 555-1234
Fax: (555) 555-5678

PATIENT NAME	CHART #	DATE		
Tim Camon			☐ MEDI-MEDI ☐ SELF PAY ☐ MEDICARE	☐ MEDICAL ☐ PRIVATE ☐ HMO___

☐	CPT/Md	DESCRIPTION	FEE
	OFFICE VISIT - NEW PATIENT		
	99202	Focused Ex.	
	99203	Detailed Ex.	
	99204	Comprehensive Ex.	
	99205	Complex Ex.	
	OFFICE VISIT - ESTABLISHED PATIENT		
	99212	Focused Ex.	
	99213	Expanded Ex.	
	99214	Detailed Ex.	
	99215	Complex Ex.	
	PREVENTATIVE MEDICINE - NEW PATIENT		
	99381	< 1 year old	
	99382	1-4 year old	
	99383	5-11 year old	
	99384	12-17 year old	
√	99385	18-39 year old	*$85.00*
	99386	40-64 year old	
	99387	65 + year old	
	PREVENTATIVE MEDICINE - ESTABLISHED PATIENT		
	99391	< 1 year old	
	99392	1-4 year old	
	99393	5-11 year old	
	99394	12-17 year old	
	99395	18-39 year old	
	99396	40-64 year old	
	99397	65 + year old	
√	*93000*	*ECG Interp*	*$50.00*

☐	CPT/Md	DESCRIPTION	FEE
	LAB STUDIES		
	36415	Venipucture	
√	81000	Urinalysis	*$78.00*
	81003	- w/o Micro	
	84703	HCG (Urine, Pregnancy)	
	82948	Glucose	
	82270	Hemoccult	
√	85025	CBC -diff.	*$120.00*
	85018	Hemoglobin	
	88174	Pap Smear	
	87210	KOH/ Saline Wet Mount	
	87430	Strep Antigen	
	87070	Throat Culture	
	80053	Chem profile	
	80061	Lipid profile	
	82465	Cholesterol	
	99000	Handling fee	
	X-RAY		
	70210	Sinuses	
	70360	Neck Soft Tissue	
	71010	CXR (PA only)	
	71020	Chest 2V	
	72040	C-Spine 2V	
	72100	Lumbrosacral	
	73030	Shoulder 2V	
	73070	Elbow 2V	
	73120	Hand 2V	
	73560	Knee 2V	
	73620	Foot 2V	
	74000	KUB	

☐	CPT/Md	DESCRIPTION	FEE
	PROCEDURES		
	92551	Audiometry	
	29705	Cast Removal Full Arm/Leg	
	2900__	Casting (by location)	
	92567	Ear Check	
	69210	Ear Wax Rem. 1 2	
	93000	EKG	
	93005	EKG tracing only	
	93010	EKG Int. and Rep	
	11750	Excision Nail	
	94375	Respiratory Flow Volume	
	93224	Holter up to 48 hours	
	10060	I & D Abscess Simple	
	10061	I & D Abscess Comp.	
	94761	Oximetry w/Exercise	
	94726	Plethysmography	
	94760	Pulse Oximetry	
	11100	Skin Bx	
	94010	Spirometry	
	99173	Visual Acuity	
	17110	Wart destruction up to 14	
	17111	Wart destruction 15 lesions +	
	11042	Wound Debrid.	

☐	CPT/Md	DESCRIPTION	FEE
	INJECTIONS		
	90655	Influenza 6-35 months	
	90656	Influenza 3 years +	
	90732	Pneumoccal	
	J0295	Ampicillin, 1.5 gr	
	J2001	Liocaine for IV infusion 10mg	
	J1885	Toradol 15mg	
	90720	DTP - HIB	
	90746	HEP B - HIB	
	90707	MMR	
	86580	PPD	
	90732	Pneumovax	
	90716	Varicella	
	82607	Vitamin B12 Inj.	
	90712	Polio oral use (OPV)	
	90713	Polio injection (IPV)	
	90714	Td preservative free 7 yrs +	
	90718	Td 7 years +	
	95115	Allergy inj., single	
	95117	Allergy inj., multiple	
	OTHER		

DIAGNOSTIC CODES (ICD-9-CM)

☐	Code	Description	☐	Code	Description	☐	Code	Description	☐	Code	Description
	789.0__	Abdominal Pain		564.0	Constipation		784.0	Headache		782.1	Rash or ezanthem
	682.__	Abscess/Cellulitis		692.6	Contact dermatitis due to plants		414.9	Heart Dis., Coronary		714.0	Rheumatoid Arthritis
	995.3	Allergic Reaction		692.9	Contact dermatitis, NOS		599.70	Hematuria	√	V70.0	Routine general exam
	331	Alzheimer's		V25.09	Contraceptive management		455.6	Hemorrhoids		V76.10	Screen, breast
	285.__	Anemia, other & unspec		923.10	Contusion, forearm		573.3	Hepatitus, NOS		V76.2	Screen, cervix
	280.9	Anemia-iron deficiency		434.91	CVA		V03.81	HIB		V76.44	Screen, prosate
	281.0	Anemia-pernicious		266.2	Deficiency, folic acid B12		V65.44	HIV counseling		V76.47	Screen, vagina
	285.9	Anemia-unspecified		311	Depression		401.1	Hypertension, benign		216.5	Sebaceous cyst
	413.9	Angina, pectoris, oyher/unspecified		250.01	Diabetes, type I, juvenile type		401.9	Hypertension, unspecified		706.2	Sebaceous cyst
	300.00	Anxiety state, NOS		787.91	Diarrhea		401.0	Hypertension, malignant		786.05	Shortness of Breath
	300.4	Anxiety reaction		780.4	Dizziness		V04.81	Influenza		701.9	Skin tag
	716.90	Arthritis, NOS		V06.1	DTP		271.3	Lactose intolerance		845.00	Strain, ankle
	493.20	Asthma; chronic obstruction		V06.3	DTP + polio		573.9	Liver Disease		307.81	Tension headache
	493.00	Asthma; extrinic		536.8	Dyspepsia		724.5	Low Back Pain		V06.5	Tetanus - distheria (Td)
	493.10	Asthma; intrinsic		788.1	Dysuria		346.9	Migraine		305.1	Tobacco dependence
	493.90	Asthmas; unspecified		782.3	Edema		V06.4	MMR		788.41	Urinary frequency
	427.31	Atrial fibulation		530.81	Esophageal reflux		278.01	Obesity/Morbid		599.0	Unrinary tract infection, NOS
	724.5	Backache, unspecified		530.11	Esophagitis reflux		715.90	Osteoarthritis		V05.3	Viral hepatitis
	790.6	Blood chemistry		530.10	Esophagitis, unspecified		719.43	Pain in joint, forearm		368.40	Visual field defect, unspecified
	E906.3	Cat bite		780.6	Fever		625.4	PMS		V20.2	Well Child Exam
	786.50	Chest Pain		789.07	Generalized abdominal pain		486	Pneumonia			
	428.0	CHF		V72.3	Gynecological examiniation		V25.01	Prescription of oral contraceptivess			

DIAGNOSIS: (IF NOT CHECKED ABOVE)		RECEIVED BY:	TODAY'S FEE	*$333.00*
PROCEDURES: (IF NOT CHECKED ABOVE)	RETURN APPOINTMENT INFORMATION: (DAYS) (WKS.) (MOS.) (PRN)	☐ CASH ☐ CREDIT CARD ☐ CHECK # ________	AMOUNT RECEIVED	—
			BALANCE	*$333.00*

Figure C.104 Encounter form (Superbill) for Tim Camon (Appendix A: Day 8).

Goode Medical Clinic
1234 Larsen Avenue
Saint Paul, Minnesota 55316

Phone: (555) 555-1234
Fax: (555) 555-5678

PATIENT NAME	CHART #	DATE		
Lynn Stone			☐ MEDI-MEDI ☐ SELF PAY ☐ MEDICARE	☐ MEDICAL ☐ PRIVATE ☐ HMO____

✓	CPT/Md	DESCRIPTION	FEE	✓	CPT/Md	DESCRIPTION	FEE	✓	CPT/Md	DESCRIPTION	FEE	✓	CPT/Md	DESCRIPTION	FEE
OFFICE VISIT - NEW PATIENT				**LAB STUDIES**				**PROCEDURES**				**INJECTIONS**			
	99202	Focused Ex.			36415	Venipuncture			92551	Audiometry			90655	Influenza 6-35 months	
	99203	Detailed Ex.			81000	Urinalysis			29705	Cast Removal Full Arm/Leg			90656	Influenza 3 years +	
	99204	Comprehensive Ex.			81003	- w/o Micro			2900__	Casting (by location)			90732	Pneumoccal	
	99205	Complex Ex.			84703	HCG (Urine, Pregnancy)			92567	Ear Check			J0295	Ampicillin, 1.5 gr	
OFFICE VISIT - ESTABLISHED PATIENT					82948	Glucose			69210	Ear Wax Rem. 1 2			J2001	Liocaine for IV infusion 10mg	
	99212	Focused Ex.			82270	Hemoccult			93000	EKG			J1885	Toradol 15mg	
✓	99213	Expanded Ex.	*$48.00*		85025	CBC -diff.			93005	EKG tracing only			90720	DTP - HIB	
	99214	Detailed Ex.			85018	Hemoglobin			93010	EKG Int. and Rep			90746	HEP B - HIB	
	99215	Complex Ex.			88174	Pap Smear			11750	Excision Nail			90707	MMR	
PREVENTATIVE MEDICINE - NEW PATIENT					87210	KOH/ Saline Wet Mount			94375	Respiratory Flow Volume			86580	PPD	
	99381	< 1 year old			87430	Strep Antigen			93224	Holter up to 48 hours			90732	Pneumovax	
	99382	1-4 year old			87070	Throat Culture			10060	I & D Abscess Simple			90716	Varicella	
	99383	5-11 year old			80053	Chem profile			10061	I & D Abscess Comp.			82607	Vitamin B12 Inj.	
	99384	12-17 year old			80061	Lipid profile			94761	Oximetry w/Exercise			90712	Polio oral use (OPV)	
	99385	18-39 year old			82465	Cholesterol			94726	Plethysmography			90713	Polio injection (IPV)	
	99386	40-64 year old			99000	Handling fee			94760	Pulse Oximetry			90714	Td preservative free 7 yrs +	
	99387	65 + year old		**X-RAY**					11100	Skin Bx			90718	Td 7 years +	
PREVENTATIVE MEDICINE - ESTABLISHED PATIENT					70210	Sinuses			94010	Spirometry			95115	Allergy inj., single	
	99391	< 1 year old			70360	Neck Soft Tissue			99173	Visual Acuity			95117	Allergy inj., multiple	
	99392	1-4 year old			71010	CXR (PA only)			17110	Wart destruction up to 14					
	99393	5-11 year old			71020	Chest 2V			17111	Wart destruction 15 lesions +					
	99394	12-17 year old			72040	C-Spine 2V			11042	Wound Debrid.		**OTHER**			
	99395	18-39 year old			72100	Lumbrosacral									
	99396	40-64 year old			73030	Shoulder 2V									
	99397	65 + year old			73070	Elbow 2V									
					73120	Hand 2V									
					73560	Knee 2V									
					73620	Foot 2V									
					74000	KUB									

DIAGNOSTIC CODES (ICD-9-CM)

✓	Code	Description	✓	Code	Description	✓	Code	Description	✓	Code	Description
	789.0__	Abdominal Pain		564.0	Constipation		784.0	Headache		782.1	Rash or ezanthem
	682.__	Abscess/Cellulitis		692.6	Contact dermatitis due to plants		414.9	Heart Dis., Coronary		714.0	Rheumatoid Arthritis
	995.3	Allergic Reaction		692.9	Contact dermatitis, NOS		599.70	Hematuria		V70.0	Routine general exam
	331	Alzheimer's		V25.09	Contraceptive management		455.6	Hemorrhoids		V76.10	Screen, breast
	285.__	Anemia, other & unspec		923.10	Contusion, forearm		573.3	Hepatitus, NOS		V76.2	Screen, cervix
	280.9	Anemia-iron deficiency		434.91	CVA		V03.81	HIB		V76.44	Screen, prosate
	281.0	Anemia-pernicious		266.2	Deficiency, folic acid B12		V65.44	HIV counseling		V76.47	Screen, vagina
✓	285.9	Anemia-unspecified		311	Depression		401.1	Hypertension, benign		216.5	Sebaceous cyst
	413.9	Angina, pectoris, oyher/unspecified		250.01	Diabetes, type I, juvenile type		401.9	Hypertension, unspecified		706.2	Sebaceous cyst
	300.00	Anxiety state, NOS		787.91	Diarrhea		401.0	Hypertension, malignant		786.05	Shortness of Breath
	300.4	Anxiety reaction		780.4	Dizziness		V04.81	Influenza		701.9	Skin tag
	716.90	Arthritis, NOS		V06.1	DTP		271.3	Lactose intolerance		845.00	Strain, ankle
	493.20	Asthma; chronic obstruction		V06.3	DTP + polio		573.9	Liver Disease		307.81	Tension headache
	493.00	Asthma; extrinic		536.8	Dyspepsia		724.5	Low Back Pain		V06.5	Tetanus - distheria (Td)
	493.10	Asthma; intrinsic		788.1	Dysuria		346.9	Migraine		305.1	Tobacco dependence
	493.90	Asthmas; unspecified		782.3	Edema		V06.4	MMR		788.41	Urinary frequency
	427.31	Atrial fibulation		530.81	Esophageal reflux		278.01	Obesity/Morbid		599.0	Unrinary tract infection, NOS
	724.5	Backache, unspecified		530.11	Esophagitis reflux		715.90	Osteoarthritis		V05.3	Viral hepatitis
	790.6	Blood chemistry		530.10	Esophagitis, unspecified		719.43	Pain in joint, forearm		368.40	Visual field defect, unspecified
	E906.3	Cat bite		780.6	Fever		625.4	PMS		V20.2	Well Child Exam
	786.50	Chest Pain		789.07	Generalized abdominal pain		486	Pneumonia			
	428.0	CHF		V72.3	Gynecological examiniation		V25.01	Prescription of oral contraceptivess			

DIAGNOSIS: (IF NOT CHECKED ABOVE)		RECEIVED BY:	TODAY'S FEE	*$48.00*
		☐ CASH	AMOUNT RECEIVED	—
PROCEDURES: (IF NOT CHECKED ABOVE)	RETURN APPOINTMENT INFORMATION: (DAYS) (WKS.) (MOS.) (PRN)	☐ CREDIT CARD ☐ CHECK # ________	BALANCE	*$48.00*

Figure C.105 Encounter form (Superbill) for Lynn Stone (Appendix A: Day 9).

Goode Medical Clinic
William B. Goode, MD

Patient Registration Information

Account # :
Insurance # :
Co-Payment: $

Please PRINT AND complete ALL sections below!

PATIENT'S PERSONAL INFORMATION Marital Status ☒ Single ☐ Married ☐ Divorced ☐ Widowed Sex: ☐ Male ☒ Female

Name: London (last name) Karen (first name) S. (initial)

Street address: 8945 Peach St. (Apt # D) City: Minneapolis State: MN Zip: 55000

Home phone: (555) 555-4321 Work phone: (555) 555-5678 Social Security # 369 - XX - 1478

Date of Birth: 05 (month) / 18 (day) / 1983 (year)

Employer / Name of School Pine Trees, Inc. ☒ Full Time ☐ Part Time

PATIENT'S / RESPONSIBLE PARTY INFORMATION

Responsible party: self Date of Birth:

Relationship to Patient: ☒ Self ☐ Spouse ☐ Other Social Security # - -

Responsible party's home phone: ( )

Address: (Apt #) City: State: Zip:

Employer's name: Phone number:( )

Address: City: State: Zip:

Name of Parent/Guardian:

PATIENT'S INSURANCE INFORMATION Please present insurance cards to receptionist.

PRIMARY insurance company's name: Blue Cross/Blue Shield

Insurance address: 1355 Insurance Carrier Loop City: Minneapolis State: MN Zip: 55401

Name of insured: Karen London Date of Birth: 5-18-83 Relationship to insured: ☒ Self ☐ Spouse ☐ Other ☐ Child

Insurance ID number: KL-51423-PT Group number: 09877

Does your insurance cover medication? Yes

EMERGENCY CONTACT

Name of person not living with you: Amy London Relationship: sister

Address: 987 Apple Avenue City: Minneapolis State: MN Zip: 55000

Phone number: (555) 555-4880 (cell)

Assignment of Benefits • Financial Agreement

I hereby give lifetime authorization for payment of insurance benefits to be made directly to Goode Medical Clinic ,and any assisting physicians, for services rendered. I understand that I am financially responsible for all charges whether or not they are covered by insurance. In the event of default, I agree to pay all costs of collection, and reasonable attorney's fees. I hereby authorize this healthcare provider to release all information necessary to secure the payment of benefits.
I further agree that a photocopy of this agreement shall be as valid as the original.

Date: XX/XX/XXXX Your Signature: Karen London

FORM # 58-8423 • BIBBERO SYSTEMS, INC.• PETALUMA, CA.• TO ORDER CALL TOLL FREE :800-BIBBERO (800-242-2376) • FAX (800) 242-9330 (REV.7/94)

Figure C.106 Registration form for Karen London (Appendix A: Day 9).

Goode Medical Clinic

1234 Larsen Avenue
Saint Paul, Minnesota 55316

Phone: (555) 555-1234
Fax: (555) 555-5678

PATIENT NAME	CHART #	DATE		
Karen London			☐ MEDI-MEDI ☐ SELF PAY ☐ MEDICARE	☐ MEDICAL ☐ PRIVATE ☐ HMO____

✓	CPT/Md	DESCRIPTION	FEE	✓	CPT/Md	DESCRIPTION	FEE	✓	CPT/Md	DESCRIPTION	FEE	✓	CPT/Md	DESCRIPTION	FEE
OFFICE VISIT - NEW PATIENT				**LAB STUDIES**				**PROCEDURES**				**INJECTIONS**			
	99202	Focused Ex.			36415	Venipucture			92551	Audiometry			90655	Influenza 6-35 months	
✓	99203	Detailed Ex.	*$80.00*		81000	Urinalysis			29705	Cast Removal Full Arm/Leg			90656	Influenza 3 years +	
	99204	Comprehensive Ex.			81003	- w/o Micro			2900__	Casting (by location)			90732	Pneumoccal	
	99205	Complex Ex.			84703	HCG (Urine, Pregnancy)			92567	Ear Check			J0295	Ampicillin, 1.5 gr	
OFFICE VISIT - ESTABLISHED PATIENT					82948	Glucose			69210	Ear Wax Rem. 1 2			J2001	Liocaine for IV infusion 10mg	
	99212	Focused Ex.			82270	Hemoccult			93000	EKG			J1885	Toradol 15mg	
	99213	Expanded Ex.			85025	CBC -diff.			93005	EKG tracing only			90720	DTP - HIB	
	99214	Detailed Ex.			85018	Hemoglobin			93010	EKG Int. and Rep			90746	HEP B - HIB	
	99215	Complex Ex.			88174	Pap Smear			11750	Excision Nail			90707	MMR	
PREVENTATIVE MEDICINE - NEW PATIENT					87210	KOH/ Saline Wet Mount			94375	Respiratory Flow Volume			86580	PPD	
	99381	< 1 year old			87430	Strep Antigen			93224	Holter up to 48 hours			90732	Pneumovax	
	99382	1-4 year old			87070	Throat Culture			10060	I & D Abscess Simple			90716	Varicella	
	99383	5-11 year old			80053	Chem profile			10061	I & D Abscess Comp.			82607	Vitamin B12 Inj.	
	99384	12-17 year old			80061	Lipid profile			94761	Oximetry w/Exercise			90712	Polio oral use (OPV)	
	99385	18-39 year old			82465	Cholesterol			94726	Plethysmography			90713	Polio injection (IPV)	
	99386	40-64 year old			99000	Handling fee			94760	Pulse Oximetry			90714	Td preservative free 7 yrs +	
	99387	65 + year old		**X-RAY**					11100	Skin Bx			90718	Td 7 years +	
PREVENTATIVE MEDICINE - ESTABLISHED PATIENT					70210	Sinuses			94010	Spirometry			95115	Allergy inj., single	
	99391	< 1 year old			70360	Neck Soft Tissue			99173	Visual Acuity			95117	Allergy inj., multiple	
	99392	1-4 year old			71010	CXR (PA only)			17110	Wart destruction up to 14					
	99393	5-11 year old			71020	Chest 2V			17111	Wart destruction 15 lesions +					
	99394	12-17 year old			72040	C-Spine 2V			11042	Wound Debrid.		**OTHER**			
	99395	18-39 year old			72100	Lumbrosacral									
	99396	40-64 year old			73030	Shoulder 2V									
	99397	65 + year old			73070	Elbow 2V									
					73120	Hand 2V									
					73560	Knee 2V									
					73620	Foot 2V									
					74000	KUB									

DIAGNOSTIC CODES (ICD-9-CM)

Code	Description	Code	Description	Code	Description	Code	Description
789.0__	Abdominal Pain	564.0	Constipation	784.0	Headache	782.1	Rash or ezanthem
682.__	Abscess/Cellulitis	692.6	Contact dermatitis due to plants	414.9	Heart Dis., Coronary	714.0	Rheumatoid Arthritis
995.3	Allergic Reaction	692.9	Contact dermatitis, NOS	599.70	Hematuria	V70.0	Routine general exam
331	Alzheimer's	V25.09	Contraceptive management	455.6	Hemorrhoids	V76.10	Screen, breast
285.__	Anemia, other & unspec	923.10	Contusion, forearm	573.3	Hepatitus, NOS	V76.2	Screen, cervix
280.9	Anemia-iron deficiency	434.91	CVA	V03.81	HIB	V76.44	Screen, prosate
281.0	Anemia-pernicious	266.2	Deficiency, folic acid B12	V65.44	HIV counseling	V76.47	Screen, vagina
285.9	Anemia-unspecified	311	Depression	401.1	Hypertension, benign	216.5	Sebaceous cyst
413.9	Angina, pectoris, oyher/unspecified	250.01	Diabetes, type I, juvenile type	401.9	Hypertension, unspecified	706.2	Sebaceous cyst
300.00	Anxiety state, NOS	787.91	Diarrhea	401.0	Hypertension, malignant	786.05	Shortness of Breath
300.4	Anxiety reaction	780.4	Dizziness	V04.81	Influenza	701.9	Skin tag
716.90	Arthritis, NOS	V06.1	DTP	271.3	Lactose intolerance	845.00	Strain, ankle
493.20	Asthma; chronic obstruction	V06.3	DTP + polio	573.9	Liver Disease	307.81	Tension headache
493.00	Asthma; extrinic	536.8	Dyspepsia	724.5	Low Back Pain	V06.5	Tetanus - distheria (Td)
493.10	Asthma; intrinsic	788.1	Dysuria	346.9	Migraine	305.1	Tobacco dependence
493.90	Asthmas; unspecified	782.3	Edema	V06.4	MMR	788.41	Urinary frequency
427.31	Atrial fibulation	530.81	Esophageal reflux	278.01	Obesity/Morbid	599.0	Unrinary tract infection, NOS
724.5	Backache, unspecified	530.11	Esophagitis reflux	715.90	Osteoarthritis	V05.3	Viral hepatitis
790.6	Blood chemistry	530.10	Esophagitis, unspecified	719.43	Pain in joint, forearm	368.40	Visual field defect, unspecified
E906.3	Cat bite	780.6	Fever	625.4	PMS	V20.2	Well Child Exam
786.50	Chest Pain	789.07	Generalized abdominal pain	486	Pneumonia		
428.0	CHF	V72.3	Gynecological examiniation	V25.01	Prescription of oral contraceptivess		

DIAGNOSIS: (IF NOT CHECKED ABOVE)		RECEIVED BY:	TODAY'S FEE	*$80.00*
490 Bronchitis		☐ CASH	AMOUNT RECEIVED	_____
PROCEDURES: (IF NOT CHECKED ABOVE)	RETURN APPOINTMENT INFORMATION: (DAYS) (WKS.) (MOS.) (PRN)	☐ CREDIT CARD ☐ CHECK # ________	BALANCE	*$80.00*

Figure C.107 Encounter form (Superbill) for Karen London (Appendix A: Day 9).

Blue Cross Blue Shield of MN
1355 Insurance Carrier Loop
Minneapolis, MN 55401
(763)555-0426

Remittance advice

Page: 1 of 1

Goode Medical Clinic
1612 Southwest Blvd.
St. Paul, MN 55100

Federal Tax ID #: 23-XX-12345
Check number: 56789

Patient name	DOS	Procedure code	Units	Total charge	Allowable	Provider responsibility	Co-pay	Amount paid
Carter, Tiffany	02/11/2013	99213	1	48.00	46.00	2.00	0	46.00

Total charges $48.00 Total provider responsibility $2.00 Total co-pay 0 Total paid $46.00

Figure C.108 Remittance Advice—Blue Cross and Blue Shield (Appendix A: Day 9).

First Med EGHP Claims
1324 Insurance Carrier Loop
Minneapolis, MN 55401
(763)345-9124

Remittance advice

Page: 1 of 1
Date: XX/XX/XX
Group Practice ID#: 567XX
Check number: 90123

Goode Medical Clinic
1612 Southwest Blvd.
St. Paul, MN 55100

Patient name	DOS	Procedure code	Units	Total charge	Allowable	Provider responsibility	Co-pay	Amount paid
Brooks, Louise	02/12/2013	99203	1	80.00	76.00	4.00	0	76.00
Camon,Tim	02/12/2013	99385	1	85.00	36.00	49.00	0	36.00
	02/12/2013	82023	1	120.00	50.00	70.00	0	50.00
	02/12/2013	81001	1	78.00	43.00	35.00	0	35.00
	02/12/2013	93000	1	50.00	27.00	23.00	0	23.00

Total charges $413.00 Total provider responsibility $181.00 Total co-pay 0 Total paid $232.00

Figure C.109 Remittance Advice—First Med Insurance for patients Brooks and Camon (Appendix A: Day 9).

Blue Cross Blue Shield of MN
1355 Insurance Carrier Loop
Minneapolis, MN 55401
(763)555-0426

Remittance advice

Page: 1 of 1

Goode Medical Clinic
1612 Southwest Blvd.
St. Paul, MN 55100

Group Practice ID #: 567XX
Check number: 36542

Patient name	DOS	Procedure code	Units	Total charge	Allowable	Provider responsibility	Co-pay	Amount paid
Rose, Cody	02/12/2013	99203	1	80.00	76.00	4.00	0	76.00

Total charges $80.00 Total provider responsibility $4.00 Total co-pay 0 Total paid $76.00

Figure C.110 Remittance Advice—Blue Cross and Blue Shield for Cody Rose (Appendix A: Day 10).

Goode Medical Clinic

1234 Larsen Avenue
Saint Paul, Minnesota 55316

Phone: (555) 555-1234
Fax: (555) 555-5678

PATIENT NAME	CHART #	DATE		
Mike Johnson			☐ MEDI-MEDI ☐ SELF PAY ☐ MEDICARE	☐ MEDICAL ☐ PRIVATE ☐ HMO_____

✓	CPT/Md	DESCRIPTION	FEE	✓	CPT/Md	DESCRIPTION	FEE	✓	CPT/Md	DESCRIPTION	FEE	✓	CPT/Md	DESCRIPTION	FEE
OFFICE VISIT - NEW PATIENT				**LAB STUDIES**				**PROCEDURES**				**INJECTIONS**			
	99202	Focused Ex.			36415	Venipucture			92551	Audiometry			90655	Influenza 6-35 months	
	99203	Detailed Ex.			81000	Urinalysis			29705	Cast Removal Full Arm/Leg			90656	Influenza 3 years +	
	99204	Comprehensive Ex.			81003	- w/o Micro			2900__	Casting (by location)			90732	Pneumoccal	
	99205	Complex Ex.			84703	HCG (Urine, Pregnancy)			92567	Ear Check			J0295	Ampicillin, 1.5 gr	
OFFICE VISIT - ESTABLISHED PATIENT					82948	Glucose			69210	Ear Wax Rem. 1 2			J2001	Liocaine for IV infusion 10mg	
	99212	Focused Ex.			82270	Hemoccult			93000	EKG			J1885	Toradol 15mg	
✓	99213	Expanded Ex.	*$48.00*		85025	CBC -diff.			93005	EKG tracing only			90720	DTP - HIB	
	99214	Detailed Ex.			85018	Hemoglobin			93010	EKG Int. and Rep			90746	HEP B - HIB	
	99215	Complex Ex.			88174	Pap Smear			11750	Excision Nail			90707	MMR	
PREVENTATIVE MEDICINE - NEW PATIENT					87210	KOH/ Saline Wet Mount			94375	Respiratory Flow Volume			86580	PPD	
	99381	< 1 year old			87430	Strep Antigen			93224	Holter up to 48 hours			90732	Pneumovax	
	99382	1-4 year old			87070	Throat Culture			10060	I & D Abscess Simple			90716	Varicella	
	99383	5-11 year old			80053	Chem profile			10061	I & D Abscess Comp.			82607	Vitamin B12 Inj.	
	99384	12-17 year old			80061	Lipid profile			94761	Oximetry w/Exercise			90712	Polio oral use (OPV)	
	99385	18-39 year old			82465	Cholesterol			94726	Plethysmography			90713	Polio injection (IPV)	
	99386	40-64 year old			99000	Handling fee			94760	Pulse Oximetry			90714	Td preservative free 7 yrs +	
	99387	65 + year old		**X-RAY**					11100	Skin Bx			90718	Td 7 years +	
PREVENTATIVE MEDICINE - ESTABLISHED PATIENT					70210	Sinuses			94010	Spirometry			95115	Allergy inj., single	
	99391	< 1 year old			70360	Neck Soft Tissue			99173	Visual Acuity			95117	Allergy inj., multiple	
	99392	1-4 year old			71010	CXR (PA only)			17110	Wart destruction up to 14					
	99393	5-11 year old			71020	Chest 2V			17111	Wart destruction 15 lesions +					
	99394	12-17 year old			72040	C-Spine 2V			11042	Wound Debrid.		**OTHER**			
	99395	18-39 year old			72100	Lumbrosacral									
	99396	40-64 year old			73030	Shoulder 2V									
	99397	65 + year old			73070	Elbow 2V									
					73120	Hand 2V									
					73560	Knee 2V									
					73620	Foot 2V									
					74000	KUB									

DIAGNOSTIC CODES (ICD-9-CM)

✓	Code	Description	✓	Code	Description	✓	Code	Description	✓	Code	Description
	789.0__	Abdominal Pain		564.0	Constipation		784.0	Headache		782.1	Rash or ezanthem
	682.__	Abscess/Cellulitis		692.6	Contact dermatitis due to plants		414.9	Heart Dis., Coronary		714.0	Rheumatoid Arthritis
	995.3	Allergic Reaction		692.9	Contact dermatitis, NOS		599.70	Hematuria		V70.0	Routine general exam
	331	Alzheimer's		V25.09	Contraceptive management		455.6	Hemorrhoids		V76.10	Screen, breast
	285.__	Anemia, other & unspec		923.10	Contusion, forearm		573.3	Hepatitus, NOS		V76.2	Screen, cervix
	280.9	Anemia-iron deficiency		434.91	CVA		V03.81	HIB		V76.44	Screen, prosate
	281.0	Anemia-pernicious		266.2	Deficiency, folic acid B12		V65.44	HIV counseling		V76.47	Screen, vagina
	285.9	Anemia-unspecified		311	Depression		401.1	Hypertension, benign		216.5	Sebaceous cyst
	413.9	Angina, pectoris, oyher/unspecified		250.01	Diabetes, type I, juvenile type	✓	401.9	Hypertension, unspecified		706.2	Sebaceous cyst
	300.00	Anxiety state, NOS		787.91	Diarrhea		401.0	Hypertension, malignant		786.05	Shortness of Breath
	300.4	Anxiety reaction		780.4	Dizziness		V04.81	Influenza		701.9	Skin tag
	716.90	Arthritis, NOS		V06.1	DTP		271.3	Lactose intolerance		845.00	Strain, ankle
	493.20	Asthma; chronic obstruction		V06.3	DTP + polio		573.9	Liver Disease		307.81	Tension headache
	493.00	Asthma; extrinic		536.8	Dyspepsia		724.5	Low Back Pain		V06.5	Tetanus - distheria (Td)
	493.10	Asthma; intrinsic		788.1	Dysuria		346.9	Migraine		305.1	Tobacco dependence
	493.90	Asthmas; unspecified		782.3	Edema		V06.4	MMR		788.41	Urinary frequency
	427.31	Atrial fibulation		530.81	Esophageal reflux		278.01	Obesity/Morbid		599.0	Unrinary tract infection, NOS
	724.5	Backache, unspecified		530.11	Esophagitis reflux		715.90	Osteoarthritis		V05.3	Viral hepatitis
	790.6	Blood chemistry		530.10	Esophagitis, unspecified		719.43	Pain in joint, forearm		368.40	Visual field defect, unspecified
	E906.3	Cat bite		780.6	Fever		625.4	PMS		V20.2	Well Child Exam
	786.50	Chest Pain		789.07	Generalized abdominal pain		486	Pneumonia			
	428.0	CHF		V72.3	Gynecological examiniation		V25.01	Prescription of oral contraceptivess			

DIAGNOSIS: (IF NOT CHECKED ABOVE)		RECEIVED BY:	TODAY'S FEE	*$48.00*
PROCEDURES: (IF NOT CHECKED ABOVE)	RETURN APPOINTMENT INFORMATION:	☐ CASH ☐ CREDIT CARD ☐ CHECK # __________	AMOUNT RECEIVED	———
	(DAYS) (WKS.) (MOS.) (PRN)		BALANCE	*$48.00*

Figure C.111 Encounter form (Superbill) for Mike Johnson (Appendix A: Day 10).

Goode Medical Clinic
William B. Goode, MD

Patient Registration Information

Account # : ____
Insurance # : ____
Co-Payment: $ ____

Please PRINT AND complete ALL sections below!

PATIENT'S PERSONAL INFORMATION Marital Status ❑ Single ❑ Married ☒ Divorced ❑ Widowed Sex: ☒ Male ❑ Female

Name: *Johnson* (last name) *Matthew* (first name) *T.* (initial)

Street address: *9351 Pine Street* (Apt # *268*) City: *Minneapolis* State: *MN* Zip: *55000*

Home phone: (*555*) *555-5431* Work phone: (*555*) *555-3144* Social Security # *321* - *XX* - *6541*

Date of Birth: *10* (month) / *05* (day) / *55* (year)

Employer / Name of School *Morning Newspaper* ☒ Full Time ❑ Part Time

PATIENT'S / RESPONSIBLE PARTY INFORMATION

Responsible party: *self* Date of Birth: ____

Relationship to Patient: ☒ Self ❑ Spouse ❑ Other ____ Social Security # ____-____-____

Responsible party's home phone: (____) ____

Address: ____ (Apt # ____) City: ____ State: ____ Zip: ____

Employer's name: ____ Phone number:(____) ____

Address: ____ City: ____ State: ____ Zip: ____

Name of Parent/Guardian: ____

PATIENT'S INSURANCE INFORMATION Please present insurance cards to receptionist.

PRIMARY insurance company's name: *Blue Cross/ Blue Shield*

Insurance address: *1355 Insurance Carrier Loops* City: *Minneapolis* State: *MN* Zip: *55401*

Name of insured: *Matt Johnson* Date of Birth: *10-5-55* Relationship to insured: ☒ Self ☐ Spouse ☐ Other ☐ Child

Insurance ID number: *MJ-43512-MN* Group number: *44566*

Does your insurance cover medication? *Yes*

EMERGENCY CONTACT

Name of person not living with you: *Mickey Johnson* Relationship: *brother*

Address: *1111 Able Street* City: *Minneapolis* State: *MN* Zip: *55000*

Phone number: (*555*) *555-8819 (home)* *555-555-2563 (cell)*

Assignment of Benefits • Financial Agreement

I hereby give lifetime authorization for payment of insurance benefits to be made directly to *Goode Medical Clinic*, and any assisting physicians, for services rendered. I understand that I am financially responsible for all charges whether or not they are covered by insurance. In the event of default, I agree to pay all costs of collection, and reasonable attorney's fees. I hereby authorize this healthcare provider to release all information necessary to secure the payment of benefits.
I further agree that a photocopy of this agreement shall be as valid as the original.

Date: *XX/XX/XXXX* Your Signature: *Matthew Johnson*

FORM # 58-8423 • BIBBERO SYSTEMS, INC.• PETALUMA, CA.• TO ORDER CALL TOLL FREE :800-BIBBERO (800-242-2376) • FAX (800) 242-9330 (REV.7/94)

Figure C.112 Registration form for Matt Johnson (Appendix A: Day 10).

Goode Medical Clinic
1234 Larsen Avenue
Saint Paul, Minnesota 55316

Phone: (555) 555-1234
Fax: (555) 555-5678

PATIENT NAME	CHART #	DATE		
Matt Johnson			☐ MEDI-MEDI ☐ SELF PAY ☐ MEDICARE	☐ MEDICAL ☐ PRIVATE ☐ HMO____

☐	CPT/Md	DESCRIPTION	FEE
OFFICE VISIT - NEW PATIENT			
	99202	Focused Ex.	
✓	99203	Detailed Ex.	*$80.00*
	99204	Comprehensive Ex.	
	99205	Complex Ex.	
OFFICE VISIT - ESTABLISHED PATIENT			
	99212	Focused Ex.	
	99213	Expanded Ex.	
	99214	Detailed Ex.	
	99215	Complex Ex.	
PREVENTATIVE MEDICINE - NEW PATIENT			
	99381	< 1 year old	
	99382	1-4 year old	
	99383	5-11 year old	
	99384	12-17 year old	
	99385	18-39 year old	
	99386	40-64 year old	
	99387	65 + year old	
PREVENTATIVE MEDICINE - ESTABLISHED PATIENT			
	99391	< 1 year old	
	99392	1-4 year old	
	99393	5-11 year old	
	99394	12-17 year old	
	99395	18-39 year old	
	99396	40-64 year old	
	99397	65 + year old	

☐	CPT/Md	DESCRIPTION	FEE
LAB STUDIES			
	36415	Venipucture	
	81000	Urinalysis	
	81003	- w/o Micro	
	84703	HCG (Urine, Pregnancy)	
	82948	Glucose	
	82270	Hemoccult	
	85025	CBC -diff.	
	85018	Hemoglobin	
	88174	Pap Smear	
	87210	KOH/ Saline Wet Mount	
	87430	Strep Antigen	
	87070	Throat Culture	
	80053	Chem profile	
	80061	Lipid profile	
	82465	Cholesterol	
	99000	Handling fee	
X-RAY			
	70210	Sinuses	
	70360	Neck Soft Tissue	
	71010	CXR (PA only)	
	71020	Chest 2V	
	72040	C-Spine 2V	
	72100	Lumbrosacral	
	73030	Shoulder 2V	
	73070	Elbow 2V	
	73120	Hand 2V	
	73560	Knee 2V	
	73620	Foot 2V	
	74000	KUB	

☐	CPT/Md	DESCRIPTION	FEE
PROCEDURES			
	92551	Audiometry	
	29705	Cast Removal Full Arm/Leg	
	2900__	Casting (by location)	
	92567	Ear Check	
	69210	Ear Wax Rem. 1 2	
	93000	EKG	
	93005	EKG tracing only	
	93010	EKG Int. and Rep	
	11750	Excision Nail	
	94375	Respiratory Flow Volume	
	93224	Holter up to 48 hours	
	10060	I & D Abscess Simple	
	10061	I & D Abscess Comp.	
	94761	Oximetry w/Exercise	
	94726	Plethysmography	
	94760	Pulse Oximetry	
	11100	Skin Bx	
	94010	Spirometry	
	99173	Visual Acuity	
	17110	Wart destruction up to 14	
	17111	Wart destruction 15 lesions +	
	11042	Wound Debrid.	

☐	CPT/Md	DESCRIPTION	FEE
INJECTIONS			
	90655	Influenza 6-35 months	
	90656	Influenza 3 years +	
	90732	Pneumoccal	
	J0295	Ampicillin, 1.5 gr	
	J2001	Liocaine for IV infusion 10mg	
	J1885	Toradol 15mg	
	90720	DTP - HIB	
	90746	HEP B - HIB	
	90707	MMR	
	86580	PPD	
	90732	Pneumovax	
	90716	Varicella	
	82607	Vitamin B12 Inj.	
	90712	Polio oral use (OPV)	
	90713	Polio injection (IPV)	
	90714	Td preservative free 7 yrs +	
	90718	Td 7 years +	
	95115	Allergy inj., single	
	95117	Allergy inj., multiple	
OTHER			

DIAGNOSTIC CODES (ICD-9-CM)

Code	Description	Code	Description	Code	Description	Code	Description
789.0__	Abdominal Pain	564.0	Constipation	784.0	Headache	782.1	Rash or ezanthem
682.__	Abscess/Cellulitis	692.6	Contact dermatitis due to plants	414.9	Heart Dis., Coronary	714.0	Rheumatoid Arthritis
995.3	Allergic Reaction	692.9	Contact dermatitis, NOS	599.70	Hematuria	V70.0	Routine general exam
331	Alzheimer's	V25.09	Contraceptive management	455.6	Hemorrhoids	V76.10	Screen, breast
285.__	Anemia, other & unspec	923.10	Contusion, forearm	573.3	Hepatitus, NOS	V76.2	Screen, cervix
280.9	Anemia-iron deficiency	434.91	CVA	V03.81	HIB	V76.44	Screen, prosate
281.0	Anemia-pernicious	266.2	Deficiency, folic acid B12	V65.44	HIV counseling	V76.47	Screen, vagina
285.9	Anemia-unspecified	311	Depression	401.1	Hypertension, benign	216.5	Sebaceous cyst
413.9	Angina, pectoris, oyher/unspecified	250.01	Diabetes, type I, juvenile type	401.9	Hypertension, unspecified	706.2	Sebaceous cyst
300.00	Anxiety state, NOS	787.91	Diarrhea	401.0	Hypertension, malignant	786.05	Shortness of Breath
300.4	Anxiety reaction	780.4	Dizziness	V04.81	Influenza	701.9	Skin tag
716.90	Arthritis, NOS	V06.1	DTP	271.3	Lactose intolerance	845.00	Strain, ankle
493.20	Asthma; chronic obstruction	V06.3	DTP + polio	573.9	Liver Disease	307.81	Tension headache
493.00	Asthma; extrinic	536.8	Dyspepsia	724.5	Low Back Pain	V06.5	Tetanus - distheria (Td)
493.10	Asthma; intrinsic	788.1	Dysuria	346.9	Migraine	305.1	Tobacco dependence
493.90	Asthmas; unspecified	782.3	Edema	V06.4	MMR	788.41	Urinary frequency
427.31	Atrial fibulation	530.81	Esophageal reflux	278.01	Obesity/Morbid	599.0	Unrinary tract infection, NOS
724.5	Backache, unspecified	530.11	Esophagitis reflux	715.90	Osteoarthritis	V05.3	Viral hepatitis
790.6	Blood chemistry	530.10	Esophagitis, unspecified	719.43	Pain in joint, forearm	368.40	Visual field defect, unspecified
E906.3	Cat bite	780.6	Fever	625.4	PMS	V20.2	Well Child Exam
786.50	Chest Pain	789.07	Generalized abdominal pain	486	Pneumonia		
428.0	CHF	V72.3	Gynecological examiniation	V25.01	Prescription of oral contraceptivess		

DIAGNOSIS: (IF NOT CHECKED ABOVE)
490 Bronchitis

PROCEDURES: (IF NOT CHECKED ABOVE)

RETURN APPOINTMENT INFORMATION:
(DAYS) (WKS.) (MOS.) (PRN)

RECEIVED BY:
☐ CASH
☐ CREDIT CARD
☐ CHECK
#________

TODAY'S FEE	*$80.00*
AMOUNT RECEIVED	———
BALANCE	*$80.00*

Figure C.113 Encounter form (Superbill) for Matt Johnson (Appendix A: Day 10).

Blue Cross Blue Shield of MN
1355 Insurance Carrier Loop
Minneapolis, MN 55401
(763)555-0426

Remittance advice

Goode Medical Clinic
1612 Southwest Blvd.
St. Paul, MN 55100

Page: 1 of 1
Date: XX/XX/XX
Group Practice ID#: 567XX
Check number: 45678

Patient name	DOS	Procedure code	Units	Total charge	Allowable	Provider responsibility	Co-pay	Amount paid
Stone, Lynn	02/13/2013	99213	1	48.00	46.00	2.00	0	46.00
London, Karen	02/13/2013	99203	1	80.00	76.00	4.00	0	76.00
Johnson, Mike	02/14/2013	99213	1	48.00	46.00	2.00	0	46.00
Johnson, Matthew	02/14/2013	99203	1	80.00	76.00	4.00	0	76.00

Total charges $256.00 Total provider responsibility $12.00 Total co-pay 0 Total paid $244.00

Figure C.114 Remittance Advice—Blue Cross and Blue Shield for patients Stone, London, Mike Johnson, and Matt Johnson (Appendix A: Day 11).

Glossary

accounts payable: Money owed by a business for unpaid purchases

accounts receivable: Money owed to a business by others

accrual-basis accounting: Method in which revenues are recorded when services are performed and expenses are recorded when incurred, not when they are paid

aging report: Printout that shows unpaid charges as current or delinquent, based on the number of days they have *aged* (been outstanding)

assets: Items of value owned by a business

backup: Process of copying computer files and storing them on a disk or another electronic device for safekeeping

basic accounting equation: Formula that expresses how financial transactions affect a business (Assets = Liabilities + Owners' Equity)

BillFlash: Able to bill and send statements to patients through this online service

capitation fee: Fixed prepayment made to a provider by an insurance carrier for supplying services to a patient during a specified period, regardless of how many times the patient is seen by the provider

case: Group of transactions related to a specific medical condition for which a patient seeks treatment

cash-basis accounting: Method in which revenues and expenses are not recorded until they are actually paid

cash flow: Money coming into and going out of a business

chart number: Set of digits or letters assigned to a patient's medical record for identification purposes

clearinghouse: Company that provides services to medical practices, which include verifying and transmitting claims to insurance carriers

cluster scheduling: Method that schedules similar procedures together at the same time or same day of the week

collection: Process of obtaining payment for services rendered, usually involving accounts that are past due an extended period

collection agency: Organization that acts as a third party to collect unpaid debts

collection letter: Correspondence sent to a patient to remind him or her of an overdue payment

collection list: Tool used to follow-up on unpaid accounts by creating reminders

Collection Tracer Report: Feature that tracks the quantities and dates of collection letters sent

consultation appointment: Office visit in which a patient or provider seeks the advice or opinion of another provider

copayment: Small, fixed fee paid by the patient or guarantor each time the patient visits the provider

Current Procedural Terminology (CPT): Numerical codes used to designate procedures or services performed in a health care setting

cycle billing: System in which a portion of patient statements are prepared at regular time intervals throughout a month rather than all at once

day sheet: List of all transactions in chronological order for a given day or range of days

deductible: Amount that must first be paid by the insurance policyholder before the insurance carrier will begin to issue payments for medical services

double-booking: Scheduling two patients in the same time slot for the same provider

e-health: Broad term used to describe the exchange of information and services in the health care industry by means of the Internet and other electronic technologies

electronic data interchange (EDI): Process of exchanging information, such as business transactions, in a standardized format from one computer to another

electronic health record (EHR): Electronic version of a patient's medical records

emergency appointment: Office visit requested by a patient that requires a quick response from the medical office staff; takes priority over other appointments

encounter form: Document used by a provider during a medical examination to indicate the patient's type of illness or injury and the medical procedures performed; also called a *superbill*

e-prescribing: Using the Internet to send providers' medical prescriptions to patients' local pharmacies

Evaluation and Management (E/M) codes: Procedure codes used to identify the level of service performed by a provider

explanation of benefits (EOB): Report sent by an insurance carrier to a patient containing details on how benefits were paid

fee-for-service plan: Type of insurance in which the carrier pays specific amounts for specific medical services covered in the policy

Final Draft: Medisoft's word processor

front desk: Area of the medical office where patients check in for their appointments

guarantor: Person who is responsible for paying the patient's bill

health insurance: Protection for patients against the financial consequences of illness, injuries, and disabilities

Health Insurance Portability and Accountability Act (HIPAA): Federal legislation that provides guidelines for transmitting electronic data and protecting patients' privacy

health maintenance organization (HMO): Type of managed care system that hires providers who agree to be paid on a regular, fixed payment per patient instead of on a fee-for-service basis

information technology (IT): Use of computers, the Internet, and other electronic or digital resources to locate, process, transmit, and store data

International Classification of Diseases–Ninth Revision–Clinical Modifications (ICD-9-CM): System used to code patient diagnoses and to facilitate the payment of health care services

ledger: Report that shows a group of financial accounts with a detailed list of all the transactions related to each account

liabilities: Debts and other financial obligations of a business

managed care: System of prepaid health plans that provides health care services at a negotiated cost

Medicaid: Joint federal and state government program that pays health care benefits for people with low incomes or limited resources

medical information cycle: Series of steps performed before, during, and after a patient has been seen by a provider

medical practice management software: Computer programs used to schedule patient appointments, submit electronic claims to insurance companies, and perform basic accounting procedures

Medicare: Federal health insurance program, primarily for people aged 65 and older and those who are disabled

Medisoft: Type of medical practice management software widely used in medical offices

menu bar: Long, rectangular bar at the top of the main Medisoft window that displays menu names

modified wave scheduling: Variation of the wave scheduling method in which patients are scheduled at regular intervals within a given hour

modifier: Two-digit code used to clarify or modify a CPT code's description, usually to indicate some alteration to the procedure performed

new patient appointment: Office visit scheduled for someone being seen at the practice for the first time

no-show: Patient who does not show up for a scheduled appointment

once-a-month billing: System in which all patient statements are prepared once a month at the same time

open office hours: Scheduling system in which patients are seen in the order they arrive at the medical office, with the exception that patients with a serious or life-threatening condition will be given priority

owners' equity: Financial stake that the business owners, business partners, or shareholders have in a business

patient notes: Information recorded in the patient's record about conditions and treatments

patient registration form: Document containing personal, financial, and insurance information needed to complete insurance claims for a patient

payment plan: Agreement that allows a patient to pay a specified dollar amount at regular time intervals to reduce his or her debt; may include interest and late fees

physical: Routine examination to determine a patient's overall health

policyholder: Person who purchased a health insurance plan

practice analysis: Report that shows the charges, payments, and adjustments made during a specified time period for procedures performed in a medical office

preferred provider organization (PPO): Type of managed care organization that uses the fee-for-service concept by predetermining a list of charges for all services

premium: Periodic payment made to an insurance carrier to maintain health care insurance coverage

preoperative appointment: Office visit scheduled for a patient prior to surgery

primary care provider (PCP): Physician or other provider who is selected by a patient enrolled in a managed care plan and who is responsible for coordinating the patient's health care treatment

provider: General term referring to someone who charges for health care services

remittance advice (RA): Report sent from a payer to a practice, often electronically, showing how insurance benefits were paid for patients

Report Designer: Medisoft tool that allows you to modify existing reports and to create new ones

resource: Item in Office Hours, such as a room or piece of equipment, which can be associated with a particular patient's appointment or provider's activity

risk management: Process of identifying practices that may put the medical office at risk and correcting those practices

routine appointment: Office visit scheduled for an established patient to follow-up a previous diagnosis or treat new acute symptoms

scheduling matrix: Pattern of working and nonworking hours for the medical office

side bar: Optional, navigational feature that allows quick access to the most frequently used Medisoft menu items

sliding fee scale: System of charging for services based on the patient's income and family size

statement: Document that shows the amount a patient owes to the medical office

stream scheduling: Method in which each patient is scheduled in a predetermined time slot, based on status and need; is sometimes referred to as *individual scheduling*

telemedicine: Use of telecommunications technology to provide types of medical care that do not require a patient to physically visit a provider

third-party payer: Public or private organization that pays health care expenses for patients who have received services from providers

tickler: Time-sensitive reminder note added to a collection list

time study: Data collected during a certain time period to determine whether changes should be made to a system in current use

toolbar: Row of buttons with icons that allow quick access to many Medisoft features

triage: Process of prioritizing patients according to the severity of their conditions

TRICARE: Health care plan that provides benefits for members of the U.S. military and their dependents; administered by the U.S. Department of Defense

voice recognition: Process that transforms spoken language into digital information that a computer can use

walk-in: Patient who arrives at the medical office without an appointment

wave scheduling: Method in which a group of patients is scheduled at the top of the hour and seen in the order of arrival

workers' compensation: Insurance that protects employees against lost wages and medical costs resulting from work-related illnesses and injuries

write-off: Accounts receivable item that is uncollectable and therefore recorded as a loss or expense in the financial records; also called a *bad debt*

Index

A

B

C

D

E

M

N

O

P

Q

R

S